Differentiation, Examination and Treatment of Movement Disorders in Manual Therapy

For Lollo, Linus and Fanja

For Regula

For Butterworth-Heinemann:

Commissioning Editor: Heidi Harrison
Development Editor: Robert Edwards, Siobhan Campbell
Production Manager: Cheryl Brant
Design: George Ajayi

Differentiation, Examination and Treatment of Movement Disorders in Manual Therapy

Robert Pfund, PT OMT, MAppSc (PT)

Physiotherapist, Master of Applied Science (Physiotherapy), Orthopaedic Manipulative Therapist IFOMT, Instructor OMT – Kaltenborn–Evjenth Concept

Fritz Zahnd, PT

Orthopaedic Manipulative Therapist IFOMT, Health & Fitness Instructor ACSM, Senior Instructor OMT – Kaltenborn–Evjenth Concept

BUTTERWORTH HEINEMANN

ELSEVIER

EDINBURGH LONDON NEW YORK OXFORD PHILADELPHIA ST LOUIS SYDNEY TORONTO 2006

BUTTERWORTH
HEINEMANN
ELSEVIER

ISBN 0 7506 8794 0

British Library Cataloguing in Publication Data
A catalogue record for this book is available from the British Library

Library of Congress Cataloging in Publication Data
A catalog record for this book is available from the Library of Congress

Notice
Medical knowledge is constantly changing. Standard safety precautions must be followed, but as new research and clinical experience broaden our knowledge, changes in treatment and drug therapy may become necessary or appropriate. Readers are advised to check the most current product information provided by the manufacturer of each drug to be administered to verify the recommended dose, the method and duration of administration, and contraindications. It is the responsibility of the practitioner, relying on experience and knowledge of the patient, to determine dosages and the best treatment for each individual patient. Neither the Publisher nor the editors/contributor assumes any liability for any injury and/or damage to persons or property arising from this publication.

The Publisher

Printed in The Netherlands

Contents

About the authors

Robert Pfund, PT OMT, MAppSc (PT) Physiotherapist, Master of Applied Science (Physiotherapy), Orthopaedic Manipulative Therapist IFOMT, Instructor OMT – Kaltenborn–Evjenth Concept

Fritz Zahnd, PT, Orthopaedic Manipulative Therapist IFOMT, Health & Fitness Instructor ACSM, Senior Instructor OMT – Kaltenborn–Evjenth Concept

ROBERT PFUND

Having finished his professional training as a masseur and medical bath attendant in 1981, Robert Pfund started to study physiotherapy, and soon discovered a major interest in manual therapy. First contacts with the Kaltenborn–Evjenth concept inspired him to attend courses in orthopaedic medicine, offered by Dos Winkel. Afterwards, he began a professional training in orthopaedic manual therapy (OMT) according to the Kaltenborn–Evjenth concept, which he finished in 1993 with the OMT-II exam. To learn the second major manual-therapeutic concept, he went to Australia in the years 1994–1996, where he received his Graduate Certificate in Advanced Manipulative Physiotherapy and then his degree of a Master of Science in Physiotherapy at the University of South Australia in Adelaide.

His combined knowledge of both the Kaltenborn–Evjenth concept and the Maitland concept provided him with the basis to develop an excellent synthesis of manual-therapeutic strategies for everyday practical work. By attending courses of the Neuro-orthopedic Institute, he extended his knowledge on the various pain mechanisms and the strategies about management of patients with chronic neuromusculoskeletal pain.

Since 1996, he has been working in a collective practice in Kempten, Germany. Exclusively patients suffering from orthopaedic–traumatic disorders, predominantly patients with chronic neuromusculoskeletal pain, consult this practice. Apart from his manual-therapeutic activities, Robert Pfund is also active in the field of training therapy, which constitutes the second major aspect of his daily work.

He teaches orthopaedic manual therapy and device-supported physiotherapy at several national and international education institutions. He is a member of the German Association for Orthopedic Manual Therapy (DGOMT), the German Association for the Study of Pain (DGSS), as well as the International Association for the Study of Pain (IASP).

FRITZ ZAHND

In 1974, Fritz Zahnd gained his physiotherapy degree at the University Hospital of Zurich, Switzerland. After 4 years of work in his own practice, he attended, from 1981 to 1983, together with his wife, a postgraduate education in orthopaedic manual therapy (OMT) and medical training therapy in Norway, offered by the renowned manual therapists Freddy Kaltenborn and Olaf Evjenth. Back from Norway, he opened the first practice for manual therapy and medical training therapy in Zurich, which he ran, together with his wife, up to 1995. At the same time, he was trained to become a teacher in OMT (1984–1986). He has taught manual therapy and medical training therapy since 1986, in Switzerland and in foreign countries.

Fritz Zahnd is one of the founders and a former president of the Swiss Union of Manual Therapy, Kaltenborn–Evjenth Concept (AMT). In addition, he is one of the founders and former member of the board of the Swiss Association for Orthopedic Manipulative Physiotherapy (SVOMP), of which, today, he is a member of the training commission. Under his presidency, Switzerland became a member of the International Federation of Orthopaedic Manipulative Therapy (IFOMT), a subgroup of the World Confederation of Physical Therapy (WCPT).

Having sold his practice in 1995, he attended, in 1996, the supplementary studies for training fitness and health, at the Sports Institute of the University of Basel, and, at the same time, received the Health and Fitness Instructors Certificate of the American College of Sports Medicine (ACSM). In 2001, he graduated as a therapist for cardiac rehabilitation at the Swiss Working Group for Cardiac Rehabilitation (SAKR).

Apart from his activities as a teacher, he works in the practice with two colleagues as a manual and training therapist and as a personal trainer. He is a member of the Swiss Association of Manipulative Physiotherapy (SVOMP) and of the International Association for the Study of Pain (IASP).

The authors studied physiotherapy together at St Thomas' Hospital, London, where the methods of Dr James Cyriax were taught. From that original inspiration they have continued to develop their clinical practice encompassing a wider scope of physiotherapy skills, but always building on the solid, logical base provided by orthopaedic medicine.

Both now work in private practice and combine this with a teaching commitment to the Society of Orthopaedic Medicine, supporting the development of collaborative partnerships with higher education institutions and multidisciplinary working. As course principals they are involved in advancing education in orthopaedic medicine, and are particularly interested in empowering students to learn through clinical reasoning and reflective practice.

Foreword

This innovative text and DVD-ROM by Robert Pfund and Fritz Zahnd is the first of its kind. The authors have produced a resource that successfully integrates principles of manual therapy examination and management with superb video images of procedures. The format of text combined with video provides unparalleled opportunity to learn both the underlying clinical reasoning and the technical execution of the selected manual therapy procedures.

As evident throughout this book, contemporary manual therapy is multidimensional in its focus, inclusive of concepts and procedures from historically different approaches, and guided by clinical reasoning that is critical, reflective, open-minded and collaborative. In recognition of the biopsychosocial continuum with which patient presentations present, the authors set the scene by discussing the key concepts related to pain mechanisms. The procedures and associated reasoning within the book are then put forward as being appropriate for a pain state that is judged to be predominantly nociceptive. This is a critical clarification typically not addressed in manual therapy texts. It enables and even encourages therapists to appreciate the significant impact psychosocial circumstances can have on patients' presentations and places the procedures covered in the book into a specific context of relevance. The procedures featured throughout the book are not put forward as the answer to all pain states, rather they are recommended for use when the patient's disability and associated impairments are hypothesized to be emanating from the somatic or neurogenic tissues capable of eliciting such symptoms.

The multidimensional focus of this book is also evident through its inclusion of joint, neural and muscle/soft tissue system examination and management procedures. The authors share a wealth of academic and clinical experience that is grounded in the biomedical sciences and practised through an integrated, reasoning-based approach born out of their initial Orthopaedic Manual Therapy Kaltenborn and Evjenth training and further developed through inclusion of theory and procedures from other manual therapy approaches. A unique product of the authors' strong science and clinical base is their integration of this knowledge in guiding the clinical reasoning associated with their recommendations for selection and progression of procedures. Readers are encouraged to consider the underlying physiology reflected in the patient's presentation with particular regard to the stage of tissue healing. This biomedical judgement is then balanced with attention to the specific characteristics of the physical impairments identified to form a hypothesis on which treatment selection and progression can be based. Guidelines and not recipes are suggested.

A particular strength of this book is its capacity to assist readers' continued development of their own clinical reasoning. Clinical reasoning, or the thinking and decision-making associated with clinical practice, requires an organization of knowledge that is contemporary with clear links to its clinical significance. The biomedical theory covered at the start of this book reflects the current state of knowledge in these topics with detailed discussion of the associated clinical implications. Readers' organization of clinical knowledge is then further promoted through the presentation of differentiating physical examination procedures available to narrow down the incriminating physical impairment of a given disability.

In addition to its ability to promote clinical reasoning and not simply examination and management procedures, a feature of this book that the authors must be congratulated for including is its attention to self-management. Patient self-management is essential for long-term success with manual therapy. As implied throughout this book, manual therapy examination and initial treatments are critical to advance the hypotheses formed through the subjective examination. Skilled assessment of physical dysfunction enables therapists to determine the principal impairments and to hypothesize to some extent about the source of the symptoms and factors contributing to the development and maintenance of the patient's disabilities and impairments. Once the pain mechanisms have been established to be predominantly nociceptive and the disabilities and associated impairments analysed, trial treatments directed toward improving or correcting those impairments then serve as a further test of the evolving hypotheses regarding the source and cause of the patient's physical problems. Here the authors take their book to another level by including specific self-management procedures directed to the specific impairments identified through the differential examination. The visual and auditory presentation of these self-management procedures through videotape then provides the reader with a unique learning opportunity whereby they can immediately switch between examination and management, including self-management, procedures to reinforce their understanding and application. While not specifically referred to as such, this represents a collaborative approach to clinical reasoning. That is, the authors promote a view that patients should not be passive recipients of health care. Instead, through a process of collaboration, therapist and patient reach a shared understanding of the problem that includes a shared responsibility for the management. While the patient may rely on the therapist to establish the nature of the problem and the management recommended, the therapist then relies on the patient to participate through self-management. Self-management includes preparedness to consider and learn new health beliefs and behaviours and to continue with self-management physical exercises as demonstrated throughout the book.

The interactive and flexible presentation of this book/DVD-ROM along with the philosophy of promoting therapists' clinical reasoning and patient self-management provide an effective application of adult learning that should foster readers' deeper understanding of the theory discussed and procedures demonstrated. Readers are certain to learn much from this book.

Mark A. Jones BSc (Psych), PT, Grad Dip Advan Manip The, MAppSc
Senior Lecturer, Director, Master of Musculoskeletal and Sports Physiotherapy, Physiotherapy International Coordinator, University of South Australia

Preface

During the last 20 years, manual therapy (MT) has changed fundamentally. At the time when we, the authors, studied manual therapy as a postgraduate training, the discipline was shaped by a few prominent personalities in this field, the originators of MT concepts, the founders of the International Federation of Orthopaedic Manipulative Therapy, IFOMT. We had the luck and at the same time the handicap to be trained by Freddy Kaltenborn and Olaf Evjenth, the originators of one of the two major MT concepts. Luck this was because it is not only a unique experience but also a privilege to learn the art from the master himself. A handicap it was since the exclusivity of the master's views, formed in years of trying to convince the 'unbelieving', was directly transferred to his disciples.

Luck it was, as it meant that we were conveyed invaluable, truly solid practical foundations, the basis of our conviction still held today that biomechanically correct performance of a passive movement is the most adequate and most easily dosed stimulus to improve movement function with a peripheral nociceptive dysfunction of the movement apparatus. A handicap it was since it significantly slowed down our own initiatives to advance concepts by freely taking up and testing emerging ideas, both of ourselves and of others.

Further development or co-development of manual-therapeutic concepts has, however, become indispensable in the context of the changing health-political situation of the last decade. Today, manual therapists work in an environment where, on the one hand, notions like health reform and global budgeting, and, on the other hand, an improved understanding of chronic processes and the inclusion of psycho-socio-economic factors into the understanding of clinical presentations of movement disorders have become relevant.

This book is meant to help people active in the field of manual therapy to learn and modify current MT concepts.

- It presupposes a basic training in manual therapy.
- It discusses problem situations with predominantly peripheral nociceptive presentations. Limiting the range of described therapeutic strategies in this way seems necessary to allow the reader to still get the general idea.
- It discusses some typical examples without claiming to be comprehensive. Rather, examples are understood as a means to demonstrate a system by which to solve clinical problems.
- It is not structured according to body regions but instead starts from the localization of symptoms. In this respect, it meets the needs of practical situations.
- By means of video clips on the CD enclosed, the reader will get a more vivid impression of how to perform examination

and treatment techniques, information which could not have been conveyed by pictures alone.

The book has been compiled on the basis of the authors' personal experiences and their many contacts and discussions with other manual therapists. The production of the enclosed, qualitatively excellent CD-ROM would not have been possible without the instructive and fascinating cooperation of the physician and media instructor Christof Daetwyler. We thank him for his commitment and his patience in realizing our project.

No less patience and staying power was required from our model patient, Lollo Ernst, both during shooting sessions and due to the many changes in schedules and frequent delays, which often interfered with the timetables of her family life. We thank her for her support and her always positive vibrations.

Moreover, we thank all those who have encouraged, confused, irritated, and inspired us, above all our patients and our teachers Freddy Kaltenborn and Olaf Evjenth.

Making mistakes may have its positive aspects, too, provided you are prepared to learn from them. That is what we did.

As this book (the German language edition) was published in two volumes, we had the chance to modify things in the second volume to improve value and practical usefulness of the book. We thank all the readers of volume 1 for their suggestions.

For easier 'navigation' within the book, the table of contents has been improved.

In the practical part, the description of a manoeuvre has been completed by adding the number of the respective film. So the film can be found more quickly on the CD. The print quality of the photographs has been improved as well.

We were pleased to hear that, in spite of the mistakes we made, volume 1 has proved useful for many readers – which their feedback confirms to us. Volume 1 has been well accepted, both as a textbook and as a manual for practice.

Together with the video films on the CD, the innovative concept of the book – not being organized in a technical way according to regions, but in a process-oriented way – contributes positively to problem solution in practice. For that reason, we have taken the introductory chapter of volume 1 on theoretical foundations as the introduction to volume 2, too. This allows the reader to use both volumes independently of each other – according to particular interests and necessities – without missing necessary information.

Two things, on the other hand, were maintained from volume 1 without modification: the structure of the book, and the technical aspects of its contents. The structure, because we want volume 2 to be organized according to the same red thread, the approach of proceeding from symptom, via identification of localization and type of problem, to treatment. And second, the technical aspects of the contents, describing procedures not as being restricted to individual concepts. Over and again we have learned in our practical work that it is not one method or technique which, on principle, would be superior to others and which hence would lead to better, or faster, results. Different methods may produce similarly positive results. What is important is that the method and its technical-practical implementation are adequate for the clinical presentation of the problem as well as for the patient's uniqueness with all its physical and psychosocial aspects. It is this openness towards different methods, and a readiness to consider them in an unbiased way, that we would like to convey in this book.

Such an approach is supported by two leading experts in manual therapy, Gwendolyn Jull and Ann Moore, who, in the editorial to *Manual Therapy* (2002; 7:63-115) wrote:

> *[...] as current evidence points towards efficacy of various approaches, the debate of superiority of approaches on factional grounds seems to lose significance and becomes redundant. Perhaps the more relevant debate that should lead MT's practice*

and research in this 21st century is what is the commonality of effect of various manipulative therapy procedures. [...] The clinical challenge is to have expertise in a variety of approaches and to be able to select which patient is responsive to which approach for most expedient and effective treatment.

Whatever concept or combination is used, success will depend on skills and clinical reasoning. The present book is meant to contribute to improving both. On the one hand, reasoning and problem solution can be learned only by consequently reflecting on considerations that led to the application of certain measures. And such reflection has to be frank and true, it must not be biased by some desired hypothesis.

On the other hand, the craft has to be learned, and technical skills have to be exercised and improved during countless hours. Such abilities cannot be acquired by studying reference lists or databases, they are developed only by exercising, by thousands of repetitions of individual movements. It is the combination of both, exemplified to us by the founders of individual treatment concepts with different focuses, which has made manual therapy and physiotherapy the valuable disciplines they are today. We thus want to emphasize their importance.

Today, the academic aspect of medical professions is the talk of the town. Undoubtedly, it is of prime importance to gain more or less 'evidence-based' data, which will clarify our work. But with such enthusiasm, the basis of our profession, the craft of physiotherapy, must not be forgotten or neglected. No study, however perfect, will help patients with back pain to 'function' again in such a way that they can resume their everyday lives. This is only achieved by the therapist's actual practical work.

Manual therapy is a combination of solid analytical conclusions and artisan skills. These are the constituents on which today's relevance of our profession is based, and only by equally advancing both will we be able to further develop our profession.

Whether we want it or not – the world is continuing to turn around, and manual therapy with it. We are asked to contribute our best to keep manual therapy part of this development.

Fritz Zahnd and Robert Pfund

Chapter 1

Fundamentals

CHAPTER CONTENTS

INTRODUCTION: PAIN AND SYMPTOMS

Various differentiation tests are employed in manual therapy to get more information about possibly affected structures or areas of the movement apparatus. Common tests are those based on active and passive movement (e.g., angular and translatory movement), specific palpation, resistance tests, or the tests for specific provocation and alleviation according to the Kaltenborn–Evjenth concept (Evjenth and Gloeck 1996). The latter aim at reproducing or reducing a patient's typical pain.

All techniques serve to identify sensitive responses to mechanical stimuli. It has to be queried, though, whether tissues detected in this way are always damaged. This is of great importance since often certain treatment strategies are chosen on the basis of hypotheses formed after differentiation tests. For a more detailed discussion of this question, possible pain mechanisms will now be described and then related to the different clinical presentations.

In manual therapy, potential pain mechanisms are classified so as to better understand responses to certain clinical tests as well as symptom behaviour. Such classification helps to optimize possible clinical strategies and improve patient management (Butler 1994, 1998, Jones 1995, Gifford and Butler 1997, Gifford 1998). The various mechanisms always occur in combinations, and in different presentations different mechanisms may predominate.

Potential pain mechanisms

- Peripheral nociceptive
- Peripheral neurogenic
- Central
- Affective
- Motor/autonomic.

We refer to a *peripheral nociceptive pain mechanism* when the primary lesion is located in tissue supplied by nociceptors. For this reason, those movements are painful in differentiation tests that increase the load on injured or damaged structures. Pain is caused by stimulation of specific nociceptors in the periphery.

In a *peripheral neurogenic pain mechanism*, the underlying cause is the primary lesion or the dysfunction in the peripheral nervous system itself.

Central pain mechanisms are involved when pain is produced in the spinal cord (dorsal horn) or in higher centres of the central nervous system (CNS) due to increased sensitivity in these areas. This means that the cause of pain does not lie in the area of the tissues mechanically provoked through the test – although certain movements will be painful in differentiation tests – but in an altered processing of mechanical afferents within the CNS.

If emotions are of predominant relevance in provoking pain, we talk about *affective pain mechanisms*.

Motor or *autonomic mechanisms* can be observed with all these forms and include the autonomic and motor reactions to painful states.

For a more detailed explanation and description of the different pain mechanisms – which is not the aim of this book – readers are referred to the specific literature (Harkins et al. 1984, Merskey and Bogduk 1994, Jones 1995, Gifford and Butler 1997, Gifford 1998, Butler 1998).

The length of time symptoms have already been present provides important hints about the potential predominance of certain pain mechanisms (Gifford and Butler 1997, Gifford 1998, Harding et al. 1998, Butler 1998). In this respect, a distinction is made between acute and chronic presentations.

In an *acute presentation* (e.g., trauma), the painful condition has usually persisted less than 3 months, and the history shows that symptoms are continually improving, in line with the healing times to be expected (Lederman 1997, van den Berg 1998). In an acute presentation, peripheral mechanisms are predominant (Jones 1995, Cohen 1996, Gifford and Butler 1997, Gifford 1998).

A *chronic presentation*, on the other hand, has already lasted for more than 3–6 months and, during this period, has shown neither any distinct improvement nor any rapidly occurring relapses (Gifford and Butler 1997, Waddell 1998). Underlying pain mechanisms are predominantly of a central nature (Jones 1995, Cohen 1996, Gifford and Butler 1997, Gifford 1998).

In each painful presentation (be it acute or chronic), there is an underlying increased sensitivity to certain stimuli. A painful presentation has always to be understood as a combination of different pain mechanisms. For this reason, it always involves changes both in the peripheral and in the CNS. An acute presentation shows predominantly peripheral mechanisms, whereas in a chronic presentation, central mechanisms are of major relevance (Cohen 1995, 1996, Jones 1995, Gifford and Butler 1997, Gifford 1998). This predominance seems to be of crucial importance in deciding whether conclusions regarding directly injured or damaged structures can be drawn from differentiation tests (Zusman 1994, Gifford 1999).

Increased sensitivity is referred to, according to its clinical appearance, as hyperalgesia, allodynia, or hyperpathia. *Hyperalgesia* is a painful condition originating from an increased response to a stimulus which is normally painful (e.g., pressure or pull on tissues).

Allodynia is produced by a stimulus which normally is not painful, e.g., soft touch, whereas *hyperpathia* is characterized by an abnormal pain reaction. This reaction may be increased by repeated stimuli and, in contrast to hyperalgesia, usually shows an increased threshold (Merskey and Bogduk 1994). In clinical language, allodynia and hyperalgesia are very often subsumed under the common term of *hyperalgesia*. In the authors' experience, hyperalgesia is the most frequently occurring form of pain problem in manual therapy practice (Cohen 1996).

As different mechanisms within the nervous system are thought to underlie hyperalgesia, a distinction needs to be made between primary and secondary hyperalgesia (Lewis 1935, 1942).

Primary hyperalgesia is characterized by a prolonged increased sensation of pain, where nociceptors in the respective painful area show increased sensitivity. Because of this decreased threshold of the nociceptors, mechanical, thermal, and chemical stimuli of lower intensities are able to induce the transmission of afferent input to the CNS. Nociceptors are stimulated when tissue is damaged or is in danger of being damaged (Merskey and Bogduk 1994). In primary hyperalgesia, an increased peripheral sensitivity can be observed. Clinically, this is evident as a painful reaction to a differentiation test that is able to identify injured tissues (Gifford and Butler 1997).

Although *secondary hyperalgesia* also shows prolonged increased sensation of pain, the painful stimulus is not directly related to injured tissue. In contrast to primary hyperalgesia, nociceptors in the injured area show normal sensitivity (Cohen 1995, Gifford and Butler 1997). The painful reaction to a mechanical stimulus, e.g., a differentiation test, is caused by a change in receptor properties in the dorsal horn, which allows thickly myelinated afferents (mechanoreceptors) to provoke pain (Dubner and Basbaum 1994, Meyer et al. 1994). Clinically, this manifests as a painful reaction to some movement, similar to the reaction to a differentiation test, but in contrast to primary hyperalgesia, this reaction does not allow any direct conclusions about injured or damaged tissues.

Both forms of hyperalgesia usually occur in combination, but here again the issue of predominance seems to be of crucial importance. Thus, in a patient with acute pain who suffered from an inversion trauma a week before, usually increased peripheral sensitivity will be predominant. The reproduction of this sensitivity by a differentiation test allows conclusions about the location of the injured tissue. In contrast, in a patient with chronic pain who underwent lumbar disc surgery 1.5 years ago and has suffered from unchanged pain ever since, positive manual differentiation tests cannot be used in the same way to identify injured or damaged tissue, because of presumed central sensitivity.

All positive manual differentiation tests investigating a painful reaction to a mechanical stimulus will identify a hyperalgesic area. Due to the differing predominance of pain mechanisms in acute or chronic conditions (increased peripheral or central sensitivity), this hyperalgesic area is, however, not always identical with the area of injured or damaged tissue. This means that although in a chronic presentation with predominantly central pain mechanisms manual differentiation tests will identify sensitive tissue, they will not reveal anything about the origin of that sensitivity. Predominantly peripheral nociceptive presentations seem to be the only group of conditions where manual differentiation tests may serve to identify injured or damaged tissue (Gifford and Butler 1997, Gifford 1998).

In the authors' view, tests for specific provocation and alleviation occupy a particular position among manual differentiation tests. In these tests, a mechanical stimulus in a small, clearly defined area of the movement apparatus will increase pain during provocation, but will relieve it in the alleviation test. If increased central sensitivity predominates, as in secondary hyperalgesia, the information provided by provocation and alleviation tests seems to be questionable. As has been mentioned before, in this case thick-fibre afferents (mechanoreceptors) are able to provoke pain due to changes within the CNS (particularly the dorsal horn). These changes also lead to an enlargement of the representation field and to a prolonged response to afferent stimuli (Dubner and Busbaum 1994, Cohen 1995, Gifford and Butler 1997).

If, in an area as precisely defined as a facet joint of the cervical spine, the flexion movement of a vertebra provokes pain, whereas the extension movement is able to alleviate that pain, there is probably no centrally increased sensitivity. Otherwise, we would expect any form of movement to provoke pain. In this example of the cervical spine, a predominantly peripherally increased sensitivity (peripheral nociceptive mechanism) is clearly more probable.

But similar to the *Apgar score* (a score to evaluate a neonate's physical condition based on respiration, heart rate, muscle tonus, colour of the skin, and reflexes), further indications are necessary to support a hypothesis based on the results of specific provocation and alleviation:

- traumatic causes
- temporal development of complaints
- reproducibility of test results
- reproducibility of treatment results
- technological procedures
- temperature test (in superficial structures only).

To infer, for example, an injury of the anterior talofibular ligament, a particular type of trauma (e.g., an inversion trauma) has to have occurred, and the temporal development of complaints has to match with normal healing times (Lederman 1997, van den Berg 1998). Moreover, during one or more sessions, test and treatment results should be consistent as far as possible, i.e. loading of the ligament should reproducibly increase pain whereas unloading should decrease it. This, however, presupposes reliable test and measurement procedures so as to avoid false positive or false negative results. Technological procedures, such as imaging diagnostics, may also provide supportive information for a clinical hypothesis.

Quite clearly it has to be pointed out, however, that very often tissue changes occur without showing any symptoms, which still very often leads to mistaken therapeutic measures (Milgrom et al. 1995, Beattie 1996). If, for instance, the painful area in the region of the lateral malleolus shows mechanical and thermal hypersensitivity, this suggests a predominantly peripheral nociceptive mechanism, since with a predominantly central mechanism, mechanical sensitivity would be increased but thermal sensitivity would not (Meyer et al. 1994, Cohen 1996). If all mentioned aspects (including specific provocation and alleviation) point to a lesion of the anterior talofibular ligament, the assumed hypothesis has to be judged as probable.

The fewer indications there are to confirm a hypothesis, the less probable it is. Any individual manual differentiation test, however elaborate and/or convincing it may be, will not suffice alone to confirm or reject a hypothesis.

Note: With respect to the hypotheses formed on the basis of differentiation tests which are discussed below, we therefore explicitly emphasize the fact that it is only with peripheral nociceptive presentations that specific findings may be interpreted as hints of an injury or damage in a certain area or a certain structure. Information from the anamnesis (patient's medical history), further examination, and treatment is always essential to support a particular hypothesis.

EXAMINATION OF THE MOVEMENT APPARATUS

INTRODUCTION

In most medical disciplines, physical examination is performed according to regions. After the medical history has been obtained, whole regions or organ systems are systematically screened for changes and/or functional disorders, according to suspected origins of symptoms. With such a way of proceeding, the therapist risks mistakenly interpreting a detected change or functional disorder as the cause of the symptoms. The more visible (imaging procedures) or measurable (measurement of torque, electrodiagnostics, laboratory measurements) the identified changes, the greater the therapist's conviction that he or she has discovered the symptom-provoking disorder. 'Solid' data ascertained in this way are seen as practical proof of the source of the symptom-provoking disorder (Jones 1997a, 1997b).

Most people become aware of functional disorders of the movement apparatus only if the latter are associated with pain or prevent them from correctly performing some important task (work or leisure). The neuromusculoskeletal system has many compensatory mechanisms at its disposal to remain free of signs and symptoms in spite of permanent or temporary functional disorders. Only decompensation, which may be due to different events (emotional stress, micro-trauma, trauma, prolonged stress), leads to awareness of the disorder and to the affected person seeking help.

As it can be assumed that most people live with well-compensated disorders of their movement apparatus, examination must not simply aim at revealing some compensated functional disorder. The likelihood that treatment of this compensated disorder might resolve the patient's relevant problem is not very great. It is necessary instead to detect, localize, analyse, and resolve by means of adequate treatment the causal problem which has become manifest through decompensation and causes symptoms. Treatment has to aim at alleviating symptoms, restoring function, and – if possible – eliminating the cause. Measures taken serve to support the healing process and re-establish the ability to compensate. Due to the complexity underlying a decompensation process, there are obviously several possibilities for restoring the compensation capacity.

The concept or mental process underlying an approach of analysing and treating health problems (also neuromusculoskeletal ones) is referred to as the *clinical reasoning process (CRP)* (Fig. 1.1). This concept is the basis for the investigator's or therapist's reflection and action. Of elementary importance in CRP is constant interaction of the components of gathering data, forming hypotheses, and testing them. Such interaction has to occur at each level of the overall process of problem solution. The quality of manual therapy has been crucially improved during recent years as a result of raising awareness about and training in clinical reasoning processes, which, at the same time, means abandoning the blind and stubborn pursuit of some technical routine in clinical practice (Jones 1997a, 1997b, 2004).

This is the background against which the approaches presented below of area localization, general movement tests, specific provocation and alleviation, specific mobility tests, and further additional tests (e.g., palpation, neurological tests) should be seen (Fig. 1.2). Deliberately, no chronological sequence has been chosen for this discussion. The authors rather want to convey the fact that there is constant interaction among the individual components of the whole examination process. Each individual step (e.g., testing specific mobility) is only performed for the reason of testing some hypothesis and not simply to execute another step in a rigid examination scheme. In the authors' view, a chronological representation of the individual components of the whole examination carries the risk that therapists might see an activity as being accomplished once it has been performed and might start from the assumption that all

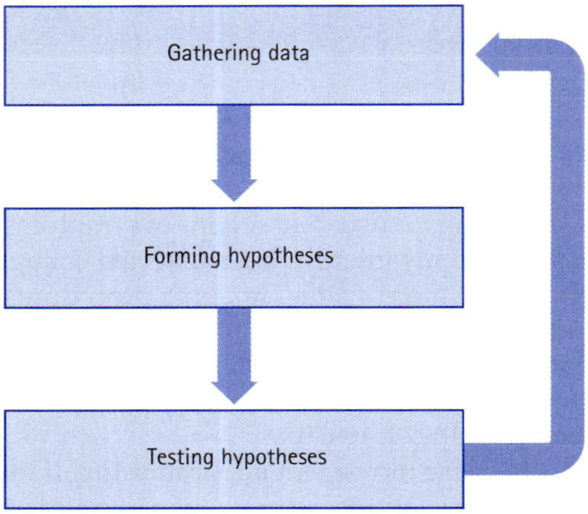

Figure 1.1 The clinical reasoning process – 1.

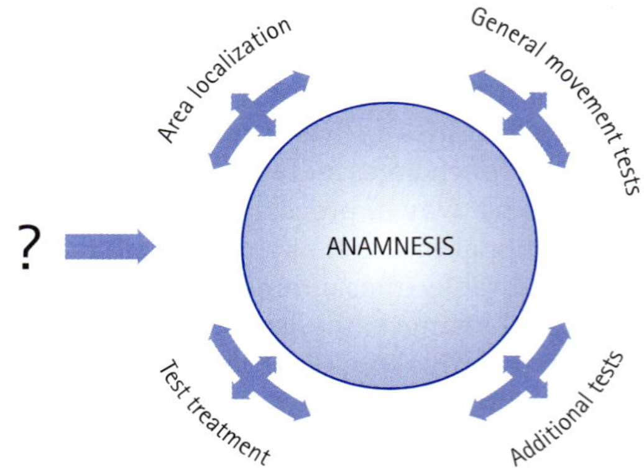

Figure 1.2 The clinical reasoning process – 2.

information was already available. Instead, anamnesis, for instance, is never finished – which a chronological arrangement might suggest. Rather, it has to be constantly present to test currently emerging hypotheses by means of specific questions and thus provide the basis for further steps in a physical (objective) examination (e.g., area localization).

As discussed in the first section of this chapter, successful and accurate localization of symptoms by the described test procedures is conditional on the fact that underlying mechanisms are peripheral nociceptive in nature. With other pain mechanisms (neurogenic, central, or autonomic/motor), the results of these test procedures seem questionable (Gifford 1999). Therefore, the following observations on functional examination are valid only for peripheral nociceptive problems.

ANAMNESIS – INITIAL INQUIRY AND INSPECTION AT REST

The anamnesis serves to ascertain all data that might relate to (one ore more) functional disorder(s). It allows early identification of situations that require caution, or contraindications for movement, and enables planning of the subsequent physical examination. Data are gathered via (verbal and non-verbal) communication with the patient. Successful communication is based on the following conditions:

- communication partners have to know with whom they communicate (introduction)
- the patient has to feel that he or she is taken seriously (empathy)
- communication has to take place in a language that the patient can easily understand (no technical jargon)
- the atmosphere in which communication takes place has to be as agreeable as possible (regarding illumination, temperature, environment, silence)
- the patient has to know in advance the maximum amount of time available for the examination (no unrealistic schedules).

The anamnesis makes it possible to identify clinical patterns and to form hypotheses about the type and origin of functional disorders, to classify such hypotheses according to categories, and to test and modify them in the course of further examination and treatment

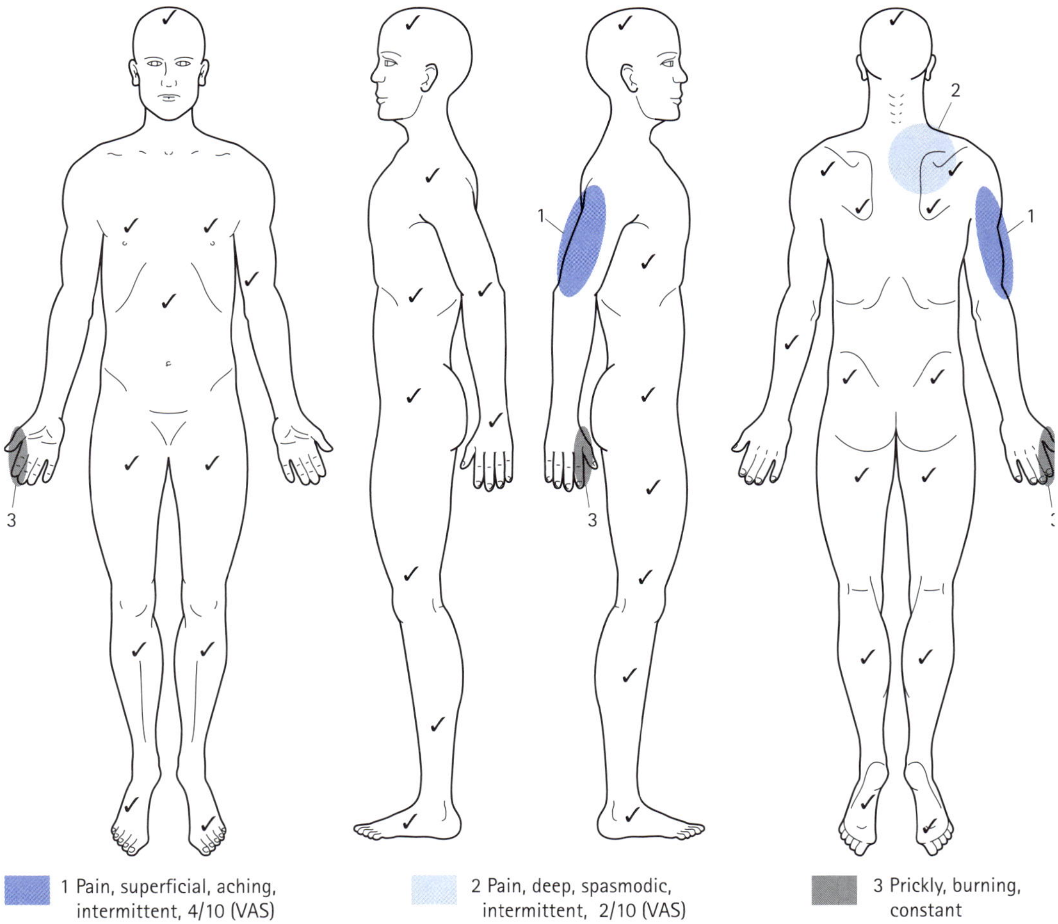

Figure 1.3 Body tables; 1 marks the main problem, 2 and 3 mark further symptoms. VAS, visual analogue scale.

steps. Furthermore, it helps to gather signs which, as comparable signs, may later serve for reassessment.

The following approach is recommended:

- describing the patient's main problem at the current point in time as well as its relevance for the patient
- documenting on a body chart (Fig. 1.3) the localization and spread of all symptoms. All symptom areas should be recorded, even if the patient does not consider them to be directly related to the current complaints:
  - numbering the different symptoms (localization of symptoms)
  - identifying links (interactions) between individual symptom areas
  - denoting symptom-free areas
- describing the type of the symptoms (character, intermittent/constant, superficial/deep)
- qualifying and quantifying individual symptoms in the course of 24 hours (symptom behaviour)

- marking data that are suitable for reassessment, e.g.:
  - sequence of appearance of symptoms (major and minor problems)
  - day/night
  - better/worse (movement, rest, position, time until pain is felt, other factors such as stress, nutrition, or medicaments)
  - mechanical/non-mechanical problem
  - stiffness
  - need for rest vs. movement
  - changes in signs and symptoms with activities of daily living
  - classification of each symptom according to severity, irritability, and nature
- recording the history of the symptoms
  - first appearance (when?)
  - kind of first appearance (how?)
  - due to trauma or spontaneously (details)
  - current development
  - treatment up to now as well as its effects
- specific questions:
  - general state, other diseases, accidents, surgeries, medicaments, imaging procedures
  - eventually family anamnesis and social anamnesis, health development
  - understanding the functional disorder in the context of the patient's activities and his or her social environment (ICF)
  - determining whether something has been overlooked or whether the patient still wants to ask something, clarifying open questions
- cause of the problem, according to the patient's judgement
- patient's expectations regarding therapy.

After the anamnesis, a summary statement of the patient's main problem and secondary problems should be formulated. In this respect, the following categories should be considered:

- activity capability/restriction, and participation capability/restriction
- patients perspectives on their experience
- pathobiological mechanisms
- physical impairments and associated structure/tissue sources
- contributing factors
- precautions and contraindications
- management and treatment
- prognosis.

This will yield the relevant working hypotheses. Subsequently, it has to be considered how these hypotheses could be tested in the course of treatment and what further data might lead to a modification of the initial hypotheses. It is hence obvious that the patient inquiry as described is not completed once and for all.

The whole process of problem solution is an interaction of communication (anamnesis), clinical test procedures, and reassessments. During functional examination and treatment, too, further anamnestic information has to be gathered which might contribute to confirmation or rejection of a relevant working hypothesis.

(Further information on this subject can be found in Frisch 1995, Greenman 1996, Hengeveld 1998, Jones 1995, Maitland 1994, 1996.)

FUNCTIONAL OR PHYSICAL EXAMINATION

Planning the examination

Functional examination is planned on the basis of the information from the anamnesis. Although standardized examination procedures exist, it is, in most cases, not sensible to automatically pursue such schemes. There is always the question what might be altered in the standardized procedure. Answers to this question will be provided by the actual clinical presentation, but will need further substantiation.

As a manual therapy examination includes movement of and load on various structures, the following questions arise with respect to the planning of the examination:

- Are there current situations that require caution or are there even contraindications with respect to movement (severity, irritability, nature or expected course of healing, stability, and development of the problem, different structures, eventual pathologies)?
- What is to be examined?
  - Are there safety tests which, in view of the actual presentation, have to be performed at the beginning of the examination, e.g., tests regarding nervous system, stability, or blood circulation?
- How should the examination be performed?
  - How far are symptoms to be reproduced?
  - Which symptoms must not be reproduced?
- Which signs and symptoms from the anamnesis might serve as comparable signs?

Examination tools

- *Inspection*
- *Active movement:* angular/rotatory movements
- *Passive movement:*
  - angular/rotatory movements (the same as with active movement)
  - accessory movements (passive movements which the patient cannot actively perform in isolation): (a) angular/rotatory movements (e.g., gapping, PAIVM – passive accessory intervertebral movements); (b) translatory movements (e.g., traction, compression, gliding)
- *Muscle tests:*
  - resistance (strength and pain, isometric, concentric, eccentric, different starting positions)
  - length (resistance and pain with increasing distance between origin and attachment)
- *Neurological examination:*
  - function (sensitivity, peripheral and central reflexes, strength of key muscles, motor function)
  - neurodynamics (mobility and tension tolerance)
- *Palpation:*
  - tissue palpation (tissue texture abnormalities)
  - movement palpation (as additional information with simultaneously performed active and/or passive movement)
- *Complementary apparative examinations, e.g.:*
  - imaging procedures
  - electrodiagnostics
  - laboratory examinations.

INSPECTION AT REST AND WITH MOVEMENT

Inspection begins immediately with the patient's first visit and is maintained during the whole process of examination and treatment. Posture, everyday and evasive movements, body shape (contours), and skin are assessed. Inspection also serves to gain information about the patient's emotional state.

ACTIVE MOVEMENT

Angular/rotatory

Normal active movement strains all structures involved in movement and presupposes normal function of these structures as well as of their control and feeder systems (nervous system, cardiopulmonary system).

The test of active movement serves to assess movement quantity and quality. Movements are to be performed by the patient himself/herself and without guiding assistance by the examiner. The test examines the anatomical and physiological movements in a joint or an articular complex (body section). If active movements induce symptoms and/or change them, active movement testing can also be used as a means of symptom localization and reassessment.

PASSIVE MOVEMENT

Angular/rotatory movements

With passive movement, stress due to muscular activities (e.g., compression and shear forces in the joint, active centring of joint surfaces) is largely excluded. Nevertheless, muscles and nervous system are not completely free of stress, since they are moved and can be put under tensile stress and/or compression. Movement directions are identical with those of active movements.

Passive movements are performed by the examiner, and possibly without any help from the patient. They serve to assess movement quantity (range) and quality through the whole range (resistance) as well as quality of the end of movement (end feel). Passive range of movement (ROM) should be greater than active ROM. Changes in the symptoms are noted.

Accessory movements

Angular/rotatory (e.g., PAIVM, gapping)

The test of these movements yields additional information about mobility and stability. Aspects assessed are the resistance-free movement range, the onset of first resistance as well as its further behaviour, the influence of movement on the symptoms, the range of the whole movement, and the quality at the end of movement.

Translatory (e.g., traction, compression, gliding)

The test of translatory movements serves to assess quantity and quality of the arthrokinematic movement components of the joint as well as their influence on the symptoms. The test is intended to help distinguish intra-articular from extra-articular problems.

MUSCLE TESTS

Resistance tests (pain and strength)

At first, muscles are tested in synergies, isometrically against resistance. If possible, an attempt is made not only to test the main function of a muscle but also to isolate the muscle within a synergy, via its side functions in potentially other starting positions. In this way, it may be possible to assign muscular disorders to a particular muscle. If need be, muscles can also be tested concentrically and/or eccentrically against resistance.

Length tests

The length (flexibility) of muscles is evaluated by the maximally possible distance between origin and attachment. It is very important in this test to prevent other, potentially sensitive structures (e.g., nerves), which are equally lengthened with this movement, from limiting the manoeuvre and thus leading to a false positive result.

NEUROLOGICAL EXAMINATION

Function

Sensitivity

Generally, only sensitivity to touch is tested. To this end, respective skin areas are touched by a brush, a cotton pad, or slightly with a finger, and changes observable by comparison of both sides as well as their spread and their borders (dermatome, peripheral nerve) are noted.

Reflexes (peripheral and central)

The quantity and side differences of the tendon reflexes as well as the occurrence of pathological reflexes (e.g., Babinski's reflex) are assessed.

Strength of key muscles

The strength of the key muscles is isometrically tested by comparison of both sides. To be able to judge the patient's strength, the patient's resistance has to be broken.

Motor function

Motor function is assessed by means of ataxia tests (e.g., finger–nose trial: deviation of speed and path of movement from the harmonic ideal) and other coordination tests.

Neurodynamics

Different movements of the movement apparatus serve to test, by comparison of both sides, mobility, adaptability, and tensile tolerance of the nervous system. To this end, standardized procedures are used, e.g., upper limb neurodynamic tests 1–3 (ULNT 1–3), straight leg raise (SLR), prone knee bend (PKB), and the slump test (Butler 2000).

PALPATION

Tissue palpation – palpation at rest

Palpation serves to assess invisible tissue changes due to functional disorders as well as their exact localization in a structure that is already known to be responsible for a disorder. In this context, temperature, turgor, elasticity and plasticity, displaceability, tonus, and adequate sensation to pressure and pull are evaluated (Zahnd and Mühlemann 1998).

Movement palpation

With the help of movement palpation, quality and quantity of movement in joints and also in adjacent tissues are assessed. Qualities such as crepitus, joint cracking, jumping of tendons and ligaments are noted.

COMPLEMENTARY APPARATIVE EXAMINATIONS

Imaging, electrodiagnostics, laboratory examinations

These examinations, which normally are not performed by the manual therapist himself/herself, may complement manual therapy examination results if necessary and serve to further test a hypothesis.

Table 1.1 Categories of examination tools and their information content

Category	Information
Safety tests	Warning about dangerous situations
Provocation and alleviation of symptoms	Identification of the symptom-provoking area (generally and specifically)
Mobility tests	Quantity and quality of movement
Tests relating to the nervous system	Function and mobility of the nervous system
Resistance tests	Quantity of strength and pain
Palpation	Changes in texture and sensitivity of tissues
Reassessment	Changes in signs and symptoms

Way of proceeding in examinations

GENERAL ASPECTS

The choice of examination tools and their selective application is sometimes difficult. Frequently, all available examination tools are employed one after another in a standardized way. This means that information might be gathered that is irrelevant for the actual presentation. Providing such 'unnecessary' information means, on the one hand, a loss of time, and on the other hand, it may cause confusion. The choice of examination tools has to be related to the question of what information is needed to test a relevant hypothesis. In this respect, it is helpful to classify examination tools according to their information content into different categories (Table 1.1) and apply them accordingly.

So, for instance, it is of little use to ask the patient whether, in a test of joint play, pain is provoked, since this is not the information that the test is designed to provide. A test of joint play serves uniquely for evaluating quantity and quality of movement. It is not an appropriate choice, however, for identification of the symptom-provoking area.

STANDARD WAY OF PROCEEDING

The standard way of proceeding provides only a framework which is to ensure that no details remain unnoticed. This, however, does not mean that a therapist has to stick to this way of proceeding in any case. The actual presentation and the therapist's clinical experience will determine which examination tools will be necessary to test relevant working hypotheses.

The way of proceeding is as follows:

1. functional demonstration
2. area localization
3. functional examination of affected or probably affected areas
   - general movement tests
     - active
     - passive
   - additional tests
     - symptomatic movement combinations
     - specific provocation and alleviation (angular or translatory (accessory))
     - specific mobility, angular or translatory (accessory)
     - resistance

- ○ palpation
- ○ neurology
- ○ data not ascertained by manual therapy means, such as imaging procedures, laboratory results

4. interpretation of the assessments
5. treatment (test treatment)
6. reassessment
7. adaptation of treatment.

Functional demonstration

This part of the physical examination tries to clarify whether symptoms occur or are changed with or after movements or with certain postures. The exact position and/or the quantity or quality of the movement which influences (provokes, increases, or decreases) the symptoms is noted.

The patient is asked to demonstrate in which position or with which movement the symptoms occur or change.

Note: With irritable presentations or symptoms that are judged as dangerous, this examination step is not performed.

Area localization

Ideally, the patient can demonstrate the symptom-provoking or symptom-changing movement or position (see 'Functional demonstration'). If this is not the case, passive manoeuvres (e.g., overpressure) may have to be used as well. Specific manual therapy differentiation tests are used in area localization to first provoke symptoms and then alleviate them. To this end, an attempt is made first to localize the region from which symptoms are provoked (e.g., cervical spine, thoracic spine, shoulder girdle) (Fig. 1.4).

Note: These considerations only refer to peripheral nociceptive mechanisms.

The patient demonstrates the symptom-provoking or symptom-reducing movement or position. According to the current hypothesis (localization and type of pain, inspection, symptom behaviour, history, clinical patterns), a differentiation has to be made among all regions in question. To this end, specific movements are employed which only move one of the sections in question into the pain-provoking or pain-reducing direction, respectively, whereas all other sections in question should remain immobile or be moved in the opposite direction by the test movement.

The starting position for these manoeuvres is the position which the patient just experiences as still pain-free. If possible, the movement should be performed actively, so that additionally the patient's ability to perform an isolated movement can be assessed. Only if the patient is not able to execute these movements correctly will the therapist assist or move passively. Then, it should be tried in the same way to alleviate symptoms by means of an isolated movement, starting from a position at the border of provoking symptoms. If in this way the patient's symptoms can be provoked and alleviated, the origin of symptom provocation should be presumed to be in the tested area.

With this way of proceeding it is possible to identify the area where the symptoms come from. If no symptom-provoking or symptom-changing movement or position is known, all potential

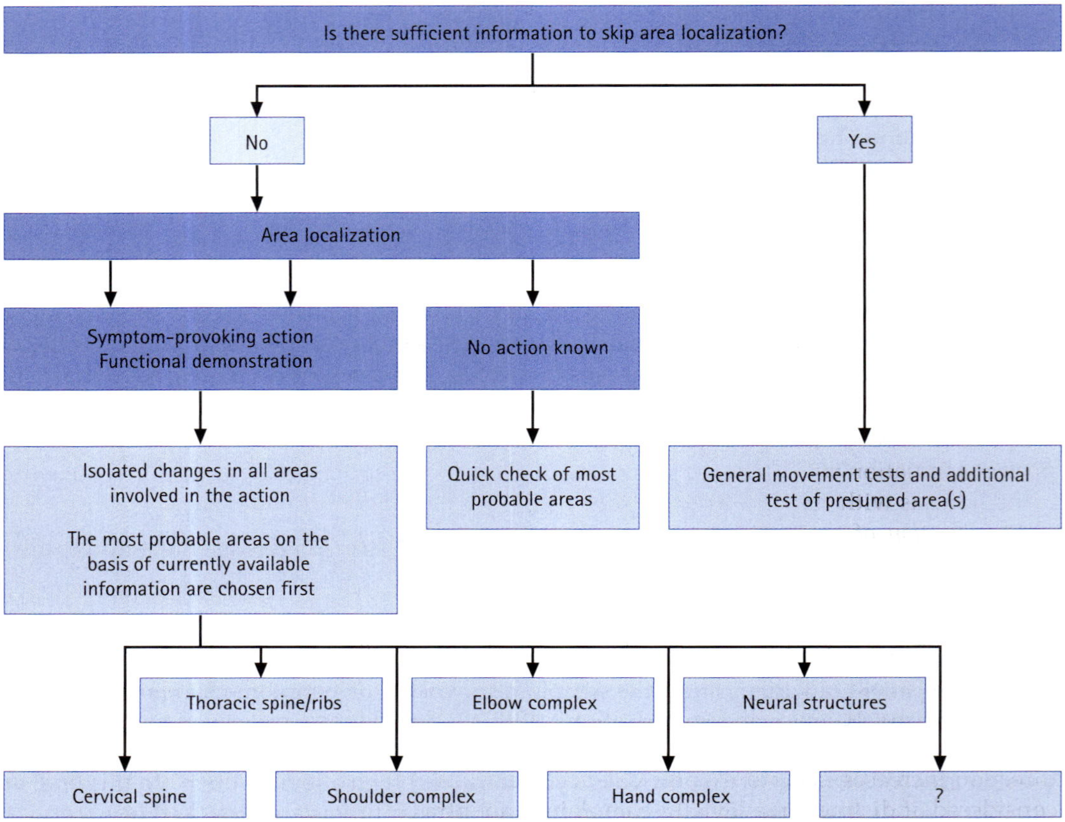

Figure 1.4 Area localization, with symptoms in the upper half of the body, overview.

regions according to the current hypothesis are checked by means of different test movements (quick check), trying to reproduce the symptoms described by the patient. Once the region is identified, systematic further differentiation within that region (additional tests) will follow.

Functional examination

General movement tests (active and passive)

Standardized examination protocols and their interpretation are described in the literature in detail, but not consistently (Cyriax 1982, Kaltenborn 1992, 1999, Maitland 1994, 1996, Frisch 1995). General movement tests include active and passive angular/rotatory movements. The examination of all other movements (e.g., accessory movements, resistance tests) is assigned to the additional tests.

Additional tests

Symptomatic movement combinations

In the spine, the affected region is moved according to the *combined movements* described by B. Edwards (1992), so as to find that combination of movements which most distinctly reproduces the patient's specific symptom. Interpretation of the identified symptom-provoking movement combinations influences the current hypothesis (e.g., regular/irregular pattern or coupled/non-coupled movement, facet problem vs. disc problem; Edwards 1992, Kaltenborn 1992).

Specific provocation and alleviation

The region suspected on the basis of area localization can be differentiated further by specific provocation/alleviation – now mostly by means of passive test movements.

Goals of specific provocation and alleviation:

- isolation of a joint/segment within an articular complex
- identification of the symptom-provoking or symptom-reducing movement direction within the affected joint/segment.

Isolation of a joint/segment within an articular complex: In a symptom-provoking articular complex, the aim is to move only one joint of this complex into the pain-provoking or pain-reducing direction. All other joints of this complex are supposed to be moved by the test movement into the opposite direction or remain immobile. The starting position for these manoeuvres is that joint position at which the patient's specific symptoms just begin. For the purpose of provocation, the starting position is just still symptom-free, whereas for the purpose of alleviation it is just at the beginning of symptom provocation. The way of proceeding is the same as with area localization (see p. 13).

Identification of the symptom-provoking or symptom-reducing movement direction within the affected joint/segment: Then, in the now identified symptom-provoking joint, an attempt is made, by means of accessory movements, to find the specific movement direction which allows provocation or alleviation of symptoms. At first, those accessory movements are employed which seem to be reasonable in a biomechanical sense. So, for instance, with a symptom-provoking flexion in segment C4, a ventrocranial push of C4 will increase the symptoms (provocation), whereas a ventrocranial push of C5 will reduce them (alleviation). Furthermore, if in a symptom-provoking position an accessory movement in a distraction direction increases symptoms, an extra-articular cause for symptom provocation has to be considered; if distraction alleviates complaints, an intra-articular cause is probable.

If the search were restricted only to 'biomechanically reasonable' movements, however, this would impose a limitation. As many alternatives as possible should be looked at, even if, at that point in time, the context still remains unclear (de Bono 1992).

Specific provocation and alleviation serves to localize the symptom-provoking movement disorder and to identify the symptom-provoking movement direction, but not to identify the symptom-provoking structure.

Structural differentiation in complex sections of the movement apparatus by means of isolated tests is very much questioned (Ure et al. 1993, Leroux et al. 1995, Pfund et al. 1998a,b). Nevertheless, this is tried again and again in many ways. Such attempts will, however, at best be suitable for gaining additional information to confirm or weaken an existing hypothesis.

Note: To form a hypothesis, the therapist has to draw on the data of the whole examination as well as on the continuity of the presentation over several sessions.

Specific mobility

When, by specific provocation and alleviation, the symptomatic joint in an articular complex has been identified, a test of specific mobility serves to find out whether the joint moves normally, too little or too much. The result of this test will influence the type and dosage of treatment.

Specific mobility is tested by means of accessory/translatory movements (e.g., joint play), and at the spine additionally by means of angular movements (Kaltenborn 1992, Maitland 1994).

The contralateral side of the body is used as reference for judging quantity and quality of movement (it has to be checked first whether this side is symptom-free and free of previous injuries). Along the spine, neighbouring segments serve as reference.

For the description of the procedures listed below, which also are part of the examination but have been discussed comprehensively elsewhere, the reader is referred to the relevant literature:

- specific palpation (Zahnd and Mühlemann 1998)
- neurological examination (Mumenthaler 1988)
- examination of the muscles (Cyriax 1982, Evjenth and Hamberg 1984).

Interpretation of the assessments

A functional or motor disorder (somatic dysfunction) manifests in the form of altered mobility, pain, and tissue changes. These three components usually do not exist in isolation, and interact with each other. For that reason, during reassessment it has always to be tested, too, how a change in mobility influences the other two components (Greenman 1996).

Quantity of movement

Mobility is assessed in comparison with the unaffected side and/or the mobility seen as normal in the respective regions. Reduced mobility is referred to as *hypomobility*, increased mobility as *hypermobility*. These notions merely refer to the quantity of movement.

With painful movement disorders, interpretation of findings is more difficult. For instance, hypomobility due to pain (defensive spasm) may hide normal mobility or even hypermobility.

(As to consequences regarding treatment, see 'Means of treatment' and 'Dosage of manual therapy treatment techniques', below).

Quality of movement (resistance)

Resistance is a quality of movement, which is assessed during the passive mobility test. It may yield important hints regarding the movement-limiting structure (*end feel*, Cyriax 1982), the acuteness of the respective movement disorder (acute vs. chronic), and the size of the neutral zone (Panjabi 1992a,b). All this, in turn, has consequences for treatment (see 'Dosage of manual therapy treatment techniques').

Tissue changes

As has been mentioned already, the dysfunction of a joint causes changes in the tissues related to this function in some way or other. No tissue is exempt from this process. Usually, the problem is some hypofunction and its consequences.

As hypofunction is associated with decreased loading capacity, the loading capacity of all affected tissues will be lower (Kannus et al. 1992). Reduced loading capacity, in turn, increases the chance of injuries due to overload, which closes the vicious circle. This has to be taken into account when, in treatment planning, the dosage of treatment techniques is determined.

Tissue changes are tested in manual therapy by the additional test of palpation. This test serves to assess changes in temperature, humidity, turgor, displaceability, tonus, mass, layering, and sensitivity (Zahnd and Mühlemann 1998).

Test treatment

The test treatment is not only the first treatment but also, together with reassessment, another means of testing the current hypothesis. Depending on the clinical presentation, it may influence the momentary dysfunction or a predominating contributing factor. It may take the form of pain treatment or of a treatment to take load off a nerve root, to improve mobility, or to stabilize hypermobility. It can often be observed that test treatments use several measures. This is a mistake insofar as it will be difficult or impossible to judge which measure has improved or worsened the situation. For that reason, a test treatment should employ only one measure, chosen as the most appropriate one in the current situation. This is usually a treatment in a symptom-provoking area or the treatment of a contributing factor. Immediately afterwards, a reassessment is performed. The trial treatment of areas with negative provocation tests can still positively influence the symptoms. Only reassessment of signs and symptoms will tell.

Reassessment

Reassessment is one of the most important aspects of manual therapy approaches. With this tool, which involves checking changes in the comparable signs that have been gained from the anamnesis and physical examination, the influence of movement stimuli on the movement disorder with all its components can be checked. In this respect, it is important to assess – in an objective way, unbiased by previous theoretical considerations or favoured hypotheses – potential improvement, worsening, or invariability of the suitable signs and symptoms chosen as comparable signs.

Reassessment makes it possible to check a working hypothesis and to change it if necessary, to select treatment measures, and to adapt their dosage. At the same time, it enables patients to check any changes in their condition and to influence the development of their problem themselves in a more purposeful way. In this way, patients are integrated into the treatment process and take responsibility and control, too.

Reassessment is used at several points in the course of examination and treatment. As examination movements may already positively or negatively influence a patient's condition, comparable signs are always checked after examination of one component (e.g., the neural component) and before transition to the next one (e.g., the joint component). This provides a good check of the state of the problem during the examination and may already lead to the detection of movements or movement directions which might positively or negatively influence the disorder.

Next, reassessment is used after the test treatment (see p. 16). Directly before the next treatment, development signs are again looked at, and then are checked anew after each specific treatment measure. Changes in development signs have to be reproducible with continuous use of treatment measures. In this way, random changes are excluded. Even if the theoretical considerations that underlie the respective choice and dosage of a treatment measure seem quite sound, a negative reassessment will sooner or later have to lead to a change in treatment and/or a re-evaluation of the problem. Only in this way will it be possible to treat purposefully, specifically, and at an adequate dosage.

TREATMENT

Several disciplines (medicine, physiotherapy, psychology, occupational therapy, and sociology) are involved in examination and treatment of disorders of the movement apparatus. Treatment goals are defined in close accordance with the ICF classification (International Classification of Functioning, Disability and Health, WHO 2001). Hence treatment results cannot be judged independently of this holistic aspect. Each discipline uses different, similar or identical procedures to reach particular goals.

From this array of available tools, manual therapy has chosen some specific examination techniques as well as stabilizing and mobilizing treatment techniques. The examples described in the present book are used to discuss various specific ways of examination as well as mobilizing measures.

It is explicitly emphasized, however, that for comprehensive patient management all other possibilities of manual therapy in particular and of physiotherapy in general (e.g., training, ergonomics, activities of daily living) will have to be considered as well.

GOALS OF TREATMENT (according to ICF)

- Improvement and/or restitution of pain-free functional and structural abilities (intactness)
- Improvement and/or restitution of activities of daily life
- Improvement and/or restitution of ability to participate.

MEANS OF TREATMENT

For each of the areas described in this book, the following treatment techniques will be discussed using examples of frequently occurring clinical presentations:

- relaxation techniques
- mobilization techniques
  - active
  - passive
- self-exercise/instruction.

The measures described are a selection of treatment options of manual therapy and are taken from the above categories. Selection of the respective treatment options depends on the clinical presentation and the individual therapist's clinical experience. When hypermobility is assessed, passively or actively stabilizing measures will be applied, according to severity, whereas with hypomobility, mobilizing techniques will be employed. If pain is predominant in a clinical presentation, manual therapy techniques applied do not differ from mobilization techniques with respect to kind and direction of treatment but with respect to dosage (strength, amplitude, site in the trajectory).

In principle, the patient's active cooperation is sought as soon as possible, because active movement incorporates all physiological stimuli necessary both for maintaining and for improving normal function. Such efforts are complemented by passive techniques. Active cooperation presupposes a learning process of varying duration on the part of the patient and solid control on the part of the therapist. If the necessary stimuli cannot be applied via active procedures, cannot be dosed exactly, and/or if there is the danger of damage, exclusively passive procedures are applied for some time.

The practical examples present different treatment measures. Techniques proposed for each example do not claim to be comprehensive. Rather, any technique is always an individual procedure resulting from the unique combination of therapist and patient. To bring some structure into this seemingly infinite continuity of possibilities, different manual therapy concepts follow different rules of treatment. If, however, these rules do not lead to the desired goal, they lose their validity. In that situation, new kinds of solutions beyond the frames of these rules have to be searched for to match the uniqueness of an individual presentation as far as possible.

RELAXATION TECHNIQUES

By relaxation techniques, we mean several types of contraction with subsequent relaxation as well as combinations of touch and movement. Relaxation techniques aim at improving restricted or painful mobility by means of relaxation. The following techniques are used:

- hold–relax techniques
  - co-contraction against distraction
  - movement-directed contraction
- soft tissue techniques
  - passive
  - assistive.

HOLD-RELAX TECHNIQUES

In the authors' clinical experience, the relaxation time after contraction and before further movement into the restricted or painful direction seems to be very important. It can be assumed that this time is necessary to consciously experience the change between tension and relaxation. In the authors' view, it is only this process of conscious experience, combined with the repetition of the active process, which provides the possibility of actively controlling muscle tension in the affected area.

The relaxation technique described by Lewit (1987) uses contraction times of 10–30 seconds and a respective duration of relaxation. According to Lewit, the strength of contraction is not proportionally related to the intensity of relaxation. Rather, a slight contraction will lead to a more intense relaxation. This largely corresponds with the authors' clinical experience, notwithstanding certain cases where a stronger contraction may be successful. This may be the case, for instance, when the method proves ineffective in reassessment even after a significantly prolonged contraction time with low resistance.

Co-contraction against distraction

The muscles in a joint or an articular complex are contracted while the physiotherapist exerts a distraction force on the joint.

Movement-directed contraction

In a joint or an articular complex those muscles are contracted that induce a movement either in a restricted or painful direction or in the opposite direction, while the physiotherapist prevents that movement.

SOFT TISSUE TECHNIQUES

Only those soft tissue techniques that include simultaneous movement of joints will be described here. In the authors' view, these have the advantage of providing a greater afferent input to the CNS than other soft tissue techniques, thus being better able to positively influence the painful movement disorder.

One variant of this technique, in which the treated tissue is lengthened during movement, was called *Funktionsmassage* (massage combined with joint movement) by Olaf Evjenth (Zahnd and Mühlemann 1998). It can be performed both passively and assistively.

MOBILIZATION TECHNIQUES

Active procedures

In active procedures, the patient performs the various mobilizing movements from a defined starting position, while the therapist either fixes one joint partner or moves it into a certain position by means of accessory movements.

Active procedures include active mobilization and active mobilization with accessory movements.

ACTIVE MOBILIZATION

Active mobilization consists of an angular movement into the restricted direction with fixation of one joint partner.

ACTIVE MOBILIZATION WITH ACCESSORY MOVEMENTS

Active mobilization with accessory movements consists of an accessory movement of the moving joint partner, e.g., translatory gliding on traction and a simultaneous angular movement into the restricted direction with fixation of the other joint partner.

The technique of active mobilization with accessory movements is not a standard component of manual therapy training. Only Mulligan (1999) made an attempt to systematize this treatment technique. In clinical application, it has achieved spectacular successes, which have not been definitely explained so far, though. The following explanations might apply:

- changes in disturbed arthrokinematics
- correction of a malposition
- changes in the input to the CNS with some movement that had been experienced as painful before.

Passive procedures

Passive procedures are characterized by lacking voluntary activity on the part of the patient. They are classified into mobilizations and manipulations and are regarded as the classical procedures of manual therapy.

A distinction is made between passive angular (physiological) movements and passive accessory (e.g., translatory) movements (Kaltenborn 1992, 1999, Maitland 1994, 1996). While accessory movements in general are defined as joint movements that cannot be performed voluntarily, the definition of translatory movements is based on a mechanical model (Kaltenborn 1999). In practice, application of theoretical models is often associated with problems, and the models are often only applied to a limited extent.

It seems questionable whether purely translatory movements could be performed at sections of the movement apparatus where the bone contact necessary for performance of such movement is not possible, e.g., at the spine. For that reason, performance of a purely passive translatory movement is more likely at joints of the extremities than at the spine (Zahnd and Baumgartner 2000).

Despite such critical observations, however, treatment with passive translatory joint techniques has proved effective in everyday clinical practice for decades.

MOBILIZATIONS

Basically, there are the following possibilities for performing passive mobilization:

- in the most restricted direction
- in the least restricted direction
- in the most painful direction
- in the least painful direction
- in all directions.

Different manual therapy concepts maintain different views on the application of these options. In the authors' view, selection of treatment direction and dosage of treatment should be determined not only by biomechanical or other rules but above all by reassessment (see 'Examination of the movement apparatus').

MANIPULATIONS

Manipulation refers to any manual intervention on the body. The different use of the notions of mobilization and manipulation in the various disciplines has certainly contributed to discordance, communication difficulties, and confusion among the different schools of manual therapy. For this reason, we will quote, below, some definitions given in the literature.

Manipulation:

- The application of accurately determined and specifically directed manual forces to the body (Korr 1978; 2nd conference of the National Institute of Neurology and Communicative Disorders and Stroke (NINCDS)).
- Manipulation is the therapeutic application of manual force. Spinal manipulative therapy broadly defined includes all procedures where the hands are used to mobilize, adjust, manipulate, apply traction, massage, stimulate or otherwise influence the spine and paraspinal tissues with the aim of influencing the patient's health (Haldeman 1980, Ward and Sprafka 1981).
- Any kind of passive movement used in examination or treatment (Maitland 1994).
- A small amplitude rapid movement (not necessarily performed at the limit of a range of movement) which the patient cannot prevent taking place (Maitland 1994).
- A passive carefully regulated thrust or force delivered with controlled speed, depth and magnitude to articulations at or near the end of the passive or physiologic range of motion, but not exceeding the anatomic limits of motion, often accompanied by joint 'crack' or vacuum phenomenon and the resultant physiologic responses (Sandoz 1976, Grice 1979).

Manipulation (high velocity thrust, HVT) is a particular passive procedure. Due partly to its sensational successes, as well as its risks, it is probably one of the most discussed issues within manual therapy.

In German speaking countries, the notion of *manipulation* is most often used in Sandoz's sense, whereas in anglophone countries, Haldemann's and Maitland's definitions are preferred.

In the context of the treatment techniques described in this book, manipulation (HVT) will not be discussed.

INSTRUCTION AND SELF-EXERCISES

Instruction refers to all means of treatment that can be imparted by verbal and visual communication. This includes, for example, the instruction of exercises and ergonomic behaviours, or information given to patients relating to their relevant problems in order to improve their experience and understanding of the disease as well as their strategies for coping successfully with their dysfunctions.

Self-exercises represent an elementary part of the treatment strategy. They are intended to be used as specifically and analytically as other therapeutic procedures. Self-exercises employed in this way provide the chance to test hypotheses developed during a treatment session and thus gain a better understanding for further clinical proceedings.

Pre-prepared, standardized exercise programmes do not match the authors' idea of a specific manual therapy treatment. Even if it is reasonable to teach the patient a series of exercises to improve his or her general fitness, such exercises will not serve the analysis and specific treatment of the patient's movement problem but at best the treatment of some contributing factor.

DOSAGE OF MANUAL THERAPY TREATMENT TECHNIQUES

Theoretical foundations

Documentation of the dosage of manual therapy techniques is usually done according to tissue resistance. For documentation of the examination, treatment and reassessment during an individual session and over several sessions as well as for communication with colleagues, the dosage of the chosen treatment techniques should be recorded as exactly as possible. Information should be given about the force used, the type of movement, and the movement direction. At present, different manual therapy concepts use different notions for such a documentation. Standardization in this respect would be of great value.

To generate a common understanding and hence a common terminology, we will relate *Kaltenborn's* and *Maitland's movement grades* to tissue resistance, as shown in Figure 1.5.

The main elements are based on the work of Noyes (Noyes and Grood 1976, Frankel and Nordin 1989), which presents the force–elongation curve for the anterior cruciate ligament (Fig. 1.5). From the force–elongation curve, a load–deformation curve can be derived by representing the deformation of some material. To this end, the extent of deformation and the increase in the tension of the material are measured simultaneously and recorded. The curve achieved in this way depicts the following three parameters, which demonstrate the strength of a structure until it breaks or tears:

- the tension it can support
- the deformation it can undergo
- the energy it can absorb (area beneath the curve).

Zones of the load–deformation curve:

- toe zone
- elastic zone
- plastic zone.

TOE ZONE

The toe zone is characterized by an overproportional deformation with a small increase in tension. Above all, the matrix is put under tension. The collagenous fibres start to align (van den Berg 1998).

ELASTIC ZONE

The elastic zone is characterized by an almost linear deformation, depending on the material, while the deformation resistance increases rapidly due to the alignment of the collagenous fibres and their absorption of the stress. In the last third of the elastic zone, micro-ruptures of the tissue already occur (Noyes and Grood 1976). Clinically, these micro-lesions may cause pain, but stability is not reduced.

If a collagenous fibre is kept under constant tension within the elastic zone for a prolonged time (greatest effect after 16 hours, van den Berg 1998), the *creep* phenomenon will show (Currier and Nelson 1992). Due to the time required for such lengthening of tissue, this effect cannot be achieved with the manual therapy techniques that are normally used. The *creep* phenomenon leads to a reversible lengthening of the fibre. If the fibre is kept constantly in a lengthened state, the *relaxation* phenomenon will occur (Currier and Nelson 1992).

PLASTIC ZONE

Here, the deformation due to macro-ruptures suddenly increases if further increase in tension is attempted. If the tissue is destroyed, the tension suddenly decreases.

The three zones correlate well with clinical conditions. The first two zones correspond with normal physiological load, which can largely be tolerated without lesions occurring. Only the end of the second as well as the third zone correspond with loads that will lead to lesions of different degrees of severity (Frankel and Nordin 1989).

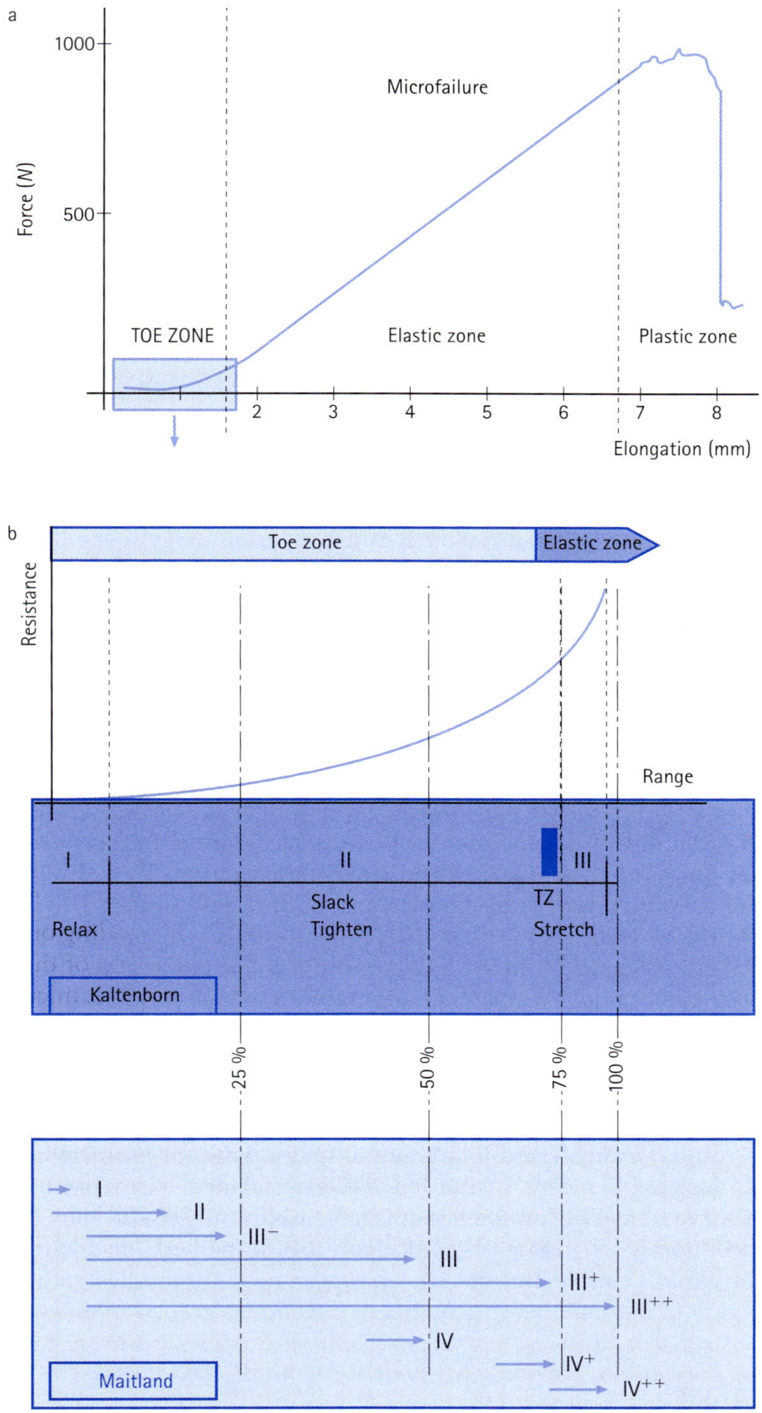

Figure 1.5a and b Model for documentation and dosage of treatment techniques. **a**, Derived from the force–elongation curve. **b**, Kaltenborn's and Maitland's movement grades are transferred to the accessible area of manual therapy load zones. The percentages depicted show the tissue resistance that can be felt. TZ, transition zone.

As the theoretical foundations for the different dosage concepts have been derived from laboratory tests on the loading capacity of collagenous fibres, and since in a living person active mechanisms will play a protective role with increasing load, manual therapy tests and treatments normally are performed only in the toe zone and at the beginning of the elastic zone (Frankel and Nordin 1989). Therefore, the end of the elastic zone as well as the plastic zone seem accessible only if protective mechanisms are eliminated (e.g., by means of anaesthesia). That is why it is always necessary to consider the loading capacity of the tissue, which differs depending on the lesion, duration of immobilization, phase of healing, age, and physical fitness.

Further information on this subject, for example on deformation with constant load, or on different tissue resistance capacities with loads of different duration, may be found in Frankel and Nordin (1989).

As can be seen in Figure 1.5b, the differences between Kaltenborn's movement grades II and III and Maitland's movement grades II–IV are obvious. Maitland's movement grades II, III, and IV are situated within the interval of Kaltenborn's movement grade II. Maitland's movement grades III^{+} and IV^{+} scarcely exceed Kaltenborn's *transition zone (TZ)*. In the latter, the end of the *slack* is reached. In the interval of Kaltenborn's movement grade III (other side of the slack), therefore, the ends of Maitland's movement grades III^{+} and IV^{+} as well as III^{++} and IV^{++} are situated. It seems clear that such different terminology will entail considerable communication difficulties. For this reason, both terms will be mentioned in the present book.

Dosage of the movement stimulus by means of tissue resistance

Difficulties in dosing the movement stimuli necessary for treatment arise where percentages of maximum tissue resistance are reported as dosage quantity. Apart from the fact that different individuals have different sensations, the maximum tissue resistance is a theoretical value, which is ascertained in in-vitro breaking tests with tissue samples (that rather rarely stem from primates) and which therefore cannot be related to some actually felt resistance.

Frankel and Nordin (1989) assume that in the test and treatment procedures used by the authors, load lies only in the toe zone of the stress–strain curve. Thus, the felt maximum resistance seems not to be relatable to the plastic area of tested tissues. This assumption is supported by laboratory tests, which show that micro-lesions will already occur before the end of the elastic zone is reached (Noyes and Grood 1976). For that reason, it is probable that already before the plastic zone is reached, involuntary protection mechanisms in the form of defensive muscle contraction or evasive movements will be activated. In this way, the parallel elastic elements of the muscle under tensile stress or the periarticular structures are protected, and reaching of the plastic zone is prevented.

The different physical resources of individual physiotherapists also make it seem improbable that set dosages could be transferred to another situation without problems. In spite of all these objections, dosage by means of the felt tissue resistance – in whatever area of the load–elongation curve it may be located – seems to be a clinically useful tool. In the authors' clinical experience, dosage by tissue resistance is a useful method for documentation and monitoring of the clinical course. But there is an urgent need for studies on intra-tester and inter-tester reliability of manual therapy treatment techniques graded in this way.

Clinical application

Due to the variability of clinical presentations of movement disorders, different treatment techniques, dosages, and progressions are chosen. Below, we will try to give some practical hints on choice and dosage of treatments. Inevitably, the representation of this subject will be one-sided now and then. The authors are well aware that described patterns often do not occur in the described form but rather in mixed forms.

PAIN CLEARLY MORE PREDOMINANT THAN RESISTANCE

Pain due to some movement manifests more clearly than resistance against that movement in an acute clinical presentation, e.g., after some tissue lesion or if that movement threatens to injure some tissues. It does not matter whether that occurs due to trauma or overload. Pain mechanisms with this type of presentation are predominantly peripheral nociceptive in nature and represent a protection mechanism against further overload, which has to be taken into account in the choice of the treatment technique.

With such presentations, therapy initially uses loads that match the stage of wound healing (see below). In principle, initially chosen techniques are meant to be performable without pain or resistance. Reassessment will show, however, whether the chosen dosage achieves the desired success. Thus it may (rarely) be the case that with a presentation where pain is more predominant than resistance, only those techniques which clearly move into tissue resistance or which are felt as very painful by the patient will lead to improvement.

RESISTANCE CLEARLY MORE PREDOMINANT THAN PAIN

If, with some movement restriction, resistance is predominating over pain, the problem is usually not an acute injury. The curve of resistance development (force–elongation curve) may differ according to momentary texture and elasticity of the tissue. Depending on the tissue that stops the movement, the end feel is of different quality. The dosage of manual therapy techniques with such presentations corresponds with the expected training-dependent tissue tolerance (see p. 27) and in most cases goes significantly into tissue resistance. Here, too, reassessment shows whether the dosage was chosen correctly. In special cases of presentations with resistance predominating over pain, only those techniques which are performed without pain and without resistance may lead to improvement .

DOSAGE AND PROGRESSION OF TREATMENT

Dosage and progression of manual therapy treatment stimuli are based on the following aspects:

- wound healing
- training state (training-dependent loading capacity of the tissue)
- reassessment (objective and reproducible assessments).

Wound healing

The amount of tissue resistance that can be built up in tissue which is dysfunctional due to a lesion depends, above all, on the healing state (Fig. 1.6). Therefore it is important for the physiotherapist to know the phases of normal wound healing (van den Berg 1998) and to conceive the treatment by taking all positive and negative influences into account as far as possible.

Phases of wound healing

- Inflammation phase: 5 days
- Proliferation phase: up to day 21
- Remodelling and maturation phase: from day 21 on.

Wound healing consists of overlapping phases of specific biochemical processes that serve to repair the injured tissue. The individual phases of wound healing require different dosages of manual therapy techniques.

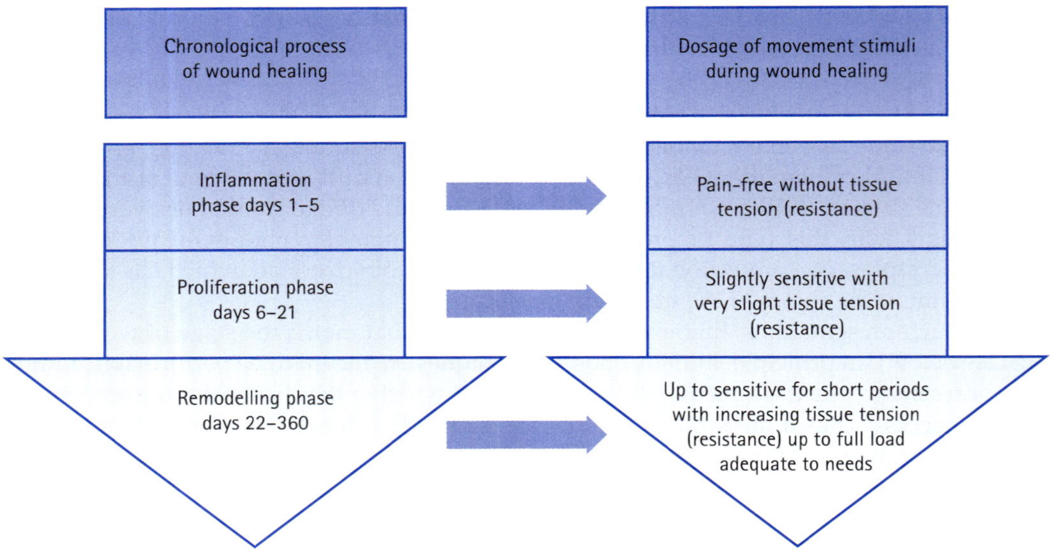

Figure 1.6 Wound healing and dosage of movement stimuli.

Usually, during the very sensitive inflammation phase (days 0–5), pain-free and resistance-free movement stimuli are applied. During the proliferation phase (days 6–21), movement up to the beginning of tissue resistance is applied, which may be associated with slight sensitivity. After completion of the proliferation phase, the intensity of the movement stimuli is slowly and continuously increased up to the full loading capacity of the tissue. Reliable information about the exact force to be used can only be provided by reassessment.

It must not be forgotten that the duration of the phases differs individually, tissue-specifically, and depends on several factors. In this respect, prognostically positive factors have to be distinguished from negative ones (e.g., age, training state, motivation, other pathologies).

Delayed wound healing, which will lead to a delayed increase in the loading capacity of the tissue, is problematic for the physiotherapist. The size of the lesion, blood supply, inflammation mediators, age, nutritional state (lack of vitamins or minerals), additional diseases (anaemia, diabetes, infectious diseases), and medications are of relevance here. Many of these factors cannot be influenced by the physiotherapist. Nevertheless, they must not be neglected, because they affect the loading capacity of the healing tissue (in relation to the time that has passed since the injury) and hence are relevant for the treatment dosage.

There are two further causes of negative wound healing, which, however, can be influenced both by the patient and by the physiotherapist, namely immobilization and bagatellization.

Even though immobilization may be necessary directly after an injury, the negative effects of prolonged immobilization cannot be overlooked (Kannus et al. 1992). In all tissues, loss of function and loading capacity will be the consequence, with loss being different for different tissues and related to the duration of immobilization. As, however, restitution of function and loading capacity, too, differ from tissue to tissue and may, for instance with joint cartilage, take a very long time, immobilization should be limited to whatever is strictly necessary. Appropriate information given to the patient by the physiotherapist is of great importance. It will reduce the patient's fear of movement and at the same time ensure the patient's cooperation, which improves the chances for a treatment success.

Bagatellization involves the opposite kind of problem. Highly motivated patients or patients driven by external factors may not be sufficiently aware that the loading capacity of the structures of their movement apparatus is reduced due to immobilization or other causes. Through continuous micro-ruptures or re-injuries they may prevent the normal progress of healing.

In view of the fact that movement stimuli of treatment and of load due to activities of everyday living may add up, it becomes clear how difficult it can be to determine the correct dosage of treatment. In this respect, theoretical dosage models unfortunately fail all too often, and only the concept of repeated reassessment is ultimately able to address this problem.

Training state of the tissue to be treated (loading capacity)

Another important issue regarding dosage of treatment is the training state of the tissue. While in the treatment of acutely injured structures it is most important to consider the phases of wound healing or the course of healing, in all other dysfunctions of the movement apparatus the training state of the tissue is of relevance.

To be effective at all, a treatment stimulus has to represent a threshold-exceeding load, which triggers an anabolic response of the biological system. Such a stimulus consists of a catabolic disturbance of homeostasis (Röthig et al. 1983). The better the training state of the tissue, the stronger the stimulus has to be so as to be able to disturb homeostasis. On the other hand, already very low stimuli may be threshold-exceeding with untrained tissues. It should be remembered in this respect that training stimuli act very specifically. This means that tissue is only trained well for tasks for which it is frequently used. If a stimulus is unusual in nature, duration, direction, speed, and amount, it will very soon become threshold-exceeding. For this reason, caution is necessary with the application of any new type of load. Tissue overload because of a physiotherapist's over-zealousness is no rare phenomenon. Although usually it only manifests as temporary increase in complaints, it has to be avoided.

For an evaluation of the training state of the tissue, the patient's age, the way tissues have been loaded so far, the duration of a potential immobilization, pathologies (metabolism), medications, and whether the patient's problem is new or recurrent, all have to be considered.

Reassessment

The concept of reassessment – as described by Maitland (1994, 1996) as a key element of his therapeutic approach – was discussed in the context of basic aspects of examination (see p. 17). With respect to dosage of manual therapy treatment, reassessment offers the only objective means of checking all theoretical basic aspects. For that reason, its relevance cannot be rated highly enough.

Clinical examples and dosage of manual therapy stimuli

Defensive spasm before pain

In some presentations, for example infected joints or joints heavily irritated after trauma, an involuntary defensive spasm occurs before sensitive structures are loaded. This prevents further movement. In this case, treatment should primarily consider the cause of the problem. To keep load on affected structures as low as possible, movement is performed only within resistance-free range (see 'Pain clearly more predominant than resistance', above). Whether angular or accessory (e.g., translatory) movements will be applied to this end has to be ascertained by means of reassessment.

Muscle shortening

Muscle tightness and muscle shortening are often reported as the reason for movement restrictions. The range of movement of one or several joints is reduced, and the end feel is soft-elastic. Muscle tightness can be felt by means of specific tissue palpation. This does not mean that the tense part of the inactive muscle would have higher action potentials than the remaining muscle.

The classical treatment for this kind of movement restriction is muscle stretching (Evjenth and Hamberg 1984). The optimum duration of a stretching exercise is still not yet known. But clinical practice shows that different forms of stretching can lead to larger movement ranges in joints. The cause of changed movement ranges is not known. Wiemann and co-workers' (1998) investigations have shown that the resting tonus of a muscle is increased rather than decreased due to stretching. The researchers could show that the resting tonus of muscles decreased with activity under aerobic metabolic conditions (biking). Moreover, their work revealed that the stretched muscle still produced its maximum force in the same angular position of the joint, that is, the muscle had not actually been lengthened (force–length curve/force production). Furthermore, the researchers showed that increased range of movement was associated with a simultaneous tonus increase of the stretched muscle. If the muscle had actually become longer, the distance between its origin and its attachment should have become extensible with tonus remaining the same (shift to the right of the force–elongation curve).

For these reasons, Wiemann et al. (1998) formulated the hypothesis that the range increase at joints after short-term stretching (different techniques and methods during a period of up to 10 weeks) is due to a greater tolerance regarding the tension felt and not to a structural lengthening of the stretched muscle. Wiemann studied healthy individuals, however, so it is not clear whether his results can be transferred to dysfunctional situations.

If the shortening of a muscle represents the functional adaptation to some habitual posture adopted for years, a correction of the problem may require measures to improve positioning (better postural alignment) and to strengthen the antagonists of the shortened muscles rather than measures to stretch the agonists. If this is done after a warm-up phase under aerobic metabolic conditions, relaxation of the shortened muscles will create optimal conditions. Of course, the momentary loading capacity of the different structures has always to be taken into account (see p. 27). For a structural adaptation of muscle length, however, it is necessary that the muscle permanently maintains the new posture and operates within it.

Entrapment problems (menisci, joint mouse)

A presentation where resistance is clearly more predominant than pain is sometimes found in entrapment problems. From a mechanical viewpoint, treatment has to bring the affected joint into a position where the entrapped structure is freed. The joint may be put into such a position passively or by active mobilizations with accessory movements. Subsequently, controlled active movements will be important, because of their good coordination-enhancing effect.

Reflex movement restriction (blocking)

Reflex movement restrictions are spontaneously emerging restrictions in which pain is more predominant than resistance. The cause for such reflex-restricted mobility or blocking is still not known. Different hypotheses about its origin have been proposed (Rahlmann 1987) but none are able to explain all clinical phenomena related to this movement disorder. Nevertheless, they yield useful treatment approaches.

In the authors' experience, such presentations can be treated very well with manipulations (HVT) or with active mobilizations with accessory movements. As such hypomobility exists only for a short time, it can be concluded that no structural tissue change is underlying, which would require a prolonged, strong mobilization technique (e.g., passive techniques of grade III according to Kaltenborn or of grade IV^{+} according to Maitland).

Summary

If manual therapy stimuli are applied with the described dosage and progression, they are, in the authors' clinical experience, very effective in everyday practice.

In general, Roux's rule has to be respected with regard to the intensity of stimuli. Roux's rule says that stimuli that are too weak will be ineffective, stimuli that are too heavy will be damaging, and only adapted stimuli will have positive effects. Accordingly, a movement stimulus is adapted if – regarding the healing process and the current training state of the tissue (loading capacity) – it is mild but nevertheless produces a positive, reproducible effect.

It seems debatable whether some model might be able to explain the effects of manual therapy in a primarily mechanical way. Probably, neurophysiological mechanisms, for example the changing of thresholds regarding the sensations of tension and of pain, in the peripheral but above all in the central nervous system, are of major relevance. Too many clinically observed phenomena cannot be explained in a satisfactory way by the mechanical, peripheralistic model. To test these hypotheses, comprehensive clinical and laboratory studies will be necessary.

This is not to say that it does not matter how joints or other structures are moved. The authors are convinced that the more that movements can be performed in a specific and biomechanically correct way, the fewer adverse effects there will be with examination and treatment techniques. And furthermore, that movement performed in this way will most closely mimic the input necessary to achieve normal movement again.

Chapter 2

Upper central back of the neck

CHAPTER CONTENTS

AREA LOCALIZATION

IDENTIFICATION OF THE POTENTIALLY AFFECTED AREA BY DEMONSTRATION OF A SYMPTOMATIC FUNCTIONAL MOVEMENT/POSITION

Based on the information gained from the anamnesis so far, the therapist tries to ascertain more details about potentially affected sections. This is done by means of area localization, which represents the beginning of the physical examination. Information gained in this way is used to check or modify the relevant hypotheses developed on the basis of the anamnesis and will determine how to proceed.

Area localization is explained by means of examples. In all three examples (different movements of the head), the patient feels pain in the upper central back of the neck. Based on clinical experience and known clinical patterns, the following areas are primarily considered as potential sources of the current complaints:

- cervical spine
- neural structures.

General question: Is there enough information available to skip area localization?	
No	Yes
⇓	⇓
Performance of area localization	• General movement tests • Additional tests • Test treatment

Example 1: Movement of the head backwards

Symptom area: upper/central back of the neck, right side
Symptom provocation: movement of the head backwards (Fig. 2.1)

With this presentation, clinical experience suggests at first the upper and lower cervical spine and the neural structures as symptom-provoking areas.

Below, examples illustrate how to differentiate between these areas. To this end, area localization is first attempted by means of active movements alone. If this is not possible, tests will be performed by means of assistive movements.

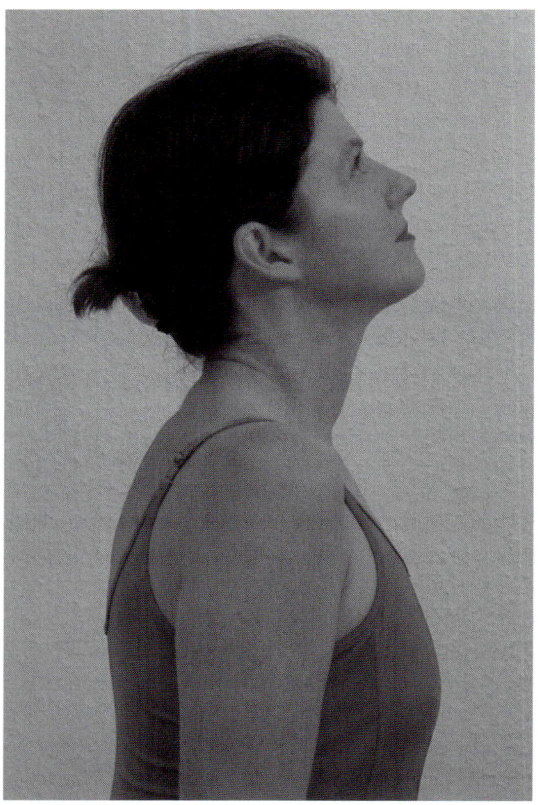

Figure 2.1 Symptom-provoking movement: movement of the head backwards provokes symptoms in the area of the upper central back of the neck.

Hypothesis 1: The symptom-provoking area is the upper cervical spine

Differentiation upper vs. lower cervical spine.

The change in symptoms can be demonstrated exactly:

- provocation of pain (Fig. 2.2a and b, film 2)
- alleviation of pain (Fig. 2.3a and b, film 3).

The result of area localization has to be verified by further specific tests – otherwise the result will remain in doubt.

Assessment			
Goal	**Provocation of pain**	**Alleviation of pain**	**Remarks**
Starting position	Movement of the head backwards to a position immediately before symptoms appear	Movement of the head backwards to a position immediately after symptoms have appeared	
Test movement	Protraction of the head (extension of the upper cervical spine with simultaneous flexion of the lower cervical spine)	Retraction of the head (flexion of the upper cervical spine with simultaneous extension of the lower cervical spine)	
Explanation	Protraction of the head increases extension in the upper cervical spine and simultaneously leads to flexion of the lower cervical spine	Retraction of the head increases extension in the lower cervical spine and simultaneously leads to flexion of the upper cervical spine	
Additional data to support the hypothesis	General and specific mobility of the affected area History, symptom behaviour, type of complaints, 24-hour behaviour Palpation Reproducibility of test results Test treatment Imaging procedures (CT, MRI)		

Hypothesis 2: The symptom-provoking area is the neural structures

Differentiation: neural structures vs. cervical spine.

The change in symptoms can be demonstrated exactly:

- provocation of pain (Fig. 2.4a and b, film 4)
- alleviation of pain (Fig. 2.5a and b, film 5).

The result of area localization has to be verified by further specific tests – otherwise the result will remain in doubt.

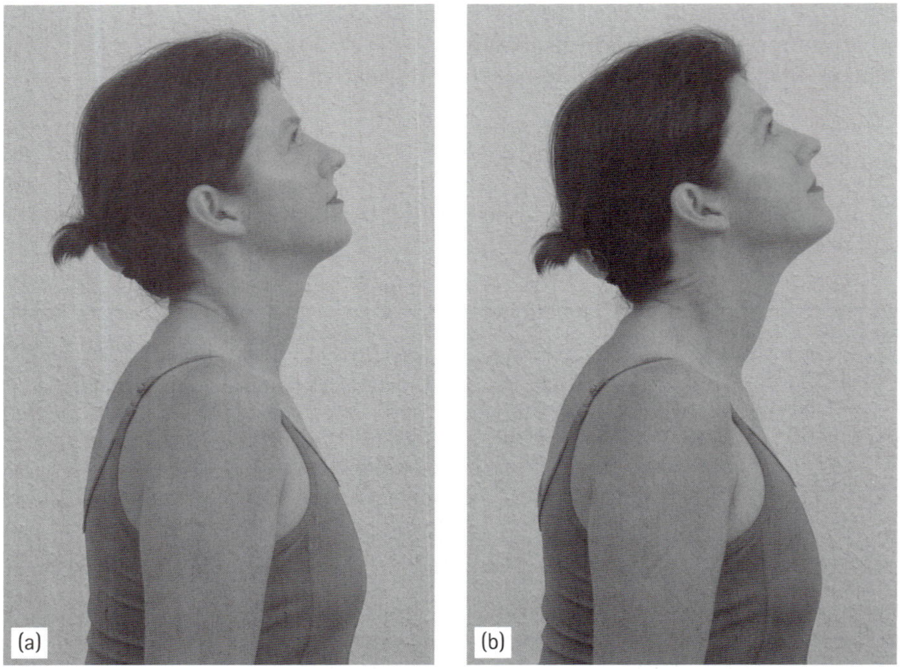

Figure 2.2a and b Area localization with symptomatic movement of the head backwards; differentiation between upper and lower cervical spine; provocation. **a**, Starting position. **b**, End position.

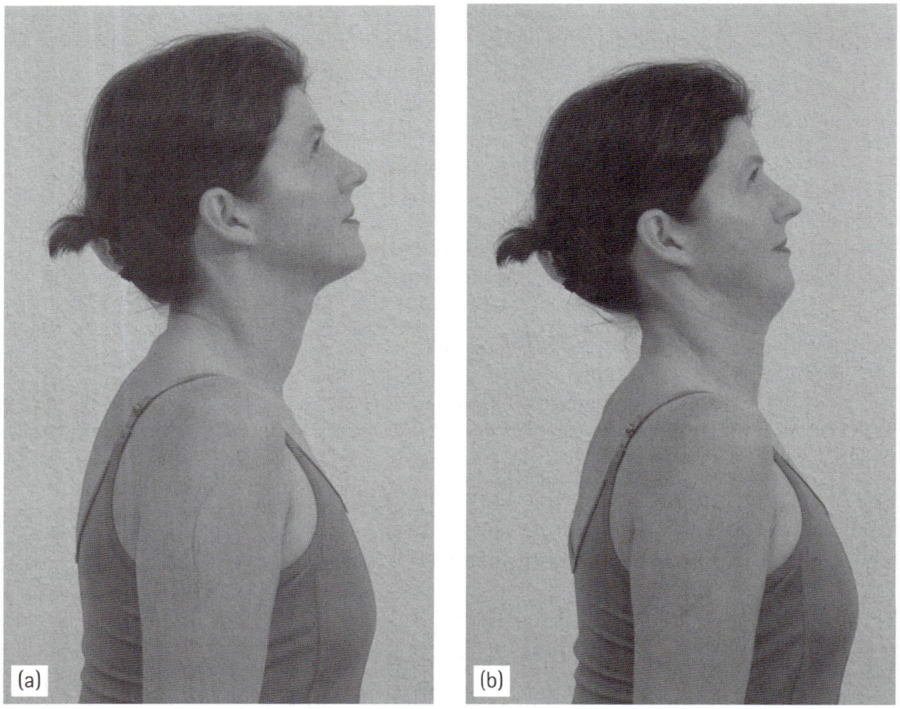

Figure 2.3a and b Area localization with symptomatic movement of the head backwards; differentiation between upper and lower cervical spine; alleviation. **a**, Starting position. **b**, End position.

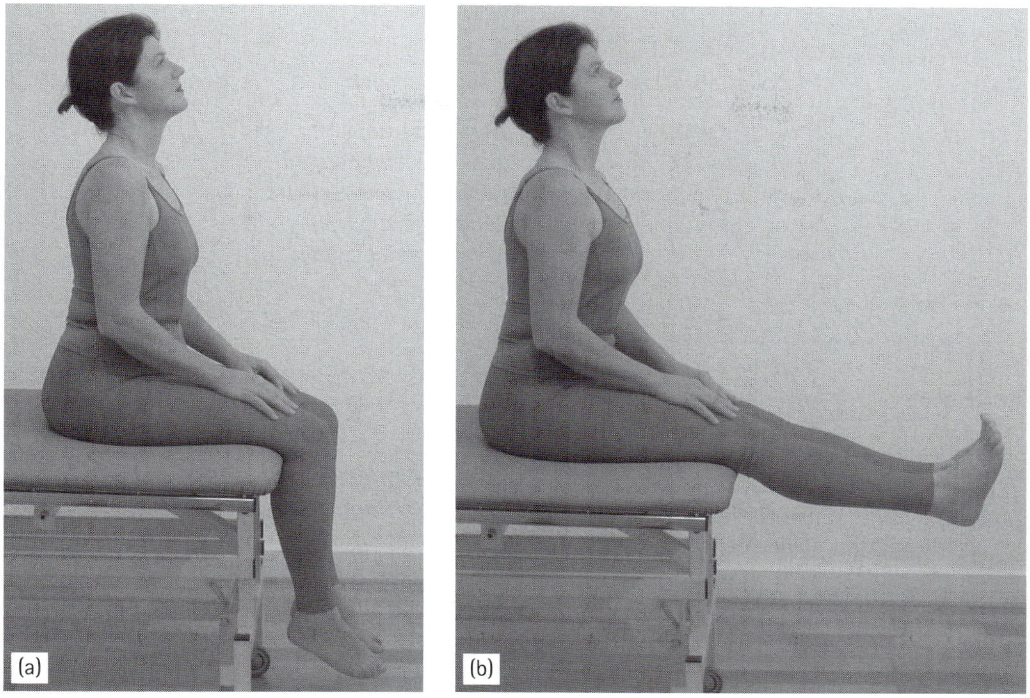

Figure 2.4a and b Area localization with symptomatic movement of the head backwards; differentiation between neural structures and cervical spine; provocation. a, Starting position. b, End position.

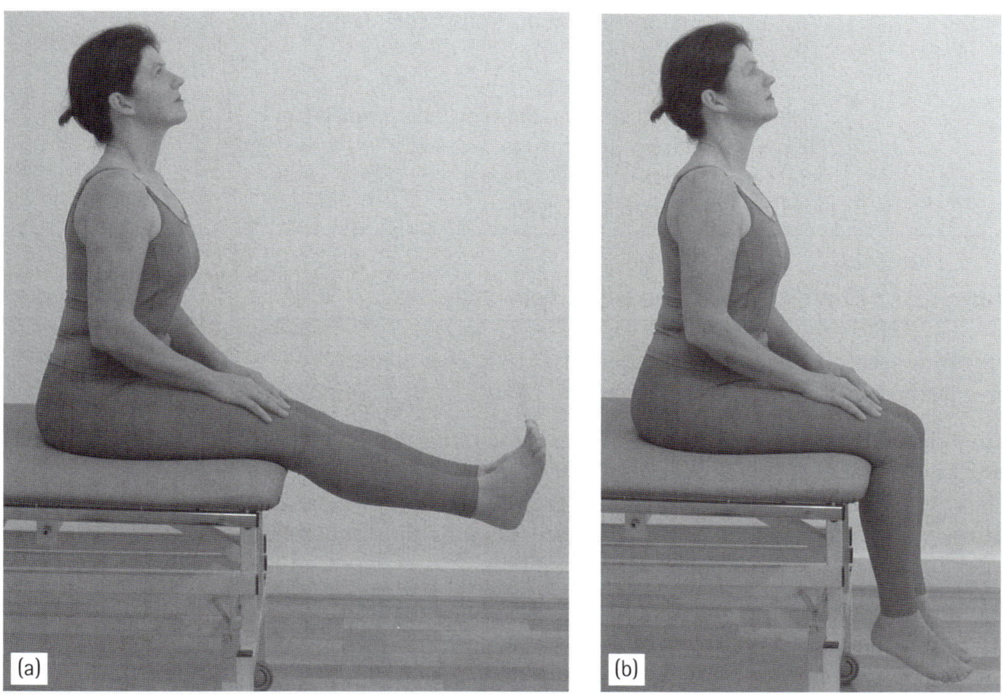

Figure 2.5a and b Area localization with symptomatic movement of the head backwards; differentiation between neural structures and cervical spine; alleviation. a, Starting position. b, End position.

Assessment			
Goal	**Provocation of pain**	**Alleviation of pain**	**Remarks**
Starting position	Movement of the head backwards to a position immediately before symptoms appear	Bilateral extension of the knees and dorsal flexion of the ankles then movement of the head backwards to a position immediately after symptoms have appeared	
Test movement	Bilateral extension of knees and dorsal flexion of ankles, in sitting	Flexion of both knees	Positions of head and spine must not change
Explanation	The test movement increases neural tension	Flexion of both knees reduces the tension of the neural structures produced by the starting position	If the typical pain is provoked or alleviated by these manoeuvres, this suggests at least an involvement of the neural structures
Additional data to support the hypothesis	General and specific mobility of the affected area Further movement of proximal and distal components to increase neural tension, not directly involved in movement of the head backwards, e.g., upper extremity movement History, symptom behaviour, type of complaints, 24-hour behaviour Palpation Nerve mobilization tests Neurodynamic tests (e.g., Spurling's test, Tinel's sign) Reproducibility of test results Test treatment Imaging procedures (CT, MRI)		

Example 2: Movement of the head forwards

Symptom area: upper/central back of the neck, right side
Symptom provocation: movement of the head forwards (Fig. 2.6)

With this clinical presentation, clinical experience suggests at first the upper and lower cervical spine and the neural structures as symptom-provoking areas.

Below, examples illustrate how to differentiate between these areas. To this end, area localization is first attempted by means of active movements alone. If this is not possible, tests will be performed by means of assistive movements.

Hypothesis 1: The symptom-provoking area is the upper cervical spine
Differentiation: upper vs. lower cervical spine.

The change in symptoms can be demonstrated exactly:

- provocation of pain (Fig. 2.7a and b, film 6)
- alleviation of pain (Fig. 2.8a and b, film 7).

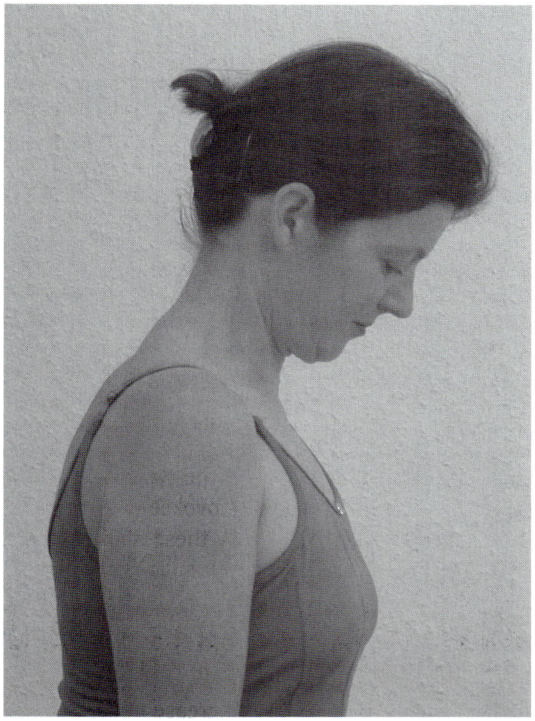

Figure 2.6 Symptom-provoking movement: movement of the head forwards provokes symptoms in the area of the upper central back of the neck.

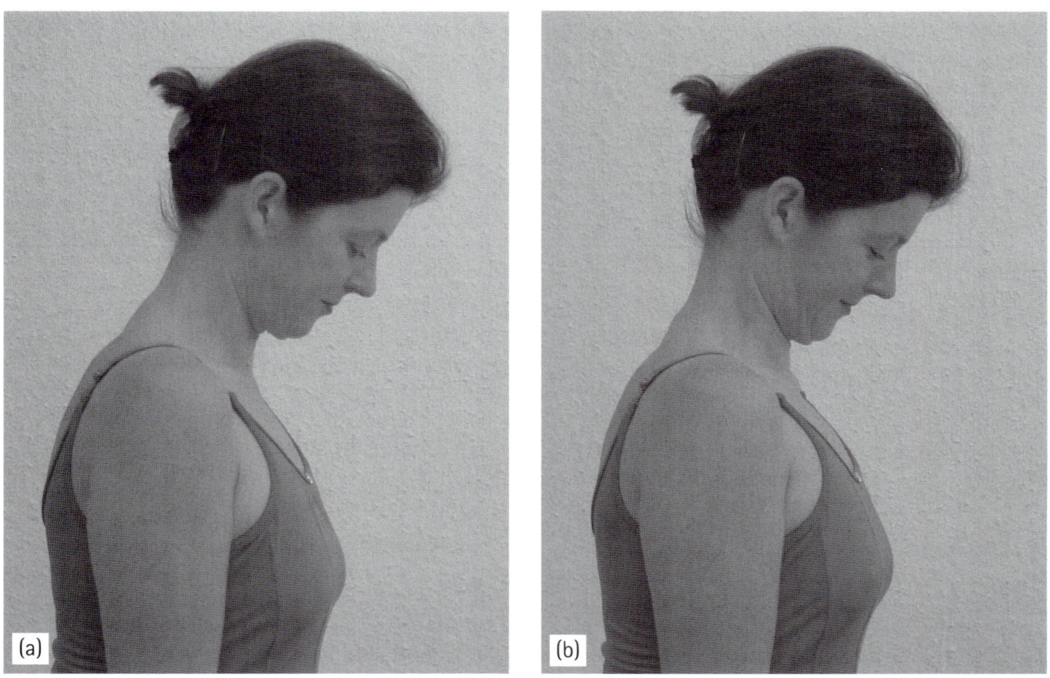

Figure 2.7a and b Area localization with symptomatic movement of the head forwards; differentiation between upper and lower cervical spine; provocation. a, Starting position. b, End position.

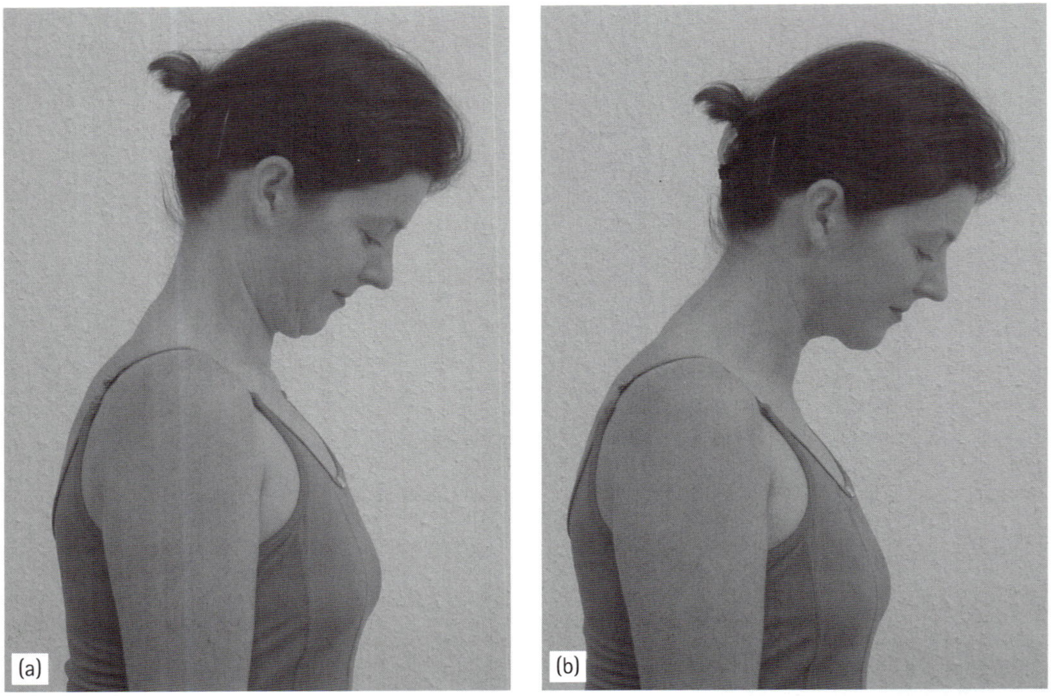

Figure 2.8a and b Area localization with symptomatic movement of the head forwards; differentiation between upper and lower cervical spine; alleviation. a, Starting position. b, End position.

The result of area localization has to be verified by further specific tests – otherwise the result will remain in doubt.

Assessment

Goal	Provocation of pain	Alleviation of pain	Remarks
Starting position	Movement of the head forwards to a position immediately before symptoms appear	Movement of the head forwards to a position immediately after symptoms have appeared	
Test movement	Retraction of the head (flexion of the upper cervical spine, with simultaneous extension of the lower cervical spine)	Protraction of the head (extension of the upper cervical spine, with simultaneous flexion of the lower cervical spine)	
Explanation	Retraction of the head leads to flexion of the upper cervical spine and simultaneously to an	Protraction of the head leads to an extension in the upper cervical spine and simultaneously	

Goal	Provocation of pain	Alleviation of pain	Remarks
	extension of the lower cervical spine	increases the flexion of the lower cervical spine	
Additional data to support the hypothesis	General and specific mobility of the affected area History, symptom behaviour, type of complaints, 24-hour behaviour Palpation Reproducibility of test results Test treatment Imaging procedures (CT, MRI)		

Hypothesis 2: The symptom-provoking area is the neural structures

Differentiation: neural structures vs. cervical spine.

The change in symptoms can be demonstrated exactly:

- provocation of pain (Fig. 2.9a and b, film 8)
- alleviation of pain (Fig. 2.10a and b, film 9).

The result of area localization has to be verified by further specific tests – otherwise the result will remain in doubt.

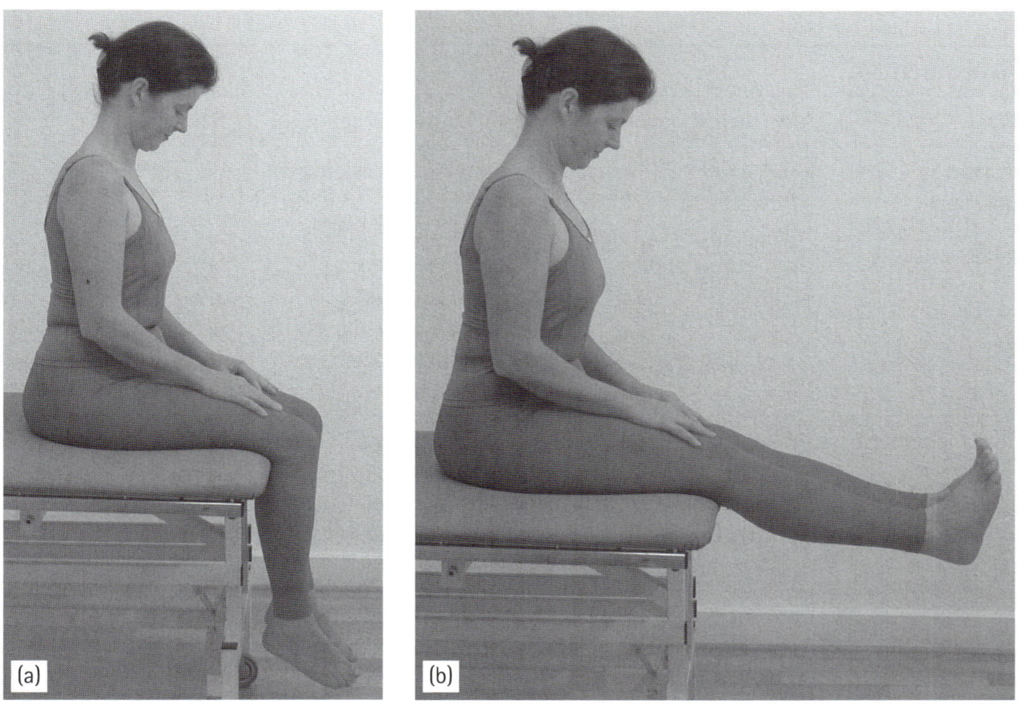

Figure 2.9a and b Area localization with symptomatic movement of the head forwards; differentiation between neural structures and cervical spine; provocation. **a**, Starting position. **b**, End position.

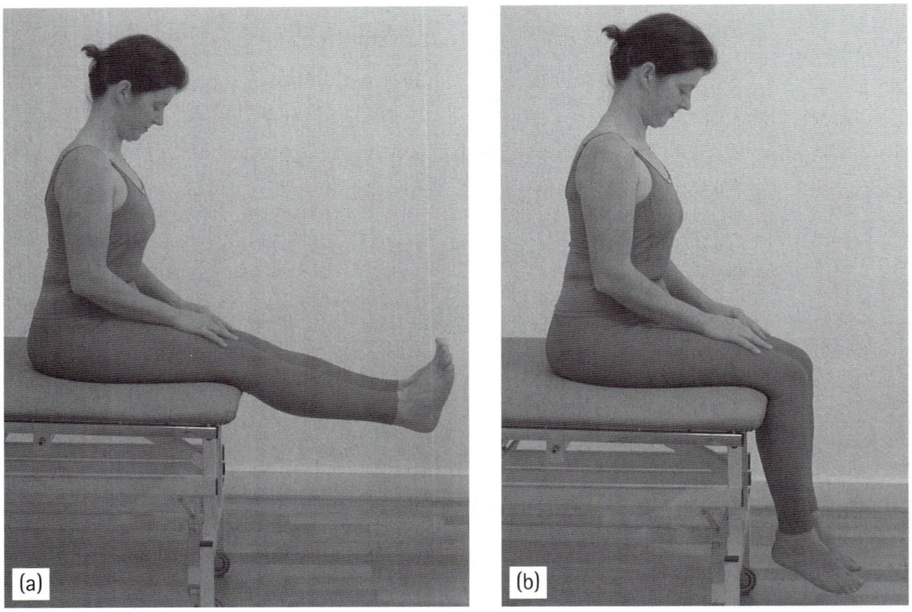

Figure 2.10a and b Area localization with symptomatic movement of the head forwards; differentiation between neural structures and cervical spine; alleviation. **a**, Starting position. **b**, End position.

Assessment			
Goal	**Provocation of pain**	**Alleviation of pain**	**Remarks**
Starting position	Movement of the head forwards to a position immediately before symptoms appear	Bilateral extension of the knees and dorsal flexion of the ankles then movement of the head forwards to a position immediately after symptoms have appeared	
Test movement	Bilateral extension of the knees and dorsal flexion of the upper ankles, in sitting	Flexion of both knees	Positions of head and spine must not change
Explanation	The test movement increases neural tension	Flexion of both knees reduces the tension of the neural structures produced by the starting position	If the typical pain is provoked or alleviated by these manoeuvres, this suggests at least an involvement of the neural structures

Goal	Provocation of pain	Alleviation of pain	Remarks
Additional data to support the hypothesis	General and specific mobility of the affected area Further movement of proximal and distal components to increase neural tension, not directly involved in movement of the head backwards, e.g., upper extremity movement History, symptom behaviour, type of complaints, 24-hour behaviour Palpation Nerve mobility tests Neurodynamic tests (e.g., Spurling's test, Tinel's sign) Reproducibility of test results Test treatment Imaging procedures (CT, MRI)		

Example 3: Turning the head to the right

Symptom area: upper/central back of the neck, right side
Symptom provocation: turning the head to the right (Fig. 2.11)

With this clinical presentation, clinical experience suggests at first the upper and lower cervical spine and the neural structures as symptom-provoking areas.

Below, examples are described of how to differentiate between these areas. To this end, area localization is first attempted by means of active movements alone. If this is not possible, tests will be performed by means of assistive movements.

Hypothesis 1: The symptom-provoking area is the upper cervical spine

Differentiation: upper vs. lower cervical spine.

The change in symptoms can be demonstrated exactly:

- provocation of pain (Fig. 2.12a and b, film 11)
- alleviation of pain (Fig. 2.13a and b, film 12).

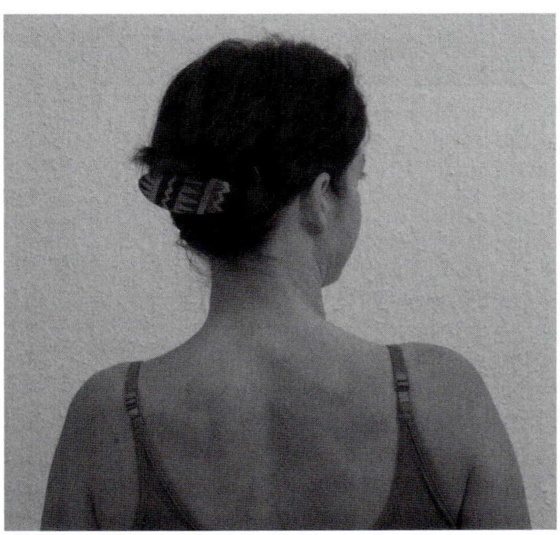

Figure 2.11 Symptom-provoking movement: turning the head to the right provokes symptoms in the area of the upper central back of the neck.

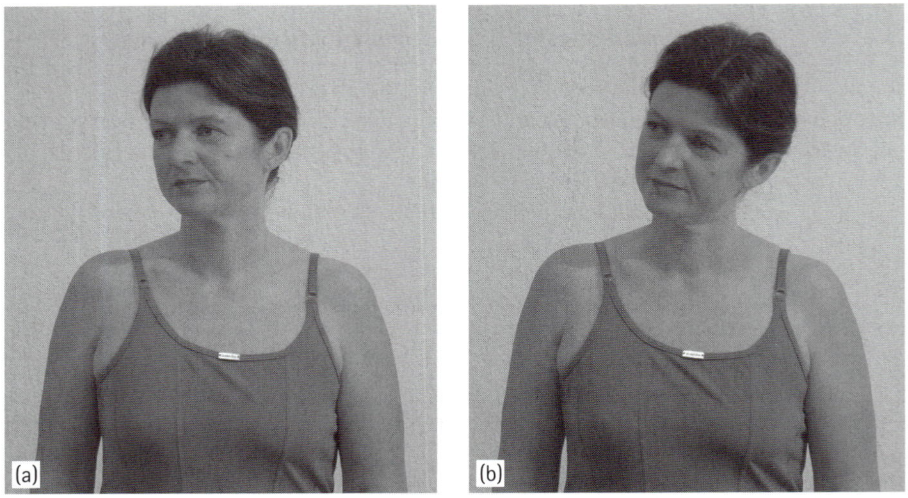

Figure 2.12a and b Area localization with symptomatic movement of the head to the right (right rotation); differentiation between upper and lower cervical spine; provocation. **a**, Starting position. **b**, End position.

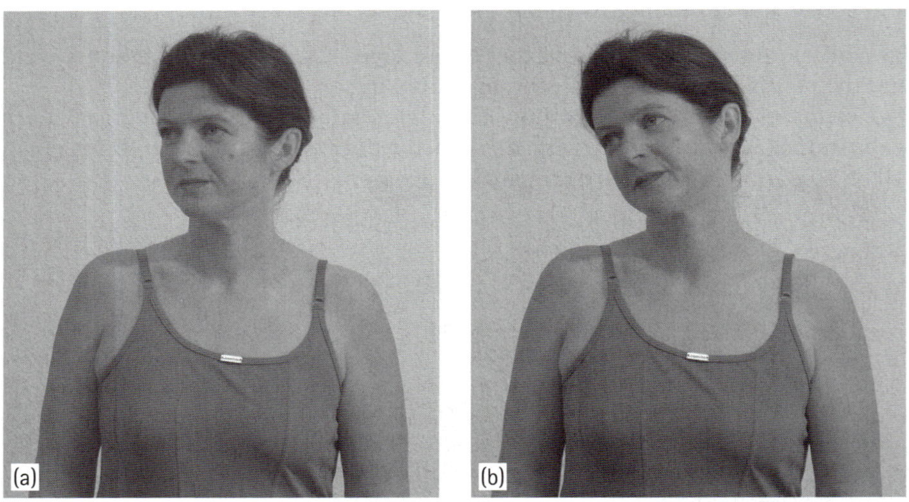

Figure 2.13a and b Area localization with symptomatic movement of the head to the right; differentiation between lower and upper cervical spine; alleviation. **a**, Starting position. **b**, End position.

Assessment

Goal	Provocation of pain	Alleviation of pain	Remarks
Starting position	Turning the head to the right to a position immediately before symptoms appear	Turning the head to the right to a position immediately after symptoms have appeared	
Test movement	Lateral flexion of head and neck to the left	Lateral flexion of head and neck to the right	Head does not change its rotated position

Goal	Provocation of pain	Alleviation of pain	Remarks
Explanation	Lateral flexion of head and neck to the left increases rotation of the upper cervical spine to the right	Lateral flexion of head and neck to the right reduces rotation of the upper cervical spine to the right	
Additional data to support the hypothesis	General and specific mobility of the affected area History, symptom behaviour, type of complaints, 24-hour behaviour Palpation Reproducibility of test results Test treatment Imaging procedures (CT, MRI)		

The result of area localization has to be verified by further specific tests – otherwise the result will remain in doubt.

Hypothesis 2: The symptom-provoking area is the neural structures
Differentiation: neural structures vs. cervical spine.

The change in symptoms can be demonstrated exactly:

- provocation of pain (Fig. 2.14a and b, film 13)
- alleviation of pain (Fig. 2.15a and b, film 14).

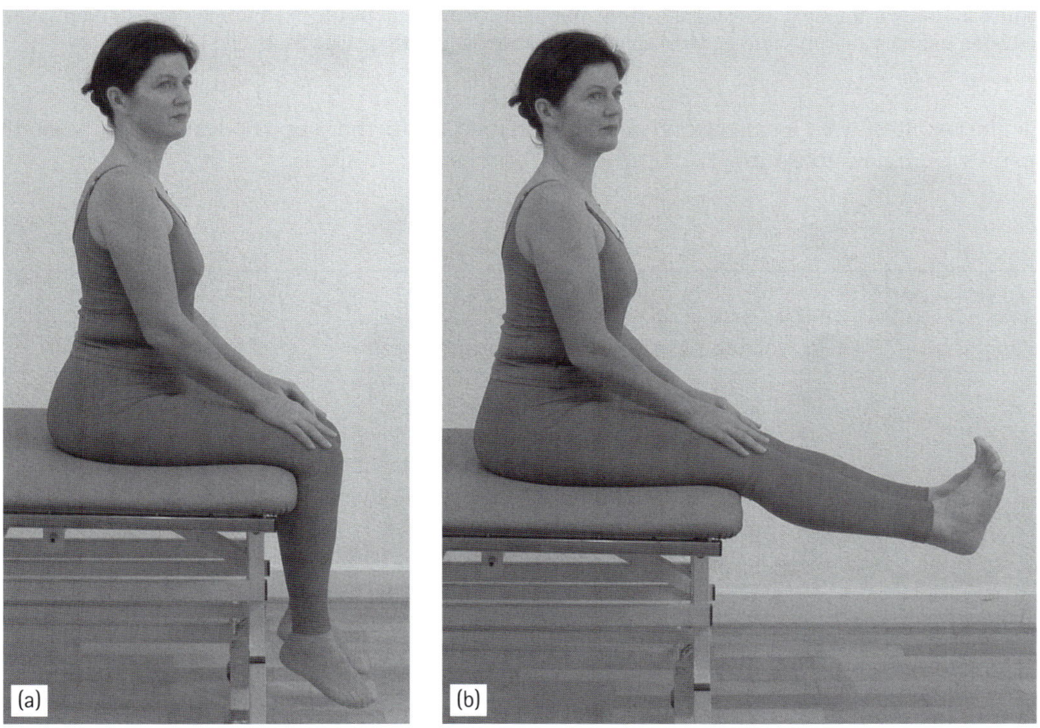

Figure 2.14a and b Area localization with symptomatic movement of the head to the right; differentiation between neural structures and cervical spine; provocation. **a**, Starting position. **b**, End position.

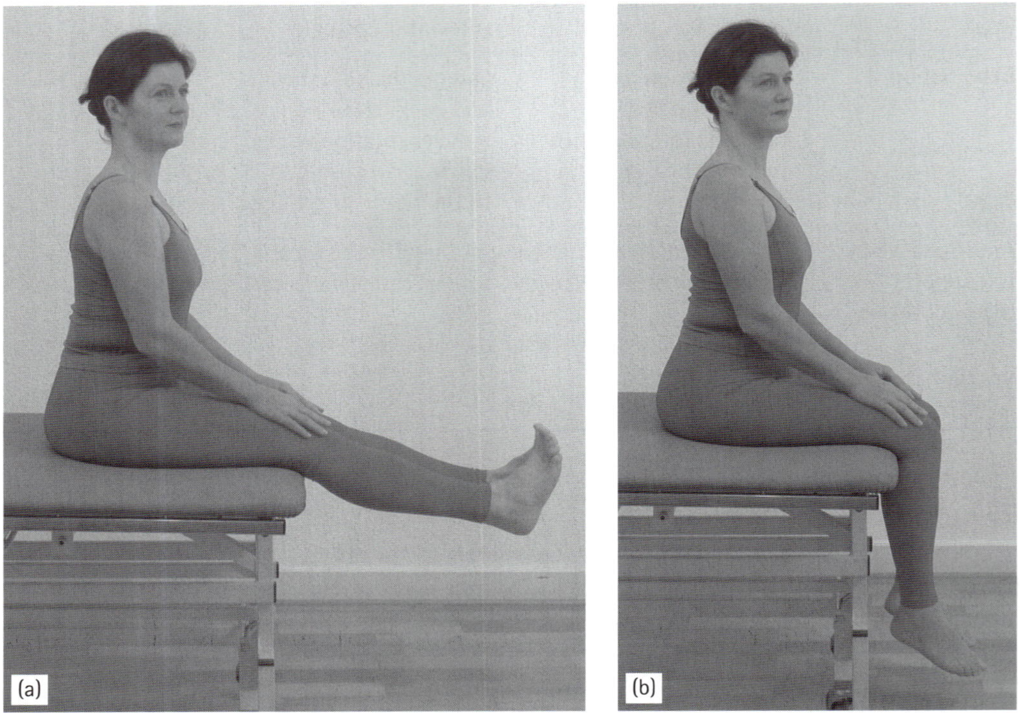

Figure 2.15a and b Area localization with symptomatic movement of the head to the right; differentiation between neural structures and cervical spine; alleviation. a, Starting position. b, End position.

The result of area localization has to be verified by further specific tests – otherwise the result will remain in doubt.

Assessment			
Goal	**Provocation of pain**	**Alleviation of pain**	**Remarks**
Starting position	Turning the head to the right to a position immediately before symptoms appear	Bilateral extension of the knees and dorsal flexion of the ankles then movement of head to the right to a position immediately after symptoms have appeared	
Test movement	Bilateral extension of the knees and dorsal flexion of the ankles, in sitting	Flexion of both knees	Head does not change its rotated position

Goal	Provocation of pain	Alleviation of pain	Remarks
Explanation	The test movement increases the tension in the neural structures	The test movement reduces the tension in the neural structures	If the typical pain is provoked or alleviated by these manoeuvres, this suggests at least an involvement of the neural structures
Additional data to support the hypothesis	General and specific mobility of the affected area History, symptom behaviour, type of complaints, 24-hour behaviour Palpation Nerve mobility tests Neurodynamic tests (e.g., Spurling's test, Tinel's sign) Test treatment Further movements of proximal or distal components that are not directly involved in the painful movement (e.g., elbow, hand, lower extremity) Reproducibility of test results Imaging procedures (CT, MRI)		

QUICK CHECK – SYMPTOMS, UPPER CENTRAL BACK OF THE NECK

If neither the area nor a symptom-provoking or symptom-reducing action is known, the quick check is used to try to load individual potential areas with specific biomechanically provocative movement combinations. The chosen movement combinations correspond with the straining and often symptom-provoking movements of the individual areas.

CERVICAL SPINE

Movement

- Extension/lateral flexion and rotation to the opposite side (Figs 2.16 and 2.17, film 15)
- Extension/lateral flexion and rotation to the same side (Figs 2.18 and 2.19, film 15).

NEURAL STRUCTURES

Tension tests

- Slump test (Fig. 2.20, film 16)
- Upper limb neurodynamic test 1 (ULNT-1; Fig. 2.21, film 17)
- Straight leg raise (SLR) (Fig. 2.22, film 18).

Note: The trial treatment of areas with negative provocation tests can still positively influence the symptoms. Reassessment of signs and symptoms will tell.

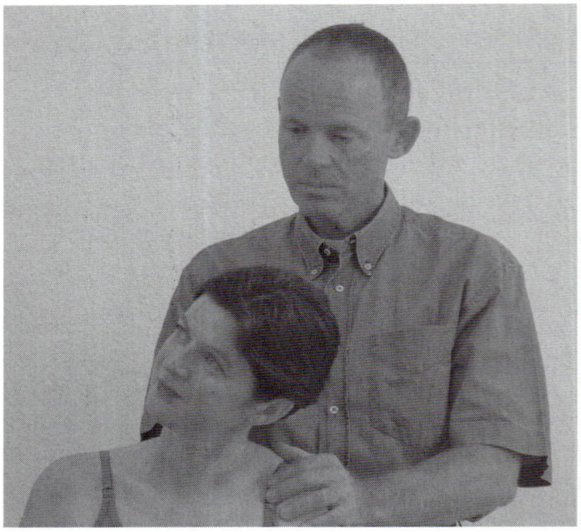

Figure 2.16 Quick check cervical spine; lateral flexion to the left with rotation to the opposite side.

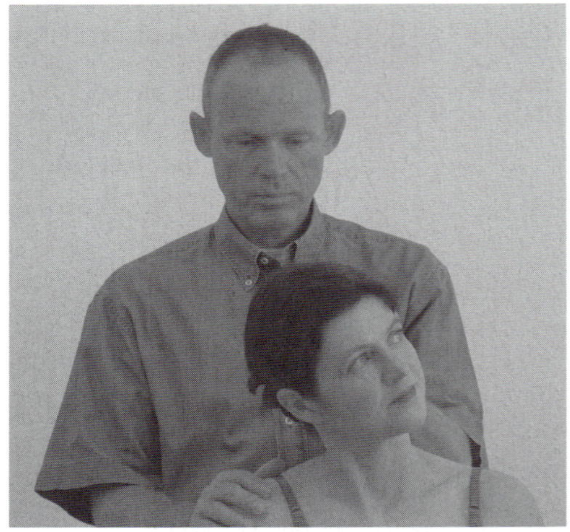

Figure 2.17 Quick check cervical spine; lateral flexion to the right with rotation to the opposite side.

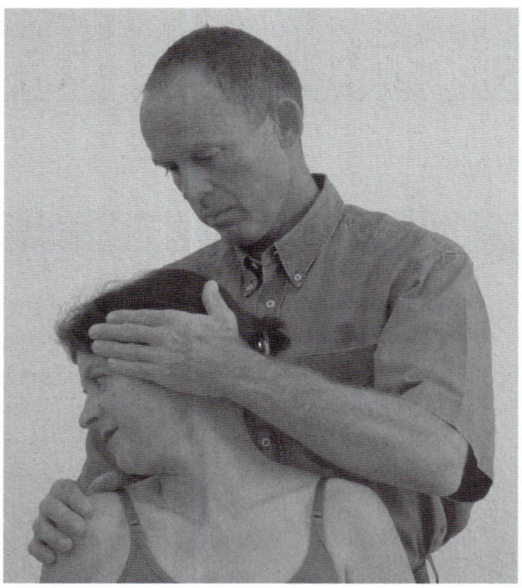

Figure 2.18 Quick check cervical spine; lateral flexion to the right with rotation to the same side.

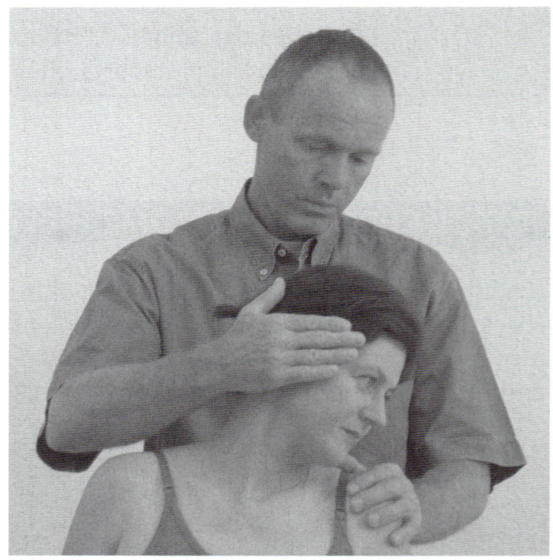

Figure 2.19 Quick check cervical spine; lateral flexion to the left with rotation to the same side.

SPECIFIC PROVOCATION AND ALLEVIATION

Specific provocation and alleviation enables differentiation within an articular complex and identification of the symptom-provoking movement direction(s).

SPECIFIC PROVOCATION AND ALLEVIATION, UPPER CERVICAL SPINE

Pain-provoking movement (Fig. 2.23)

- Turning the head to the right provokes pain in the upper central back of the neck.
- Area localization hints at the upper cervical spine.

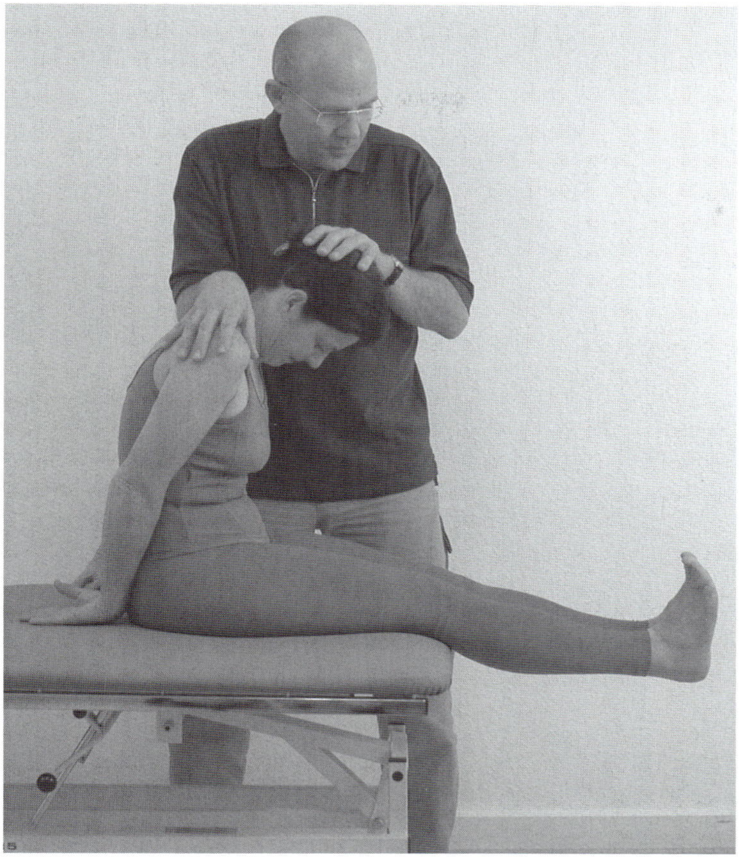

Figure 2.20 Quick check neurodynamics; slump test.

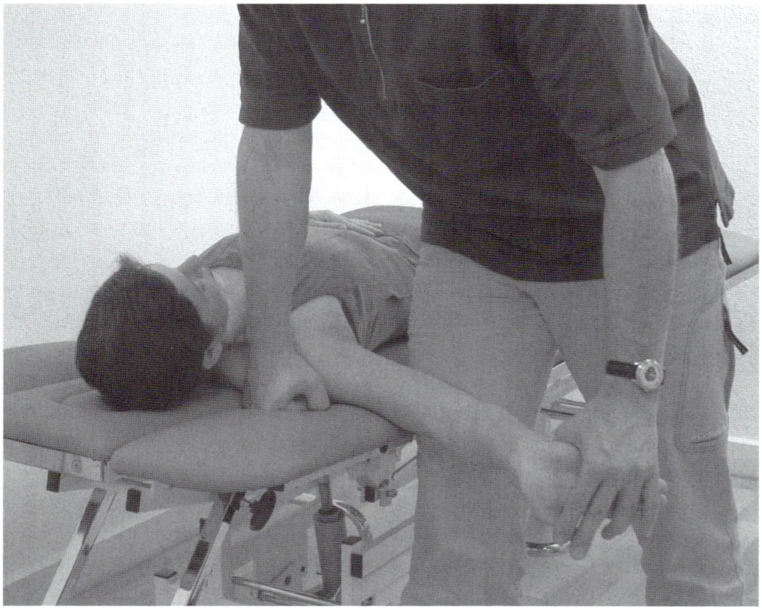

Figure 2.21 Quick check neurodynamics; upper limb neurodynamic test 1 (ULNT-1).

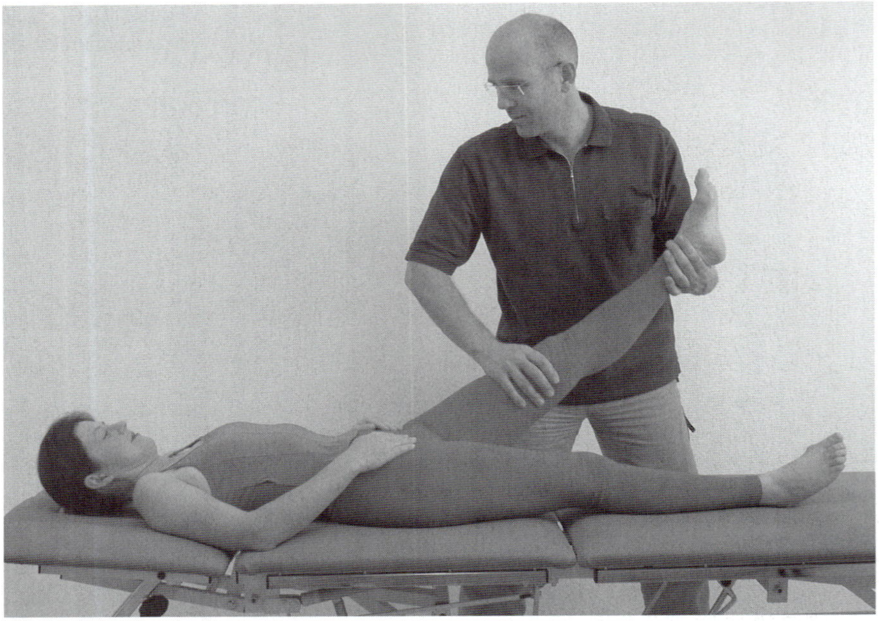

Figure 2.22 Quick check neurodynamics; straight leg raise (SLR) test.

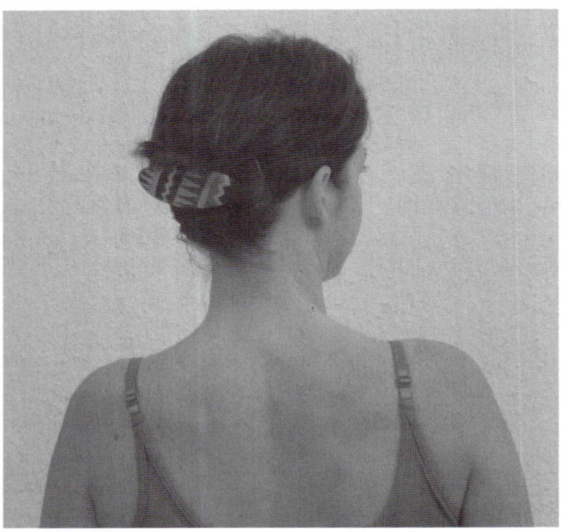

Figure 2.23 Symptom-provoking movement: turning the head to the right provokes symptoms in the area of the upper central back of the neck.

Differentiation, upper cervical spine (occiput-atlas axis)

The change in symptoms can be demonstrated exactly:

- provocation of pain (Fig. 2.24a and b, film 19)
- alleviation of pain (Fig. 2.25a and b, film 20).

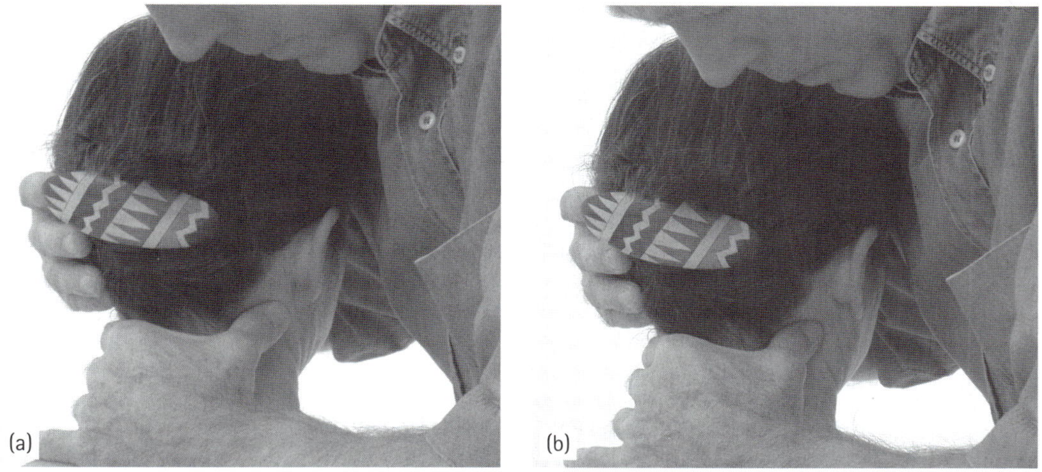

Figure 2.24a and b Specific provocation and alleviation in the area of the upper cervical spine with symptomatic movement of the head to the right; provocation. **a**, Starting position. **b**, End position.

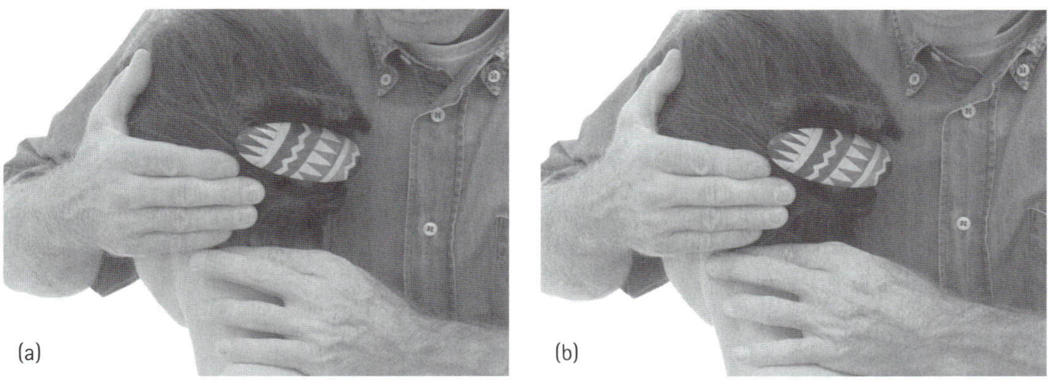

Figure 2.25a and b Specific provocation and alleviation in the area of the upper cervical spine with symptomatic movement of the head to the right; alleviation. **a**, Starting position. **b**, End position.

Assessment

Goal	Provocation of pain	Alleviation of pain	Remarks
Starting position	Turning the head to the right to a position immediately before symptoms appear	Turning the head to the right to a position immediately after symptoms have appeared	Head remains in starting position
Test movement	Pushing the vertebra in rotation to the left; the movement has to be started cranially (C1)	Pushing the vertebra in rotation to the right; the movement has to be started cranially (C1)	

Goal	Provocation of pain	Alleviation of pain	Remarks
Neural involvement	Proximal and/or distal component without change of position in the relevant area	Proximal and/or distal component without change of position in the relevant area	
Explanation	The symptoms are provoked when the caudal vertebra in the affected segment is moved into rotation to the left	The symptoms are alleviated when the caudal vertebra in the affected segment is moved into rotation to the right	
Additional data to support the hypothesis	General and specific mobility of the cervical spine History, symptom behaviour, type of complaints, 24-hour behaviour Specific palpation Neurodynamic tests (if specific provocation and alleviation indicate neural involvement) Reproducibility of test results Test treatment Imaging procedures (CT, MRI)		

GENERAL MOVEMENT TESTS

General movement tests identify individual anatomical movements and, in part, movement combinations in the suspected area. The individual manual therapy concepts have respective protocols at their disposal, which more or less have the same goals.

Information gained in this way is used to check or modify the relevant hypotheses developed on the basis of the anamnesis and it can determine further proceedings.

General question: Is there enough information available to skip general movement tests?	
No	Yes
⇓	⇓
Performance of the general movement tests	● Additional tests ● Test treatment

In view of the described clinical presentation and the results of area localization, general movement tests of the following regions seem to be useful.

Cervical spine		
	Active	Passive (assistive)
Upper cervical spine (above C2)	Flexion Extension	Flexion Extension

	Active	Passive (assistive)
in general	Rotation (to the right and left) Lateral flexion (to the right and left)	Rotation (to the right and left) Lateral flexion (to the right and left)
Lower cervical spine (below C2) in general	Flexion Extension Rotation (to the right and left) Lateral flexion (to the right and left)	Flexion Extension Rotation (to the right and left) Lateral flexion (to the right and left)

TREATMENT EXAMPLE, C2

SYMPTOMATIC MOVEMENT

Turning the head to the right is restricted by 30% as compared to turning it to the contralateral side and, in end-range positions, provokes pain (VAS 2–3/10) in the upper and central area of the back of the neck, right side.

ASSESSMENTS

Area localization

Area localization hints at a provocation of symptoms by the lower cervical spine (C2–C7). There is no contraindication for movement (e.g., no vertebrobasilar insufficiency, negative imaging procedures, no neurological involvement).

Specific provocation and alleviation

Specific provocation and alleviation hints at a provocation of symptoms by movement of C2 into rotation to the right.

Specific mobility

Specific mobility tests show hypomobility of C2, right side.

Palpation

Palpation indicates a painful change of tissue over segment C2, right side.

HYPOTHESIS

A painful rotation restriction of C2, right side, is suspected (Fig. 2.26).

RELAXATION TECHNIQUES

Hold–relax techniques

CO-CONTRACTION AGAINST DISTRACTION

Therapy technique (film 21)

- Patient's starting position: sitting.
- Therapist's starting position: standing, at the patient's left or right side , fixation of C3, contact against the lamina and the joint processes of C2 (Fig. 2.27a).
- Movement: traction above, while the patient tries to prevent distraction by means of muscle contraction (Fig. 2.27b).

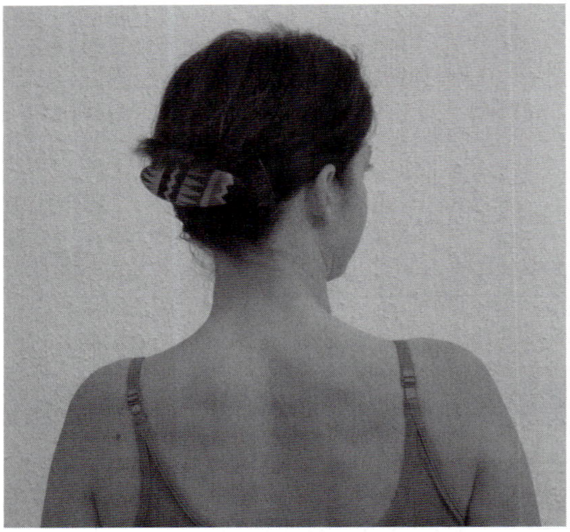

Figure 2.26 Symptom-provoking movement: turning the head to the right provokes symptoms in the area of the upper central back of the neck.

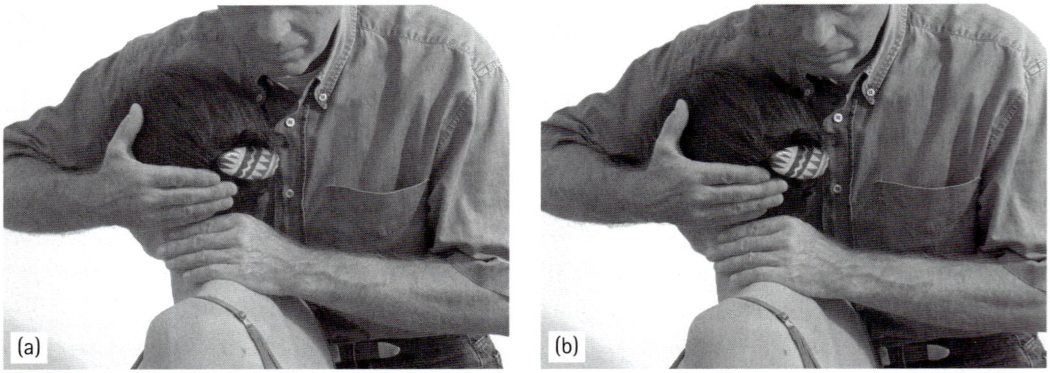

Figure 2.27a and b Hold-relax technique; C2; co-contraction against distraction; therapy technique. a, Starting position. b, End position.

Self-exercise 1 (film 22)

- Patient's starting position: sitting, cervical spine in neutral position, fixation of the skull (Fig. 2.28a).
- Movement: traction in a longitudinal direction, with simultaneous contraction of muscles working against this movement (Fig. 2.28b).

Self-exercise 2 (film 23)

- Patient's starting position: sitting, cervical spine rotated to the right before P1, fixation of the skull (Fig. 2.29a).
- Movement: traction in a longitudinal direction, with simultaneous contraction of muscles working against this movement (Fig. 2.29b).

MOVEMENT-DIRECTED CONTRACTION IN THE DIRECTION OPPOSING THE PAINFUL AND/OR RESTRICTED DIRECTION

Therapy technique (film 24)

- Patient's starting position: sitting.

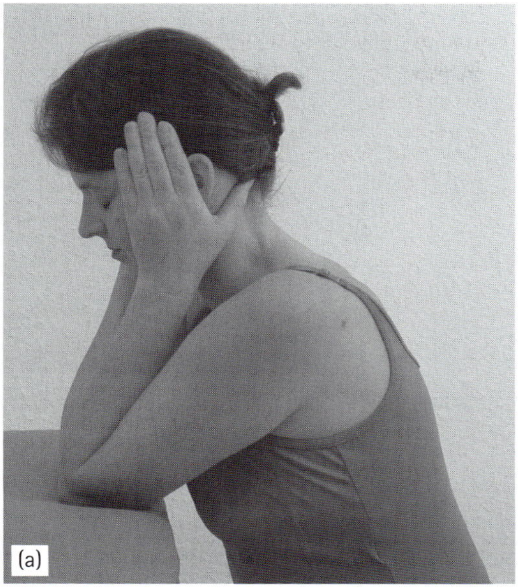

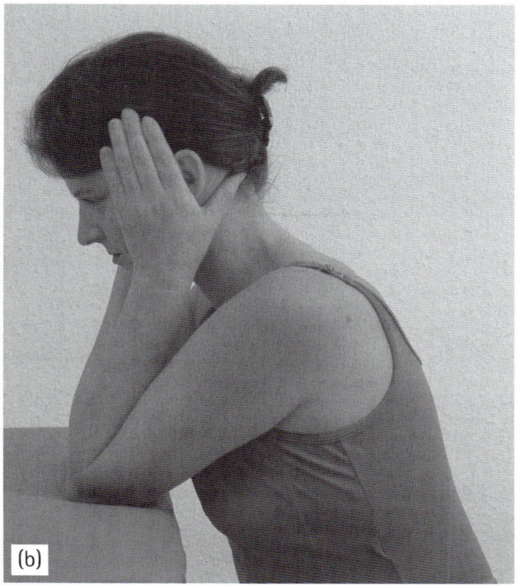

Figure 2.28a and b Hold–relax technique; C2; co-contraction against distraction; neutral position; self-exercise. **a**, Starting position. **b**, End position.

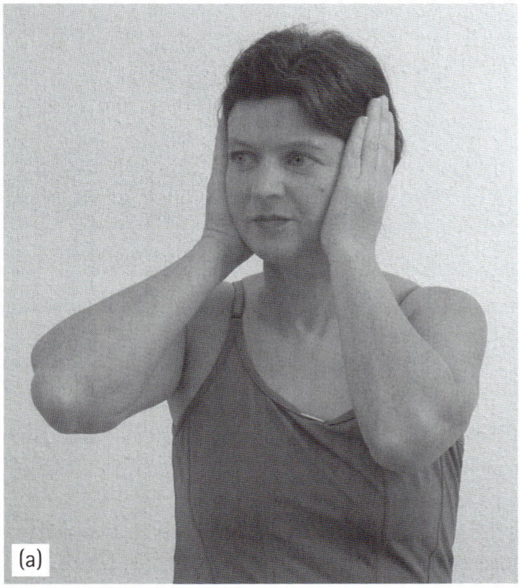

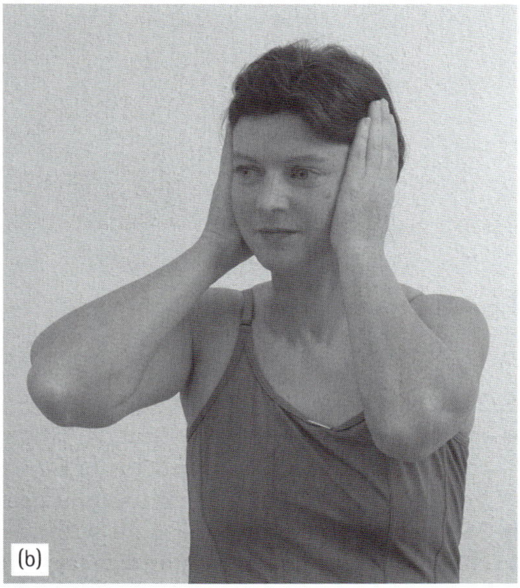

Figure 2.29a and b Hold–relax technique; C2; co-contraction against distraction; rotated to the right; self-exercise. **a**, Starting position. **b**, End position.

- Therapist's starting position: standing, at the patient's right side, fixation of C3 with thumb and index of the left hand, contact with the ulnar edge of the right hand against the lamina and the joint processes of C2, left side (Fig. 2.30a).
- Movement: rotation to the right with lateral flexion of C2 to the right, while the patient tries to prevent movement by muscle contraction (Fig. 2.30b).

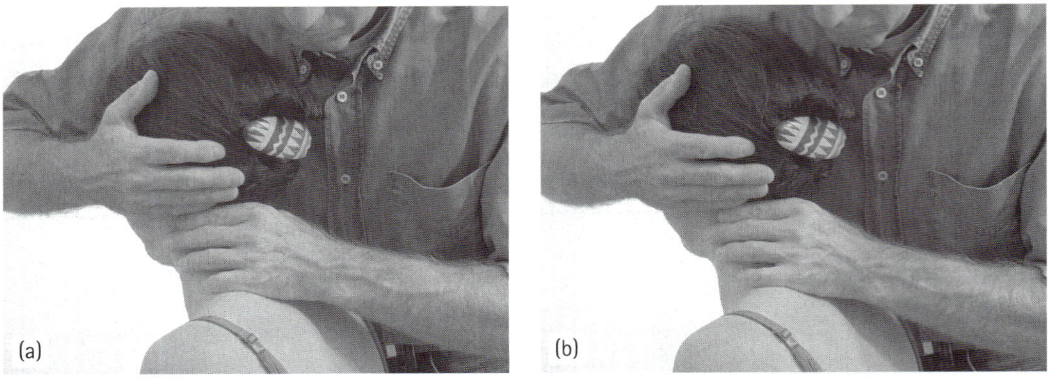

Figure 2.30a and b Hold-relax technique; C2; movement-directed contraction in the direction opposing the painful and/or restricted direction; therapy technique. a, Starting position. b, End position.

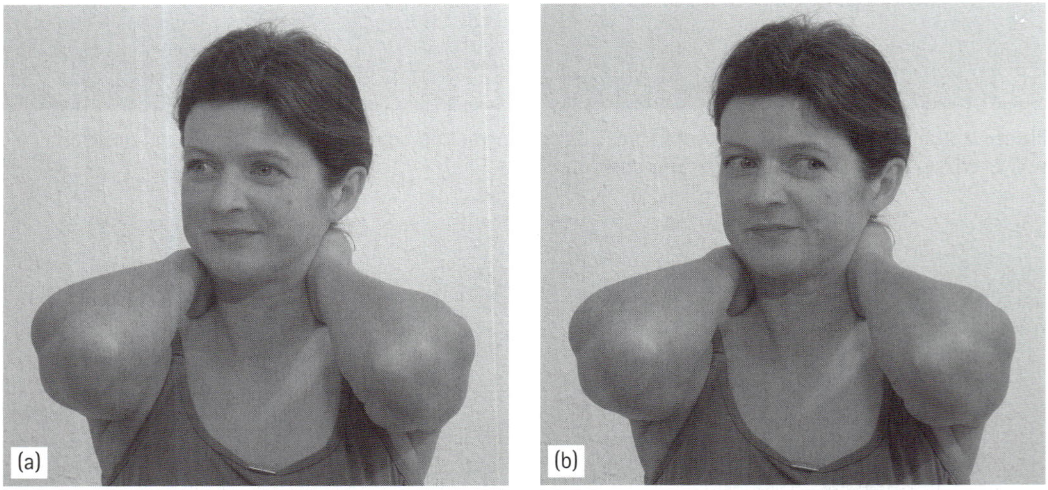

Figure 2.31a and b Hold-relax technique; C2; movement-directed contraction in the direction opposing the painful and/or restricted direction; self-exercise. a, Starting position. b, End position.

Self-exercise (flim 25)

- Patient's starting position: sitting, fixation of C3 by the ulnar edge of the right hand against the lamina and the joint process of C3, right side, contact with the ulnar edge of the left hand against the lamina and the joint process of C2, left side (Fig. 2.31a).
- Movement: rotation to the right with lateral flexion of C2 to the right, while the patient tries to prevent movement by muscle contraction (Fig. 2.31b).

MOVEMENT-DIRECTED CONTRACTION IN THE PAINFUL AND/OR RESTRICTED DIRECTION

Therapy technique (film 26)

- Patient's starting position: sitting.
- Therapist's starting position: standing, at the patient's right side, fixation at the vertebral arch of C3 with thumb and index of the left hand, contact with the ulnar edge of the right hand against the lamina and the joint processes of C2, left side (Fig. 2.32a).

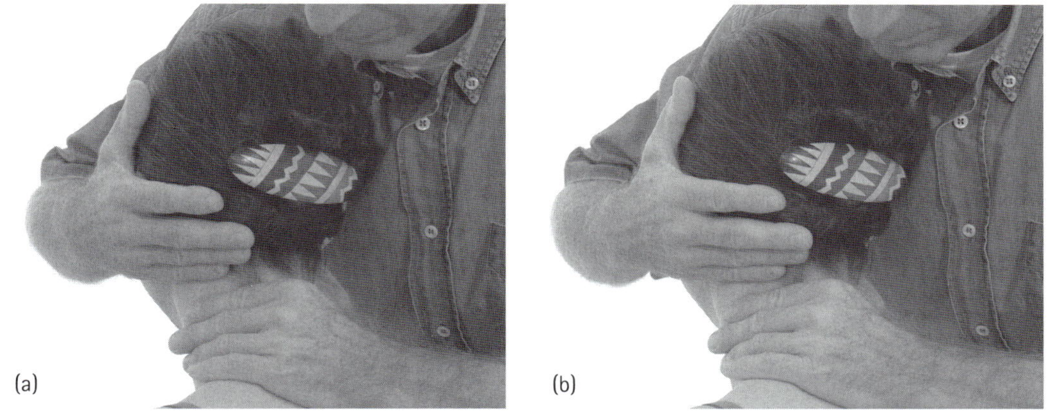

Figure 2.32a and b Hold–relax technique; C2; movement-directed contraction in the painful and/or restricted direction; therapy technique. a, Starting position. b, End position.

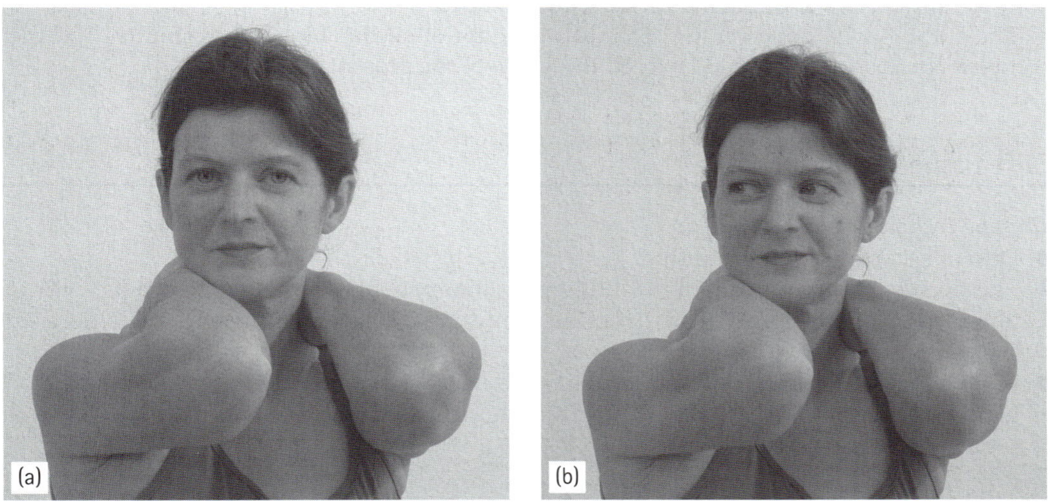

Figure 2.33a and b Hold–relax technique; C2; movement-directed contraction in the painful and/or restricted direction; self-exercise. a, Starting position. b, End position.

- Movement: rotation to the left with lateral flexion of C2 to the left, while the patient tries to prevent movement by muscle contraction (Fig. 2.32b).

Self-exercise (film 27)

- Patient's starting position: sitting, fixation of C3 by the ulnar edge of the right hand against the lamina and the joint process of C3, left side, contact with the ulnar edge of the right hand against the lamina and the joint process of C2, right side (Fig. 2.33a).
- Movement: rotation to the left with lateral flexion of C2 to the left, while the patient tries to prevent movement by muscle contraction (Fig. 2.33b).

Remarks (regarding relaxation techniques)

Goal of the technique

Reduction of the tonicity and improvement of the metabolism of the periarticular tissues involved in a painfully restricted rotation to the right of C2, right side.

Performance
Depending on irritability or the desired treatment goal, the joint to be treated is first adjusted as necessary.

Dosage (regarding the affected symptomatic structure)
Both with an acute and with a chronic presentation, the contraction should always be pain-free.

Choice of technique
The selection of the technique depends, among other things, on the therapist as well as the patient, on the therapist's clinical experience, but primarily on reassessment. This means that even if all preconditions on the part of therapist and patient seem to be met, it is, in the authors' view, of no use to continue the technique if reassessment is negative.

Contributing factors
For a satisfactory solution of the patient's current problems it is important to consider the contributing factors and include them in the treatment.

The authors will, however, not go into a description of the various possibilities and their complex contexts as this would exceed the scope of the present book.

Soft tissue techniques

Therapy technique (film 28)

- Patient's starting position: sitting.
- Therapist's starting position: standing, at the patient's left side, contact with the ulnar edge of the right hand over the lamina and the joint process of C2, left side (Fig. 2.34a).
- Movement: passive rotation to the right with lateral flexion of C2 to the right, while one hand impedes co-movement of C3 and simultaneously compresses the soft tissue around segment C2 (Fig. 2.34b).

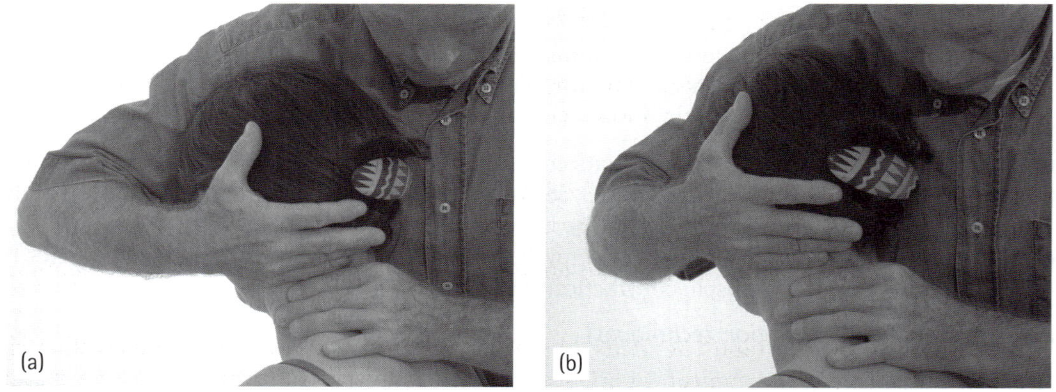

Figure 2.34a and b Soft tissue technique; C2; rotation to the right, in sitting; therapy technique. a, Starting position. b, End position.

Note: If the patient is not able to relax or if performance of the movement seems too difficult, this soft tissue technique can also be performed assistively. Application of the assistive technique leads to a simultaneous reciprocal inhibition of the treated muscles, which might facilitate relaxation.

Therapy technique, alternative 1 (film 29)

- Patient's starting position: supine.
- Therapist's starting position: standing, at the patient's head end, stabilization of C3 with one finger of the left hand over the lamina and the joint process, left side, contact with one finger of the right hand over the lamina and the joint process of C2, right side (Fig. 2.35a).
- Movement: passive rotation and lateral flexion of C2 to the left by moving C2 on its right side in a ventrocranial direction, while the other hand impedes co-movement of C3 (Fig. 2.35b).

Therapy technique, alternative 2 (film 30)

- Patient's starting position: supine.
- Therapist's starting position: standing, at the patient's head end, stabilization of C2 with one finger of the left hand over the lamina and the joint process, left side, contact with one finger of the right hand over the lamina and the joint process of C3, right side (Fig. 2.36a).
- Movement: passive rotation and lateral flexion of C2 to the right by moving C3 on its right side in a ventrocranial direction, while the other hand impedes co-movement of C2 (Fig. 2.36b).

Self-exercise (film 31)

- Patient's starting position: sitting, contact with the ulnar edge of the right hand at the lamina and at the spinous process of C3, right side (Fig. 2.37a).
- Movement: active rotation to the left with lateral flexion to the left, while the patient impedes co-movement of C3 by contact (push against the spinous process) and simultaneously manipulates the soft tissue (Fig. 2.37b).

Remarks (regarding soft tissue techniques)

Goal of the technique

Reduction of the tone and improvement of the metabolism of the periarticular tissues with painfully restricted rotation to the right of C2, right side. The technique is well suited for acute presentations where treatment has to be done with small movement amplitudes and little force.

Since there is not one vertebra fixed and the neighbouring vertebra moved, the technique is not included among the mobilization techniques, in spite of its high specificity.

Performance

Treatment is done within the symptom-free range of movement.

Dosage (regarding the affected symptomatic structure)

Both with an acute and with a chronic presentation, the movement should always be pain-free.

Choice of technique

The selection of the technique depends, among other things, on the therapist as well as the patient, on the therapist's clinical experience, but primarily on reassessment. This means that even if all preconditions on the part of therapist and patient seem to be met, it is, in the authors' view, of no use to continue the technique if reassessment is negative.

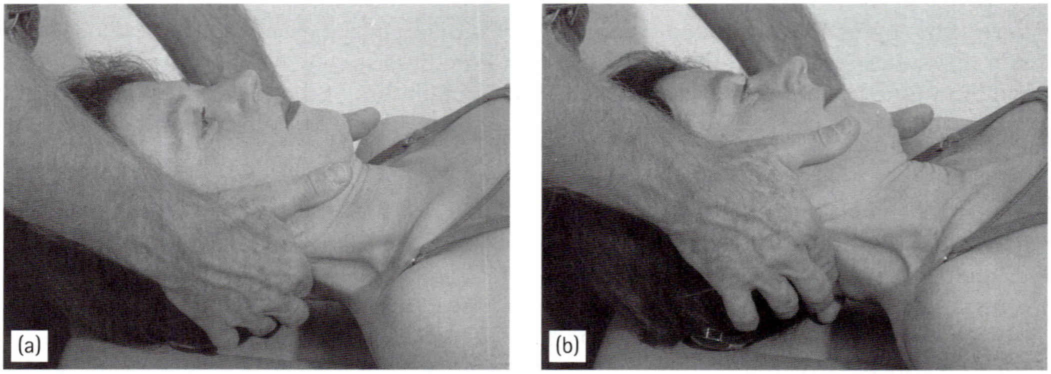

Figure 2.35a and b Soft tissue technique; C2; rotation to the left, in supine position; therapy technique. a, Starting position. b, End position.

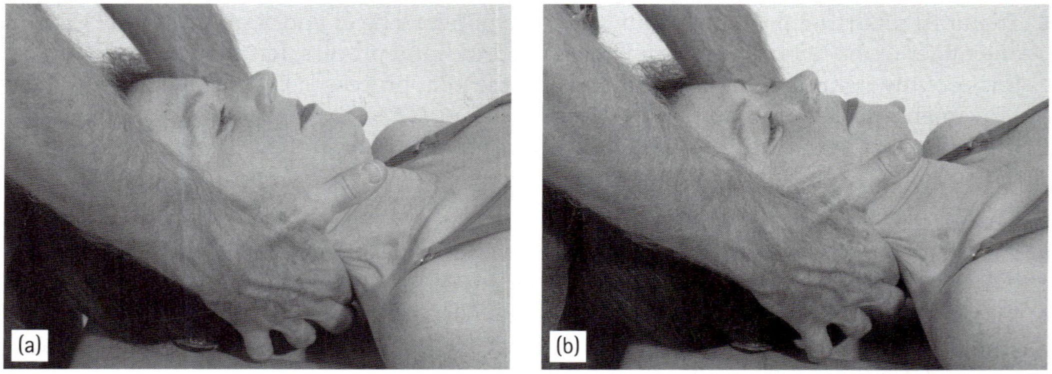

Figure 2.36a and b Soft tissue technique; C2; rotation to the right, in supine position; therapy technique. a, Starting position. b, End position.

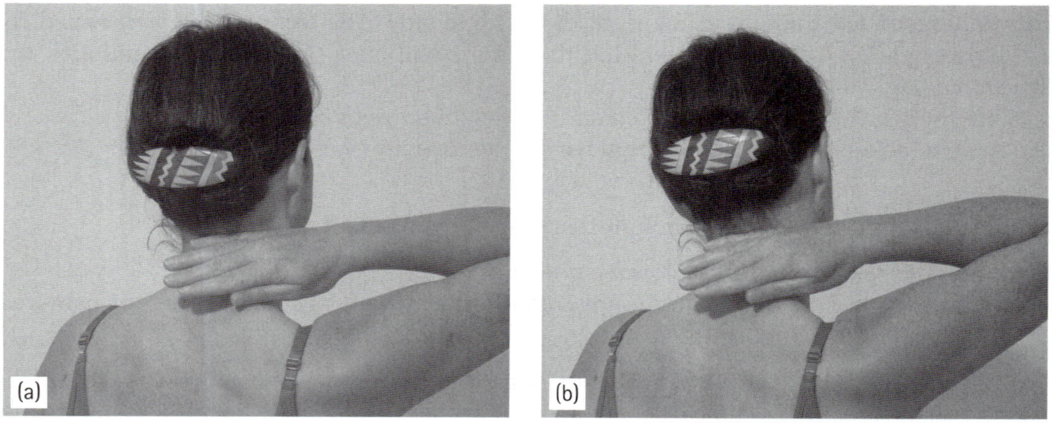

Figure 2.37a and b Soft tissue technique; C2; rotation to the left, in sitting; self-exercise (starting position). a, Starting position. b, End position.

Contributing factors

For a satisfactory solution of the patient's current problems it is essential to consider the contributing factors and include them in the treatment.

The authors will, however, not go deeper into a description of the various possibilities and their complex contexts as this would exceed the scope of the present book.

MOBILIZATION TECHNIQUES

Active techniques

ACTIVE MOBILIZATION

Coupled movement of the affected segment

Therapy technique (film 32)

- Patient's starting position: sitting.
- Therapist's starting position: standing, at the patient's left or right side, fixation of C3 with thumb and index of the left or right hand over the lamina and the joint processes (Fig. 2.38a).
- Movement: active movement above C3 into rotation to the right and lateral flexion to the right (Fig. 2.38b).

Self-exercise (film 33)

- Patient's starting position: sitting, contact with the ulnar edge of the right hand at the lamina and the joint process of C3, right side (Fig. 2.39a).
- Movement: active movement above C3 into rotation to the right and lateral flexion to the right (Fig. 2.39b).

Non-coupled movement of the affected segment

Therapy technique (film 34)

- Patient's starting position: sitting.
- Therapist's starting position: standing, at the patient's left or right side, fixation of C3 with thumb and index of the left or right hand over the lamina and the joint processes, with adjusted lateral flexion of the cervical spine to the left (Fig. 2.40a).
- Movement: active movement above into rotation to the right, with lateral flexion to the left remaining unchanged (Fig. 2.40b).

Self-exercise (film 35)

- Patient's starting position: sitting, the cervical spine bent sideways to the left, contact and fixation with the ulnar edge of the right hand at the lamina and the joint process of C3, right side (Fig. 2.41a).
- Movement: active movement above into rotation to the right, with lateral flexion of the cervical spine to the left remaining unchanged (Fig. 2.41b).

Remarks (regarding mobilization techniques)

Goal of the technique

With a painfully restricted rotation to the right of C2, right side, the described techniques serve to:

- reduce tonicity and improve the metabolism of the affected tissues
- restore pain-free function (change the input to respective centres of the central nervous system (CNS))
- restore normal function of symptomatic tissue by application of the symptom-provoking stimulus dosed according to the current load tolerance.

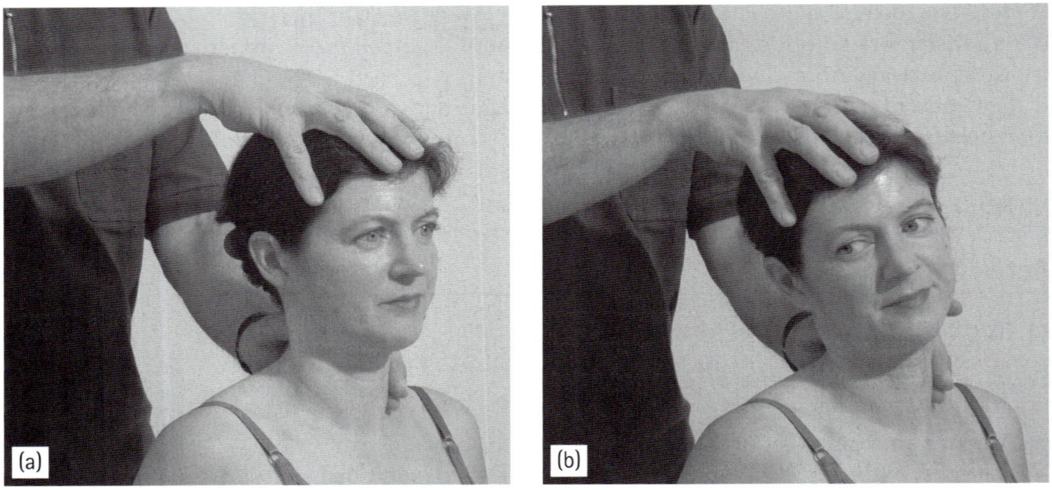

Figure 2.38a and b Active mobilization; C2; coupled movement into rotation to the right; therapy technique. **a**, Starting position. **b**, End position.

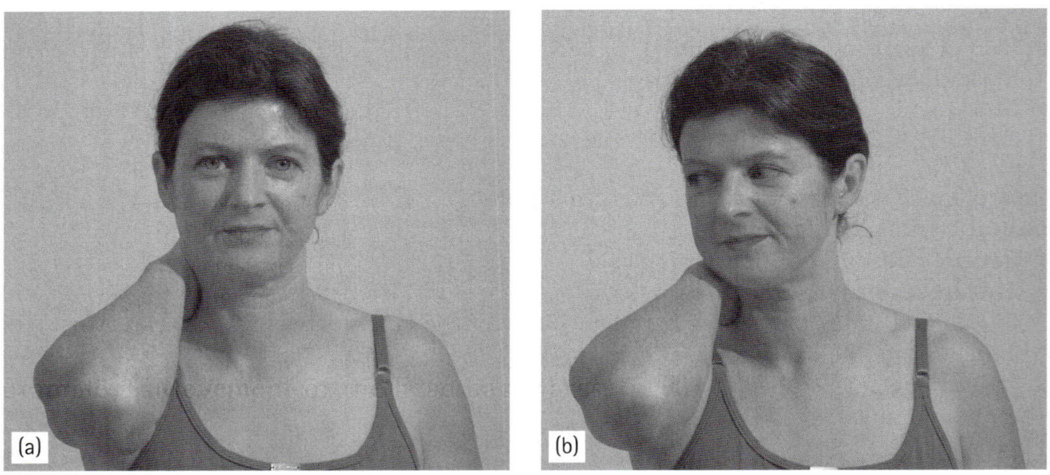

Figure 2.39a and b Active mobilization; C2; coupled movement into rotation to the right; self-exercise. **a**, Starting position. **b**, End position.

Note: The non-coupled movement (lateral flexion to the left with simultaneous rotation to the right) may, with an intra-articular problem (i.e. symptom provocation by compression of symptomatic intra-articular structures, right side) very well be used to improve mobility of neighbouring, non-symptomatic tissues inside or outside the affected articular complex (contributing factors ?). In this way, the symptom-provoking compression is avoided.

With an extra-articular problem (i.e. symptom provocation by pull on symptomatic extra-articular structures, right side), the non-coupled movement serves to restore normal function of the symptomatic tissue by application of the symptom-provoking stimulus dosed according to the current load tolerance.

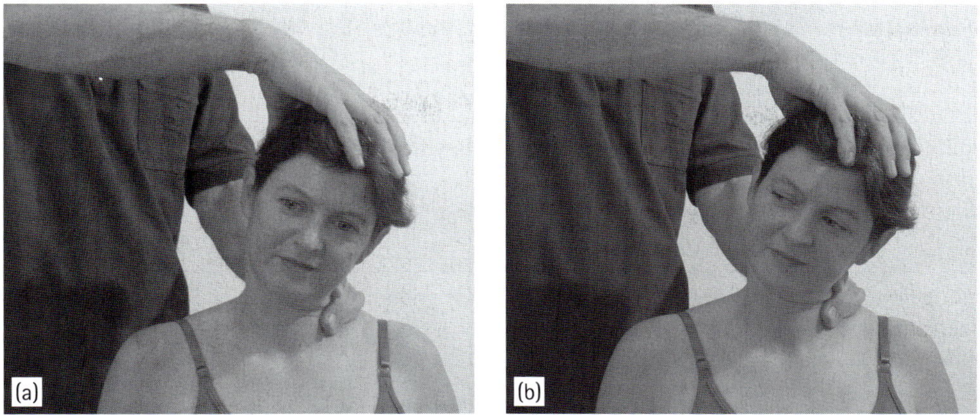

Figure 2.40a and b Active mobilization; C2; non-coupled movement into rotation to the right; therapy technique. **a**, Starting position. **b**, End position.

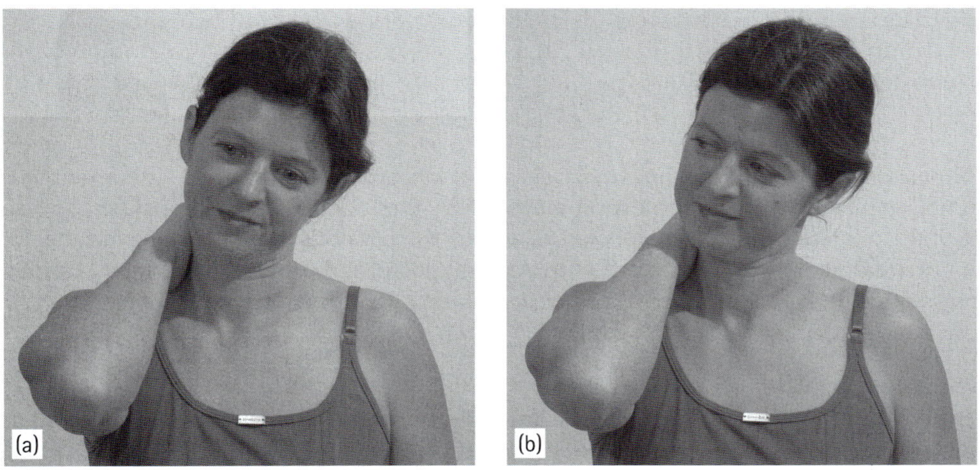

Figure 2.41a and b Active mobilization; C2; non-coupled movement into rotation to the right; self-exercise. **a**, Starting position. **b**, End position.

Performance

Depending on irritability or the desired treatment goal, the joint to be treated is adjusted as necessary before treatment. As the self-exercise is performed without 'specific fixation', an uncontrolled continuation of movement (here mainly above C2) has to be considered when the indication for this exercise is determined.

Dosage (regarding the affected symptomatic structure)

Acute presentation (predominantly peripheral pain mechanisms)			
Phase	Limitation of movement due to pain and resistance	Concept	Movement grade

Inflammation phase	No pain	Kaltenborn–Evjenth	Up to the beginning of II
	No resistance	Maitland	Up to II
Proliferation phase	Up to P1	Kaltenborn–Evjenth	Up to the 1st third of II
	Slowly progressing up to low resistance	Maitland	III^{-}
Remodelling/ organization phase	Slowly progressing up to maximum resistance	Kaltenborn–Evjenth	Up to III
	(Note: duration of turnover!)	Maitland	Up to IV^{++} or III^{++}

Note: The chances of a disturbed (delayed) course of healing and their consequences for the loading capacity of the tissue (e.g., diabetes, old age, partial or general immobilization) have to be considered.

Chronic presentation (predominantly central pain mechanisms): Since here it is assumed that pain no longer represents a protection mechanism, the therapist has to consider the training state of the treated tissue to be expected as well as the patient's personal expectations. In case of doubt, treatment is always started with very low force, and progression is made conditional on reassessment. Hence with a chronic presentation, pain does not always represent the limiting factor regarding dosage of treatment.

Choice of technique

The selection of the technique depends, among other things, on the therapist as well as the patient, on the therapist's clinical experience, but primarily on reassessment. This means that even if all preconditions on the part of therapist and patient seem to be met, it is, in the authors' view, of no use to continue the technique if reassessment is negative.

Contributing factors

For a satisfactory solution of the patient's current problems it is essential to consider the contributing factors and include them in the treatment.

The authors will, however, not go into a description of the various possibilities and their complex contexts as this would exceed the scope of the present book.

ACTIVE MOBILIZATION PLUS ACCESSORY MOVEMENTS

Rotation of the occiput to the right up to and including C2, with lateral glide to the right

Therapy technique (film 36)

- Patient's starting position: supine.
- Therapist's starting position: standing, at the patient's head end, fixation of C3 with the radial side of the right hand against the lamina and the joint process, right side. Contact

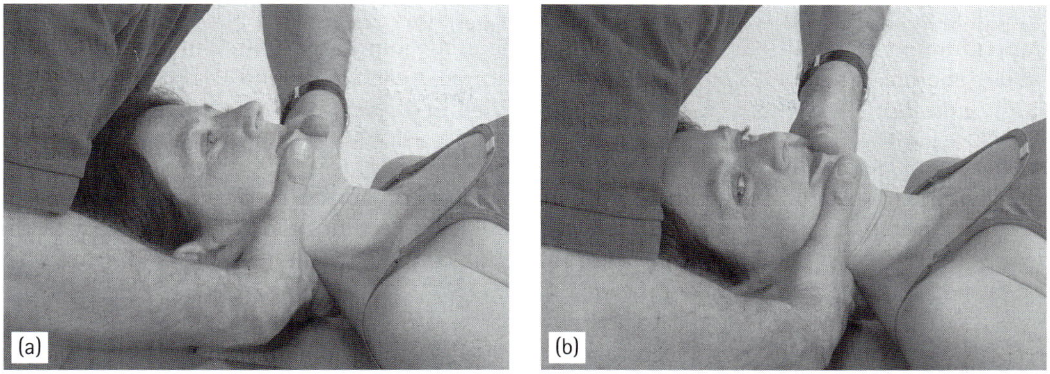

Figure 2.42a and b Active mobilization with accessory movement; C2; lateral glide to the right with active rotation to the right; therapy technique. a, Starting position. b, End position.

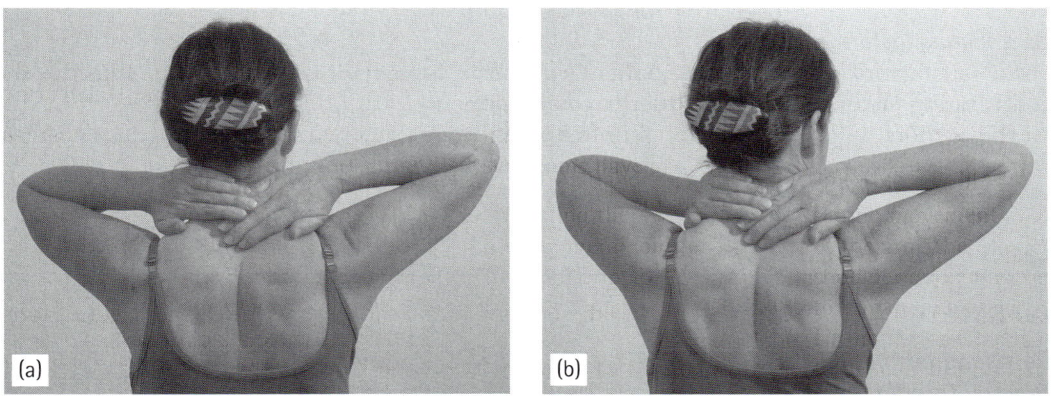

Figure 2.43a and b Active mobilization with accessory movement; C2; lateral glide to the right with active rotation to the right; self-exercise. a, Starting position. b, End position.

with the radial side of the left hand against the lamina and the joint process of C2, left side, lateral push of C2 to the right (Fig. 2.42a).

- Movement: active rotation to the right of C2 and above (Fig. 2.42b).

Self-exercise (film 37)

- Patient's starting position: sitting, fixation of C3 from the right side, contact with C2 from the left side, with simultaneous lateral push of C2 to the right (Fig. 2.43a).
- Movement: active rotation to the right of C2 and above (Fig. 2.43b).

Remarks (regarding active mobilization plus accessory movements)

Goal of the technique

With a painfully restricted rotation to the right of C2, right side, this technique serves to:

- reduce tonicity and improve the metabolism of the affected tissues
- restore pain-free function (change the input to respective centres of the CNS)
- restore normal function of symptomatic tissue by application of the symptom-provoking stimulus dosed according to the current load tolerance.

Performance

Depending on irritability or desired treatment goal, the joint to be treated is adjusted appropriately before treatment. Due to the great anatomical variability and the individual pathology, lateral push may have to be slightly modified in direction in some cases.

Dosage (regarding the affected symptomatic structure)

Both with an acute (predominantly peripheral pain mechanisms) and with a chronic presentation (predominantly central pain mechanisms), this technique should not reproduce the patient's symptoms. Dosage of the technique is determined by the expected training state of the tissue and, above all, by reassessment.

Choice of technique

The selection of the technique depends, among other things, on the therapist as well as the patient, on the therapist's clinical experience, but primarily on reassessment. This means that even if all preconditions on the part of therapist and patient seem to be met, it is, in the authors' view, of no use to continue the technique if reassessment is negative.

Contributing factors

For a satisfactory solution of the patient's current problems it is important to consider the contributing factors and include them in the treatment.

The authors will, however, not go into a description of the various possibilities and their complex contexts as this would exceed the scope of the present book.

Passive procedures

TRANSLATORY MOVEMENTS

Dorsocaudal glide

Therapy technique (film 48)

- Patient's starting position: sitting.
- Therapist's starting position: standing, at the patient's left side, fixation of C3 with thumb and index of the right hand over the laminae and the joint processes. Contact with the ulnar edge of the left hand against the joint process, the lamina, and the spinous process of C2, right side (Fig. 2.44a).
- Movement: translatory gliding movement of the right facet joint of C2 by push via the joint process, the lamina, and the spinous process of C2, right side, in a dorsocaudal direction (Fig. 2.44b).

Self-exercise (film 49)

- Patient's starting position: sitting, fixation of C3 via lamina and spinous process, left side, with the ulnar edge of the left hand (Fig. 2.45a).
- Movement: translatory gliding movement via the transverse process of C2, right side, with the ulnar edge of the right hand in a dorsocaudal direction (Fig. 2.45b).

FACET TRACTION

Therapy technique (film 50)

- Patient's starting position: sitting, lateral flexion to the left with simultaneous rotation to the right.

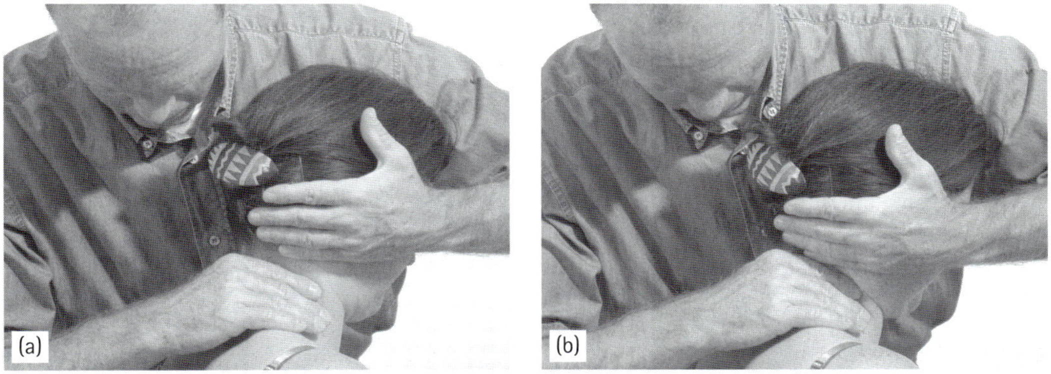

Figure 2.44a and b Passive mobilization; C2; translatory gliding; therapy technique. **a**, Starting position. **b**, End position.

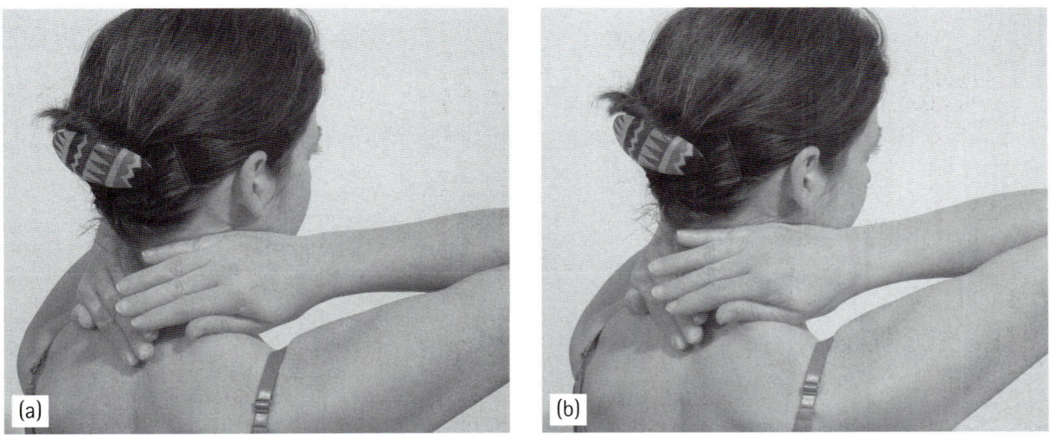

Figure 2.45a and b Passive mobilization; C2; translatory gliding; self-exercise. **a**, Starting position. **b**, End position.

- Therapist's starting position: standing, at the patient's left side, fixation of the position of cervical spine and head in lateral flexion to the left and rotation to the right, with the left forearm and the left hand (Fig. 2.46a).
- Movement: push at the joint process of C3, right side, with the radial side of the right index in a ventrocaudal direction (Fig. 2.46b).

In the demonstrated technique, the caudal vertebra of the treated segment is moved. Alternatively, this technique may also be performed via movement of the cranial vertebra.

Self-exercise (film 51)

- Patient's starting position: sitting, lateral flexion to the left with simultaneous rotation to the right, fixation of C2 at the lamina and the joint process, left side, with the ulnar edge of the left hand (Fig. 2.47a).
- Movement: pull via lamina and joint process of C3 with the ulnar edge of the right hand in a ventrocaudal direction (Fig. 2.47b).

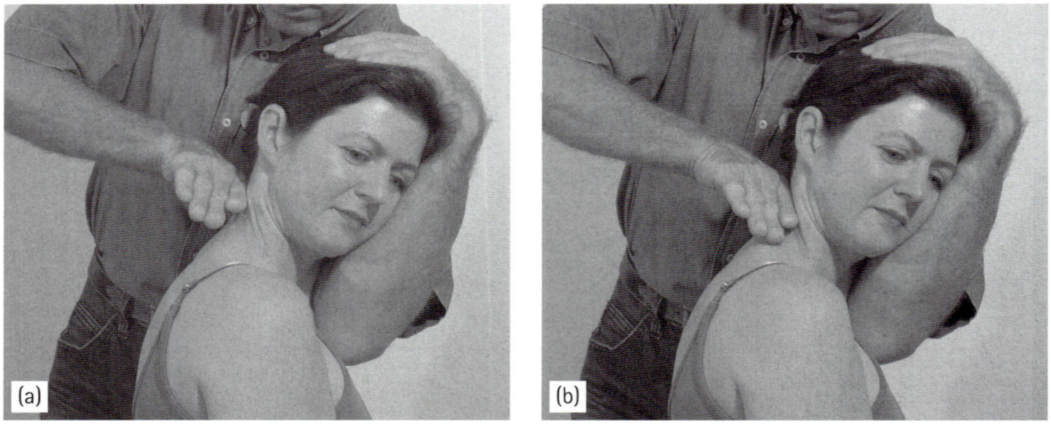

Figure 2.46a and b Passive mobilization; C2; facet traction; therapy technique. **a**, Starting position. **b**, End position.

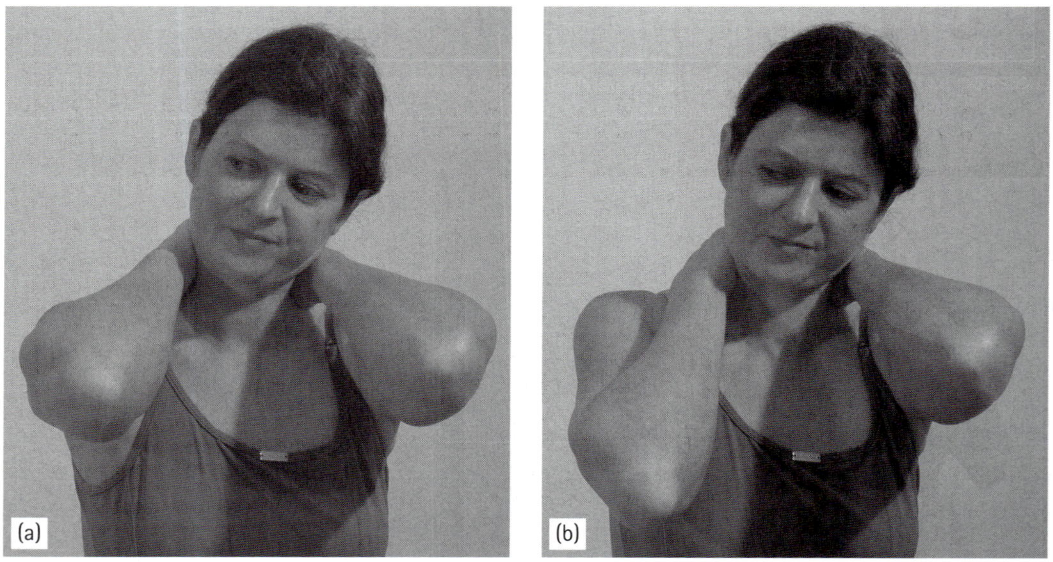

Figure 2.47a and b Passive mobilization; C2; facet traction; self-exercise. **a**, Starting position. **b**, End position.

Remarks (regarding passive procedures, translatory movements)

Goals of the technique

With a painfully restricted rotation to the right of C2, right side, the techniques serve to:

- reduce tonicity and improve the metabolism of the affected tissues
- restore pain-free function (change the input to respective centres of the CNS)
- restore normal function of symptomatic tissue by application of the symptom-provoking stimulus dosed according to the current load tolerance.

Note: Facet traction of C2, right side (non-coupled movement with lateral flexion to the left with simultaneous rotation to the right) may, with an intra-articular problem (i.e. symptom provocation by compression of symptomatic intra-articular structures, right side), very well be used to improve mobility of neighbouring, non-symptomatic tissues inside or outside the affected articular complex (supporting factors ?). In this way, the symptom-provoking compression is avoided.

With an extra-articular problem (i.e. symptom provocation by pull on symptomatic extra-articular structures, right side), it serves to restore normal function of the symptomatic tissue by application of the symptom-provoking stimulus dosed according to the current load tolerance.

Performance

Depending on irritability or desired treatment goal, the joint to be treated is adjusted appropriately before treatment.

Dosage (regarding the affected symptomatic structure)

Acute presentation (predominantly peripheral pain mechanisms)

Phase	Limitation of movement due to pain and resistance	Concept	Movement grade
Inflammation phase	No pain	Kaltenborn–Evjenth	Up to the beginning of II
	No resistance	Maitland	Up to II
Proliferation phase	Up to P1	Kaltenborn–Evjenth	Up to the 1st third of II
	Slowly progressing up to low resistance	Maitland	III^{-}
Remodelling/organization phase	Slowly progressing up to maximum resistance	Kaltenborn–Evjenth	Up to III
	(Note: duration of turnover!)	Maitland	Up to IV^{++} or III^{++}

Note: The chances of a disturbed (delayed) course of healing and their consequences for the loading capacity of the tissue (e.g., diabetes, old age, partial or general immobilization) have to be considered.

Chronic presentation (predominantly central pain mechanisms): Since here it is assumed that pain no longer represents a protection mechanism, the therapist has to consider the expected training state of the treated tissue as well as the patient's personal expectations. In case of doubt, treatment is always started with very low force, and progression is made conditional on reassessment. Hence with a chronic presentation, pain does not always represent the limiting factor regarding dosage of treatment.

Choice of technique

The selection of the technique depends, among other things, on the therapist as well as the patient, on the therapist's clinical experience, but primarily on reassessment. This means that even if all preconditions on the part of therapist and patient seem to be met, it is, in the authors' view, of no use to continue the technique if reassessment is negative.

Contributing factors

For a satisfactory solution of the patient's current problems it is important to consider the contributing factors and include them in the treatment.

The authors will, however, not go deeper into a description of the various possibilities and their complex contexts as this would exceed the scope of the present book.

ACCESSORY MOVEMENTS

Central posterior-anterior push

Therapy technique (film 38)

- Patient's starting position: prone.
- Therapist's starting position: standing, at the patient's head end (Fig. 2.48a).
- Movement: central push with the tips of both thumbs on the spinous process of C2 from posterior to anterior (Fig. 2.48b).

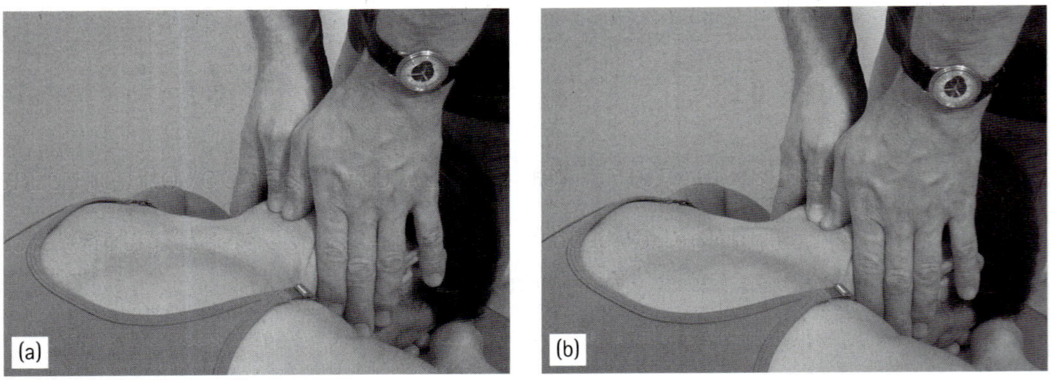

Figure 2.48a and b Passive mobilization; C2; central posterior-anterior movement; therapy technique. a, Starting position. b, End position.

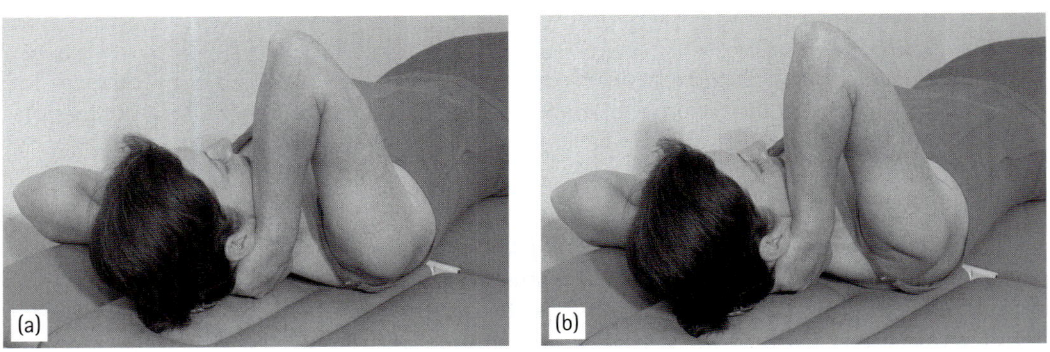

Figure 2.49a and b Passive mobilization; C2; central posterior-anterior movement; self-exercise. a, Starting position. b, End position.

Self-exercise (film 39)

- Patient's starting position: supine, with a cushion under the head, contact with the middle finger of the left hand on the spinous process of C2 (Fig. 2.49a).
- Movement: central push on the spinous process of C2 from posterior to anterior via the right hand with pressure on the middle finger of the left hand (Fig. 2.49b).

Unilateral posterior-anterior push

Therapy technique (film 40)

- Patient's starting position: prone.
- Therapist's starting position: standing, at the patient's head end (Fig. 2.50a).
- Movement: unilateral push with the tips of both thumbs on the joint process of C2 from posterior to anterior (Fig. 2.50b).

Self-exercise (film 41)

- Patient's starting position: supine, with a cushion under the head, contact with the end part of the middle finger of the right hand on the joint process of C2, right side, with simultaneous contact of the middle finger of the left hand on this finger (Fig. 2.51a).
- Movement: unilateral push on the joint process of C2 from posterior to anterior via pull of the right hand and push of the left hand (Fig. 2.51b).

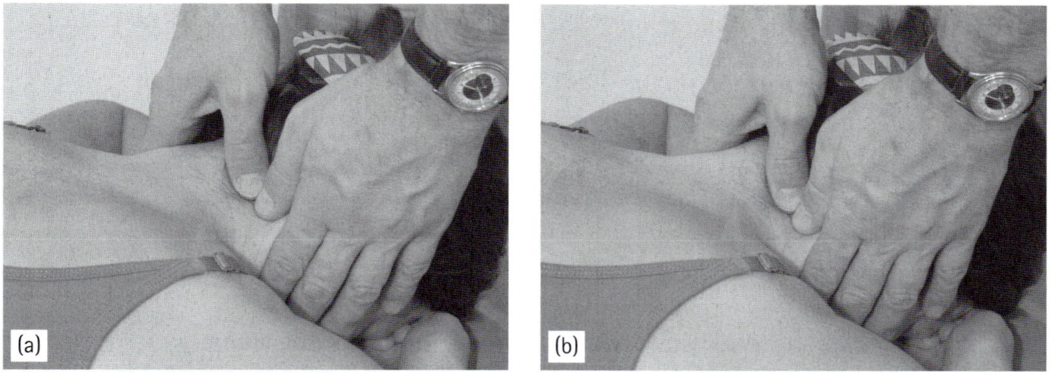

Figure 2.50a and b Passive mobilization; C2; unilateral posterior-anterior movement; therapy technique. a, Starting position. b, End position.

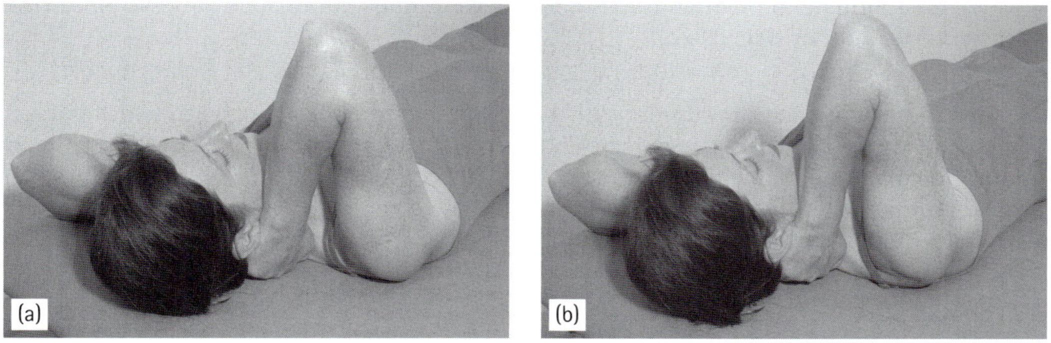

Figure 2.51a and b Passive mobilization; C2; unilateral posterior-anterior movement; self-exercise. a, Starting position. b, End position.

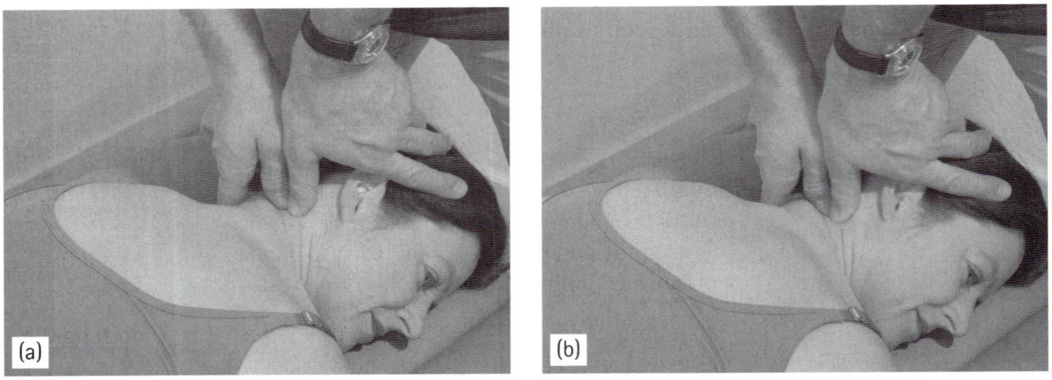

Figure 2.52a and b Passive mobilization; C2; unilateral posterior-anterior movement with previously adjusted rotation to the right; therapy technique. **a**, Starting position. **b**, End position.

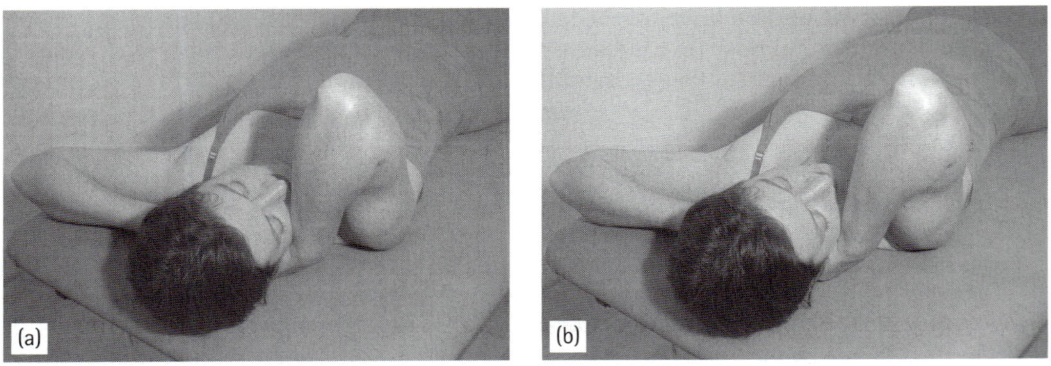

Figure 2.53a and b Passive mobilization; C2; unilateral posterior-anterior movement with previously adjusted rotation to the right; self-exercise. **a**, Starting position. **b**, End position.

Unilateral posterior-anterior push with adjusted rotation to the right

Therapy technique (film 42)

- Patient's starting position: prone, the cervical spine adjusted in rotation to the right.
- Therapist's starting position: standing, at the patient's head end (Fig. 2.52a).
- Movement: unilateral push with the tips of both thumbs on the joint process of C2 from posterior to anterior (Fig. 2.52b).

Self-exercise (film 43)

- Patient's starting position: supine, with a cushion under the head, cervical spine adjusted in rotation to the right, contact with the end part of the middle finger of the right hand on the joint process of C2, right side, with simultaneous contact of the middle finger of the left hand on this finger (Fig. 2.53a).
- Movement: unilateral push on the joint process of C2 from posterior to anterior via pull of the right hand and push of the left hand (Fig. 2.53b).

Transversal push

Therapy technique (film 44)

- Patient's starting position: side-lying.

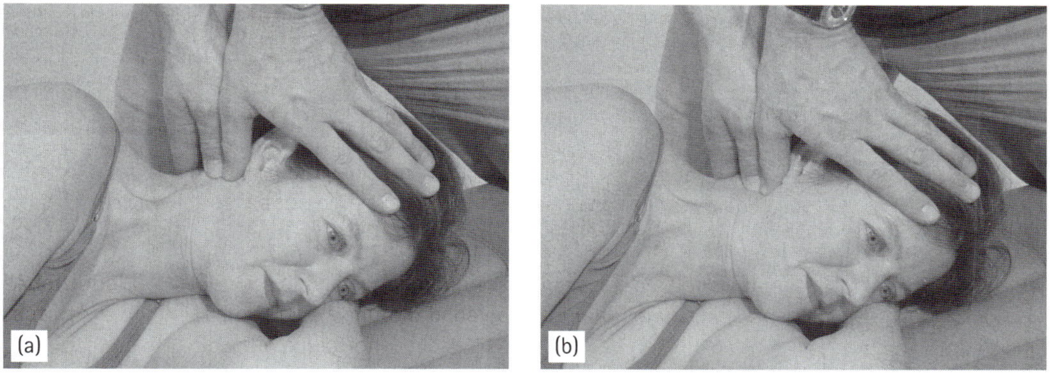

Figure 2.54a and b Passive mobilization; C2; transversal movement; therapy technique. **a**, Starting position. **b**, End position.

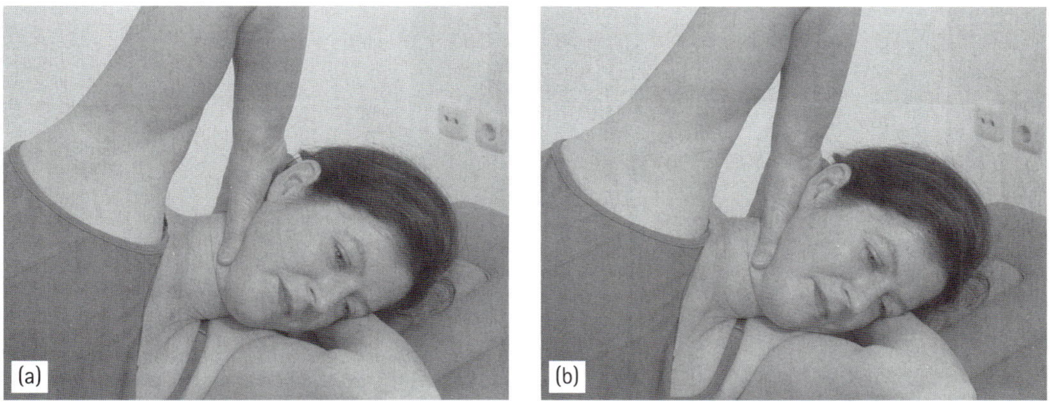

Figure 2.55a and b Passive mobilization; C2; transversal movement; self-exercise. **a**, Starting position. **b**, End position.

- Therapist's starting position: standing, at the patient's head end behind the patient (Fig. 2.54a).
- Movement: transversal push with the tips of both thumbs on the transverse process and the joint process of C2 (Fig. 2.54b).

Self-exercise (film 45)

- Patient's starting position: side-lying, with a cushion under the head, contact with the metacarpophalangeal joint 2 (MCP2) of the right hand over the transverse process and the joint process of C2 (Fig. 2.55a).
- Movement: transversal push on the transverse process of C2 via push of the right hand in a transversal direction (Fig. 2.55b).

Unilateral anterior–posterior push

Therapy technique (film 46)

- Patient's starting position: supine.
- Therapist's starting position: standing, at the patient's head end. Contact with the tips of the thumbs from anterior against the transverse process of C2, right side (Fig. 2.56a).
- Movement: unilateral push on the right transverse process of C2 from anterior to posterior, with the tips of both thumbs put one over another or with the hypothenar (Fig. 2.56b).

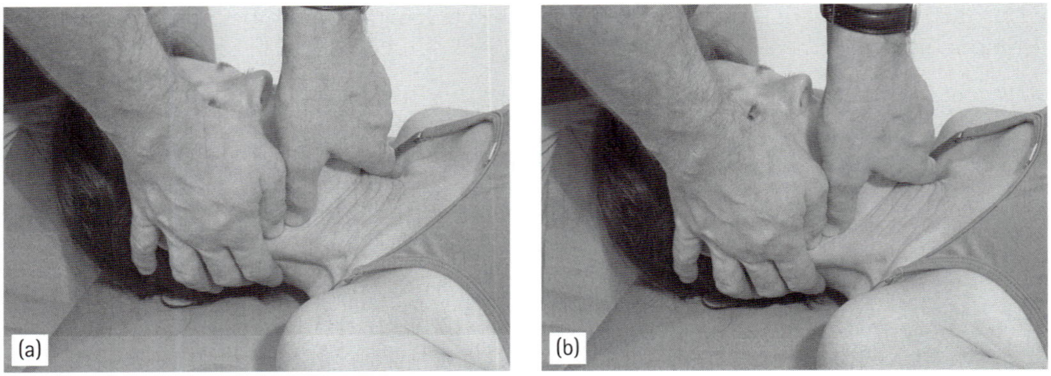

Figure 2.56a and b Passive mobilization; C2; unilateral anterior-posterior movement; therapy technique. a, Starting position. b, End position.

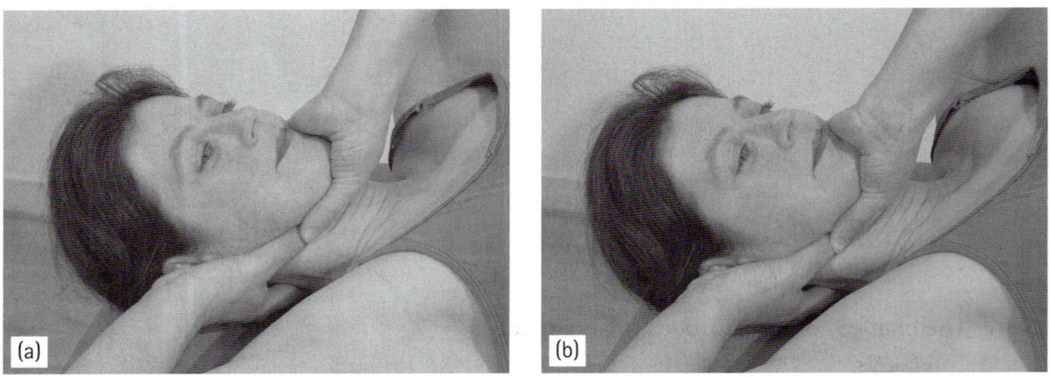

Figure 2.57a and b Passive mobilization; C2; unilateral anterior-posterior movement; self-exercise. a, Starting position. b, End position.

Self-exercise (film 47)

- Patient's starting position: supine, with a cushion under the head, contact with the right thumb on the anterior aspect of the transverse process of C2, right side. The left thumb is put over the right thumb (Fig. 2.57a).
- Movement: unilateral push on the transverse process of C2, right side, from anterior to posterior via pressure of the left thumb on the right thumb (Fig. 2.57b).

Remarks (regarding passive procedures, accessory movements)

Goals of the technique

With a painfully restricted rotation to the right of C2, right side, these techniques serve to:

- reduce tonicity and improve the metabolism of the affected tissues
- restore pain-free function (change the input to respective centres of the CNS)
- restore normal function of symptomatic tissue by application of the symptom-provoking stimulus dosed according to the current load tolerance.

Performance

Depending on irritability or desired treatment goal, the joint to be treated is adjusted as necessary before treatment. As the techniques are performed without 'specific fixation', an uncontrolled continuation of movement has to be considered when the indication for these techniques is determined.

Dosage (regarding the affected symptomatic structure)

Acute presentation (predominantly peripheral pain mechanisms)			
Phase	Limitation of movement due to pain and resistance	Concept	Movement grade
Inflammation phase	No pain	Kaltenborn–Evjenth	Up to the beginning of II
	No resistance	Maitland	Up to II
Proliferation phase	Up to P1	Kaltenborn–Evjenth	Up to the 1st third of II
	Slowly progressing up to low resistance	Maitland	III^{-}
Remodelling/ organization phase	Slowly progressing up to maximum resistance	Kaltenborn–Evjenth	Up to III
	(Note: duration of turnover!)	Maitland	Up to IV^{++} or III^{++}

Note: The chances of a disturbed (delayed) course of healing and their consequences for the loading capacity of the tissue (e.g., diabetes, old age, partial or general immobilization) have to be considered.

Chronic presentation (predominantly central pain mechanisms): Since here it is assumed that pain no longer represents a protection mechanism, the therapist has to consider the training state of the treated tissue to be expected as well as the patient's personal expectations. In case of doubt, treatment is always started with very low force, and progression is made conditional on reassessment. Hence with a chronic presentation, pain does not always represent the limiting factor regarding dosage of treatment.

Choice of technique

The selection of the technique depends, among other things, on the therapist as well as the patient, on the therapist's clinical experience, but primarily on reassessment. This means that even if all preconditions on the part of therapist and patient seem to be met, it is, in the authors' view, of no use to continue the technique if reassessment is negative.

Contributing factors

For a satisfactory solution of the patient's current problems it is essential to consider the contributing factors and include them in the treatment.

The authors will, however, not go into a description of the various possibilities and their complex contexts as this would exceed the scope of the present book.

Chapter 3

Lateral upper arm

CHAPTER CONTENTS

AREA LOCALIZATION

IDENTIFICATION OF THE POTENTIALLY AFFECTED AREA BY DEMONSTRATION OF A SYMPTOMATIC FUNCTIONAL MOVEMENT/POSITION

Based on the information gained from the anamnesis so far, the therapist tries to ascertain more details about potentially affected sections. This is done by means of area localization, which represents the beginning of the physical examination. Information gained in this way is used to check or modify the relevant hypotheses developed on the basis of the anamnesis and will determine how to proceed.

The way area localization is performed is explained by means of examples. In all four examples, the patient feels pain in the area of the lateral upper arm. Based on clinical experience and known clinical patterns, primarily the following sections are considered as potential sources of the current complaints:

- cervical spine
- thoracic spine (without example)
- shoulder complex
- neural structures.

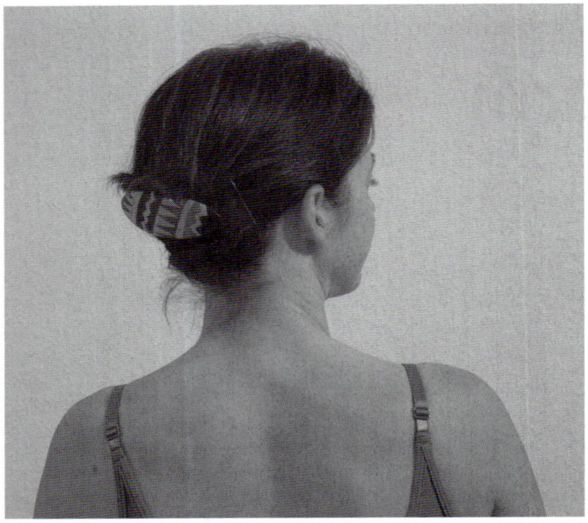

Figure 3.1 Symptom-provoking movement: turning the head to the right provokes symptoms in the area of the lateral upper arm.

General question: Is there enough information available to skip area localization?	
No	Yes
⇓	⇓
Performance of area localization	• General movement tests • Additional tests • Test treatment

Example 1: Turning the head to the right

Symptom area: lateral upper arm
Symptom provocation: turning the head to the right (Fig. 3.1)

With this presentation, clinical experience suggests primarily the cervical spine, the thoracic spine, and the neural structures as symptom-provoking areas.

Below, examples illustrate how to differentiate between these areas. To this end, area localization is first attempted by means of active movements alone. If this is not possible, tests will be performed by means of assistive movements.

Hypothesis 1: The symptom-provoking area is the cervical spine
Differentiation: cervical spine vs. thoracic spine.

The change in symptoms can be demonstrated exactly:

- provocation of pain (Fig. 3.2a and b, film 52)
- alleviation of pain (Fig. 3.3a and b, film 53).

The result of area localization has to be verified by further specific tests – otherwise the result will be open to question.

Hypothesis 2: The symptom-provoking area is the neural structures
Differentiation: neural involvement vs. cervical spine.

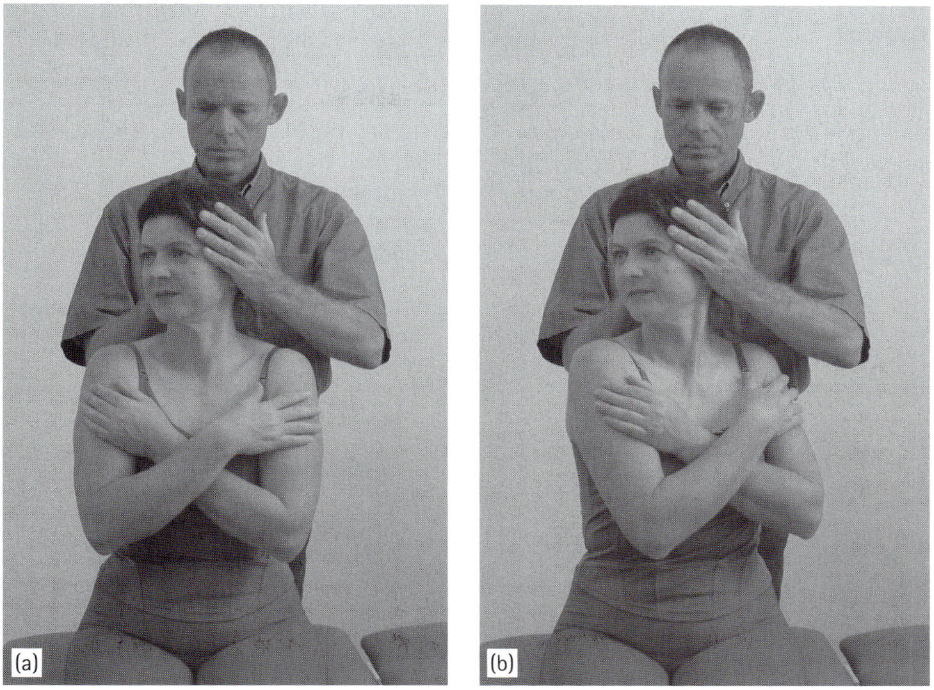

Figure 3.2a and b Area localization with symptomatic turning of the head to the right; differentiation between cervical spine and thoracic spine; provocation. a, Starting position. b, End position.

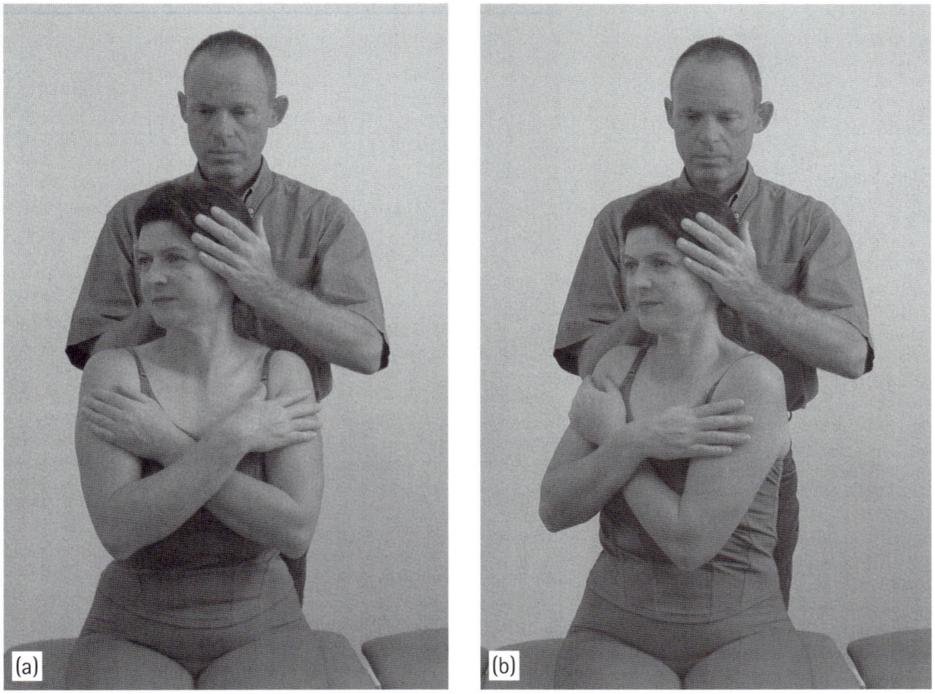

Figure 3.3a and b Area localization with symptomatic turning of the head to the right; differentiation between cervical spine and thoracic spine; alleviation. a, Starting position. b, End position.

Assessment			
Goal	**Provocation of pain**	**Alleviation of pain**	**Remarks**
Starting position	Turning the head to the right to a position immediately before symptoms appear	Turning the head to the right to a position immediately after symptoms have appeared	Head remains in starting position
Test movement	Rotation of the thoracic spine to the left	Rotation of the thoracic spine to the right	
Explanation	Rotation of the thoracic spine to the left increases the rotation of the cervical spine to the right	Rotation of the thoracic spine to the right reduces the rotation of the cervical spine to the right	
Additional data to support the hypothesis	General and specific mobility of cervical spine and thoracic spine History, e.g., symptom behaviour, type of complaints, 24-hour behaviour Palpation Reproducibility of test results Test treatment Imaging procedures (CT, MRI)		

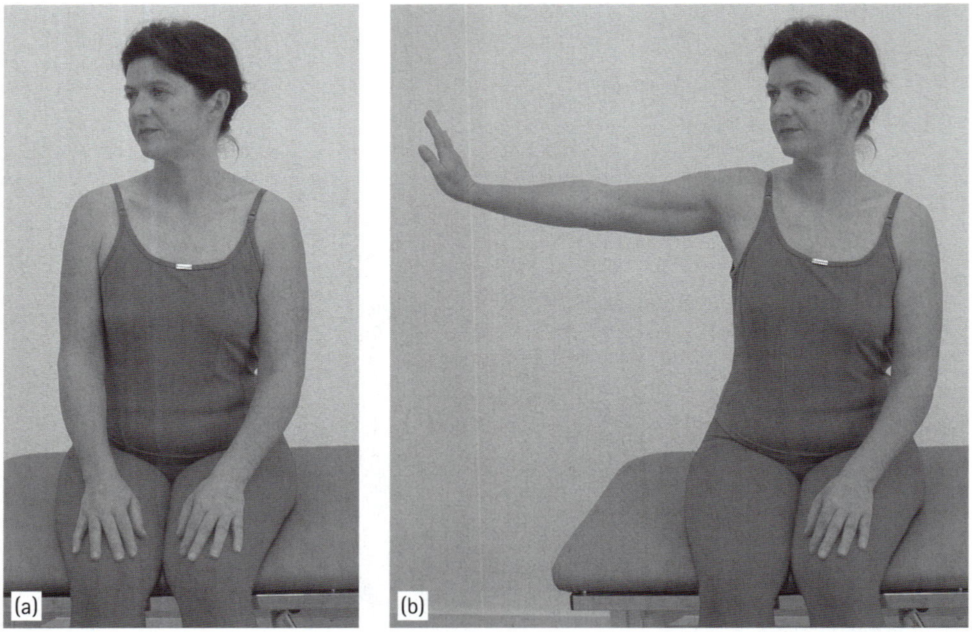

Figure 3.4a and b Area localization with symptomatic turning of the head to the right; differentiation between neural structures and cervical spine; provocation. a, Starting position. b, End position.

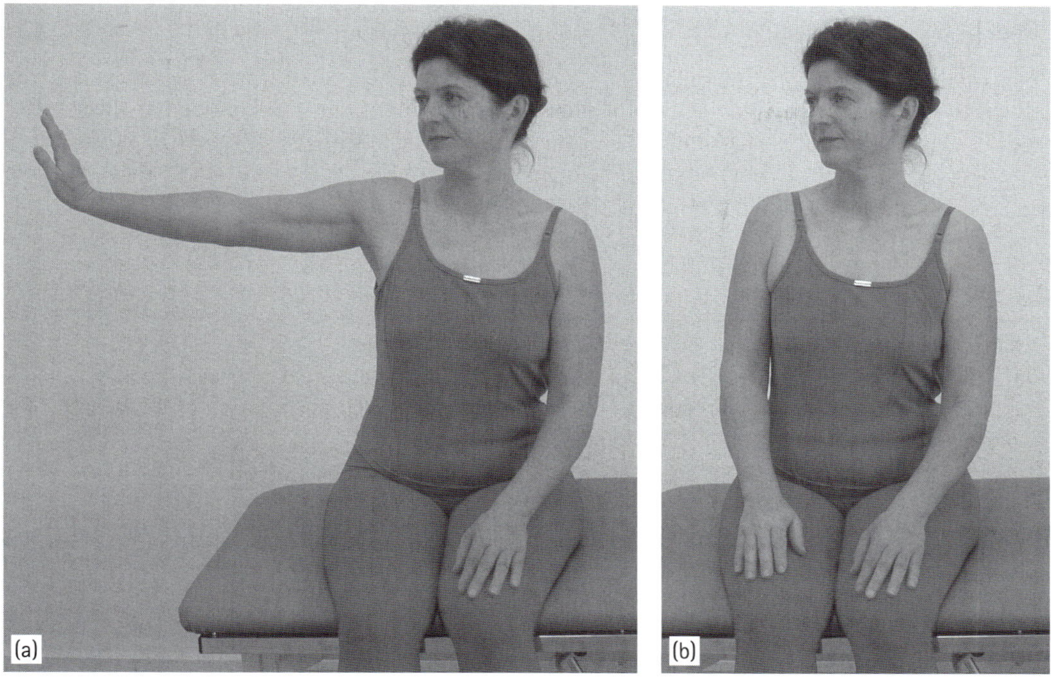

Figure 3.5a and b Area localization with symptomatic turning of the head to the right; differentiation between neural structures and cervical spine; alleviation. a, Starting position. b, End position.

The change in symptoms can be demonstrated exactly:

- provocation of pain (Fig. 3.4a and b, film 54)
- alleviation of pain (Fig. 3.5a and b, film 55).

The result of area localization has to be verified by further specific tests – otherwise the result will be open to question.

Assessment

Goal	Provocation of pain	Alleviation of pain	Remarks
Starting position	Turning the head to the right to a position immediately before symptoms appear	With the right arm adjusted first in abduction of the glenohumeral joint, extension of the elbow and dorsal flexion of the wrist, turning the head to the right	
Test movement	Abducting the glenohumeral joint of the right arm, extending the elbow, and dorsiflexing the wrist	Adducting the glenohumeral joint of the previously adjusted arm	The shoulder girdle has to remain immobile during movement. Lifting the arm has to be pain-free

Goal	Provocation of pain	Alleviation of pain	Remarks
Explanation	Abducting the right glenohumeral joint produces mechanical stress on the neural structures and the structures directly associated with them	Adducting the right glenohumeral joint from the previously adjusted position reduces the mechanical stress on the neural structures and the structures directly associated with them	If the typical pain is provoked or alleviated by these manoeuvres without moving the cervical spine, this suggests at least an involvement of the neural structures
Additional data to support the hypothesis	General and specific mobility of the affected area Further movements of proximal and distal components to increase neural tension, not directly involved in movement of the right rotation of the head, e.g., upper or lower extremity movements History, e.g., symptom behaviour, type of complaints, 24-hour behaviour Palpation Neurodynamic tests Nerve provocation tests (e.g., Spurling's test, Tinel's sign) Reproducibility of test results Test treatment Imaging procedures (CT, MRI)		

Example 2: Movement of the head forwards

Symptom area: lateral upper arm
Symptom provocation: movement of the head forwards (Fig. 3.6)

With this presentation, clinical experience suggests primarily the cervical spine, the thoracic spine, and the neural structures as symptom-provoking areas.

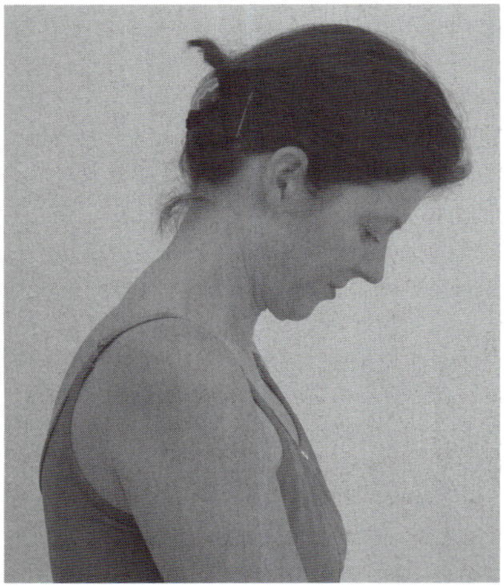

Figure 3.6 Symptom-provoking movement: movement of the head forwards provokes symptoms in the area of the lateral upper arm.

Below, examples illustrate how to differentiate between these areas. To this end, area localization is first attempted by means of active movements alone. If this is not possible, tests will be performed by means of assistive movements.

Hypothesis 1: The symptom-provoking area is the cervical spine

Differentiation: cervical spine vs. thoracic spine.

The change in symptoms can be demonstrated exactly:

- provocation of pain (Fig. 3.7a and b, film 66)
- alleviation of pain (Fig. 3.8a and b, film 67).

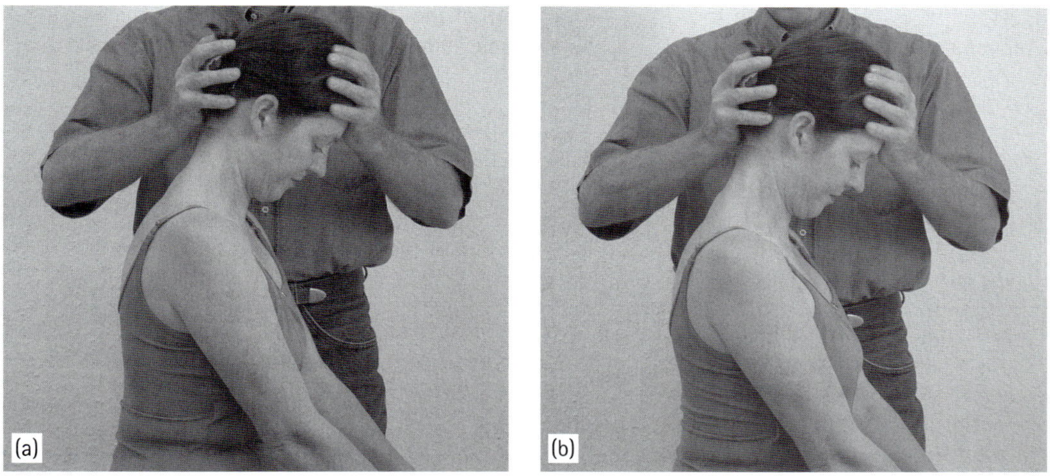

Figure 3.7a and b Area localization with symptomatic movement of the head forwards; differentiation between cervical spine and thoracic spine; provocation. **a**, Starting position. **b**, End position.

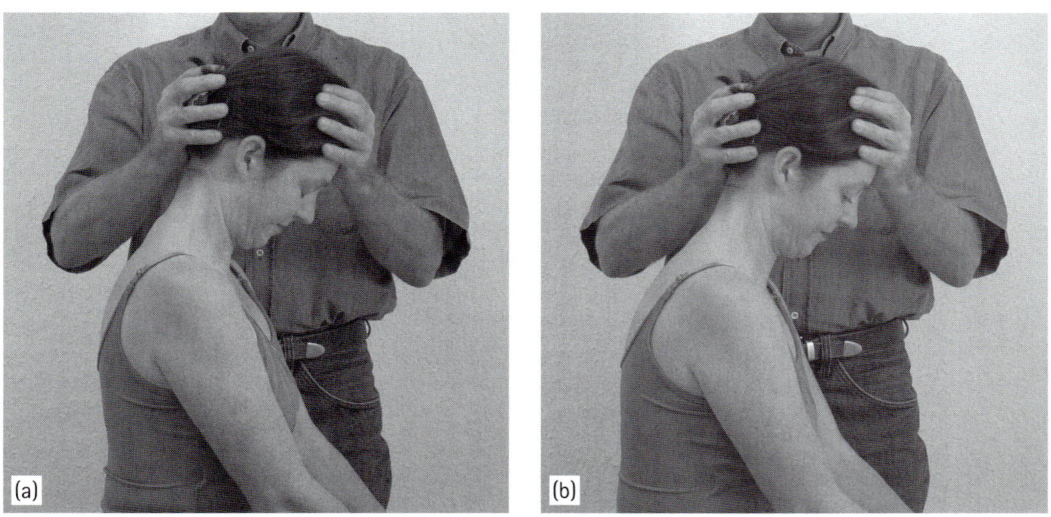

Figure 3.8a and b Area localization with symptomatic movement of the head forwards; differentiation between cervical spine and thoracic spine; alleviation. **a**, Starting position. **b**, End position.

The result of area localization has to be verified by further specific tests – otherwise the result will be open to question.

Assessment

Goal	Provocation of pain	Alleviation of pain	Remarks
Starting position	Movement of the head forwards to a position immediately before symptoms appear	Movement of the head forwards to a position immediately after symptoms have appeared	
Test movement	Extension of the thoracic spine	Flexion of the thoracic spine	The head remains in the respective starting position, fixed by the therapist
Explanation	With fixed head, extension of the thoracic spine produces an increased flexion of the cervical spine	With fixed head, flexion of the thoracic spine produces an increased extension of the cervical spine	
Additional data to support the hypothesis	General and specific mobility of cervical spine and thoracic spine History, e.g., symptom behaviour, type of complaints, 24-hour behaviour Palpation Reproducibility of test results Test treatment Imaging procedures (CT, MRI)		

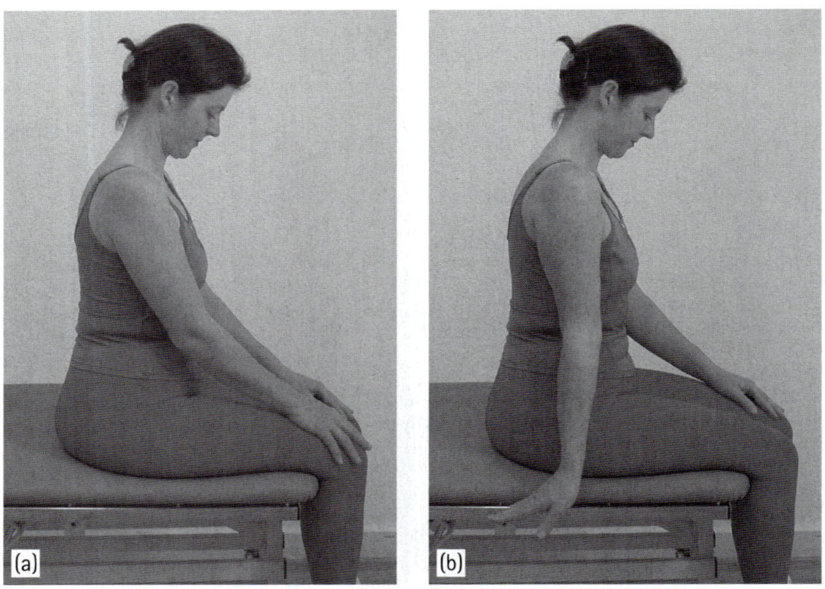

Figure 3.9a and b Area localization with symptomatic movement of the head forwards; differentiation between neural structures and cervical spine; provocation. **a**, Starting position. **b**, End position.

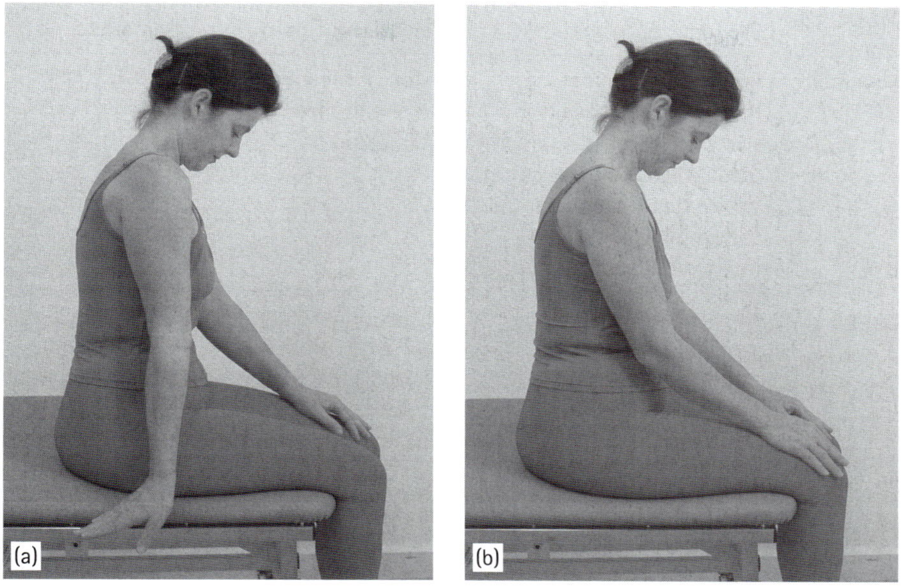

Figure 3.10a and b Area localization with symptomatic movement of the head forwards; differentiation between neural structures and cervical spine; alleviation. **a**, Starting position. **b**, End position.

Hypothesis 2: The symptom-provoking area is the neural structures

Differentiation: neural involvement vs. cervical spine.

The change in symptoms can be demonstrated exactly:

- provocation of pain (Fig. 3.9a and b, film 68)
- alleviation of pain (Fig. 3.10a and b, film 69).

The result of area localization has to be verified by further specific tests – otherwise the result will be open to question.

Assessment

Goal	Provocation of pain	Alleviation of pain	Remarks
Starting position	Movement of the head forwards to a position immediately before symptoms appear, with arm adjusted before	With the right arm adjusted in maximum supination, maximum dorsal flexion of the wrist with extended fingers, and maximum extension of the elbow, movement of the head forwards to a position immediately after symptoms have appeared	

Goal	Provocation of pain	Alleviation of pain	Remarks
Test movement	From a position of maximum supination of the forearm and maximum dorsal flexion of the wrist with extended fingers, the elbow is moved into extension	Flexion of the elbow with simultaneous volar flexion of the wrist	
Explanation	The test movement produces mechanical stress on the neural structures and the structures directly associated with them	The test movement reduces the mechanical stress on the neural structures and the structures directly associated with them	If the typical pain is provoked or alleviated by these manoeuvres, without moving the cervical spine, this suggests at least an involvement of neural structures
Additional data to support the hypothesis	General and specific mobility of the affected area Further movements of proximal and distal components to increase neural tension, not directly involved in movement of the right rotation of the head, e.g., upper or lower extremity movements History, e.g., symptom behaviour, type of complaints, 24-hour behaviour Palpation Neurodynamic tests Nerve provocation tests (e.g., Spurling's test, Tinel's sign) Reproducibility of test results Test treatment Imaging procedures (CT, MRI)		

Example 3: Movement of the head backwards

Symptom area: lateral upper arm
Symptom provocation: movement of the head backwards (Fig. 3.11)

With this presentation, clinical experience suggests primarily the cervical spine, the thoracic spine, and the neural structures as symptom-provoking areas.

Below, examples illustrate how to differentiate between these areas. To this end, area localization is first attempted by means of active movements alone. If this is not possible, tests will be performed by means of assistive movements.

Hypothesis 1: The symptom-provoking area is the cervical spine

Differentiation: cervical spine vs. thoracic spine.

The change in symptoms can be demonstrated exactly:

- provocation of pain (Fig. 3.12a and b, film 78)
- alleviation of pain (Fig. 3.13a and b, film 79).

The result of area localization has to be verified by further specific tests – otherwise the result will be open to question.

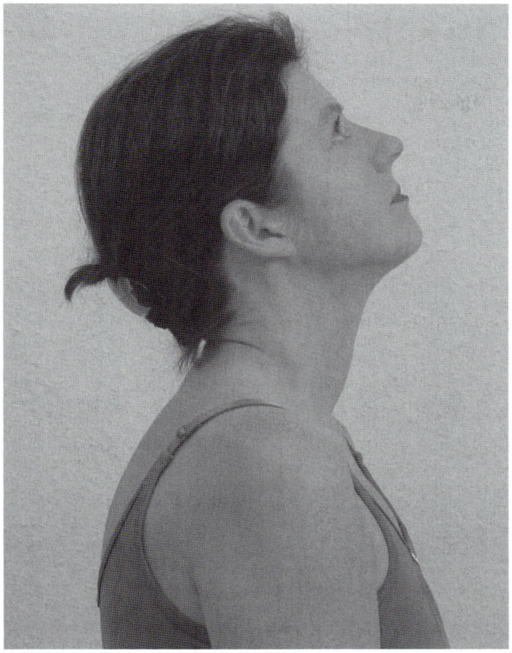

Figure 3.11 Symptom-provoking movement: movement of the head backwards provokes symptoms in the area of the lateral upper arm.

Assessment			
Goal	**Provocation of pain**	**Alleviation of pain**	**Remarks**
Starting position	Movement of the head backwards to a position before symptoms appear	Movement of the head backwards to a position immediately after symptoms have appeared	
Test movement	Flexion of the thoracic spine	Extension of the thoracic spine	The head remains in the respective starting position, fixed by the therapist
Explanation	With fixed head, flexion of the thoracic spine produces an increased extension of the cervical spine	With fixed head, extension of the thoracic spine produces an increased flexion of the cervical spine	
Additional data to support the hypothesis	General and specific mobility of cervical spine and thoracic spine History, e.g., symptom behaviour, type of complaints, 24-hour behaviour Palpation Reproducibility of test results Test treatment Imaging procedures (CT, MRI)		

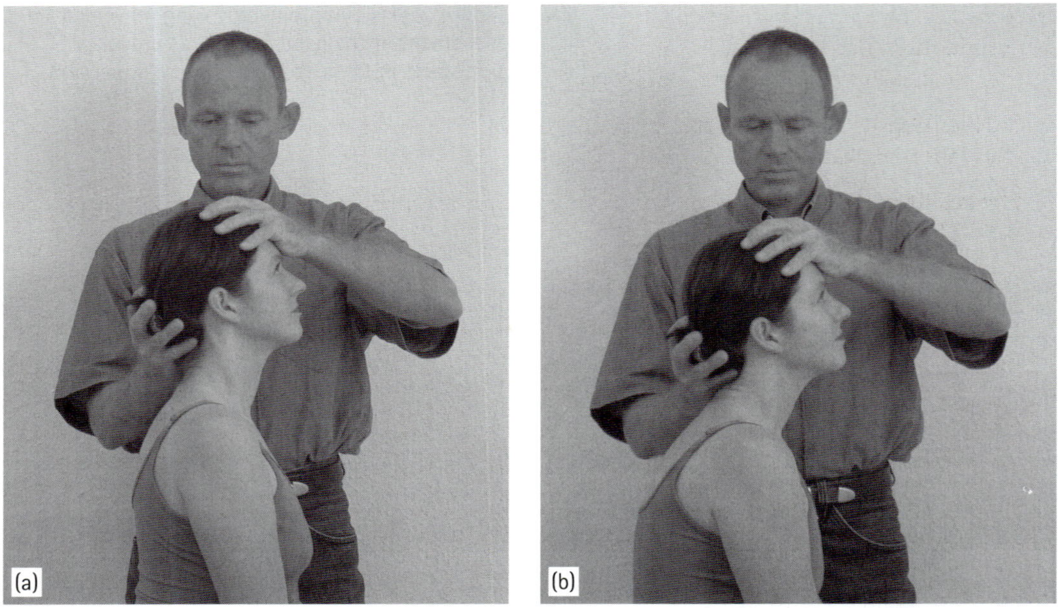

Figure 3.12a and b Area localization with symptomatic movement of the head backwards; differentiation between cervical spine and thoracic spine; provocation. **a**, Starting position. **b**, End position.

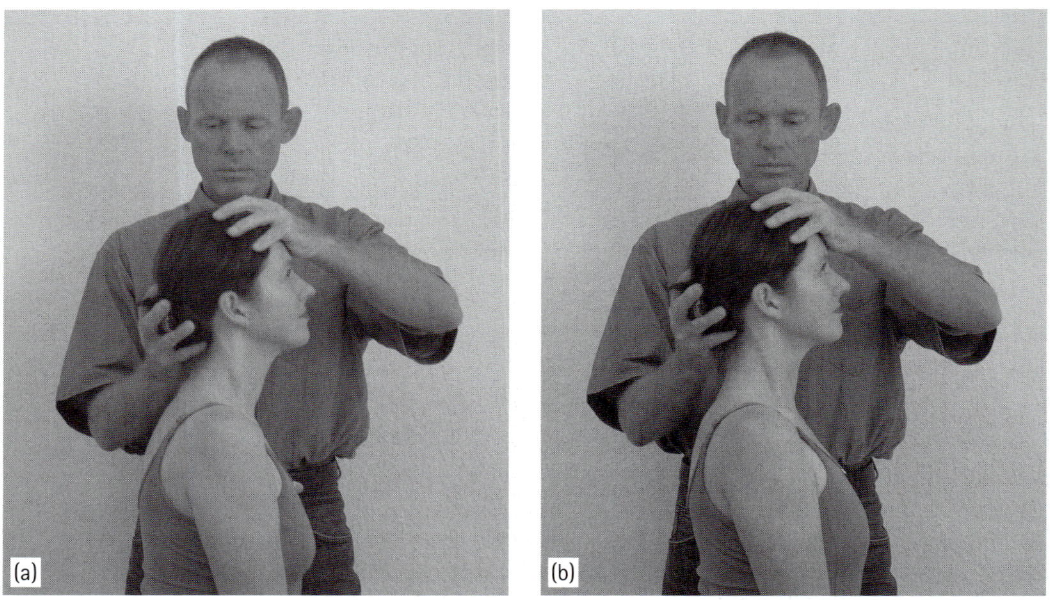

Figure 3.13a and b Area localization with symptomatic movement of the head backwards; differentiation between cervical spine and thoracic spine; alleviation. **a**, Starting position. **b**, End position.

Hypothesis 2: The symptom-provoking area is the neural structures
Differentiation: neural involvement vs. cervical spine.

The change in symptoms can be demonstrated exactly:

- provocation of pain (Fig. 3.14a and b, film 80)
- alleviation of pain (Fig. 3.15a and b, film 81).

The result of area localization has to be verified by further specific tests – otherwise the result will be open to question.

Assessment			
Goal	**Provocation of pain**	**Alleviation of pain**	**Remarks**
Starting position	Movement of the head backwards to a position immediately before symptoms appear	With the right arm first adjusted in abduction of the glenohumeral joint, extension of the elbow, and dorsal flexion of the wrist, movement of the head backwards to a position immediately after symptoms have appeared	
Test movement	Abducting the glenohumeral joint of the right arm, extending the elbow, and dorsiflexing the wrist	Adducting the glenohumeral joint of the right arm	During movement of the arm, the shoulder girdle has to remain immobile. Lifting the arm has to be pain-free
Explanation	Abducting the right glenohumeral joint produces mechanical stress on the neural structures and the structures directly associated with them	Adducting the right glenohumeral joint reduces the mechanical stress on the neural structures and the structures directly associated with them	If the typical pain is provoked or alleviated by these manoeuvres, without moving the cervical spine, this suggests at least an involvement of the neural structures
Additional data to support the hypothesis	General and specific mobility of the affected area Further movements of proximal and distal components to increase neural tension, not directly involved in the backward movement of the head, e.g., upper or lower extremity movements History, e.g., symptom behaviour, type of complaints, 24-hour behaviour Palpation Neurodynamic tests Nerve provocation tests (e.g., Spurling's test, Tinel's sign) Test treatment Reproducibility of test results		

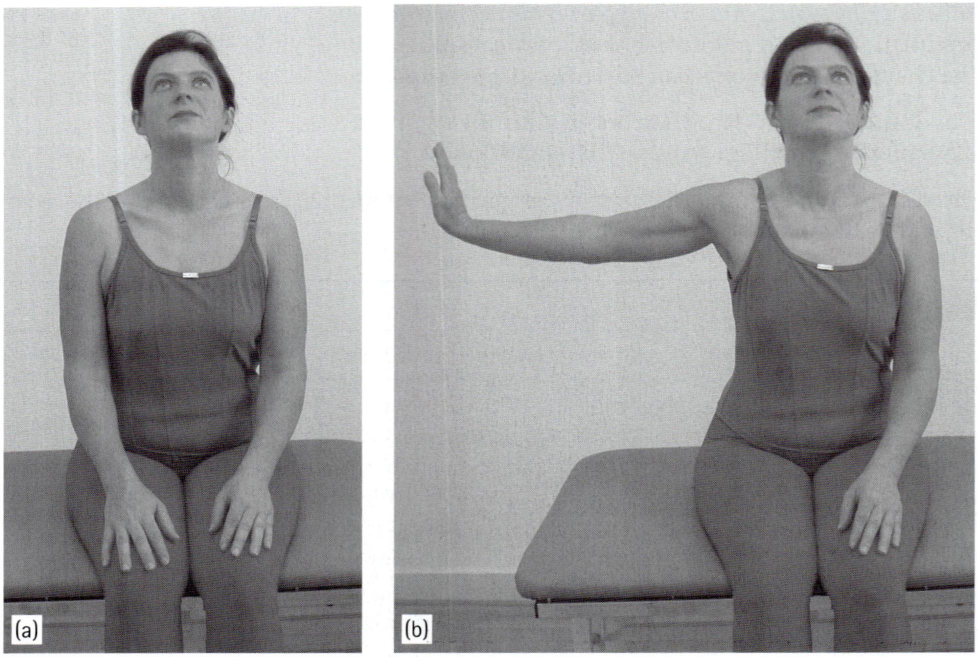

Figure 3.14a and b Area localization with symptomatic movement of the head backwards; differentiation between neural structures and cervical spine; provocation. **a**, Starting position. **b**, End position.

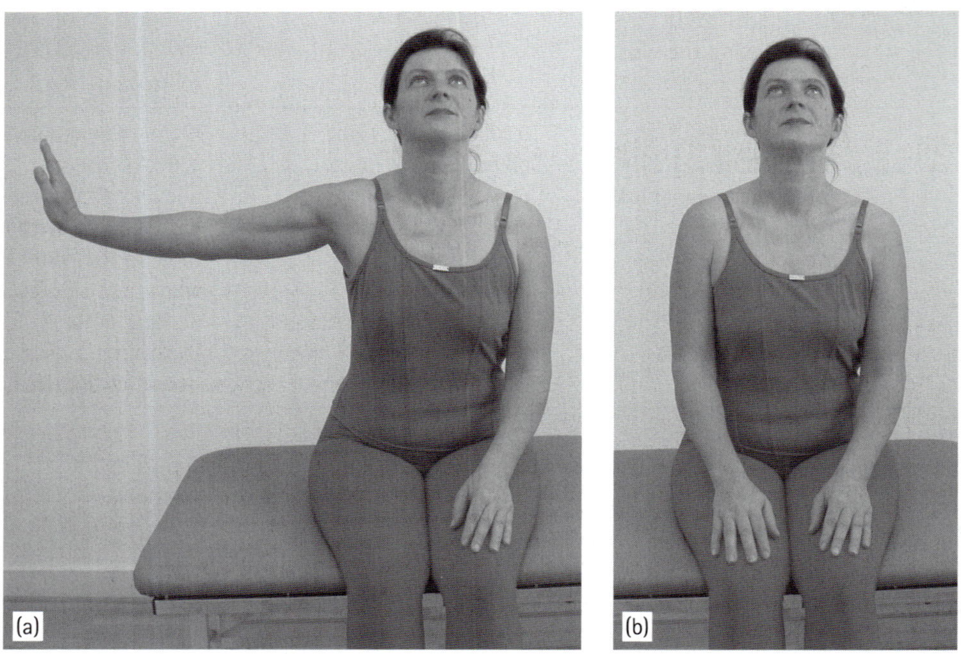

Figure 3.15a and b Area localization with symptomatic movement of the head backwards; differentiation between neural structures and cervical spine; alleviation. **a**, Starting position. **b**, End position.

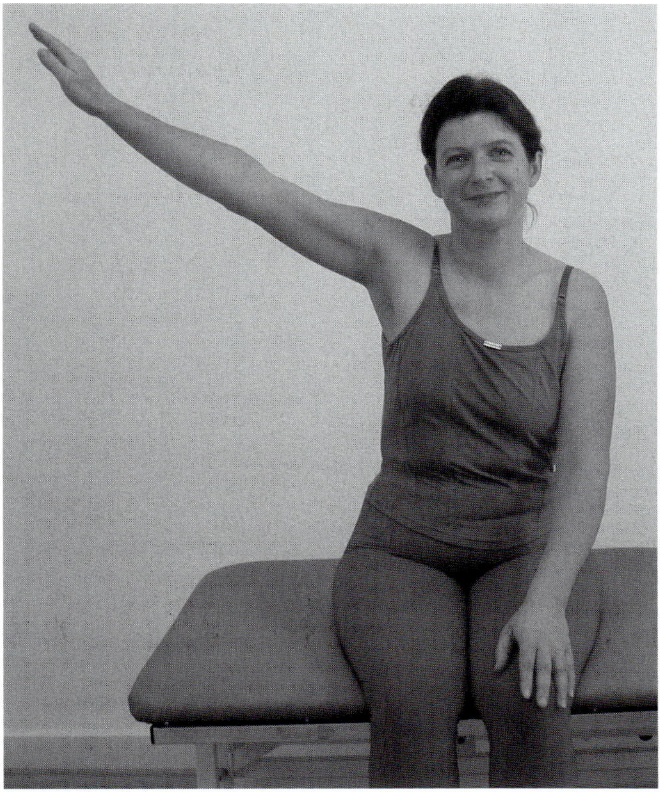

Figure 3.16 Symptom-provoking movement: movement of the arm into abduction/elevation provokes symptoms in the area of the lateral upper arm.

Example 4: Abduction/elevation of the arm

Symptom area: lateral upper arm
Symptom provocation: abduction/elevation of the arm (Fig. 3.16)

With this presentation, clinical experience suggests primarily the cervical spine, the shoulder complex, and the neural structures as symptom-provoking areas.

Below, examples illustrate how to differentiate between these areas. To this end, area localization is first attempted by means of active movements alone. If this is not possible, tests will be performed by means of assistive movements.

Hypothesis 1: The symptom-provoking area is the cervical spine

Differentiation: cervical spine vs. shoulder complex.

The change in symptoms can be demonstrated exactly:

- provocation of pain (Fig. 3.17a and b, film 92)
- alleviation of pain (Fig. 3.18a and b, film 93).

The result of area localization has to be verified by further specific tests – otherwise the result will be open to question.

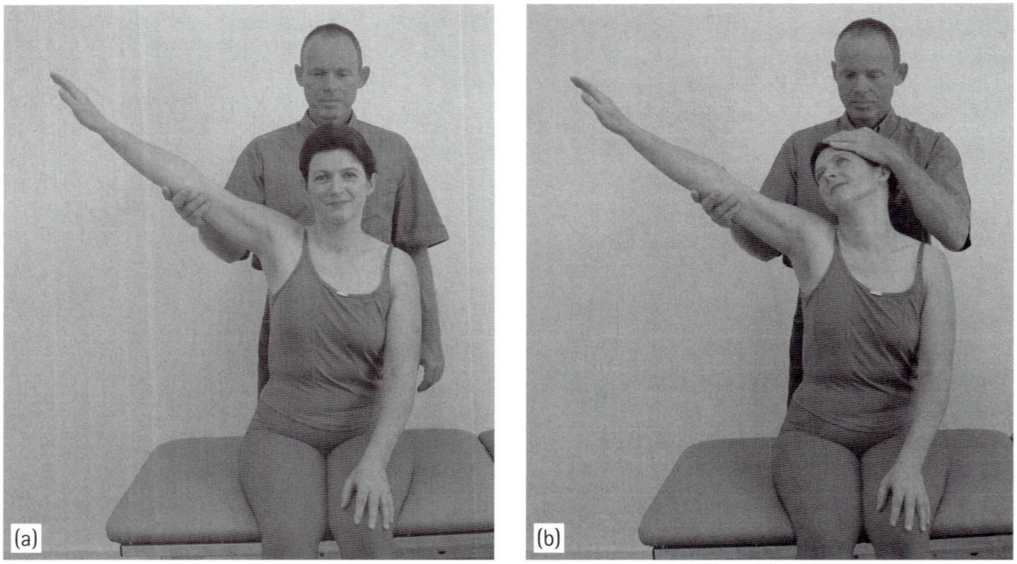

Figure 3.17a and b Area localization with symptomatic movement of the arm into abduction–elevation; differentiation between cervical spine and shoulder complex; provocation. a, Starting position. b, End position.

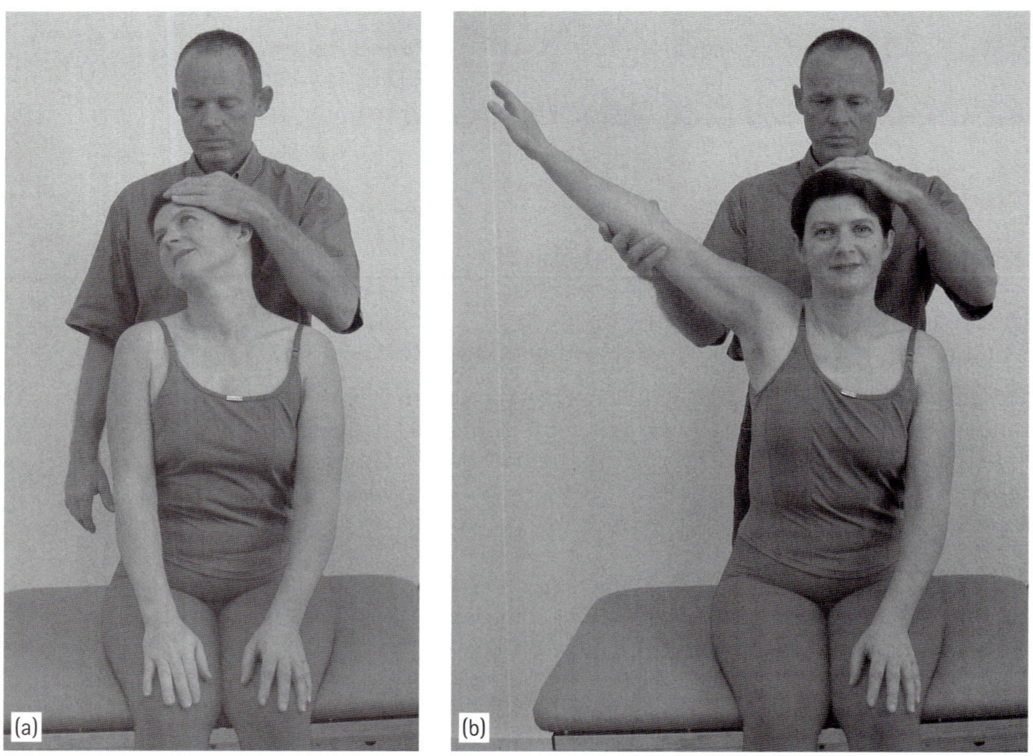

Figure 3.18a and b Area localization with symptomatic movement of the arm into abduction–elevation; differentiation between cervical spine and shoulder complex; alleviation. a, Starting position. b, End position.

Assessment			
Goal	**Provocation of pain**	**Alleviation of pain**	**Remarks**
Starting position	Lifting the right arm to a position immediately before symptoms appear	The cervical spine positioned in extension, lateral flexion to the right, and rotation to the right, the right arm lifted to a position immediately after symptoms have appeared	
Test movement	Extension, lateral flexion, and rotation of the cervical spine to the right	Guiding the cervical spine back into neutral position	The described movement directions of the cervical spine have to be understood as examples only; any other movement combination is possible, too, and has to be tested separately if need be
Explanation	If any movement of the cervical spine is able to reproduce the typical symptoms, an isolated lesion of the shoulder complex is doubtful	If any movement of the cervical spine is able to reduce the typical symptoms, an isolated lesion of the shoulder complex is doubtful	
Additional data to support the hypothesis	General and specific mobility of cervical spine and shoulder complex History, e.g., symptom behaviour, type of complaints, 24-hour behaviour Palpation Reproducibility of test results Test treatment Imaging procedures (CT, MRI)		

Hypothesis 2: The symptom-provoking area is the neural structures
Differentiation: neural involvement vs. shoulder complex.

The change in symptoms can be demonstrated exactly:

- provocation of pain (Fig. 3.19a and b, film 94)
- alleviation of pain (Fig. 3.20a and b, film 95).

The result of area localization has to be verified by further specific tests – otherwise the result will be open to question.

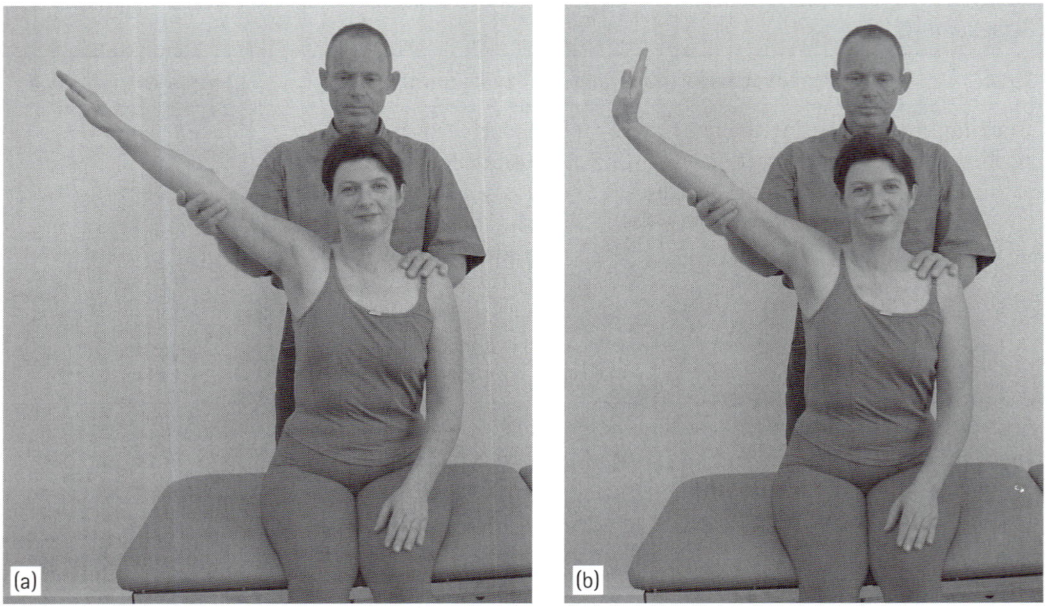

Figure 3.19a and b Area localization with symptomatic movement of the arm into abduction–elevation; differentiation between neural structures and shoulder complex; provocation. **a**, Starting position. **b**, End position.

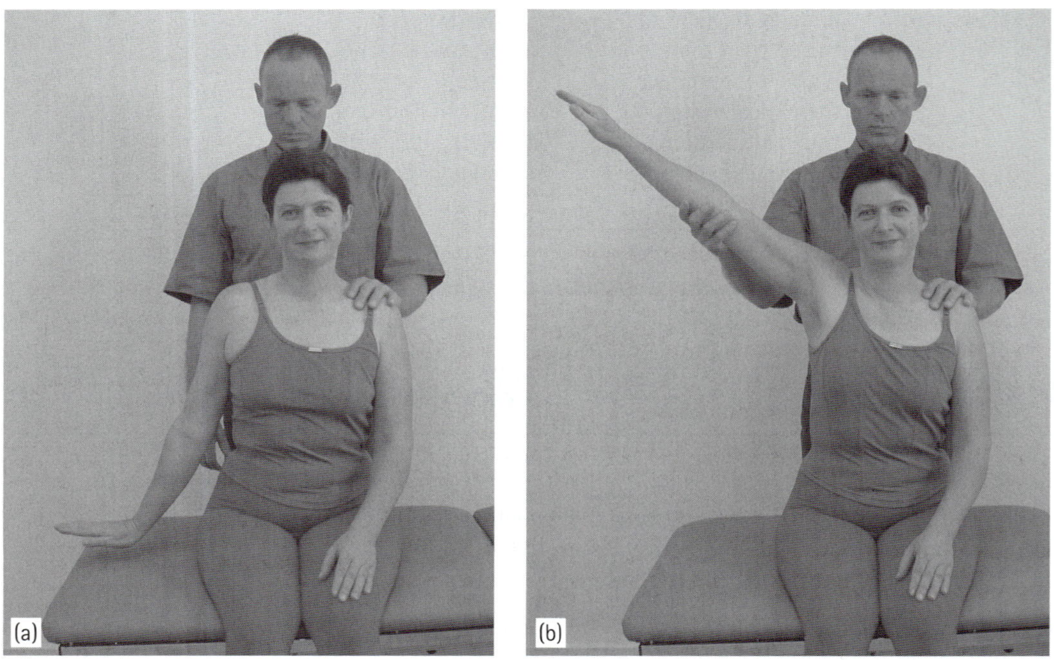

Figure 3.20a and b Area localization with symptomatic movement of the arm into abduction–elevation; differentiation between neural structures and shoulder complex; alleviation. **a**, Starting position. **b**, End position.

Assessment			
Goal	Provocation of pain	Alleviation of pain	Remarks
Starting position	Lifting the arm to a position immediately before symptoms appear	The wrist is dorsiflexed, the arm lifted to a position immediately after symptoms have appeared	
Test movement	Dorsal flexion of the wrist	Volar flexion of the wrist	Head remains in starting position
Explanation	The test movement produces mechanical stress on the neural structures and the structures directly associated with them	The test movement reduces the mechanical stress on the neural structures and the structures directly associated with them	If the typical pain can be provoked and alleviated by movements of the wrist, this suggests a dysfunction in the area of the neural structures
Additional data to support the hypothesis	General and specific mobility of the affected area Further movements of proximal and distal components to increase neural tension, not directly involved in the lifting of the arm, e.g., cervical spine or lower extremity movements History, e.g., symptom behaviour, type of complaints, 24-hour behaviour Palpation Neurodynamic tests Nerve provocation tests (e.g., Spurling's test, Tinel's sign) Reproducibility of test results Test treatment Imaging procedures (CT, MRI)		

QUICK CHECK – SYMPTOMS, LATERAL UPPER ARM

If neither the area nor a symptom-provoking or symptom-reducing action is known, the quick check is used to try to load individual potential areas with specific biomechanically provocative movement combinations. The chosen movement combinations correspond with the straining and often symptom-provoking movements of the individual sections.

CERVICAL SPINE

Movement

- Extension/lateral flexion, and rotation to the opposite side (Figs 3.21 and 3.22, film 15)
- Extension/lateral flexion, and rotation to the same side (Figs 3.23 and 3.24, film 15).

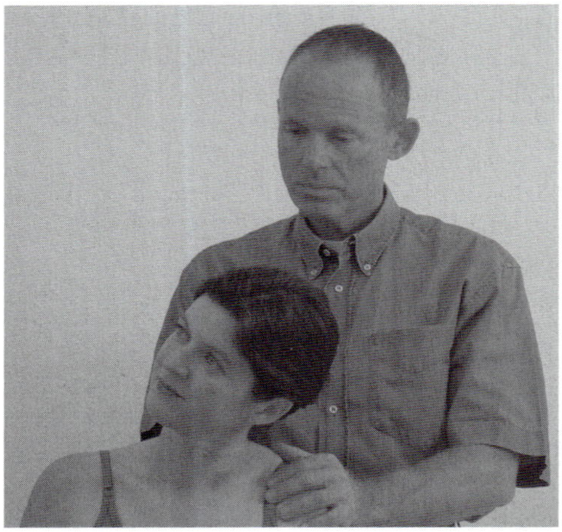

Figure 3.21 Quick check cervical spine; lateral flexion to the left with rotation to the opposite side.

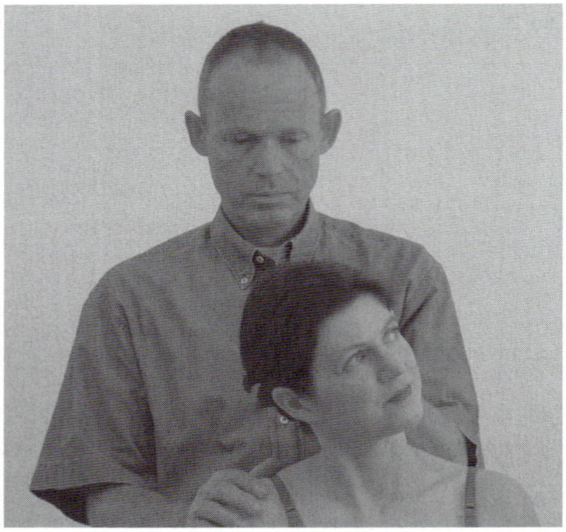

Figure 3.22 Quick check cervical spine; lateral flexion to the right with rotation to the opposite side.

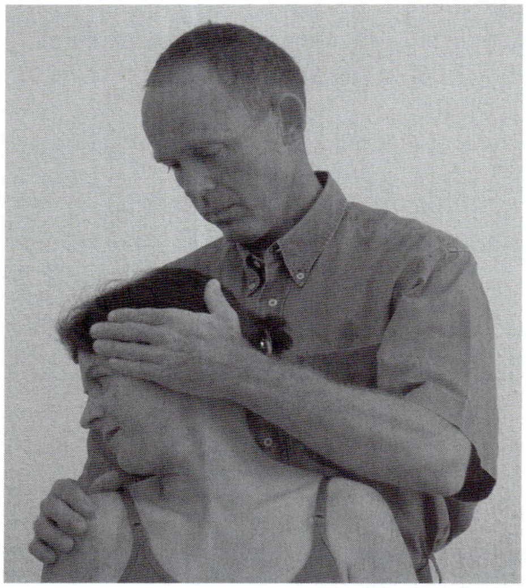

Figure 3.23 Quick check cervical spine; lateral flexion to the right with rotation to the same side.

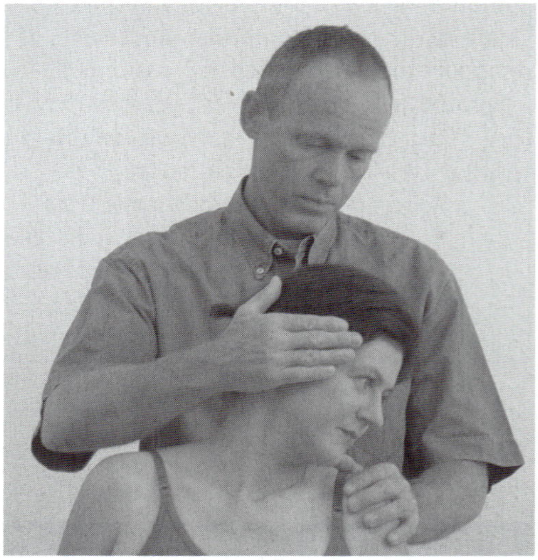

Figure 3.24 Quick check cervical spine; lateral flexion to the left with rotation to the same side.

NEURAL STRUCTURES

Tension tests

- Slump test (Fig. 3.25, film 16)
- Upper limb neurodynamic test 1 (ULNT-1; Fig. 3.26, film 17)
- Straight leg raise (SLR; Fig. 3.27, film 18).

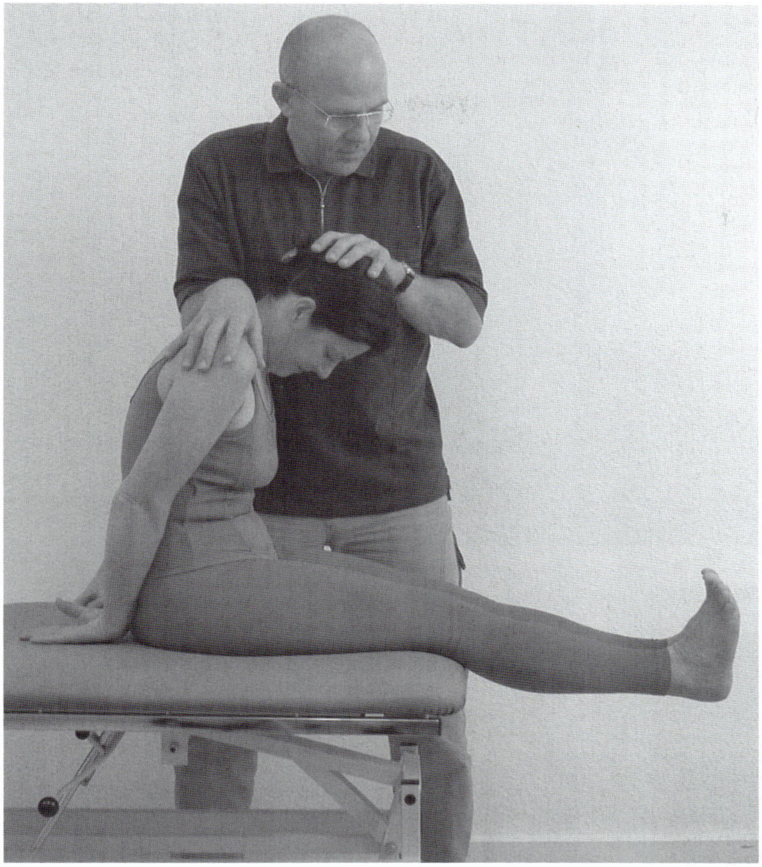

Figure 3.25 Quick check neurodynamics; slump test.

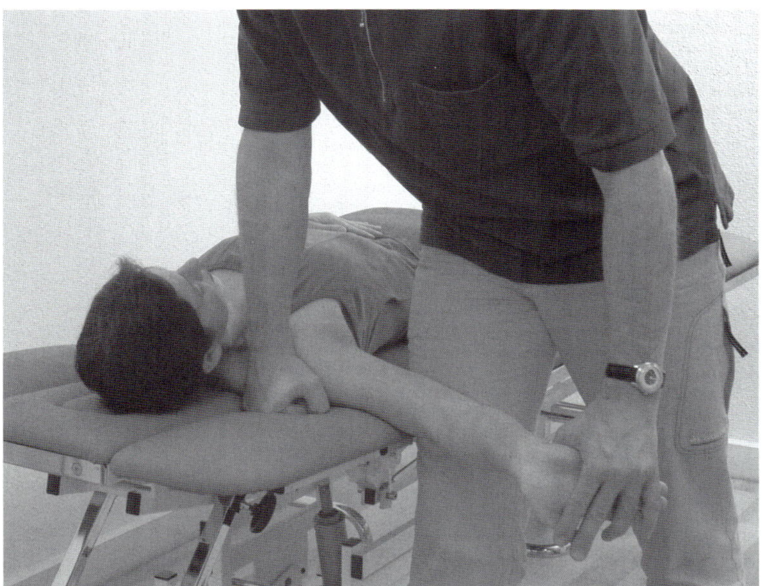

Figure 3.26 Quick check neurodynamics; upper limb neurodynamic test 1.

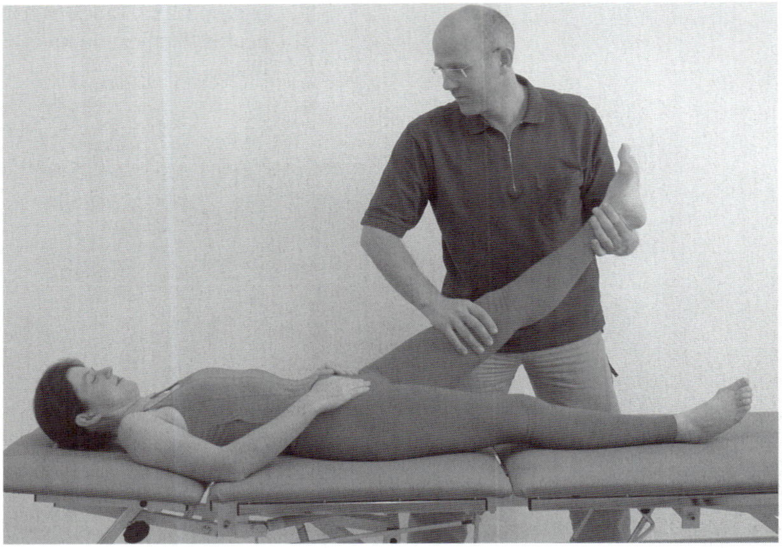

Figure 3.27 Quick check neurodynamics; straight leg raise test.

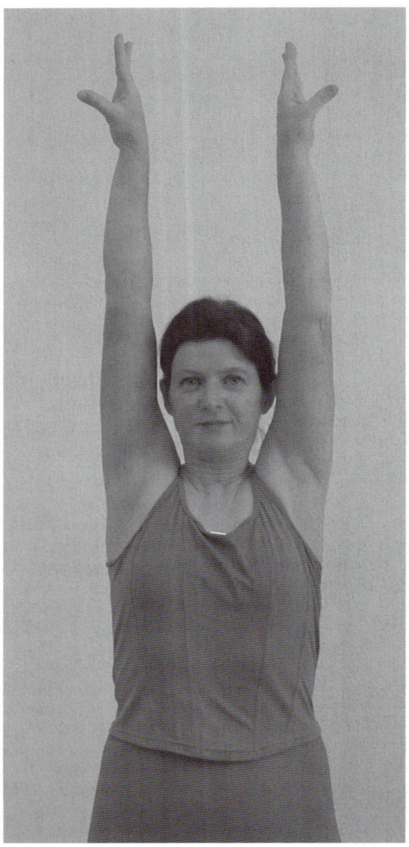

Figure 3.28 Quick check shoulder complex; abduction/elevation with simultaneous internal rotation.

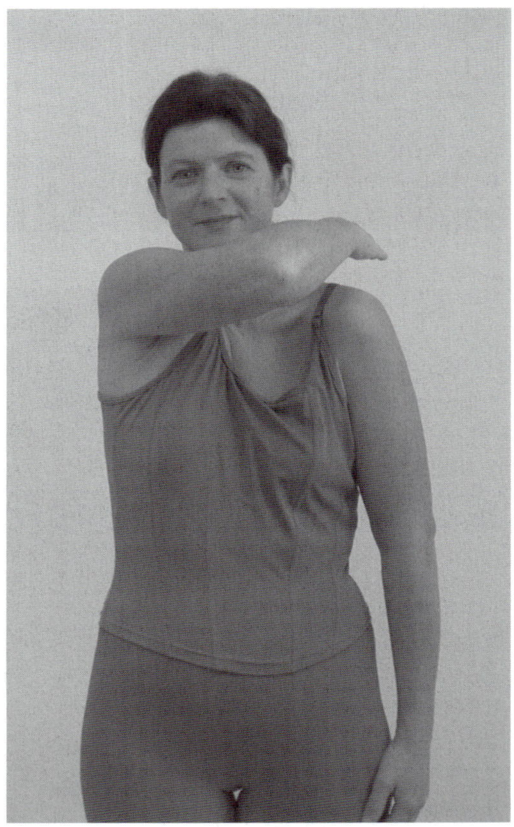

Figure 3.29 Quick check shoulder complex; horizontal adduction.

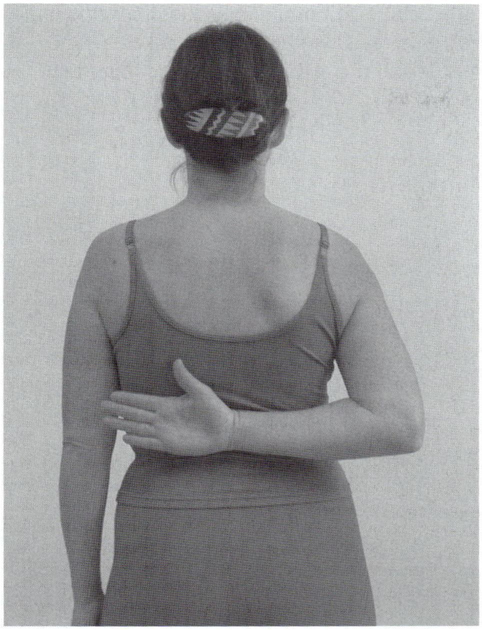

Figure 3.30 Quick check shoulder complex; extension/adduction/internal rotation.

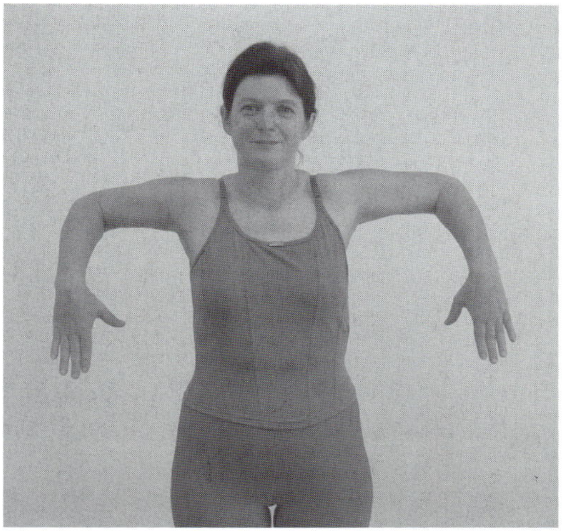

Figure 3.31 Quick check shoulder complex; internal rotation with 90° abduction.

SHOULDER COMPLEX

Movement

- Abduction/internal rotation/elevation (Fig. 3.28, film 108)
- Horizontal adduction (Fig. 3.29, film 109)
- Extension/adduction/internal rotation (Fig. 3.30, film 110)
- With 90° abduction, maximum internal rotation (Fig. 3.31, film 111).

Note: Even an area that proves negative in the quick check may possibly be symptom-provoking (another movement combination, or passive overpressure may be required).

SPECIFIC PROVOCATION AND ALLEVIATION

Specific provocation and alleviation enables differentiation within an articular complex and identification of the symptom-provoking movement direction(s).

SPECIFIC PROVOCATION AND ALLEVIATION, CERVICAL SPINE

Localization, lower cervical spine – turning the head to the right

Pain-provoking movement (Fig. 3.32)

- Turning the head to the right provokes pain in the lateral upper arm.
- Area localization hints at the lower cervical spine.

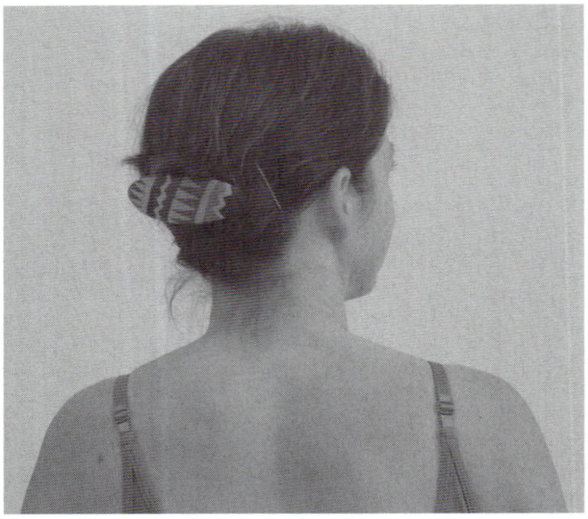

Figure 3.32 Symptom-provoking movement: turning the head to the right provokes symptoms in the area of the lateral upper arm.

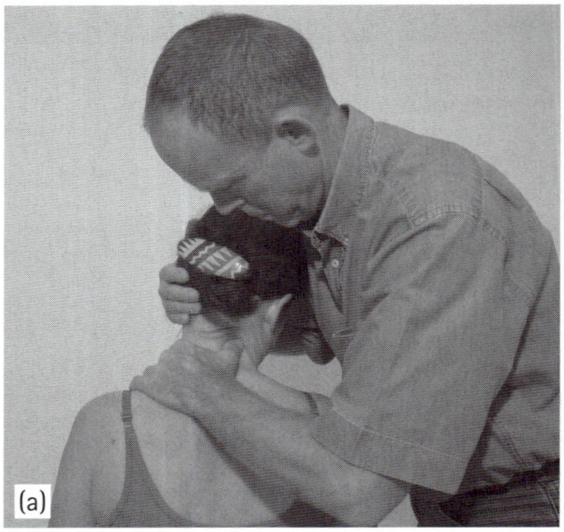

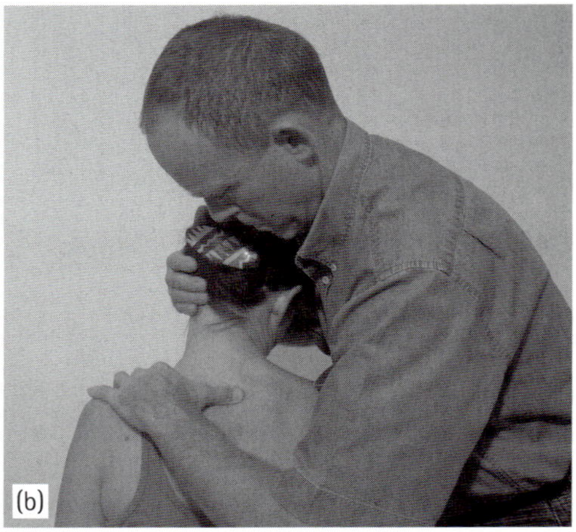

Figure 3.33a and b Specific provocation and alleviation in the area of the lower cervical spine with symptomatic movement of the head to the right; provocation. **a**, Starting position. **b**, End position.

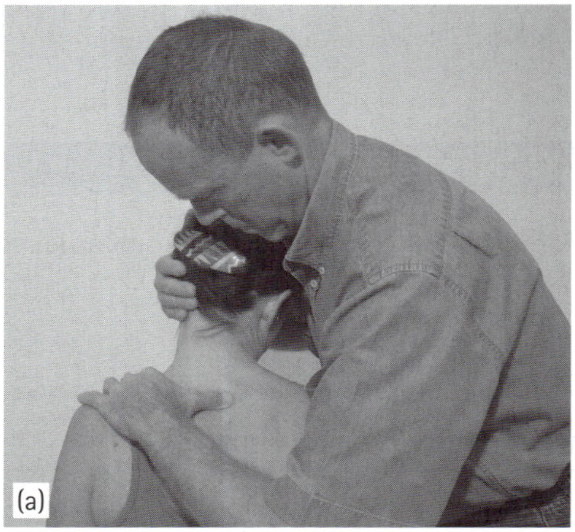

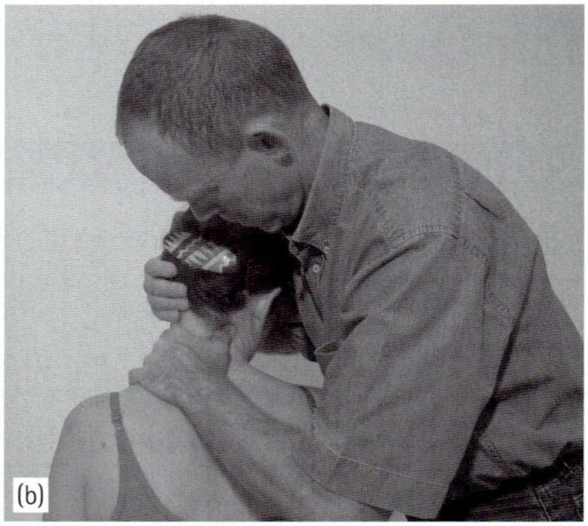

Figure 3.34a and b Specific provocation and alleviation in the area of the lower cervical spine with symptomatic movement of the head to the right; alleviation. **a**, Starting position. **b**, End position.

The change in symptoms can be demonstrated exactly:

- provocation of pain (Fig. 3.33a and b, film 56)
- alleviation of pain (Fig. 3.34a and b, film 57).

Assessment			
Goal	**Provocation of pain**	**Alleviation of pain**	**Remarks**
Starting position	Turning the head to the right to a position immediately before symptoms appear	Turning the head to the right to a position immediately after symptoms have appeared	Head remains in starting position
Test movement	Pushing the vertebra into rotation to the left; the movement has to be started cranially	Pushing the vertebra into rotation to the left; the movement has to be started caudally	If differentiation via rotation to the right is tried, the movement has to be started caudally with provocation and cranially with alleviation
Neural involvement	Proximal and/or distal component without change of position in the relevant area	Proximal and/or distal component without change of position in the relevant area	
Explanation	The symptoms are provoked when the caudal vertebra in the segment is moved	The symptoms are alleviated when the cranial vertebra in the segment is moved	
Additional data to support the hypothesis	General and specific mobility of the cervical spine History, e.g., symptom behaviour, type of complaints, 24-hour behaviour Specific palpation Neurodynamic tests (if specific provocation and alleviation indicate neural involvement) Reproducibility of test results Test treatment Imaging procedures (CT, MRI)		

Alternative technique

- Provocation of pain (Fig. 3.35a and b, film 58)
- Alleviation of pain (Fig. 3.36a and b, film 59).

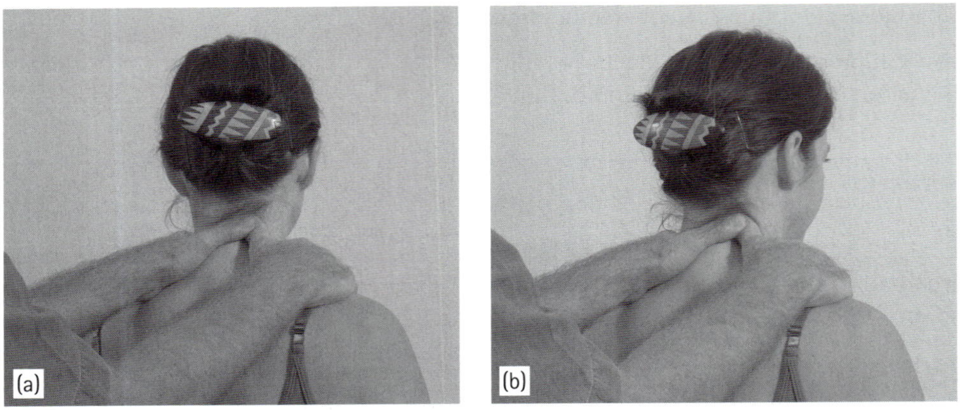

Figure 3.35a and b Specific provocation and alleviation in the area of the lower cervical spine with symptomatic movement of the head to the right; alternative technique; provocation. a, Starting position. b, End position.

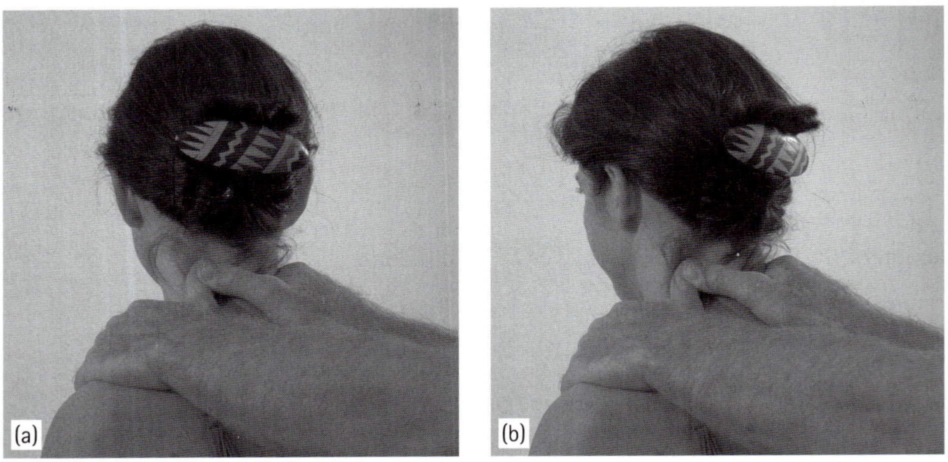

Figure 3.36a and b Specific provocation and alleviation in the area of the lower cervical spine with symptomatic movement of the head to the right; alternative technique; alleviation. a, Starting position. b, End position.

Assessment			
Goal	Provocation of pain	Alleviation of pain	Remarks
Starting position	Whole cervical spine rotated to the left	Whole cervical spine rotated to the right, to a position immediately after symptoms have appeared	
Test movement	Active rotation to the right above the fixed vertebrae; fixation has to begin cranially	Active rotation to the left above the fixed vertebrae; fixation has to begin cranially	Fixation must not be painful

Goal	Provocation of pain	Alleviation of pain	Remarks
Neural involvement	Proximal and/or distal component without change of position in the relevant area	Proximal and/or distal component without change of position in the relevant area	
Explanation	The symptoms are provoked when the symptomatic segment is rotated to the right	The symptoms are alleviated when the symptomatic segment is rotated to the right	
Additional data to support the hypothesis	General and specific mobility of the cervical spine History, e.g., symptom behaviour, type of complaints, 24-hour behaviour Specific palpation Neurodynamic tests (if specific provocation and alleviation indicate neural involvement) Reproducibility of test results Test treatment Imaging procedures (CT, MRI)		

Localization, lower cervical spine – movement of the head forwards

Pain-provoking movement (Fig. 3.37)

- Flexion of the cervical spine provokes pain in the lateral upper arm.
- Area localization hints at the cervical spine.

The change in symptoms can be demonstrated exactly:

- provocation of pain (Fig. 3.38a and b, film 70)
- alleviation of pain (Fig. 3.39a and b, film 71).

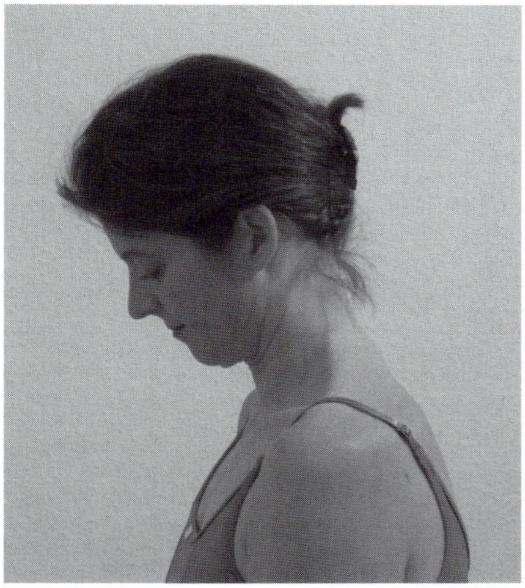

Figure 3.37 Symptom-provoking movement: movement of the head forwards provokes symptoms in the area of the lateral upper arm.

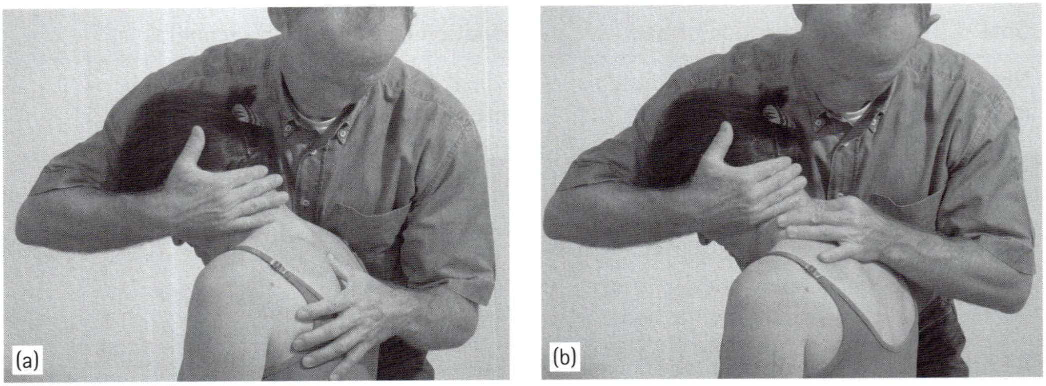

Figure 3.38a and b Specific provocation and alleviation in the area of the lower cervical spine with symptomatic movement of the head forwards; provocation. **a**, Starting position. **b**, End position.

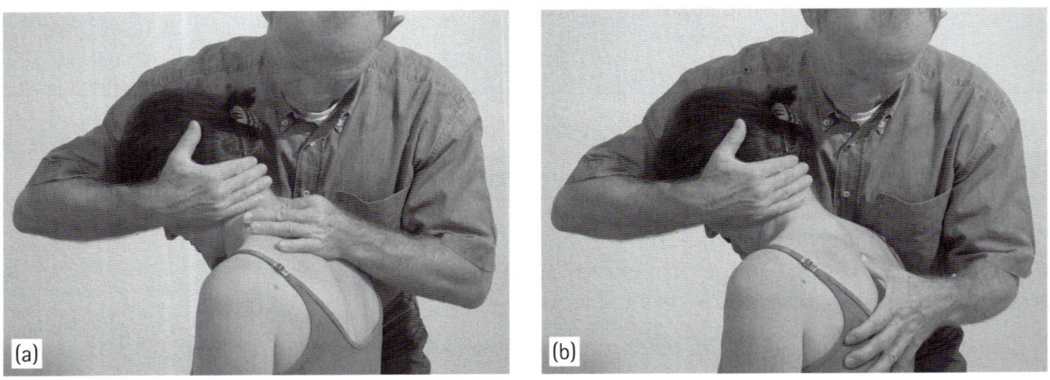

Figure 3.39a and b Specific provocation and alleviation in the area of the lower cervical spine with symptomatic movement of the head forwards; alleviation. **a**, Starting position. **b**, End position.

Assessment			
Goal	**Provocation of pain**	**Alleviation of pain**	**Remarks**
Starting position	Flexion of the cervical spine to a position immediately before symptoms appear	Flexion of the cervical spine to a position immediately after symptoms have appeared	Head remains in starting position
Test movement	Pushing the vertebra via the lamina in ventrocranial direction; the movement has to be started caudally	Pushing the vertebra via the lamina in ventrocranial direction; the movement has to be started cranially	

Goal	Provocation of pain	Alleviation of pain	Remarks
Neural involvement	Proximal and/or distal component without change of position in the relevant area	Proximal and/or distal component without change of position in the relevant area	
Explanation	The symptoms are provoked when the cranial vertebra in the segment is moved (flexion in the affected segment)	The symptoms are alleviated when the caudal vertebra in the segment is moved (extension in the affected segment)	
Additional data to support the hypothesis	General and specific mobility of the cervical spine History, e.g., symptom behaviour, type of complaints, 24-hour behaviour Specific palpation Neurodynamic tests (if specific provocation and alleviation indicate neural involvement) Reproducibility of test results Test treatment Imaging procedures (CT, MRI)		

Alternative technique

- Provocation of pain (Fig. 3.40a and b, film 72)
- Alleviation of pain (Fig. 3.41a and b, film 73).

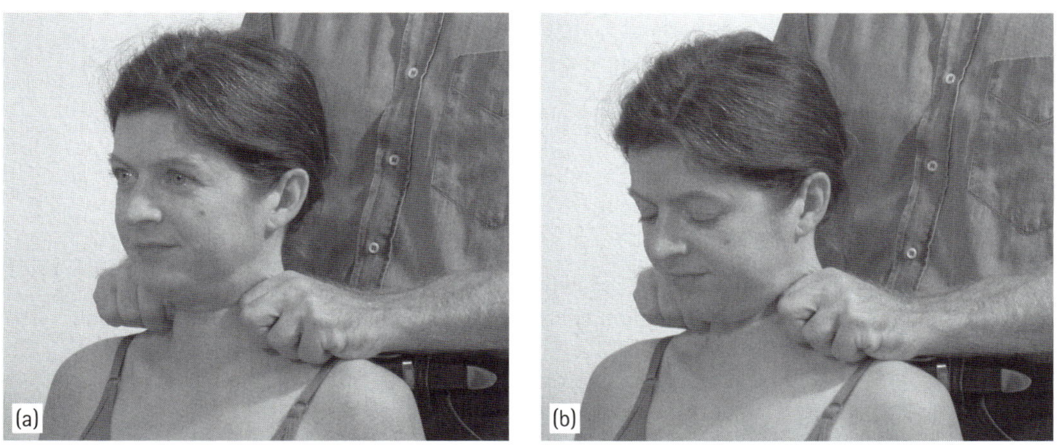

Figure 3.40a and b Specific provocation and alleviation in the area of the lower cervical spine with symptomatic movement of the head forwards; alternative technique; provocation. **a**, Starting position. **b**, End position.

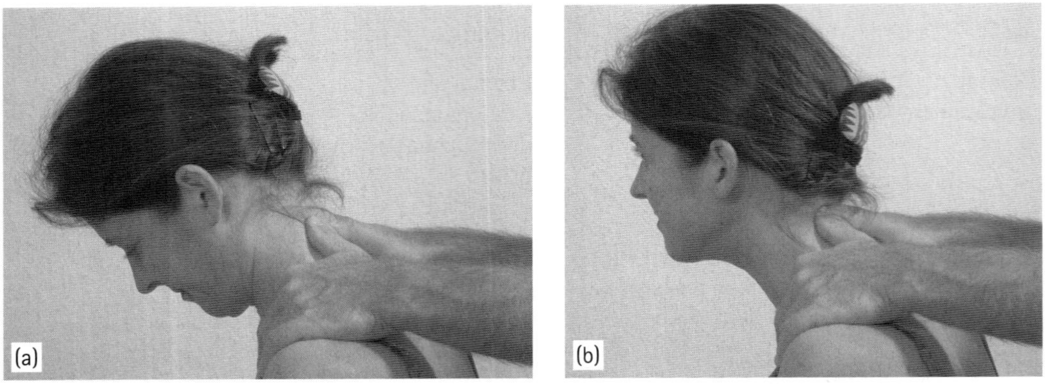

Figure 3.41a and b Specific provocation and alleviation in the area of the lower cervical spine with symptomatic movement of the head forwards; alternative technique; alleviation. **a**, Starting position. **b**, End position.

Assessment			
Goal	**Provocation of pain**	**Alleviation of pain**	**Remarks**
Starting position	Extension of the cervical spine	Flexion of the cervical spine to a position immediately after symptoms have appeared	
Test movement	Active flexion above the fixed vertebrae, fixation has to start cranially	Active extension above the fixed vertebrae, fixation has to start cranially	Fixation must not be painful
Neural involvement	Proximal and/or distal component without change of position in the relevant area	Proximal and/or distal component without change of position in the relevant area	
Explanation	The symptoms are provoked when the symptomatic segment is moved into flexion	The symptoms are alleviated when the symptomatic segment is moved into extension	
Additional data to support the hypothesis	General and specific mobility of the cervical spine History, e.g., symptom behaviour, type of complaints, 24-hour behaviour Specific palpation Neurodynamic tests (if specific provocation and alleviation indicate neural involvement) Reproducibility of test results Test treatment Imaging procedures (CT, MRI)		

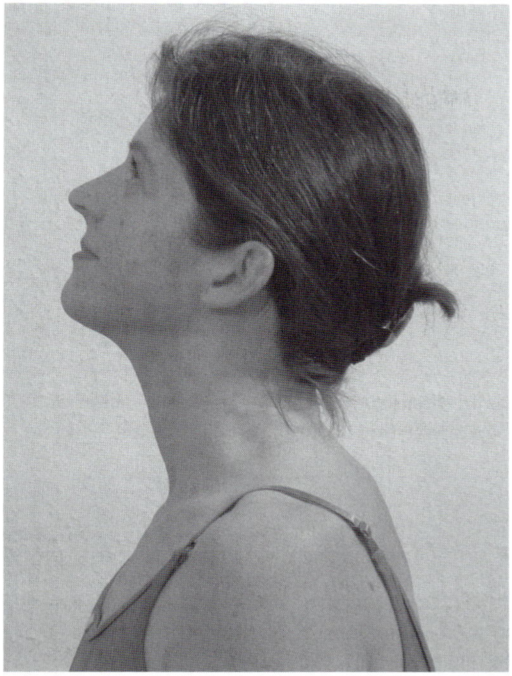

Figure 3.42 Symptom-provoking movement: moving the head backwards provokes symptoms in the area of the lateral upper arm.

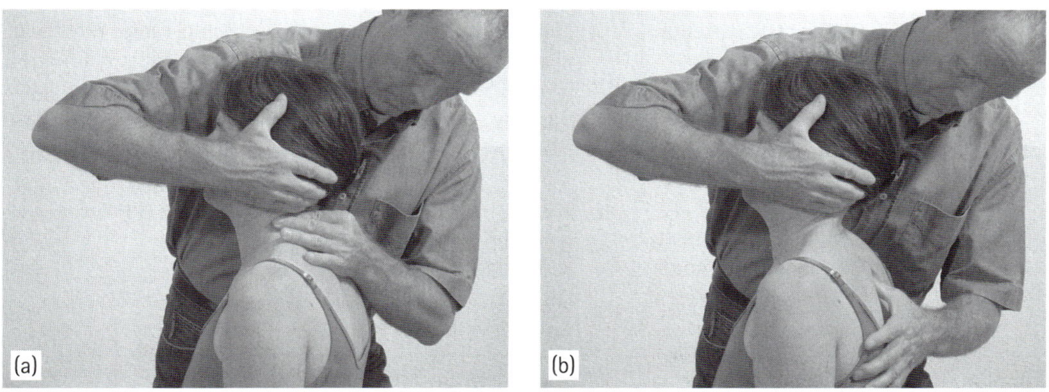

Figure 3.43a and b Specific provocation and alleviation in the area of the lower cervical spine with symptomatic movement of the head backwards; provocation. **a**, Starting position. **b**, End position.

Localization, lower cervical spine – movement of the head backwards

Pain-provoking movement (Fig. 3.42)

- Extension of the cervical spine provokes pain in the lateral upper arm.
- Area localization hints at the cervical spine.

The change in symptoms can be demonstrated exactly:

- provocation of pain (Fig. 3.43a and b, film 82)
- alleviation of pain (Fig. 3.44a and b, film 83).

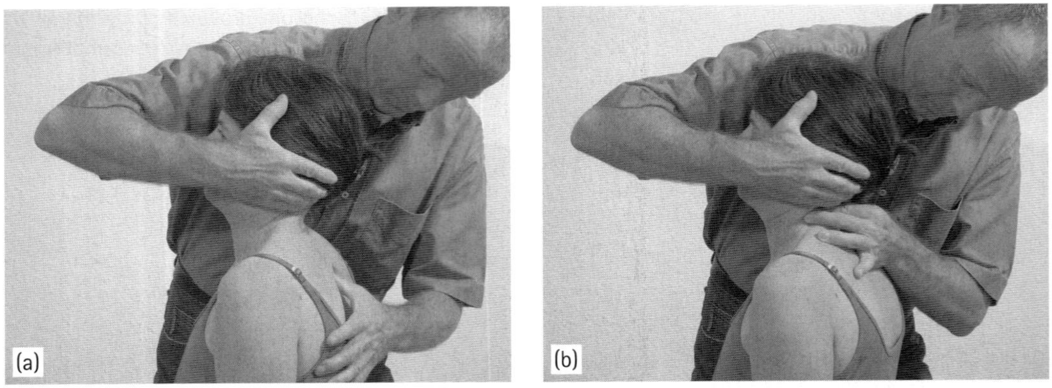

Figure 3.44a and b Specific provocation and alleviation in the area of the lower cervical spine with symptomatic movement of the head backwards; alleviation. **a**, Starting position. **b**, End position.

Assessment			
Goal	**Provocation of pain**	**Alleviation of pain**	**Remarks**
Starting position	Extension of the cervical spine to a position immediately before symptoms appear	Extension of the cervical spine to a position immediately after symptoms have appeared	Head remains in starting position
Test movement	Pushing the vertebra via the lamina in ventrocranial direction; the movement has to be started cranially	Pushing the vertebra via the lamina in ventrocranial direction; the movement has to be started caudally	With end-range extension positions, this technique is often not possible, as no direct contact to the individual vertebrae can can be made from dorsal
Neural involvement	Proximal and/or distal component without change of position in the relevant area	Proximal and/or distal component without change of position in the relevant area	
Explanation	The symptoms are provoked when the caudal vertebra in the segment is moved (extension in the affected segment)	The symptoms are alleviated when the cranial vertebra in the segment is moved (flexion in the affected segment)	
Additional data to support the hypothesis	General and specific mobility of the cervical spine History, e.g., symptom behaviour, type of complaints, 24-hour behaviour Specific palpation Neurodynamic tests (if specific provocation and alleviation indicate neural involvement) Reproducibility of test results Test treatment Imaging procedures (CT, MRI)		

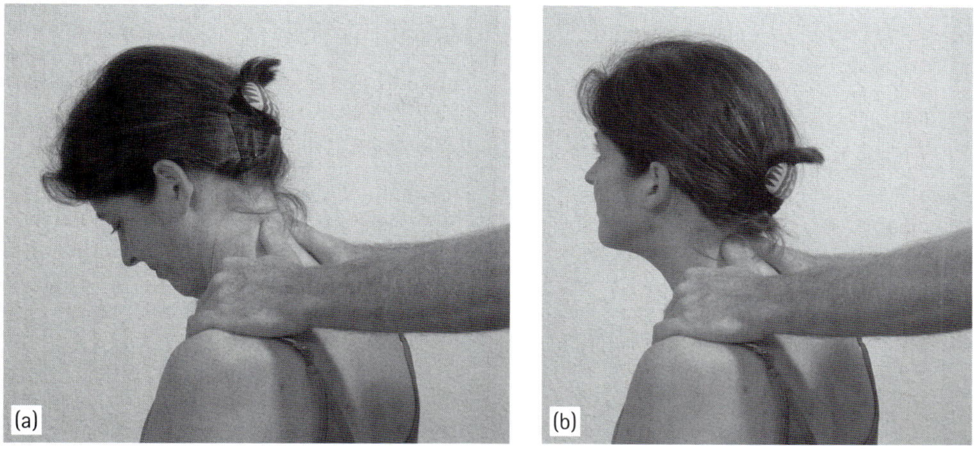

Figure 3.45a and b Specific provocation and alleviation in the area of the lower cervical spine with symptomatic movement of the head backwards; alternative technique; provocation. **a**, Starting position. **b**, End position.

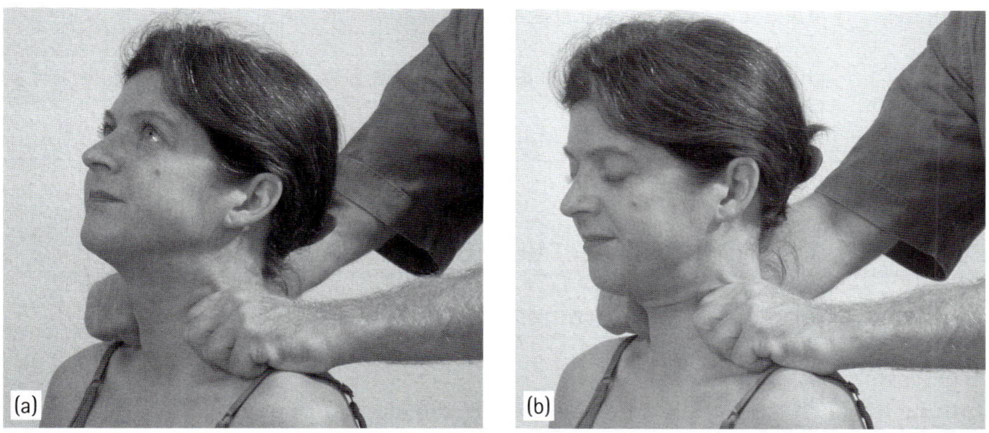

Figure 3.46a and b Specific provocation and alleviation in the area of the lower cervical spine with symptomatic movement of the head backwards; alternative technique; alleviation. **a**, Starting position. **b**, End position.

Alternative technique

- Provocation of pain (Fig. 3.45a and b, film 84)
- Alleviation of pain (Fig. 3.46a and b, film 85).

Assessment

Goal	Provocation of pain	Alleviation of pain	Remarks
Starting position	Flexion of the cervical spine	Extension of the cervical spine to a position immediately after symptoms have appeared	Head remains in starting position

Goal	Provocation of pain	Alleviation of pain	Remarks
Test movement	Active extension above the fixed vertebrae, fixation has to start cranially	Active flexion above the fixed vertebrae, fixation has to start cranially	Fixation must not be painful
Neural involvement	Proximal and/or distal component without change of position in the relevant area	Proximal and/or distal component without change of position in the relevant area	
Explanation	The symptoms are provoked when the symptomatic segment is moved into extension	The symptoms are alleviated when the symptomatic segment is moved into flexion	
Additional data to support the hypothesis	General and specific mobility of the cervical spine History, e.g., symptom behaviour, type of complaints, 24-hour behaviour Specific palpation Neurodynamic tests (if specific provocation and alleviation indicate neural involvement) Reproducibility of test results Test treatment Imaging procedures (CT, MRI)		

SPECIFIC PROVOCATION AND ALLEVIATION, THORACIC SPINE

Localization, thoracic spine – turning the head to the right

Pain-provoking movement (Fig. 3.47)

- Turning the head to the right provokes pain in the lateral upper arm.
- Area localization hints at the thoracic spine.

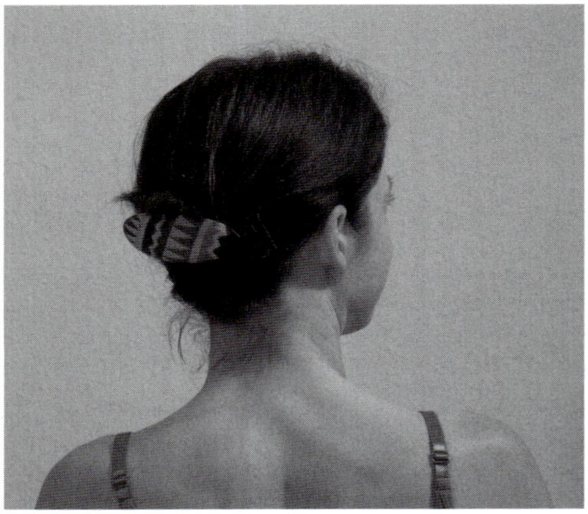

Figure 3.47 Symptom-provoking movement: turning the head to the right provokes symptoms in the area of the lateral upper arm.

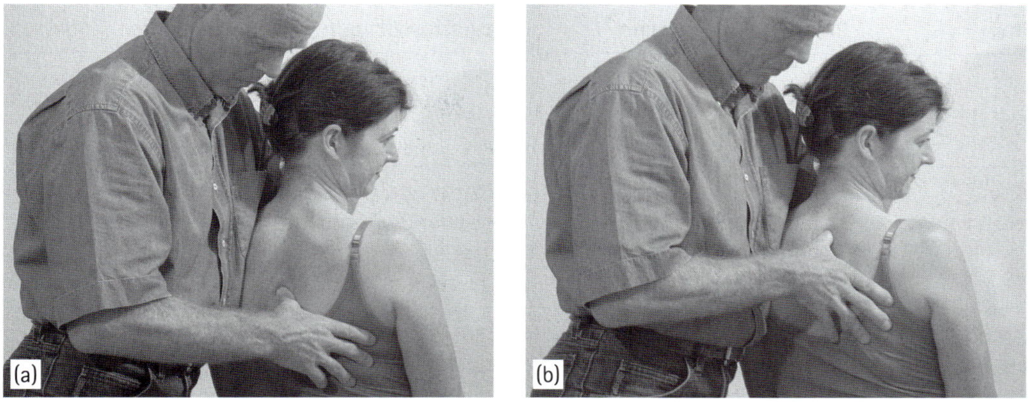

Figure 3.48a and b Specific provocation and alleviation in the area of the thoracic spine with symptomatic turning of the head to the right; provocation. **a**, Starting position. **b**, End position.

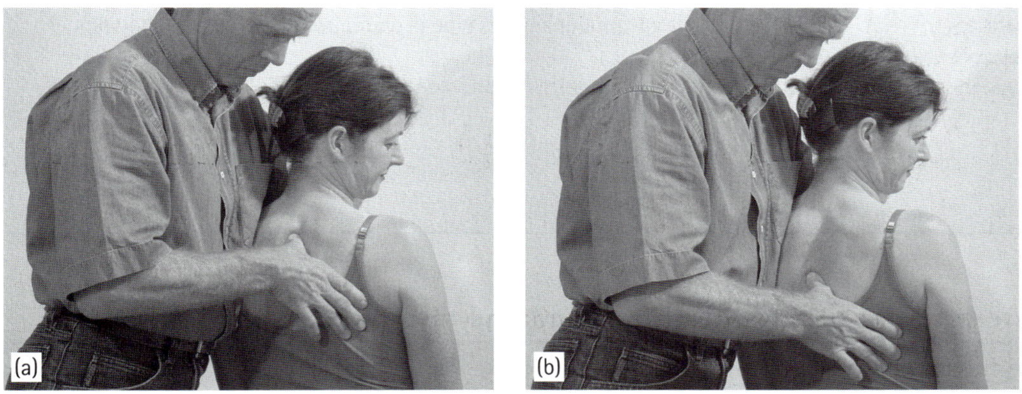

Figure 3.49a and b Specific provocation and alleviation in the area of the thoracic spine with symptomatic turning of the head to the right; alleviation. **a**, Starting position. **b**, End position.

The change in symptoms can be demonstrated exactly:

- provocation of pain (Fig. 3.48a and b, film 60)
- alleviation of pain (Fig. 3.49a and b, film 61).

Assessment

Goal	Provocation of pain	Alleviation of pain	Remarks
Starting position	Turning the head to the right to a position immediately before symptoms appear	Turning the head to the right to a position immediately after symptoms have appeared	Head remains in starting position
Test movement	Pushing the vertebra into rotation to the right; the movement has to be started caudally	Pushing the vertebra into rotation to the right; the movement has to be started cranially	If differentiation via rotation to the left is tried, provocation starts

Goal	Provocation of pain	Alleviation of pain	Remarks
			cranially, and alleviation starts caudally
Neural involvement	Proximal and/or distal component without change of position in the relevant area	Proximal and/or distal component without change of position in the relevant area	
Explanation	The symptoms are provoked when the cranial vertebra in the segment is moved	The symptoms are alleviated when the caudal vertebra in the segment is moved	
Additional data to support the hypothesis	General and specific mobility of the thoracic spine History, e.g., symptom behaviour, type of complaints, 24-hour behaviour Specific palpation Neurodynamic tests (if specific provocation and alleviation indicate neural involvement) Reproducibility of test results Test treatment Imaging procedures (CT, MRI)		

Differentiation between vertebral joints and rib within the affected segment

The change in symptoms can be demonstrated exactly:

- provocation of pain (Fig. 3.50a and b, film 62)
- alleviation of pain (Fig. 3.51a and b, film 63).

Assessment			
Goal	**Provocation of pain**	**Alleviation of pain**	**Remarks**
Starting position	Turning the head to the right to a position immediately before symptoms appear	Turning the head to the right to a position immediately after symptoms have appeared	Head remains in starting position
Test movement	Pushing the costal angle of the corresponding rib in ventral direction	Push from ventral against the corresponding rib	
Neural involvement	Proximal and/or distal component without change of position in the relevant area	Proximal and/or distal component without change of position in the relevant area	

Goal	Provocation of pain	Alleviation of pain	Remarks
Explanation	If the symptoms can be provoked in this way, this is not due to the vertebra, since in this manoeuvre it is rotated to the left	If the symptoms can be alleviated in this way, this is not due to the vertebra, since in this manoeuvre it is rotated to the right	The pain-provoking movement was rotation to the right in the affected segment
Additional data to support the hypothesis	General and specific mobility of thoracic spine and ribs History, e.g., symptom behaviour, type of complaints, 24-hour behaviour Specific palpation Neurodynamic tests (if specific provocation and alleviation indicate neural involvement) Reproducibility of test results Test treatment Imaging procedures (CT, MRI)		

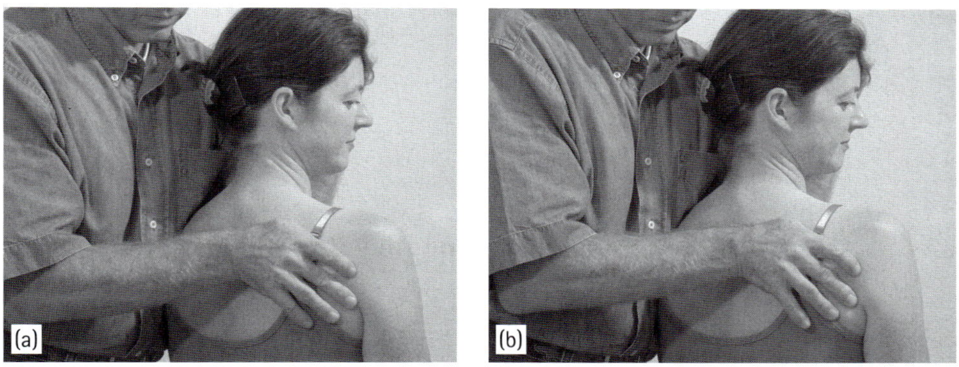

Figure 3.50a and b Specific provocation and alleviation in the area of the thoracic spine with symptomatic turning of the head to the right; differentiation between vertebra and rib; provocation. a, Starting position. b, End position.

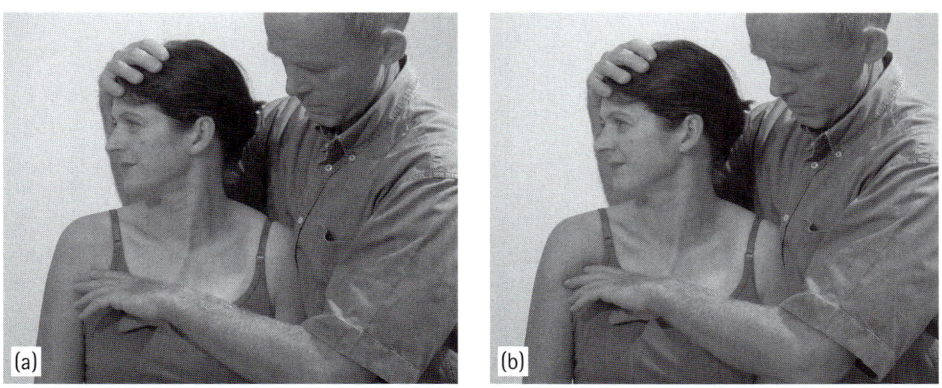

Figure 3.51a and b Specific provocation and alleviation in the area of the thoracic spine with symptomatic turning of the head to the right; differentiation between vertebra and rib; alleviation. a, Starting position. b, End position.

Localization, thoracic spine – movement of the head forwards

Pain-provoking movement (Fig. 3.52)

- Flexion of the cervical spine provokes pain in the lateral upper arm.
- Area localization hints at the thoracic spine.

The change in symptoms can be demonstrated exactly:

- provocation of pain (Fig. 3.53a and b, film 74)
- alleviation of pain (Fig. 3.54a and b, film 75).

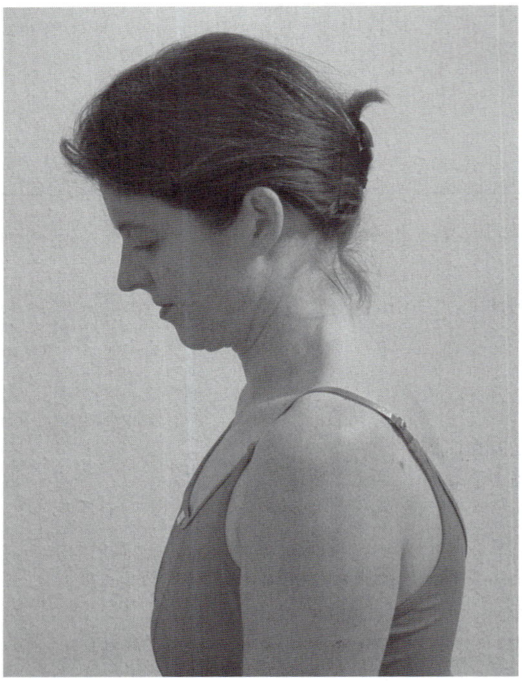

Figure 3.52 Symptom-provoking movement: movement of the head forwards provokes symptoms in the area of the lateral upper arm.

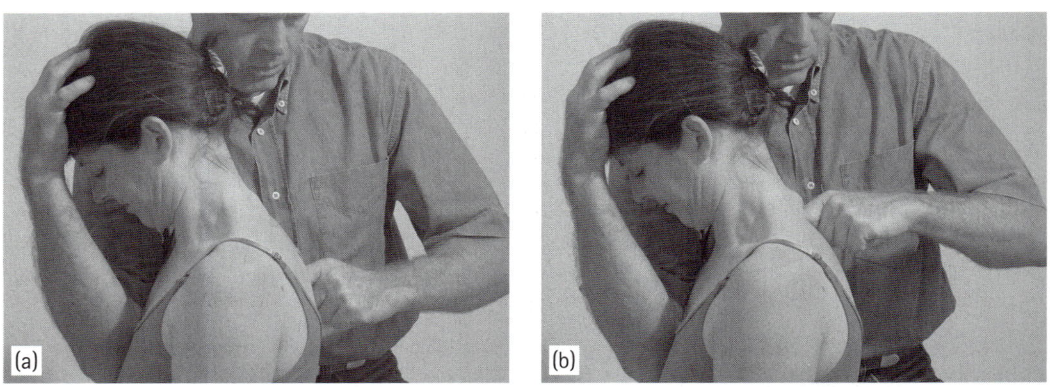

Figure 3.53a and b Specific provocation and alleviation in the area of the thoracic spine with symptomatic movement of the head forwards; provocation. **a**, Starting position. **b**, End position.

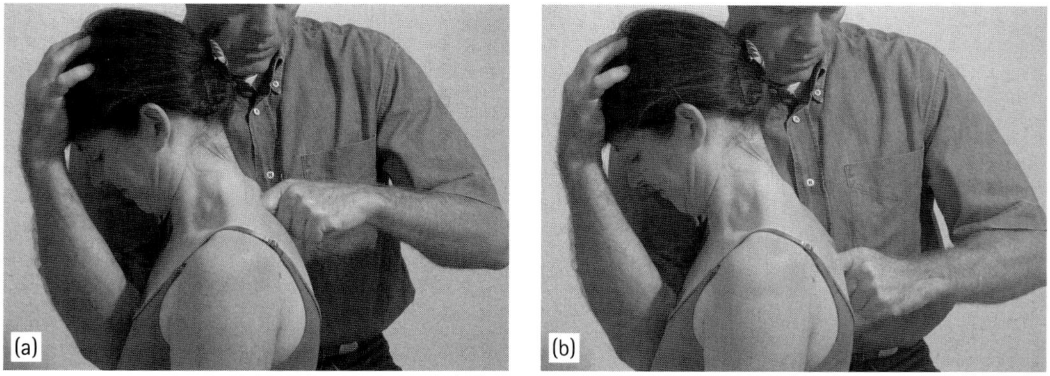

Figure 3.54a and b Specific provocation and alleviation in the area of the thoracic spine with symptomatic movement of the head forwards; alleviation. **a**, Starting position. **b**, End position.

Assessment			
Goal	**Provocation of pain**	**Alleviation of pain**	**Remarks**
Starting position	Flexion of the cervical spine to a position immediately before symptoms appear	Flexion of the cervical spine to a position immediately after symptoms have appeared	Head remains in starting position
Test movement	Pushing the vertebra via the lamina in ventrocranial direction, the movement has to be started caudally	Pushing the vertebra via the lamina in ventrocranial direction, the movement has to be started cranially	
Neural involvement	Proximal and/or distal component without change of position in the relevant area	Proximal and/or distal component without change of position in the relevant area	
Explanation	The symptoms are provoked when the cranial vertebra in the segment is moved (flexion in the affected segment)	The symptoms are alleviated when the cranial vertebra in the segment is moved (extension in the affected segment)	
Additional data to support the hypothesis	General and specific mobility of the thoracic spine History, e.g., symptom behaviour, type of complaints, 24-hour behaviour Specific palpation Neurodynamic tests (if specific provocation and alleviation indicate neural involvement) Reproducibility of test results Test treatment Imaging procedures (CT, MRI)		

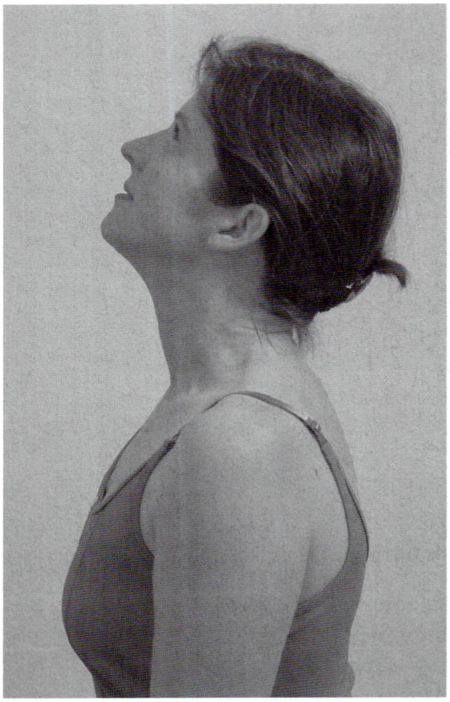

Figure 3.55 Symptom-provoking movement: movement of the head backwards provokes symptoms in the area of the lateral upper arm.

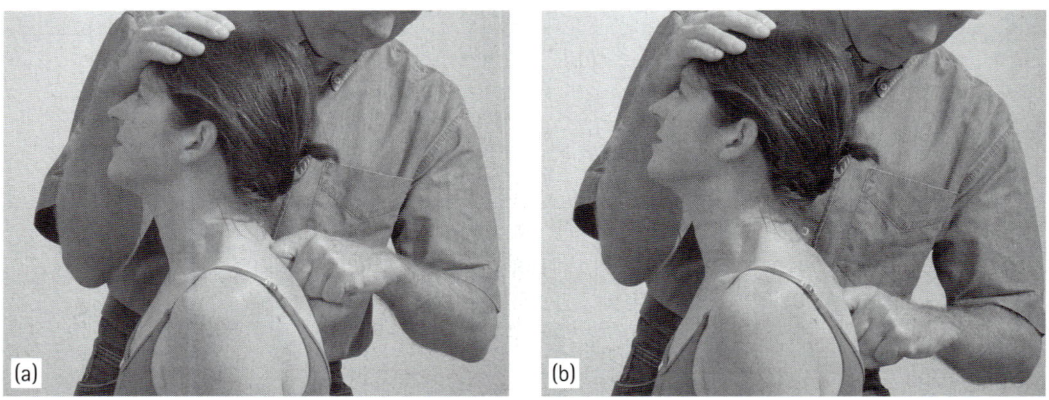

Figure 3.56a and b Specific provocation and alleviation in the area of the thoracic spine with symptomatic movement of the head backwards; provocation. **a**, Starting position. **b**, End position.

Localization, thoracic spine – movement of the head backwards

Pain-provoking movement (Fig. 3.55)

- Extension of the cervical spine provokes pain in the lateral upper arm.
- Area localization hints at the thoracic spine.

The change in symptoms can be demonstrated exactly:

- provocation of pain (Fig. 3.56a and b, film 76)
- alleviation of pain (Fig. 3.57a and b, film 77).

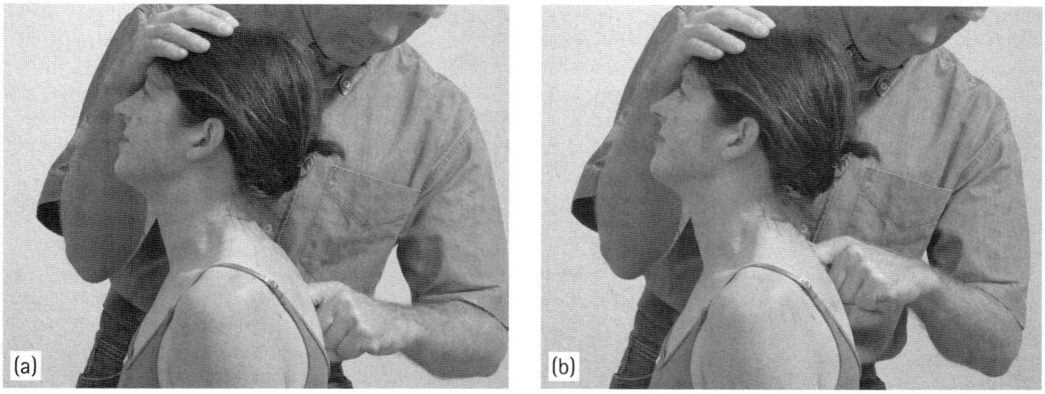

Figure 3.57a and b Specific provocation and alleviation in the area of the thoracic spine with symptomatic movement of the head backwards; alleviation. **a**, Starting position. **b**, End position.

Assessment			
Goal	**Provocation of pain**	**Alleviation of pain**	**Remarks**
Starting position	Extension of the cervical spine to a position immediately before symptoms appear	Extension of the cervical spine to a position immediately after symptoms have appeared	Head remains in starting position
Test movement	Pushing the vertebra via the lamina in ventrocranial direction, the movement has to be started cranially	Pushing the vertebra via the lamina in ventrocranial direction, the movement has to be started caudally	With end-range extension positions, this technique is often not possible, as no direct contact to the individual vertebrae can be made from dorsal
Neural involvement	Proximal and/or distal component without change of position in the relevant area	Proximal and/or distal component without change of position in the relevant area	
Explanation	The symptoms are provoked when the caudal vertebra in the segment is moved (extension in the affected segment)	The symptoms are alleviated when the cranial vertebra in the segment is moved (flexion in the affected segment)	
Additional data to support the hypothesis	General and specific mobility of the thoracic spine History, e.g., symptom behaviour, type of complaints, 24-hour behaviour Specific palpation Neurodynamic tests (if specific provocation and alleviation indicate neural involvement) Reproducibility of test results Test treatment Imaging procedures (CT, MRI)		

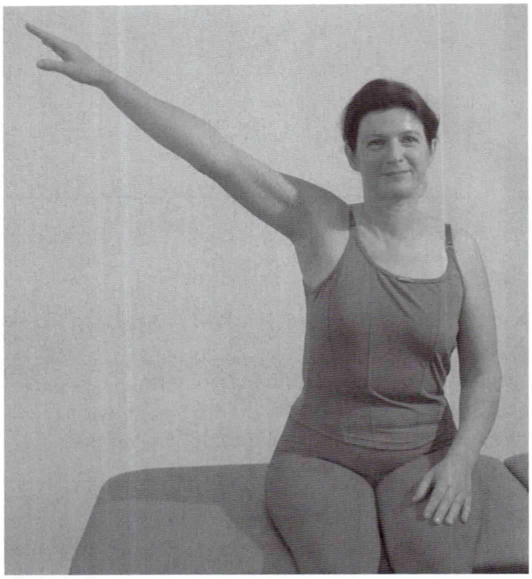

Figure 3.58 Symptom-provoking movement: movement of the arm into abduction/elevation provokes symptoms in the area of the lateral upper arm.

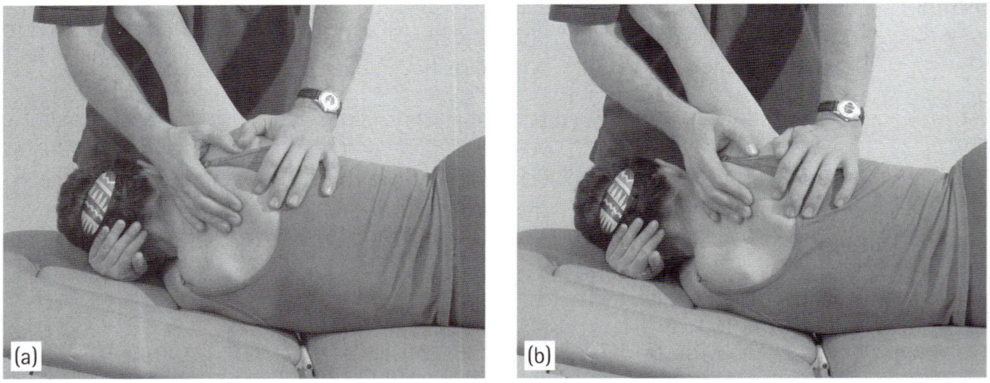

Figure 3.59a and b Specific provocation and alleviation in the area of the shoulder complex with symptomatic movement of the arm into abduction/elevation; differentiation between glenohumeral joint and acromio-clavicular joint; provocation. **a**, Starting position. **b**, End position.

SPECIFIC PROVOCATION AND ALLEVIATION, SHOULDER COMPLEX

Differentiation, glenohumeral joint vs. acromio-clavicular joint

Pain-provoking movement (Fig. 3.58)

- Abduction/elevation of the arm provokes pain in the lateral upper arm.
- Area localization hints at the shoulder complex.

The change in symptoms can be demonstrated exactly:

- provocation of pain (Fig. 3.59a and b, film 96)
- alleviation of pain (Fig. 3.60a and b, film 97).

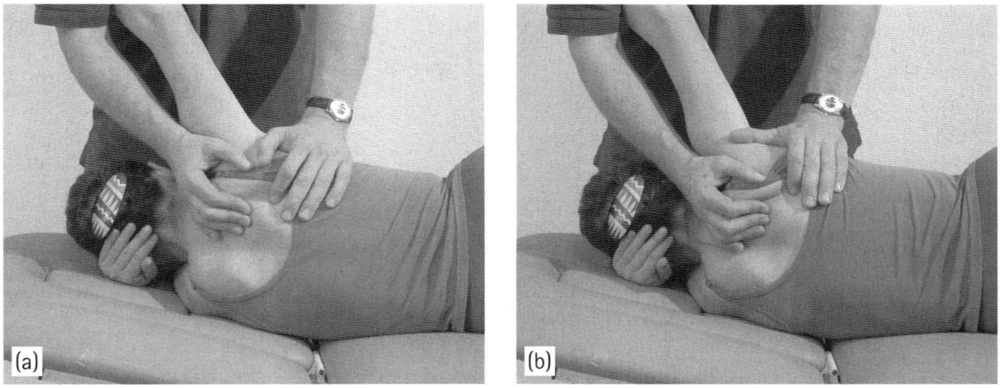

Figure 3.60a and b Specific provocation and alleviation in the area of the shoulder complex with symptomatic movement of the arm into abduction/elevation; differentiation between glenohumeral joint and acromio-clavicular joint; alleviation. **a**, Starting position. **b**, End position.

Assessment			
Goal	**Provocation of pain**	**Alleviation of pain**	**Remarks**
Starting position	Abduction/elevation of the arm to a position immediately before symptoms appear	Abduction/elevation of the arm to a position immediately after symptoms have appeared	
Test movement	Pushing the angulus inferior of the scapula in dorsomedial direction, with fixed humerus	Pushing the angulus inferior of the scapula in ventrolateral direction, with fixed humerus	The arm is not allowed to move during the test movement
Neural involvement	Proximal and/or distal component without change of position in the relevant area	Proximal and/or distal component without change of position in the relevant area	
Explanation	Augmentation of the abduction/elevation movement in the glenohumeral joint with simultaneous reduction in the shoulder girdle	Reduction of the abduction/elevation movement in the glenohumeral joint with simultaneous augmentation in the shoulder girdle	
Additional data to support the hypothesis	General and specific mobility of the shoulder complex History, e.g., symptom behaviour, type of complaints, 24-hour behaviour Specific palpation Neurodynamic tests (if specific provocation and alleviation indicate neural involvement) Reproducibility of test results Test treatment Imaging procedures (CT, MRI)		

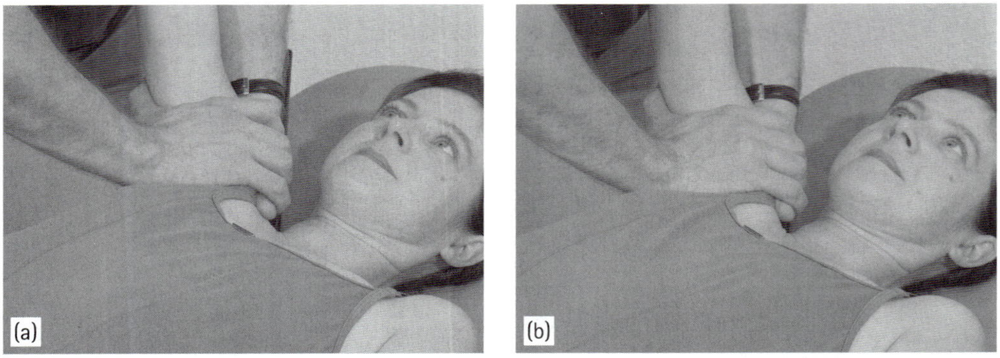

Figure 3.61a and b Specific provocation and alleviation in the area of the shoulder complex with symptomatic movement of the arm into abduction/elevation; subacromial compression; provocation. **a**, Starting position. **b**, End position.

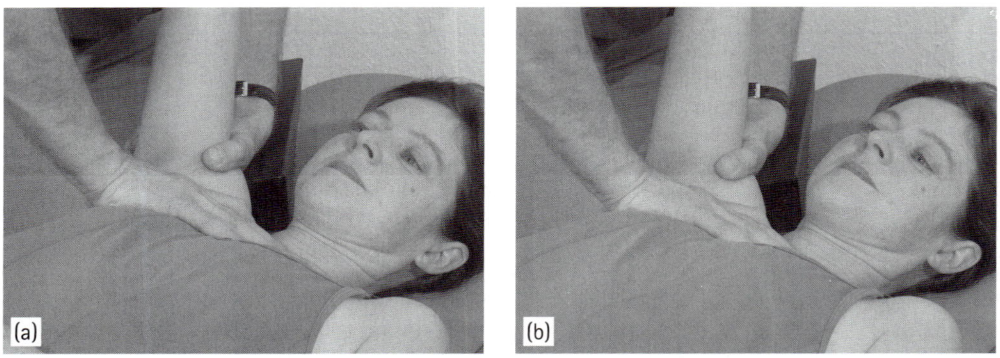

Figure 3.62a and b Specific provocation and alleviation in the area of the shoulder complex with symptomatic movement of the arm into abduction/elevation; subacromial compression; alleviation. **a**, Starting position. **b**, End position.

Localization in the subacromial space

The change in symptoms can be demonstrated exactly:

- provocation of pain (Fig. 3.61a and b, film 98)
- alleviation of pain (Fig. 3.62a and b, film 99).

Assessment

Goal	Provocation of pain	Alleviation of pain	Remarks
Starting position	Abduction/elevation of the arm to exactly the position where symptoms appear	Abduction/elevation of the arm to exactly the position where symptoms appear	
Test movement	Compression between humerus and scapula	Separation between humerus and scapula	As compression is presumed to be the

Goal	Provocation of pain	Alleviation of pain	Remarks
	(acromion); this movement may be performed both via the humerus, with the scapula fixed, and via the scapula, with the humerus fixed (example: movement of the humerus)	(acromion); this movement may be performed both via the humerus, with the scapula fixed, and via the scapula, with the humerus fixed (example: movement of the scapula)	pain-provoking event, the position where symptoms appear is used even for pain provocation, since before that position there is probably no contact of the potentially affected structures
Neural involvement	Proximal and/or distal component without change of position in the relevant area	Proximal and/or distal component without change of position in the relevant area	
Explanation	Compression in the subacromial space is increased	Compression in the subacromial space is reduced	
Additional data to support the hypothesis	General and specific mobility of the shoulder complex History, e.g., symptom behaviour, type of complaints, 24-hour behaviour Specific palpation Neurodynamic tests (if specific provocation and alleviation indicate neural involvement) Reproducibility of test results Test treatment Imaging procedures (CT, MRI)		

Differentiation in the glenohumeral joint – intra-articular vs. extra-articular (symptom provocation by an intra-articular component)

The change in symptoms can be demonstrated exactly:

- provocation of pain (Fig. 3.63a and b, film 100)
- alleviation of pain (Fig. 3.64a and b, film 101).

Assessment			
Goal	**Provocation of pain**	**Alleviation of pain**	**Remarks**
Starting position	Abduction/elevation of the arm to exactly the position where symptoms appear	Abduction/elevation of the arm to exactly the position where symptoms appear	
Test movement	Compression in the glenohumeral joint	Traction in the glenohumeral joint	As compression is presumed to be the

Goal	Provocation of pain	Alleviation of pain	Remarks
	(at a right angle to the treatment plane)	(at a right angle to thetreatment plane)	pain-provoking event, the position where symptoms appear is used even for pain provocation, since before that position there is probably no contact of the potentially affected structures
Neural involvement	Proximal and/or distal component without change of position in the relevant area	Proximal and/or distal component without change of position in the relevant area	
Explanation	Increase in compression between humeral head and glenoid cavity in the symptom-provoking position (suggests an intra-articular dysfunction)	Decrease in compression between humeral head and glenoid cavity in the symptom-provoking position (suggests an intra-articular dysfunction)	With an extra-articular dysfunction, converse findings would show with compression and traction
Additional data to support the hypothesis	General and specific mobility of the shoulder complex History, e.g., symptom behaviour, type of complaints, 24-hour behaviour Specific palpation Neurodynamic tests (if specific provocation and alleviation indicate neural involvement) Reproducibility of test results Test treatment Imaging procedures (CT, MRI)		

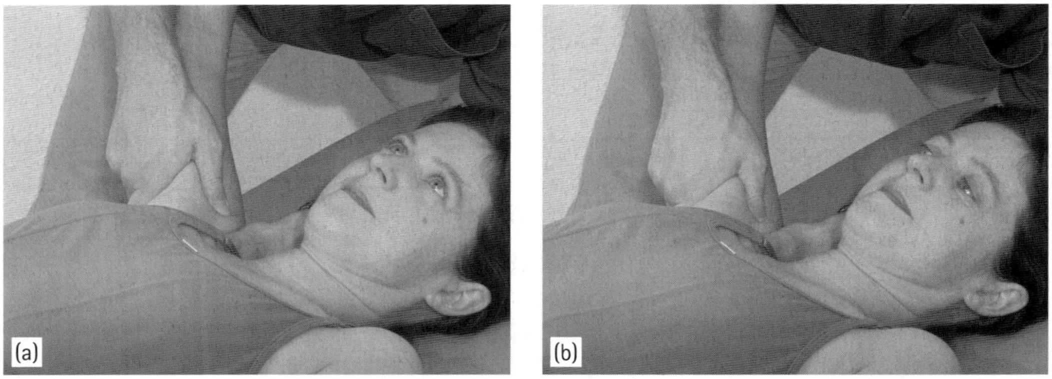

Figure 3.63a and b Specific provocation and alleviation in the area of the shoulder complex with symptomatic movement of the arm into abduction/elevation; intra-articular vs. extra-articular mechanism; provocation. **a**, Starting position. **b**, End position.

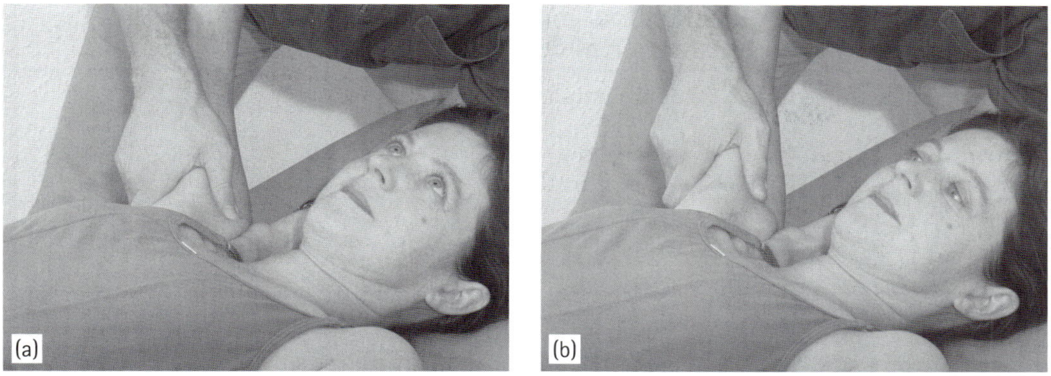

Figure 3.64a and b Specific provocation and alleviation in the area of the shoulder complex with symptomatic movement of the arm into abduction/elevation; intra-articular vs. extra-articular mechanism; alleviation. **a**, Starting position. **b**, End position.

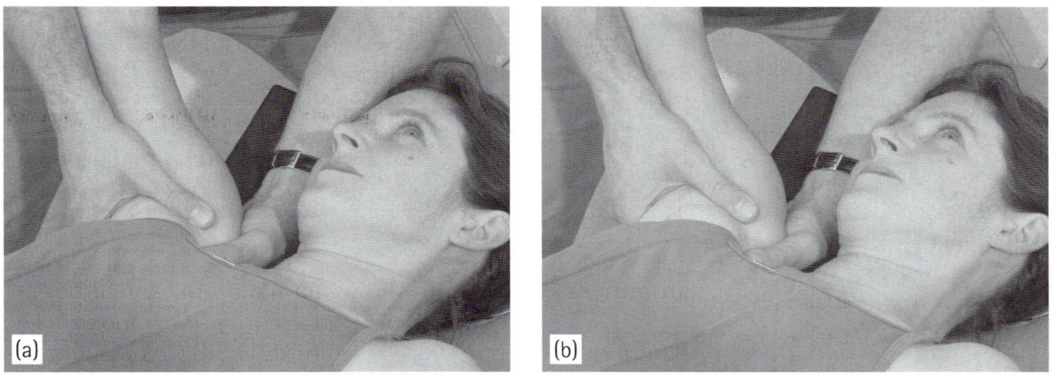

Figure 3.65a and b Specific provocation and alleviation in the area of the shoulder complex with symptomatic movement of the arm into abduction/elevation; anterior vs. posterior glide; provocation. **a**, Starting position. **b**, End position.

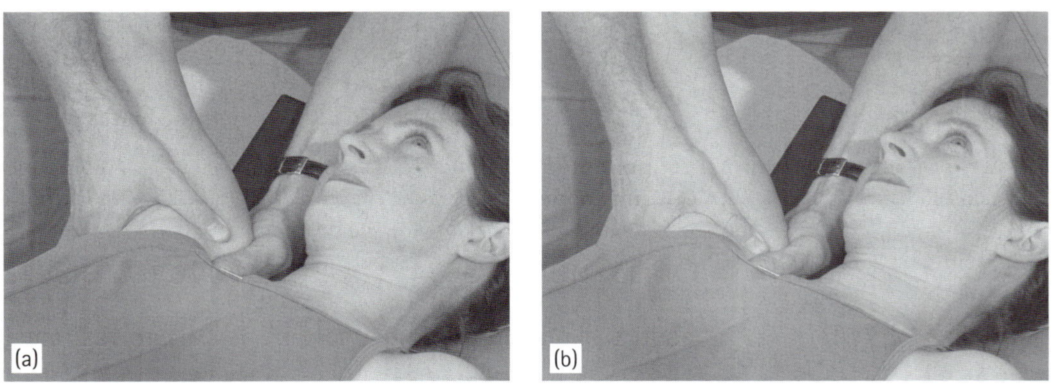

Figure 3.66a and b Specific provocation and alleviation in the area of the shoulder complex with symptomatic movement of the arm into abduction/elevation; anterior vs. posterior glide; alleviation. **a**, Starting position. **b**, End position.

Differentiation in the glenohumeral joint – anterior vs. posterior glide (symptom provocation by anterior glide)

The change in symptoms can be demonstrated exactly:

- provocation of pain (Fig. 3.65a and b, film 102)
- alleviation of pain (Fig. 3.66a and b, film 103).

Assessment			
Goal	**Provocation of pain**	**Alleviation of pain**	**Remarks**
Starting position	Abduction/elevation of the arm to a position immediately before symptoms appear	Abduction/elevation of the arm to a position immediately after symptoms have appeared	
Test movement	Humerus in anterior direction in relation to the fixed scapula	Humerus in posterior direction in relation to the fixed scapula	To test a posterior dysfunction, the manoeuvre is performed in the opposite direction
Neural involvement	Proximal and/or distal component without change of position in the relevant area	Proximal and/or distal component without change of position in the relevant area	
Explanation	Pushing the humerus in anterior direction increases the load in anterior direction	Pushing the humerus in posterior direction reduces the load in anterior direction	With the described presentation, in the authors' experience, symptoms are more often provoked by a gliding movement in anterior direction
Additional data to support the hypothesis	General and specific mobility of the shoulder complex History, e.g., symptom behaviour, type of complaints, 24-hour behaviour Specific palpation Neurodynamic tests (if specific provocation and alleviation indicate neural involvement) Reproducibility of test results Test treatment Imaging procedures (CT, MRI)		

GENERAL MOVEMENT TESTS

General movement tests identify individual anatomical movements and, in part, movement combinations in the area being investigated. The individual manual therapy concepts have respective protocols at their disposal, which more or less have the same goals.

Information gained in this way is used for checking or modifying the relevant hypotheses developed on the basis of anamnesis and area localization and will help in deciding how to proceed.

General question: Is there enough information available to skip general movement tests?	
No	Yes
⇓	⇓
Performance of the general movement tests	• Additional tests • Test treatment

In view of the described clinical presentation and the results of area localization, general movement tests of the following regions seem to be useful.

Cervical spine		
	Active	Passive (assistive)
Upper cervical spine (above C2) in general	Flexion Extension Rotation (to the right and left) Lateral flexion (to the right and left)	Flexion Extension Rotation (to the right and left) Lateral flexion (to the right and left)
Lower cervical spine (below C2) in general	Flexion Extension Rotation (to the right and left) Lateral flexion (to the right and left)	Flexion Extension Rotation (to the right and left) Lateral flexion (to the right and left)
Thoracic spine and ribs		
	Active	Passive (assistive)
Thoracic spine in general	Flexion Extension Rotation (to the right and left) Lateral flexion (to the right and left)	Flexion Extension Rotation (to the right and left) Lateral flexion (to the right and left)

	Active	Passive (assistive)
Ribs in general	Inspiration Expiration	
Movement combinations, thoracic spine and ribs in general	Symptomatic movements of the thoracic spine plus inspiration or expiration	
Shoulder complex		
	Active	Passive
Shoulder girdle	Elevation Depression Protraction Retraction	Elevation Depression Protraction Retraction
Glenohumeral joint	Flexion Extension Internal rotation External rotation Abduction Adduction	Flexion Extension Internal rotation External rotation Abduction Adduction
Movement combinations, shoulder girdle and shoulder	Abduction/Elevation Flexion/Elevation Horizontal adduction Internal rotation with abduction of 90°	Abduction/Elevation Flexion/Elevation Horizontal adduction Internal rotation with abduction of 90°

TREATMENT EXAMPLE, C5

Symptomatic movement

End-range extension of the cervical spine provokes pain (VAS 2–3/10) in area of the lateral upper arm, right side.

ASSESSMENTS

Area localization

Area localization hints at a provocation of symptoms by the cervical spine. There is no contraindication for movement (e.g., vertebrobasilar insufficiency, positive imaging procedure results, no neurological involvement).

Specific provocation and alleviation

Specific provocation and alleviation hints at a provocation of symptoms by movement of C5 into extension.

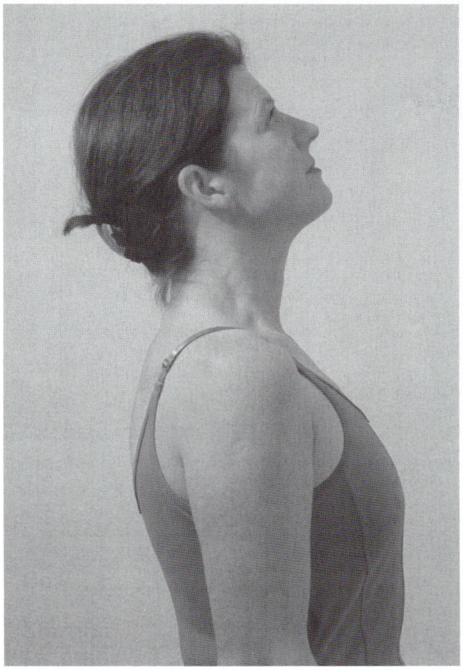

Figure 3.67 Symptom-provoking movement: movement of the head backwards provokes symptoms in the area of the lateral upper arm.

Specific mobility

Specific mobility tests show angular hypermobility of C5 in extension with translatory hypermobility (anterior–posterior) in resting position.

Palpation

Palpation indicates a painful change of tissue over segment C5.

HYPOTHESIS

The problem is a painful hypermobility of C5 in extension (Fig. 3.67).

Based on our understanding of painful hypermobility, local therapeutic procedures in the symptom-provoking area aim at decreasing sensitivity (alleviation of pain). In clinical everyday practice, all kinds of movement that do not go to the end range of the symptomatic movement have proved useful for this purpose. The choice of techniques (active and/or passive procedures) depends, among other things, on the therapist as well as the patient, on the therapist's clinical experience, but primarily on reassessment. This means that even if all preconditions on the part of therapist and patient seem to be met, it is of no use to continue the technique if reassessment is negative.

Treatment of hypermobility consists mainly in stabilizing the hypermobile segment and in reducing the load on the symptomatic joint by treating contributing factors. These may consist of shortened muscles, hypomobile, functionally related areas, habitual postures and movements, as well as insufficient local or general endurance.

Stabilization of the hypermobile segment is done primarily by improving proprioception (processing of afferent input regarding position and movement) as well as coordination (muscular control) with different forms of motor load on the segment. To this end, treatment starts at a joint position which the patient is still well able to control. End positions of the joint are avoided so as not to further stress the irritated structures. The treatment of contributing factors is an indispensable and complex process, which is often underestimated.

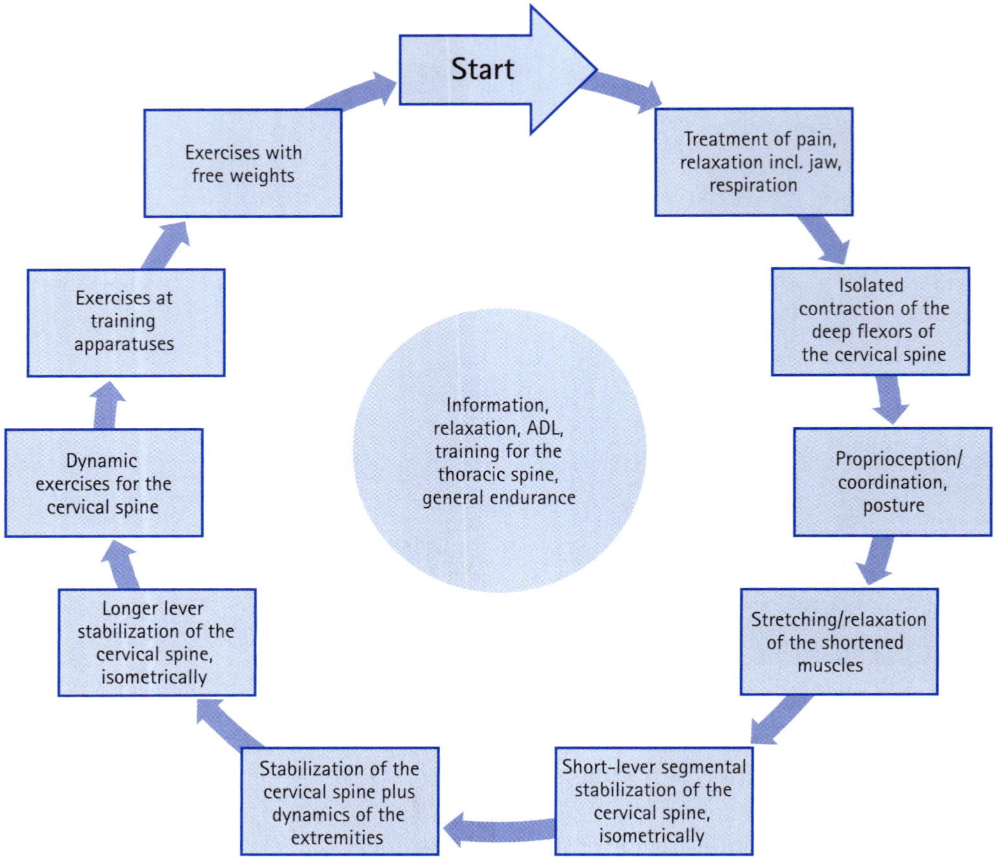

Figure 3.68 Structure of cervical stabilization training.

Apart from local, often mobilizing measures, it frequently includes a change of movement patterns.

With markedly painful presentations, it may be necessary to start or accompany treatment with some external mechanical stabilization (e.g., soft collar, tape) so as to prevent constant (even if not consciously perceived) irritation of the affected segment. The structure of a stabilization programme that has proved to be efficient in clinical practice, in the authors' experience, is represented in Figure 3.68.

Different schools put different emphasis on the measures listed in Figure 3.68. First of all, it is of crucial importance to know the patients' requirements regarding their movement apparatus and then to identify the deficits which prevent successful performance of the required movements. These deficits will have to be remedied to such a degree that the necessary stress will become tolerable again. Possibly, an improvement of the load tolerance beyond the necessary extent will reduce recurrences.

The overall management of painful hypermobility is not part of this book. Here, discussion will be restricted to the treatment of those contributing factors which, in the authors' experience, are very often clinically relevant to the hypothesis of a painful hypermobility of C5 in extension. Most often, hypomobility of the upper thoracic spine as well as of the cervico-thoracic junction is of relevance. Below, exemplary techniques to improve mobility of the cervico-thoracic junction will be described.

MOBILIZATION TECHNIQUES

Active procedures

EXTENSION OF THE CERVICO-THORACIC JUNCTION

Therapy technique (film 86)

- Patient's starting position: prone, the front fixed on the supporting surface, fixation of T2 by a wedge, extension of the head and the cervical spine by moving the headrest of the plinth up (putting chin forward) to a position shortly before symptoms appear (Fig. 3.69a).
- Movement: the patient is asked to draw the chin in (Fig. 3.69b).

Self-exercise from above (film 87)

- Patient's starting position: supine, fixation of T2 by a wedge, occiput fixed on the supporting surface, extension of the head and cervical spine to a position shortly before symptoms appear (Fig. 3.70a).
- Movement: drawing chin in (Fig. 3.70b).

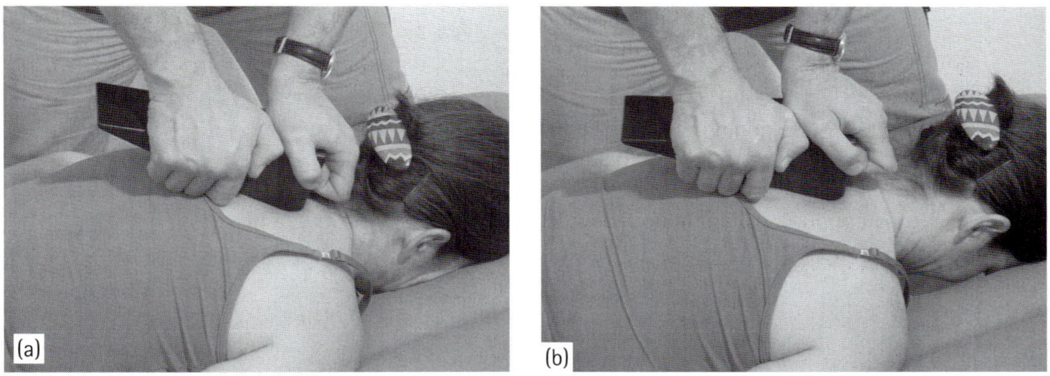

Figure 3.69a and b Active mobilization of T1 in extension; therapy technique. **a**, Starting position. **b**, End position.

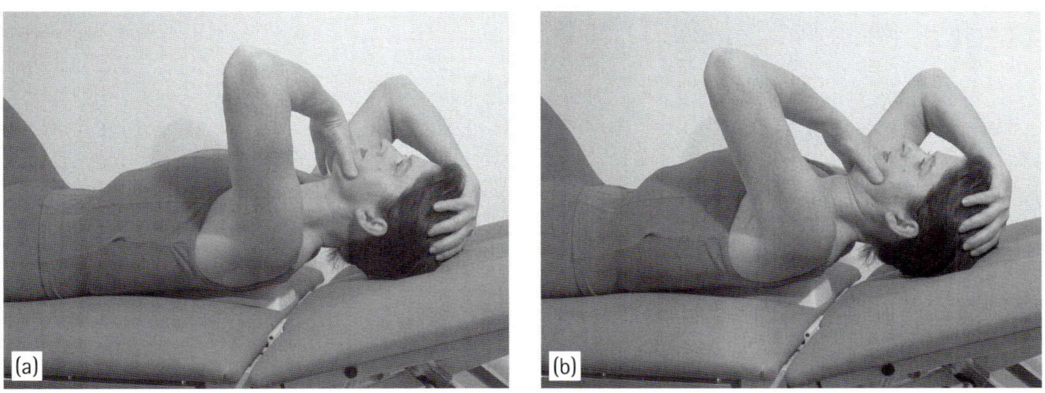

Figure 3.70a and b Active mobilization of the cervico-thoracic junction in extension (moving above); self-exercise. **a**, Starting position. **b**, End position.

Self-exercise from below (film 88)

- Patient's starting position: supine, fixation of T2 by a wedge, occiput fixed on the supporting surface, extension to a position shortly before symptoms appear (Fig. 3.71a).
- Movement: tilting the pelvis in a posterior direction (Fig. 3.71b).

Self-exercise from above and below simultaneously (film 89)

- Patient's starting position: supine, fixation of T2 by a wedge, occiput fixed on the supporting surface, extension of the head and cervical spine to a position shortly before symptoms appear (Fig. 3.72a).
- Movement: drawing chin in and tilting the pelvis in a posterior direction (Fig. 3.72b).

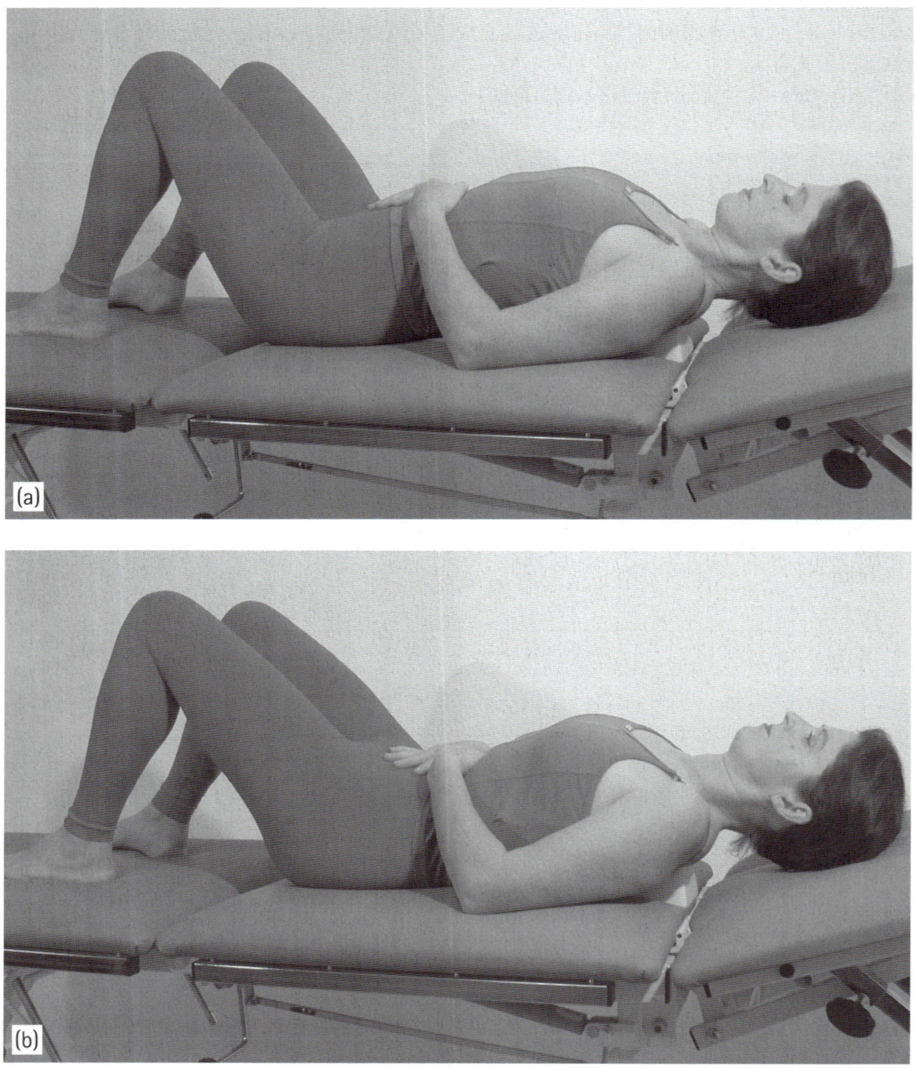

Figure 3.71a and b Active mobilization of the cervico-thoracic junction in extension (moving below); self-exercise. **a**, Starting position. **b**, End position.

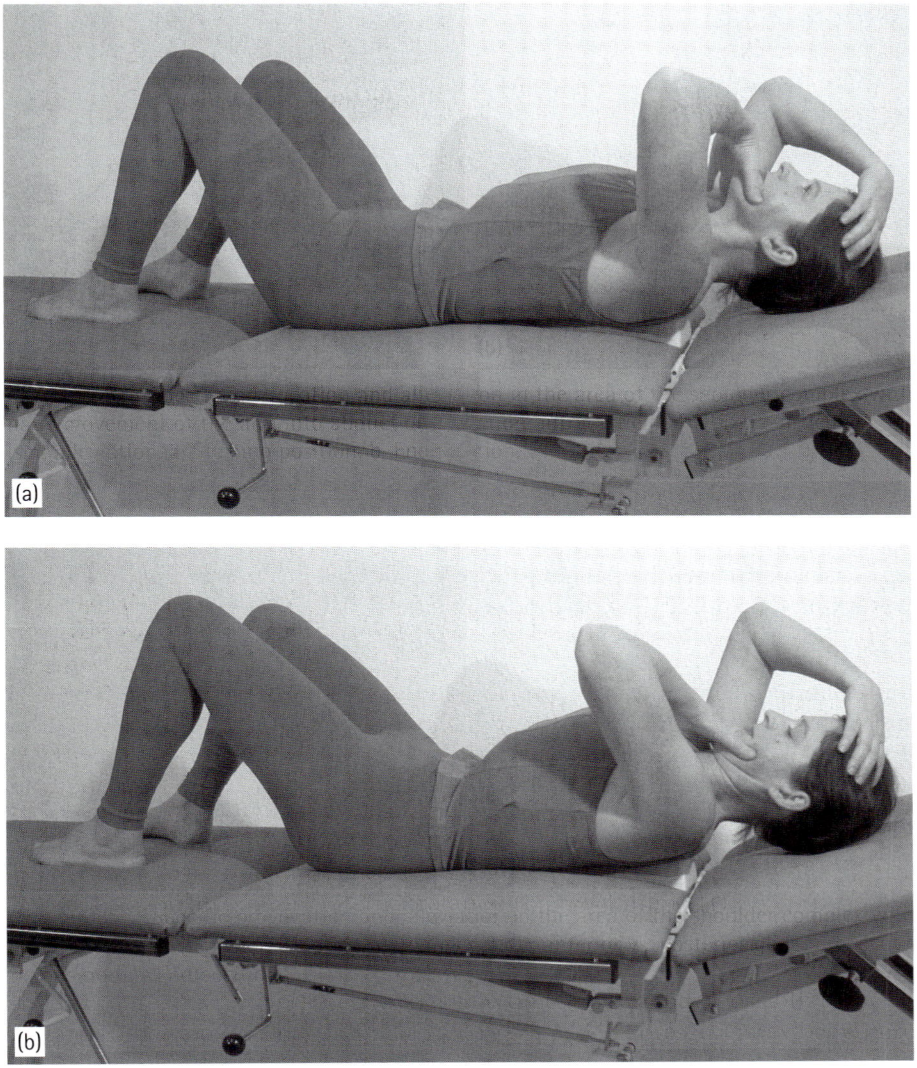

Figure 3.72a and b Active mobilization of the cervico-thoracic junction in extension (moving above and below simultaneously); self-exercise. **a**, Starting position. **b**, End position.

Remarks (regarding active procedures)

Goal of the technique

With a painful hypermobility of C5 in extension, these techniques serve to improve hypomobility of the cervico-thoracic junction by mobilization of non-symptomatic tissue.

Performance

- Therapy technique: the higher the tissue resistance to be overcome by mobilization, the more important the fixation of T2 by the wedge. Care has to be taken that the patient only draws the chin in and by no means moves the cervical spine further into extension.

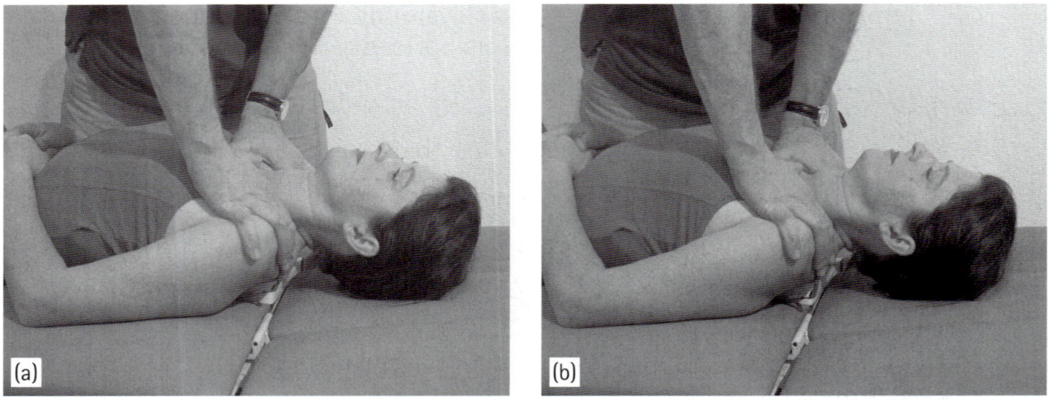

Figure 3.73a and b Mobilization of the cervico-thoracic junction in extension; therapy technique. a, Starting position. b, End position.

- Self-exercise: instructing the patient precisely about the position of the wedge for fixation (e.g., marking the appropriate position with a tape).

Dosage

As in this example a contributing factor close to the symptomatic tissue is to be treated, the symptomatic area may be put under stress due to transferred movement or inexact performance of the technique. Therefore, great care has to be taken not to reproduce the patient's symptoms. Dosage is determined by the expected training state of the tissue and, above all, by reassessment.

Choice of technique

The selection of the technique depends, among other things, on the therapist as well as the patient, on the therapist's clinical experience, but primarily on reassessment. This means that even if all preconditions on the part of therapist and patient seem to be met, it is of no use to continue the technique if reassessment is negative.

Contributing factors

For a satisfactory solution of the patient's current problems it is important to consider the contributing factors and include them in the treatment.

The authors will, however, not go deeper into a description of the various possibilities and their complex contexts as this would exceed the scope of the present book.

Passive procedures

EXTENSION OF THE CERVICO-THORACIC JUNCTION

Therapy technique (film 90)

- Patient's starting position: supine, fixation of T2 by a wedge, occiput fixed on the supporting surface, cervical spine extended to a position shortly before symptoms appear.
- Therapist's starting position: standing, at the patient's side (Fig. 3.73a).
- Movement: dorsal push via the first rib or the sternal manubrium (Fig. 3.73b).

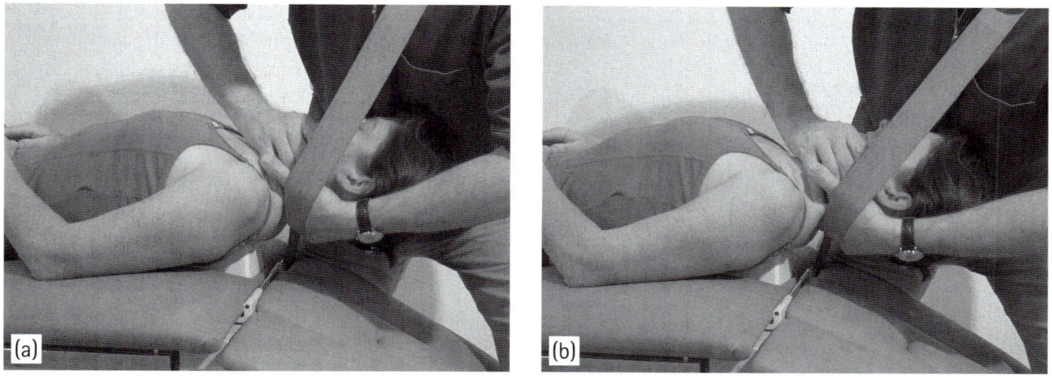

Figure 3.74a and b Mobilization of C7 by traction in the vertebral disc plane; therapy technique. a, Starting position. b, End position.

TRACTION

Therapy technique (film 91)

- Patient's starting position: supine, fixation of T2 by a wedge, pelvis fixed on the supporting surface, manual fixation of head and cervical spine up to C7 (belt), pre-positioning of T1 in extension (Fig. 3.74a).
- Movement: traction in vertebral disc plane (Fig. 3.74b).

Remarks (regarding passive procedures)

Goal of the technique

With painful hypermobility of C5 in extension, these techniques serve to improve hypomobility of the cervico-thoracic junction (contributing factor) by mobilization of non-symptomatic tissue. The extension mobilization described is used for the treatment of hypomobility of T1, the traction mobilization for the treatment of hypomobility of C7.

Performance

The higher the tissue resistance to be overcome by mobilization, the more important the fixation.

Dosage

As in this example a contributing factor close to the symptomatic tissue is to be treated, the symptomatic area may be put under stress due to transferred movement or inexact performance of the technique. Therefore, great care has to be taken not to reproduce the patient's symptoms. Dosage is determined by the training state of the tissue to be expected and, above all, by reassessment.

Choice of technique

The selection of the technique depends, among other things, on the therapist as well as the patient, on the therapist's clinical experience, but primarily on reassessment. This means that even if all preconditions on the part of therapist and patient seem to be met, it is of no use to continue the technique if reassessment is negative.

Contributing factors

For a satisfactory solution of the patient's current problems it is important to consider the contributing factors and include them in the treatment.

The authors will, however, not go into a description of the various possibilities and their complex contexts as this would exceed the scope of the present book.

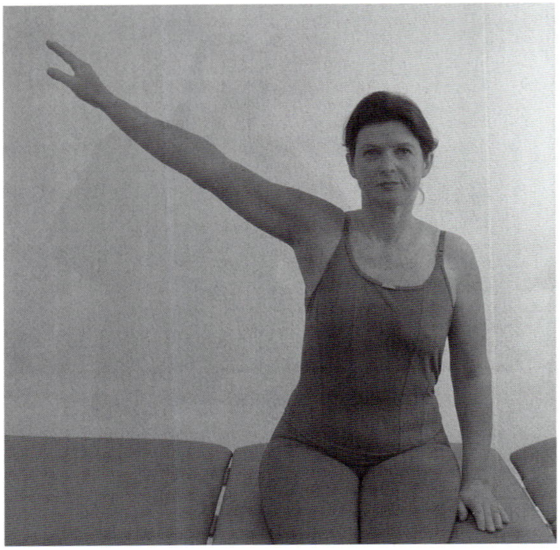

Figure 3.75 Symptom-provoking movement: the movement of the arm into abduction/elevation provokes symptoms in the area of the lateral upper arm.

TREATMENT EXAMPLE, GLENOHUMERAL JOINT

SYMPTOMATIC MOVEMENT

Abduction/elevation of the right arm is restricted by 20% as compared with the contralateral side and, in end-range positions, provokes pain (VAS 4/10) in the area of the lateral upper arm, right side.

ASSESSMENTS

Area localization

Area localization hints at symptom provocation by the shoulder complex. There is no contraindication for movement.

Specific provocation and alleviation

- Specific provocation and alleviation hints at a provocation of symptoms by the right shoulder joint.
- Symptoms are provoked by compression of the subacromial space, right side.

Specific mobility

Specific mobility tests show restricted dorsal and caudal glide.

Palpation

The presumed symptomatic area (subacromial space) is not accessible to palpation.

HYPOTHESIS

A painfully restricted abduction/elevation of the right arm due to compression of the subacromial space, right side, with simultaneous hypomobility in the glenohumeral joint (in caudal and dorsal direction) is suspected (Fig. 3.75).

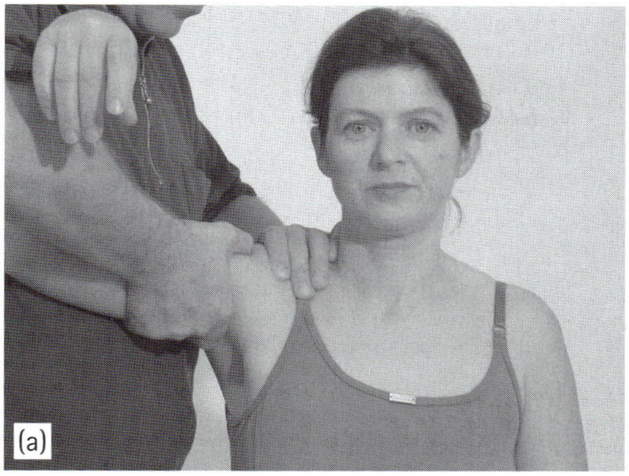

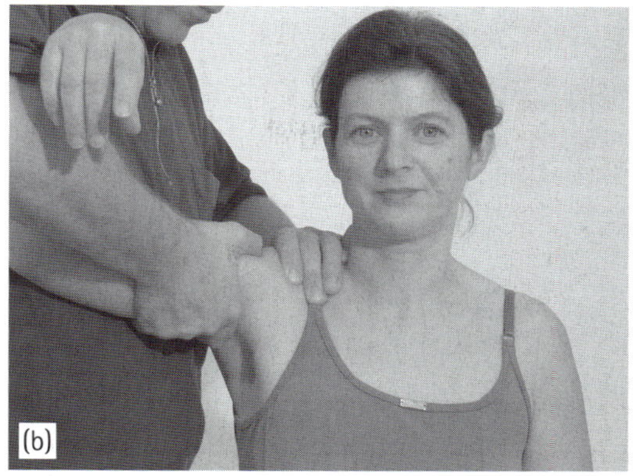

Figure 3.76a and b Co-contraction against distraction in the shoulder joint; therapy technique. a, Starting position. b, End position.

RELAXATION TECHNIQUES

Hold–relax techniques

CO-CONTRACTION AGAINST DISTRACTION

Therapy technique (film 112)

- Patient's starting position: sitting, the right arm abducted/elevated (to a position before symptoms appear).
- Therapist's starting position: standing, at the patient's right side, fixing the scapula at the lateral edge of the acromion and at the coracoid process, seizing the humerus near the joint (Fig. 3.76a).
- Movement: traction in the glenohumeral joint, while the patient tries to prevent distraction by means of muscle contraction (Fig. 3.76b).

Remarks

Goal of the technique

Reduction of the tonicity and improvement of the metabolism of the periarticular tissues with painfully restricted abduction/elevation of the right arm due to compression of the subacromial space, right side, with simultaneous hypomobility in the glenohumeral joint (in caudal and dorsal direction).

Performance

Depending on irritability or the desired treatment goal, the joint to be treated is pre-positioned as necessary before treatment.

Dosage (regarding the affected symptomatic structure)

Both with an acute and with a chronic presentation, the contraction should always be pain-free.

Choice of technique

The selection of the technique depends, among other things, on the therapist as well as the patient, on the therapist's clinical experience, but primarily on reassessment. This means that even if all preconditions on the part of therapist and patient seem to be met, it is of no use to continue the technique if reassessment is negative.

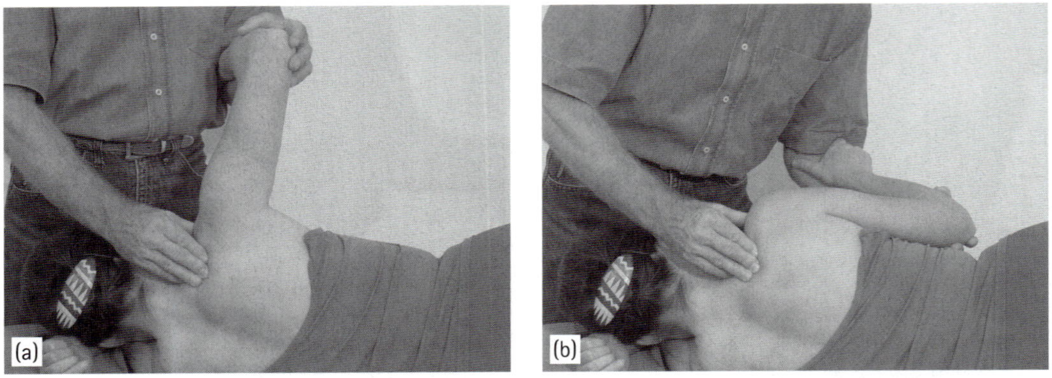

Figure 3.77a and b Massage of the supraspinatus muscle combined with joint movement; therapy technique. **a**, Starting position. **b**, End position.

Contributing factors

For a satisfactory solution of the patient's current problems it is important to consider the contributing factors and include them in the treatment.

The authors will, however, not go into a description of the various possibilities and their complex contexts as this would exceed the scope of the present book.

Soft tissue techniques

SUPRASPINATUS MUSCLE

Therapy technique (film 113)

- Patient's starting position: lying on the left side, arm abducted.
- Therapist's starting position: standing, in front of the patient (Fig. 3.77a; Zahnd and Mühlemann 1998).
- Movement: passive adduction in the glenohumeral joint while simultaneously exerting manual pressure into the supraspinous fossa, then releasing the pressure into the supraspinous fossa, and back to the starting position (Fig. 3.77b).

Note: If the patient is not able to relax or if performance of the movement seems too difficult, this soft tissue technique can also be performed assistively.

Self-exercise (film 114)

- Patient's starting position: sitting, arm abducted to a position before symptoms appear, contact with three finger tips of the left hand in the supraspinous fossa (Fig. 3.78a).
- Movement: pressure into the supraspinous fossa, active adduction of the right glenohumeral joint, then releasing the pressure into the supraspinous fossa, and back to the starting position (Fig. 3.78b).

INFRASPINATUS MUSCLE

Therapy technique (film 115)

- Patient's starting position: lying on the left side, arm abducted horizontally and externally rotated.
- Therapist's starting position: standing, in front of the patient (Fig. 3.79a; Zahnd and Mühlemann 1998).

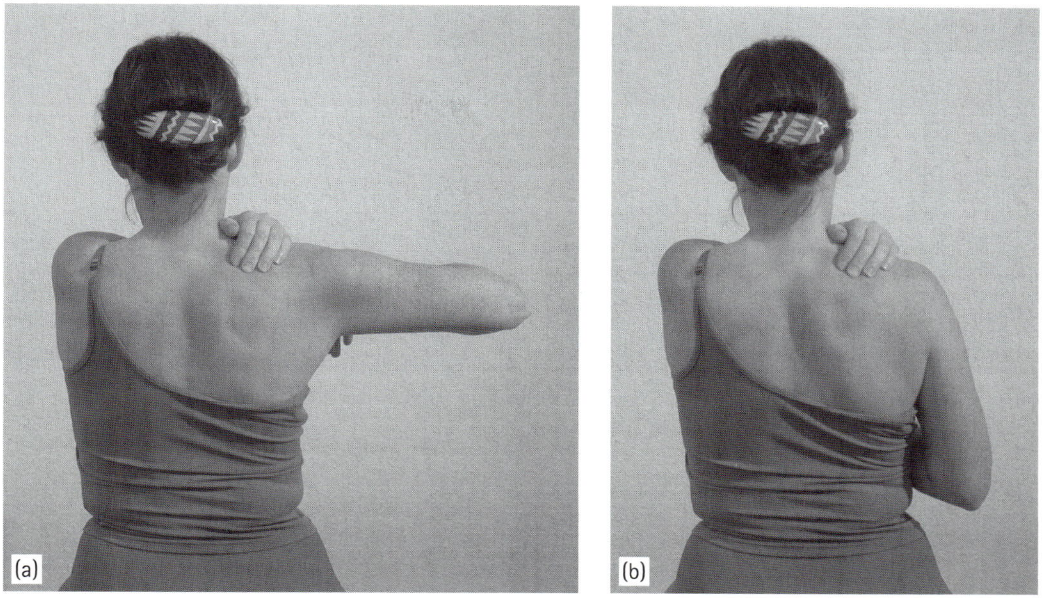

Figure 3.78a and b Massage of the supraspinatus muscle combined with joint movement; self-exercise. a, Starting position. b, End position.

- Movement: passive horizontal adduction with simultaneous internal rotation in the glenohumeral joint. Simultaneously exerting manual pressure into the infraspinous fossa, then releasing the pressure into the infraspinous fossa, and back to the starting position (Fig. 3.79b).

> *Note:* If the patient is not able to relax or if performance of the movement seems too difficult, this soft tissue technique can also be performed assistively.

Self-exercise (film 116)

- Patient's starting position: sitting, arm externally rotated, contact with three finger tips of the left hand in the infraspinous fossa (Fig. 3.80a).
- Movement: internal rotation in the right glenohumeral joint with simultaneous manual pressure into the infraspinous fossa, then releasing the pressure into the infraspinous fossa, and back to the starting position (Fig. 3.80b).

Remarks (regarding soft tissue techniques)

Goal of the technique

Reduction of the tonicity and improvement of the metabolism of the treated soft tissue with painfully restricted abduction/elevation of the right arm due to compression of the subacromial space, right side, with simultaneous hypomobility in the glenohumeral joint (in the caudal and dorsal direction).

Performance

Treatment is done within the pain-free range of movement. If, with self-exercise, movement of the arm against gravity is painful, a position has to be chosen where the movement can be performed without pain. As the treatment techniques are performed without 'specific fixation',

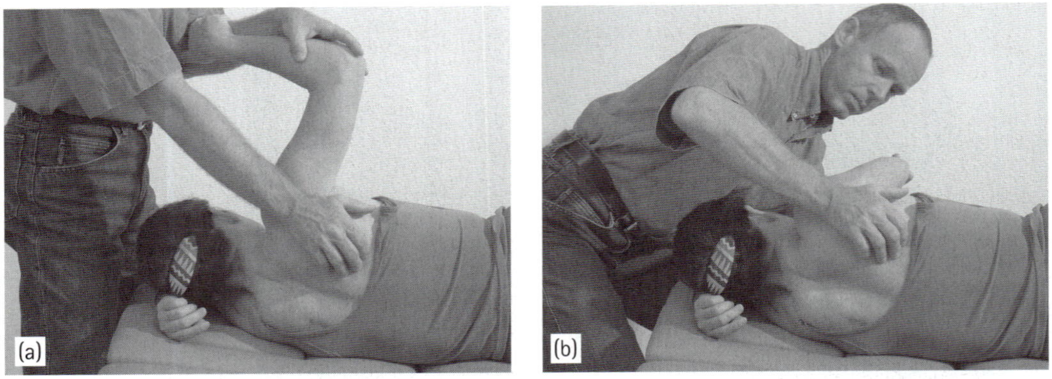

Figure 3.79a and b Massage of the infraspinatus muscle combined with joint movement; therapy technique. a, Starting position. b, End position.

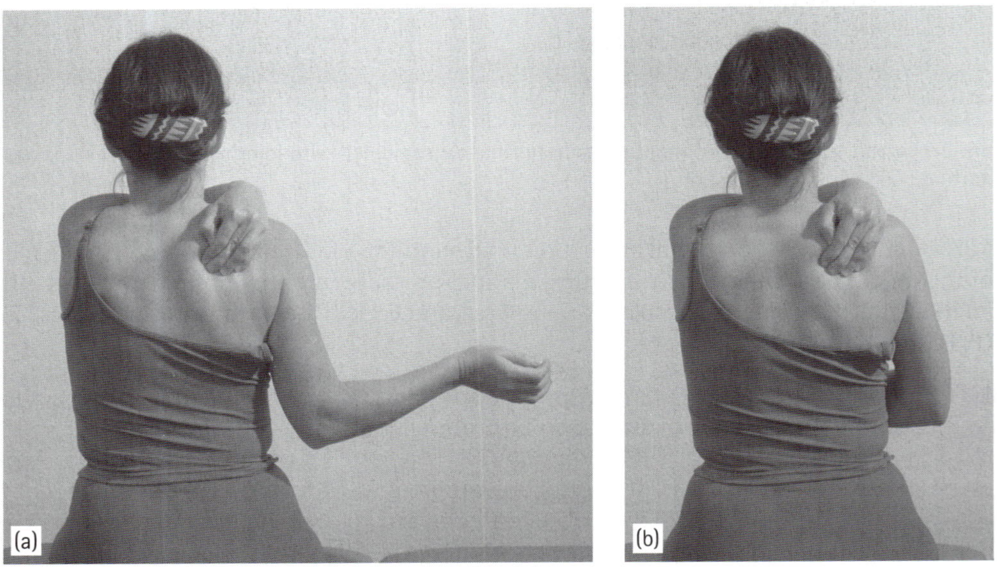

Figure 3.80a and b Massage of the infraspinatus muscle combined with joint movement; self-exercise. a, Starting position. b, End position.

an uncontrolled transferral of movement has to be considered when the indication for the technique is determined.

Choice of technique

The selection of the technique depends, among other things, on the therapist as well as the patient, on the therapist's clinical experience, but primarily on reassessment. This means that even if all preconditions on the part of therapist and patient seem to be met, it is of no use to continue the technique if reassessment is negative.

Contributing factors

For a satisfactory solution of the patient's current problems it is important to consider the contributing factors and include them in the treatment.

The authors will, however, not go into a description of the various possibilities and their complex contexts as this would exceed the scope of the present book.

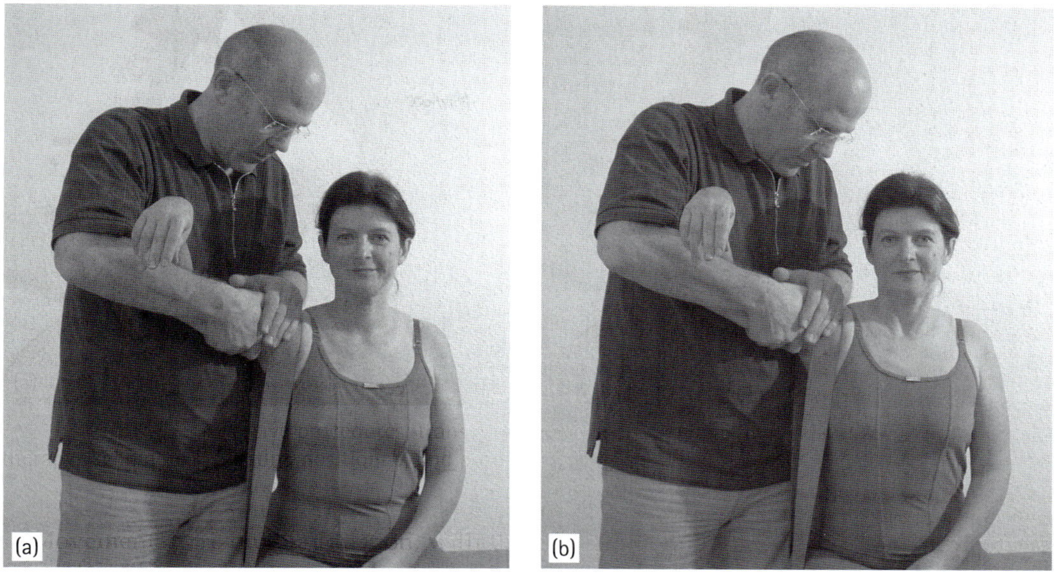

Figure 3.81a and b Active mobilization in the shoulder joint by caudal glide of the humerus; therapy technique. **a**, Starting position. **b**, End position.

MOBILIZATION TECHNIQUES

Active procedures

ACTIVE MOBILIZATION

Caudal glide of the humerus

Therapy technique (film 123)

- Patient's starting position: sitting, the arm abducted/elevated to a position shortly before symptoms appear, a belt goes round the humeral head, just laterally of the acromion, and is firmly linked to the plinth.
- Therapist's starting position: standing, at the right side behind the patient, fixation of the glenohumeral joint in a position shortly before symptoms appear (Fig. 3.81a).
- Movement: the patient is asked to pull up the shoulder girdle against the fixation of the humerus by the belt (Fig. 3.81b).

Self-exercise (film 124)

- Patient's starting position: standing, with slightly bent knees, the arm abducted/elevated to a position shortly before symptoms appear, with the elbow supported, a belt goes round the humeral head, just laterally of the acromion, and passes beneath the patient's foot (Fig. 3.82a).
- Movement: when the knees are extended, the belt becomes tense and moves the humeral head in a caudal direction; lifting of the shoulder girdle increases the gliding movement in a caudal direction (Fig. 3.82b).

Remarks

Goal of the technique

Improvement of the restricted caudal glide in the glenohumeral joint with painfully restricted abduction/elevation of the right arm due to compression of the subacromial space, right

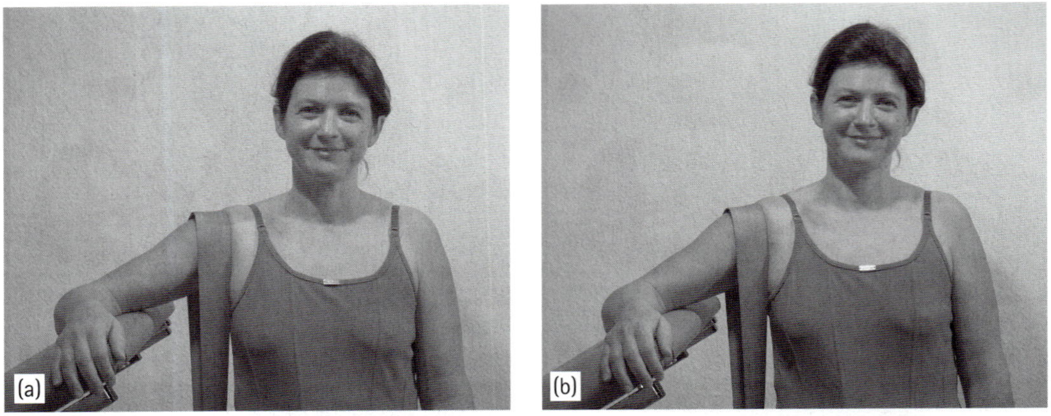

Figure 3.82a and b Active mobilization in the shoulder joint by caudal glide of the humerus; self-exercise. **a**, Starting position. **b**, End position.

side, with simultaneous hypomobility in the glenohumeral joint (in caudal and dorsal direction).

Performance

According to irritability or the desired treatment goal, the joint to be treated is pre-positioned as necessary before treatment.

Dosage (regarding the affected symptomatic structure)

As, in this example, a subacromial pathology is assumed, direct loading of the symptomatic structures by the technique is improbable. The patient's typical pain with abduction/elevation should not appear. Because of the active performance of the mobilization technique, resistance cannot be assessed. Therefore, pain and reassessment are used in determining dosage.

Choice of technique

The selection of the technique depends, among other things, on the therapist as well as the patient, on the therapist's clinical experience, but primarily on reassessment. This means that even if all preconditions on the part of therapist and patient seem to be met, it is of no use to continue the technique if reassessment is negative.

Contributing factors

For a satisfactory solution of the patient's current problems it is important to consider the contributing factors and include them in the treatment.

The authors will, however, not go into a description of the various possibilities and their complex contexts as this would exceed the scope of the present book.

ACTIVE MOBILIZATION PLUS ACCESSORY MOVEMENT

Abduction/elevation of the humerus with posterior glide

Therapy technique (film 117)

- Patient's starting position: sitting.
- Therapist's starting position: standing, on the right side behind the patient, contact with the left hand from posterior against the scapula, with the right hand from anterior against the humeral head (Fig. 3.83a).

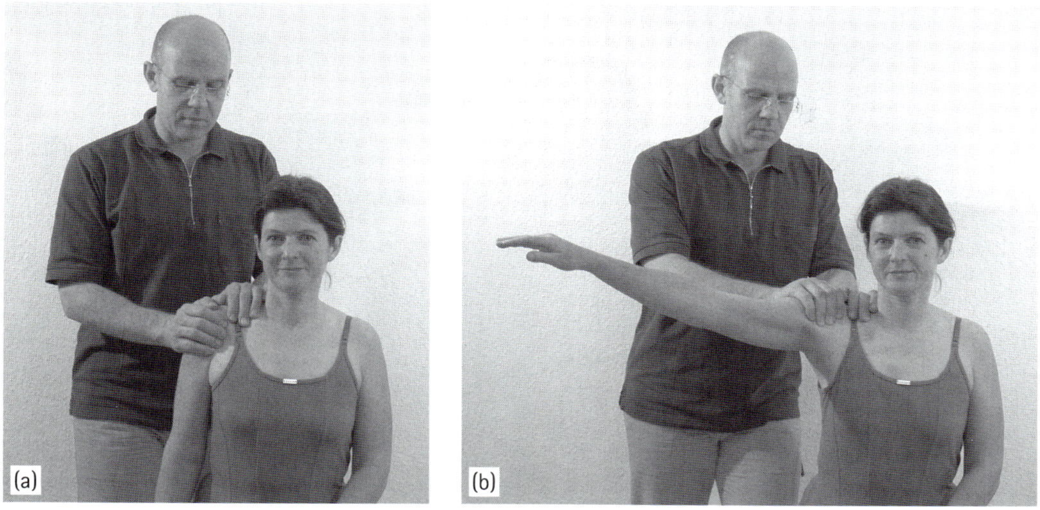

Figure 3.83a and b Active mobilization with accessory movement; abduction with posterior glide; therapy technique. a, Starting position. b, End position.

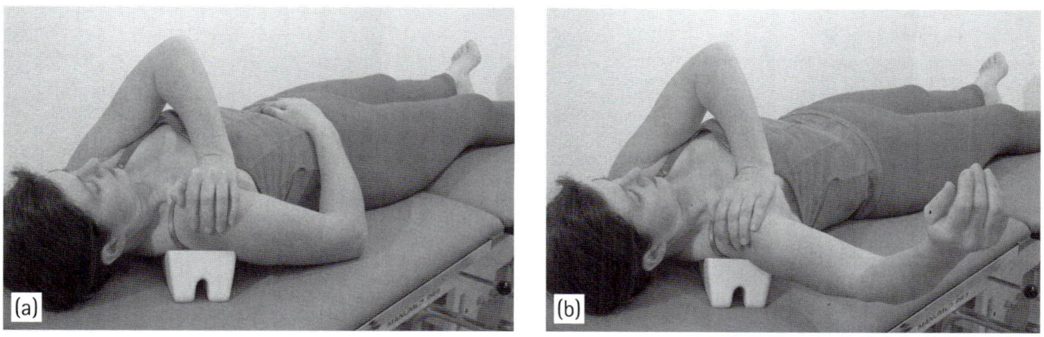

Figure 3.84a and b Active mobilization with accessory movement; abduction with posterior glide; self-exercise. a, Starting position. b, End position.

- Movement: posterior push of the humeral head with subsequent active movement of the humerus into abduction/elevation, then guiding the arm back to the starting position, and releasing the posterior push (Fig. 3.83b).

Self-exercise (film 118)

- Patient's starting position: supine, fixation of the scapula by a wedge, contact with the left hand from anterior against the humeral head (Fig. 3.84a).
- Movement: posterior push of the humeral head with subsequent active movement of the humerus into abduction/elevation, then guiding the arm back to the starting position, and releasing the posterior push (Fig. 3.84b).

Abduction/elevation of the humerus with caudal glide

Therapy technique (film 119)

- Patient's starting position: sitting.
- Therapist's starting position: standing, on the right side behind the patient, contact with the right hand cranially against the humeral head (Fig. 3.85a).

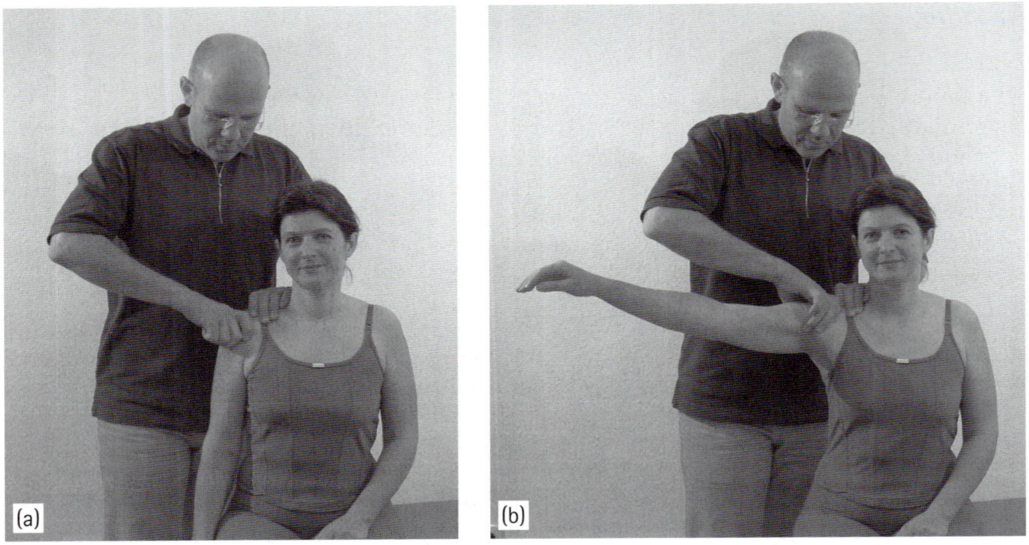

Figure 3.85a and b Active mobilization with accessory movement; abduction with caudal glide; therapy technique. a, Starting position. b, End position.

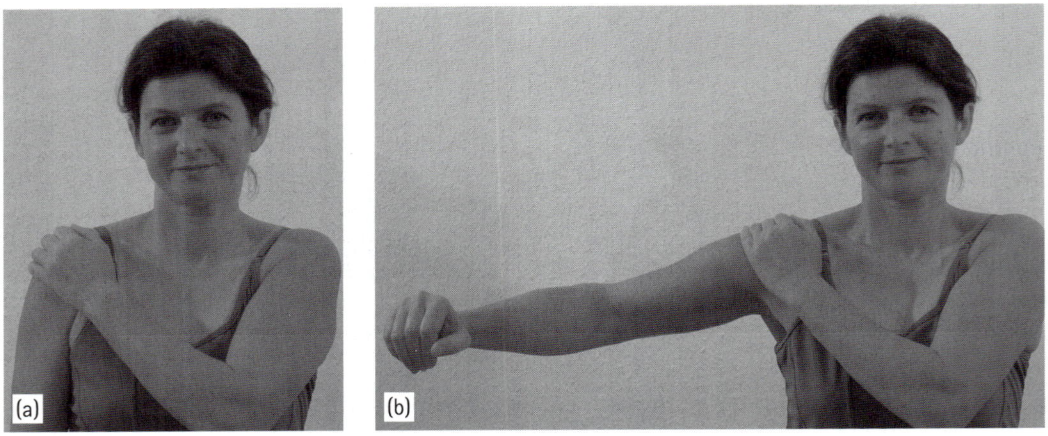

Figure 3.86a and b Active mobilization with accessory movement; abduction with caudal glide; self-exercise. a, Starting position. b, End position.

- Movement: caudal push of the humeral head with subsequent active movement of the humerus into abduction/elevation, then guiding the arm back to the starting position, and releasing the caudal push (Fig. 3.85b).

Self-exercise (film 120)

- Patient's starting position: sitting or standing, the left hand grasps the humeral head cranially (Fig. 3.86a).
- Movement: caudal push of the humeral head with subsequent active movement of the humerus into abduction/elevation, then guiding the arm back to the starting position, and releasing the caudal push (Fig. 3.86b).

Remarks (regarding active mobilization plus accessory movement)

Goal of the technique

With a painfully restricted abduction/elevation of the right arm due to compression of the subacromial space, right side, with simultaneous hypomobility in the glenohumeral joint (in caudal and dorsal direction), these techniques serve to:

- reduce tonicity and improve the metabolism of the affected tissues
- restore pain-free function (change the input to the respective centres of the central nervous system (CNS)).

Performance

In active mobilization with glide into a posterior or caudal direction, the push is performed in relation to the treatment plane (parallel to the glenoid fossa) and not to space.

Dosage (regarding the affected symptomatic structure)

Both with an acute (predominantly peripheral pain mechanism) and with a chronic presentation (predominantly central pain mechanism), this technique should not reproduce the patient's symptoms. Dosage is adjusted in line with the expected training state of the tissue and with reassessment.

Choice of technique

The selection of the technique depends, among other things, on the therapist as well as the patient, on the therapist's clinical experience, but primarily on reassessment. This means that even if all preconditions on the part of therapist and patient seem to be met, it is of no use to continue the technique if reassessment is negative.

Contributing factors

For a satisfactory solution of the patient's current problems it is important to consider the contributing factors and include them in the treatment.

The authors will, however, not go into a description of the various possibilities and their complex contexts as this would exceed the scope of the present book.

Abduction/elevation of the humerus with subacromial compression

Therapy technique (film 121)

- Patient's starting position: supine, the arm abducted/elevated to a position clearly before symptoms appear.
- Therapist's starting position: standing, at the patient's side, the therapist's hands grasp the humeral head from the axilla, and the acromion dorsocranially (Fig. 3.87a).
- Movement: after increasing the subacromial compression (hands pressed together), the patient actively moves into abduction/elevation and back to the starting position (Fig. 3.87b).

External/internal rotation of the humerus with subacromial compression

Therapy technique (film 122)

- Patient's starting position: supine, the arm abducted/elevated to a position shortly before symptoms appear.
- Therapist's starting position: standing, at the patient's side, the therapist's hands grasp the humeral head and the acromion; both thumbs are in the axilla, while the fingers rest on the acromion (Fig. 3.88a).

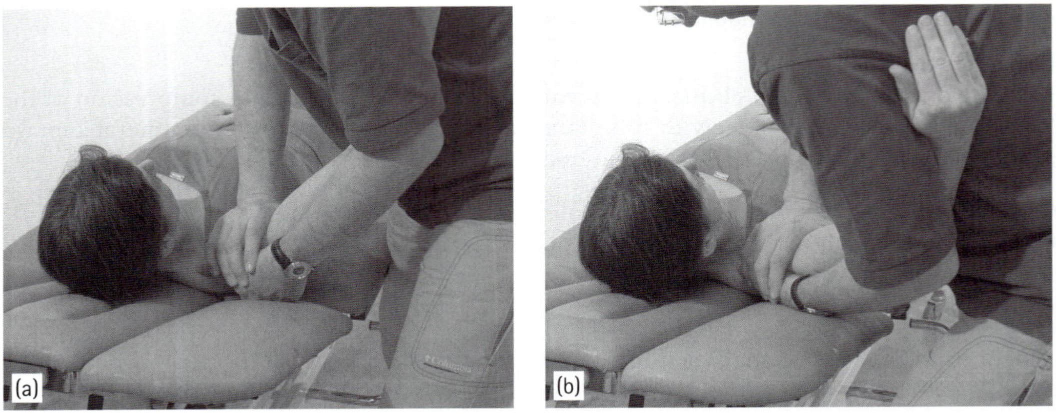

Figure 3.87a and b Active mobilization with accessory movement; abduction/elevation with subacromial compression; therapy technique. **a**, Starting position. **b**, End position.

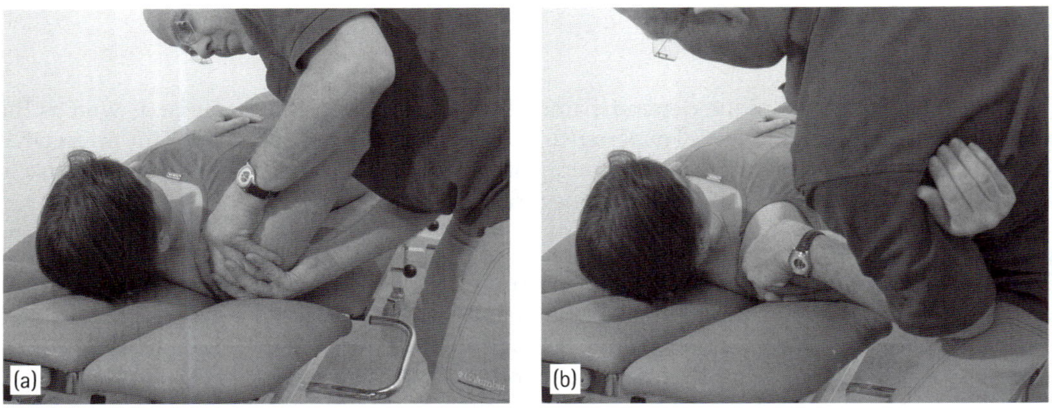

Figure 3.88a and b Active mobilization with accessory movement; external/internal rotation with subacromial compression; therapy technique. **a**, Starting position. **b**, End position.

- Movement: after increasing the subacromial compression (fingers pressed together), the patient actively moves into external/internal rotation and back to the starting position, then pressure is released (Fig. 3.88b).

Since this technique is difficult to perform as self-exercise, all exercises can be employed instead which reduce subacromial compression so far that the movement can be performed without pain. In this respect, correction of the scapula position in the direction of retraction/depression is of crucial importance.

Remarks (regarding techniques with subacromial compression)

Goal of the technique

With a painfully restricted movement of the right arm into abduction/elevation by compression of the subacromial space, right side, with simultaneous hypomobility in the glenohumeral joint (in caudal and dorsal direction), these techniques serve to:

- restore normal function of symptomatic tissue by application of the symptom-provoking stimulus dosed according to the current load tolerance.
- restore symptom-free function by changing the input to the respective centres of the CNS.

Performance

While the therapist maintains subacromial compression, the patient should move actively. If this is too painful, either compression has to be reduced or, perhaps, the movement has to be performed assistively.

Choice of technique

The selection of the technique depends, among other things, on the therapist as well as the patient, on the therapist's clinical experience, but primarily on reassessment. This means that even if all preconditions on the part of therapist and patient seem to be met, it is of no use to continue the technique if reassessment is negative.

Contributing factors

For a satisfactory solution of the patient's current problems it is important to consider the contributing factors and include them in the treatment.

The authors will, however, not go into a description of the various possibilities and their complex contexts as this would exceed the scope of the present book.

Dosage (regarding the affected symptomatic structure)

Acute presentation (predominantly peripheral pain mechanisms)

Phase	Limitation of movement due to pain and resistance	Concept	Movement grade
Inflammation phase	No pain No resistance	Kaltenborn–Evjenth Maitland	Up to the beginning of II Up to II
Proliferation phase	Up to P1 Slowly progressing up to low resistance	Kaltenborn–Evjenth Maitland	Up to the 1st third of II III^-
Remodelling/ organization phase	Slowly progressing up to maximum resistance (Note: duration of turnover!)	Kaltenborn–Evjenth Maitland	Up to III Up to IV^{++} or III^{+++}

Note: The chances of a disturbed (delayed) course of healing and the consequences for the loading capacity of the tissue (e.g., diabetes, old age, partial or general immobilization) have to be considered.

Chronic presentation (predominantly central pain mechanisms): Since here it is assumed that pain no longer represents a protection mechanism, the therapist has to consider the expected training state of the treated tissue as well as the patient's personal expectations. In case of

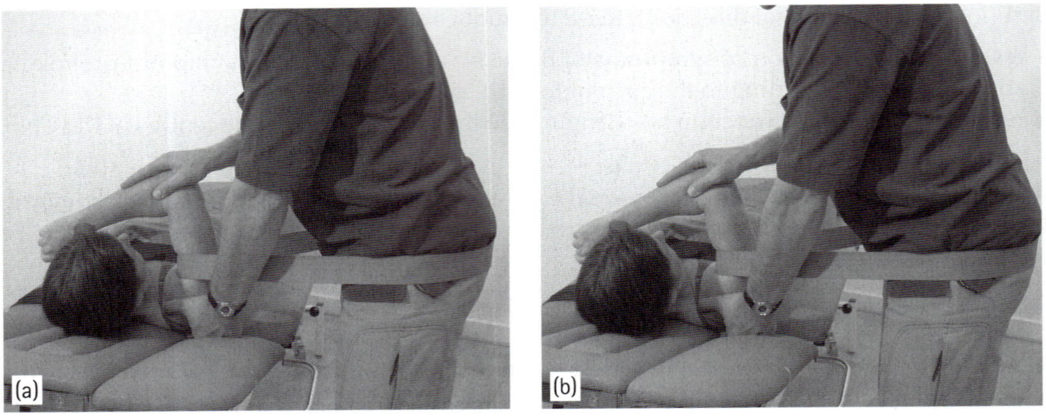

Figure 3.89a and b Passive procedures; translatory movement; traction in horizontal adduction with internal rotation; therapy technique. **a**, Starting position. **b**, End position.

doubt, treatment is always started with very low force. Progression depends on reassessment. Hence with a chronic presentation, pain does not always represent the limiting factor regarding dosage of treatment.

Passive procedures

TRANSLATORY MOVEMENTS

Traction

Therapy technique (film 126)

- Patient's starting position: supine, the arm in horizontal adduction and internal rotation, with fixed scapula (belt).
- Therapist's starting position: standing, at the patient's side, manual stabilization of the humerus distally (Fig. 3.89a).
- Movement: distraction in the glenohumeral joint which is three-dimensionally prepositioned (at a right angle to the treatment plane) (Fig. 3.89b).

Caudal glide

Therapy technique (film 125)

- Patient's starting position: supine, the arm abducted/elevated to a position shortly before symptoms appear, the humerus with stable support near the joint (wedge or sandbag).
- Therapist's starting position: standing, at the patient's side, manual stabilization of the humerus distally (Fig. 3.90a).
- Movement: push of the scapula parallel to the treatment plane in a dorsocranial direction (Fig. 3.90b).

ANGULAR MOVEMENTS

Stretching the posterior periarticular tissues of the glenohumeral joint

Therapy technique (film 127)

- Patient's starting position: supine, the arm in horizontal abduction with internal rotation.
- Therapist's starting position: standing, at the patient's contralateral side, manual stabilization of the scapula via its lateral margin on the plinth (Fig. 3.91a).

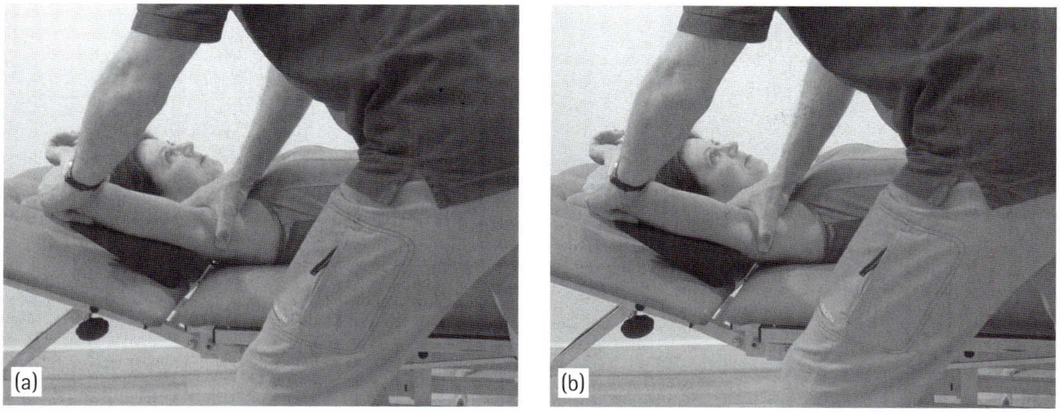

Figure 3.90a and b Passive procedures; translatory movement; caudal glide in abduction/elevation; therapy technique. a, Starting position. b, End position.

- Movement: horizontal adduction, with the glenohumeral joint pre-positioned in internal rotation (Fig. 3.91b).

Self-exercise (film 128)

- Patient's starting position: lying on the affected (right) side, the arm in horizontal adduction and internal rotation (held by the left hand), with simultaneous stabilization of the scapula on the supporting surface by the patient's own body weight (Fig. 3.92a).
- Movement: rolling the body to the right, or alternatively further moving into horizontal adduction by pulling the right upper arm with the left hand (Fig. 3.92b).

Remarks

Goal of the technique

With a painfully restricted movement of the right arm into abduction/elevation due to compression of the subacromial space, right side, with simultaneous hypomobility in the glenohumeral joint (in caudal and dorsal direction), these techniques serve to improve mobility of the glenohumeral joint by mobilization of non-symptomatic tissue.

Performance

The greater the tissue resistance to be overcome by mobilization, the more important the fixation of the scapula. It can be assumed that thereby the mobilizing effect in the respective sections of the glenohumeral joint becomes greater and that there will be no other, undesired movements.

Dosage (regarding the affected symptomatic structure)

As in this example a subacromial pathology is assumed, direct loading of the symptomatic structures by the technique is improbable. The patient's typical pain with abduction/elevation should not appear. Dosage is adjusted in line with the expected training state of the tissue and, above all, with reassessment.

Choice of technique

The selection of the technique depends, among other things, on the therapist as well as the patient, on the therapist's clinical experience, but primarily on reassessment. This means that even if all preconditions on the part of therapist and patient seem to be met, it is of no use to continue the technique if reassessment is negative.

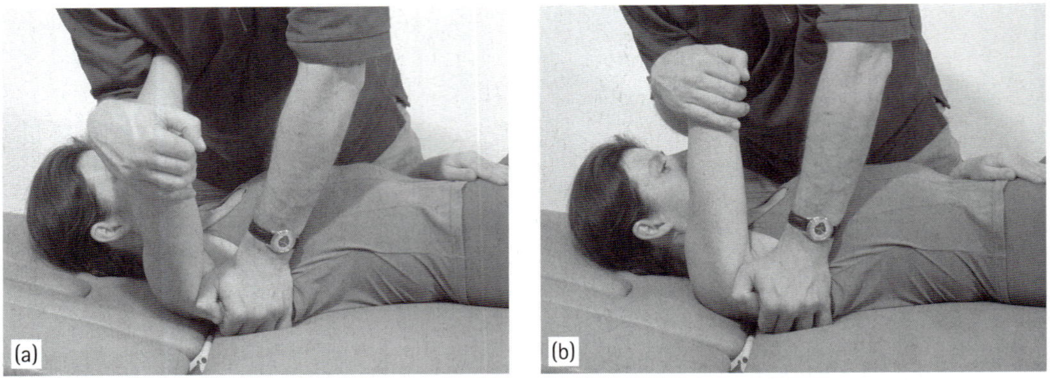

Figure 3.91a and b Passive procedures; angular movement; stretching the posterior periarticular structures of the glenohumeral joint; therapy technique. **a**, Starting position. **b**, End position.

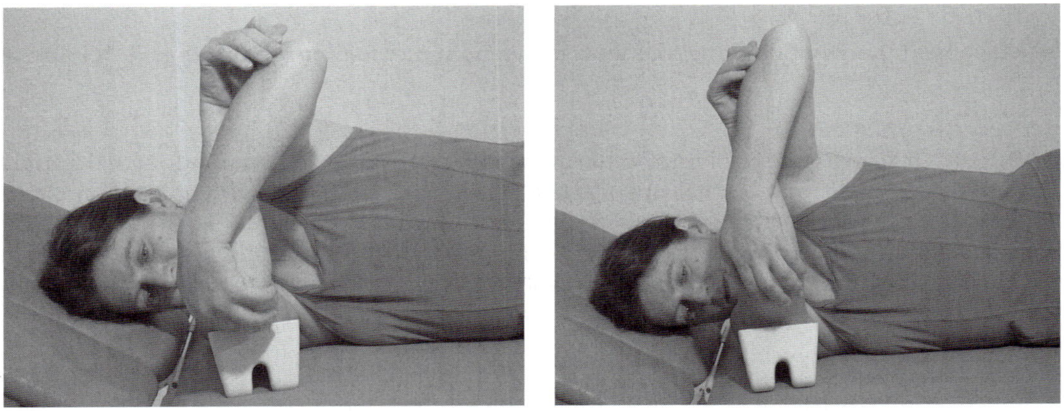

Figure 3.92a and b Passive procedures; angular movement; stretching the posterior periarticular structures of the glenohumeral joint; self-exercise. **a**, Starting position. **b**, End position.

Contributing factors

For a satisfactory solution of the patient's current problems it is important to consider the contributing factors and include them in the treatment.

The authors will, however, not go into a description of the various possibilities and their complex contexts as this would exceed the scope of the present book.

Chapter 4

Lateral elbow

CHAPTER CONTENTS

AREA LOCALIZATION

IDENTIFICATION OF THE POTENTIALLY AFFECTED AREA BY DEMONSTRATION OF A SYMPTOMATIC FUNCTIONAL MOVEMENT/POSITION

Based on the information gained from the anamnesis so far, the therapist tries to ascertain more details about potentially affected sections. This is done by means of area localization, which represents the beginning of the physical examination. Information gained in this way is used to check or modify the relevant hypotheses developed on the basis of the anamnesis and will determine how to proceed.

Area localization is explained by means of four examples, in which the patient feels pain in the area of the lateral elbow. Based on clinical experience and known clinical patterns, primarily the following sections are considered as potential sources of the current complaints:

- cervical spine
- shoulder complex
- elbow complex
- neural structures.

General question: Is there enough information available to skip area localization?	
No	Yes
⇓	⇓
Performance of area localization	• General movement tests • Additional tests • Test treatment

Example 1: Extension

Symptom area: lateral elbow
Symptom provocation: extension of the elbow (Fig. 4.1)

With this clinical presentation, clinical experience suggests primarily the cervical spine, the shoulder complex, the elbow complex, and the neural structures as symptom-provoking areas.

Below, examples illustrate how to differentiate between these areas. To this end, area localization is first attempted by means of active movements alone. If this is not possible, tests will be performed by means of assistive movements.

Hypothesis 1: The symptom-provoking area is the cervical spine
Differentiation: cervical spine vs. elbow complex.

The change in symptoms can be demonstrated exactly:

- provocation of pain (Fig. 4.2a and b, film 130)
- alleviation of pain (Fig. 4.3a and b, film 131).

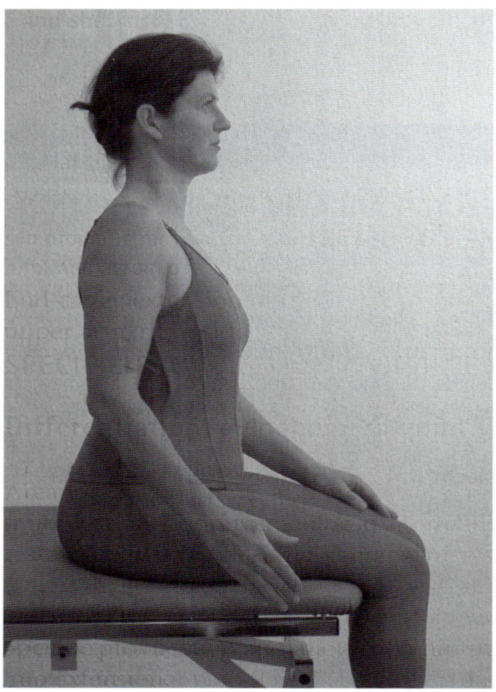

Figure 4.1 Symptom-provoking movement: movement of the elbow into extension provokes pain in the area of the lateral elbow.

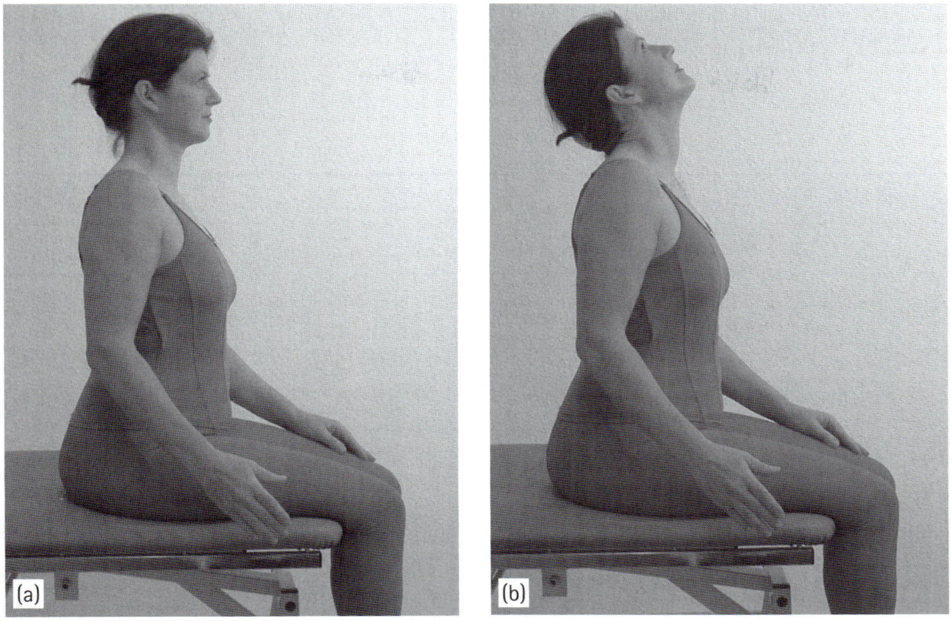

Figure 4.2a and b Area localization with symptomatic movement of the elbow into extension; differentiation between cervical spine and elbow complex; provocation. **a**, Starting position. **b**, End position.

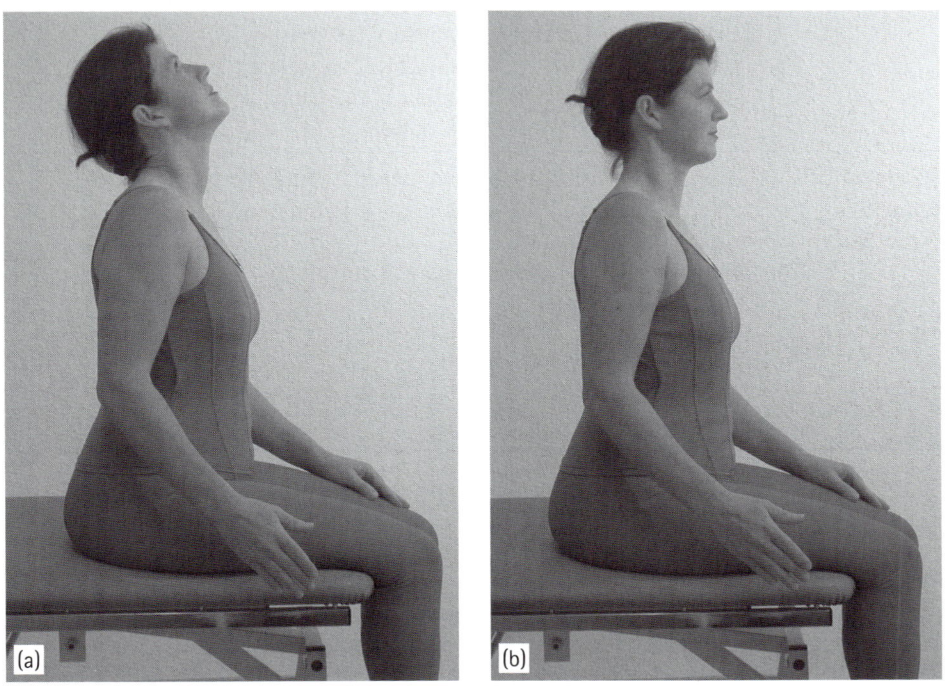

Figure 4.3a and b Area localization with symptomatic movement of the elbow into extension; differentiation between cervical spine and elbow complex; alleviation. **a**, Starting position. **b**, End position.

The result of area localization has to be verified by further specific tests; otherwise the result will be open to question.

Assessment			
Goal	**Provocation of pain**	**Alleviation of pain**	**Remarks**
Starting position	Extension of the elbow to a position immediately before symptoms appear	With the cervical spine pre-positioned in extension, extension of the elbow to a position immediately after symptoms have appeared	
Test movement	Extension of the cervical spine	Moving the cervical spine back to neutral position	Elbow remains in starting position
Explanation	If by any movement of the cervical spine (here, as an example, extension) the typical symptoms are reproduced, an isolated lesion of the elbow is doubtful	If by any movement of the cervical spine (here, as an example, moving back to neutral position) the typical symptoms are alleviated, an isolated lesion of the elbow is doubtful	
Additional data to support the hypothesis	General and specific mobility of cervical spine and elbow complex (potential positive findings have to be found under neural relaxation as well) History, symptom behaviour, type of complaints, 24-hour behaviour Palpation Reproducibility of test results Test treatment Imaging procedures (CT, MRI)		

Hypothesis 2: The symptom-provoking area is the neural structures

Differentiation: neural involvement vs. elbow complex.

The change in symptoms can be demonstrated exactly:

- provocation of pain (Fig. 4.4a and b, film 132)
- alleviation of pain (Fig. 4.5a and b, film 133).

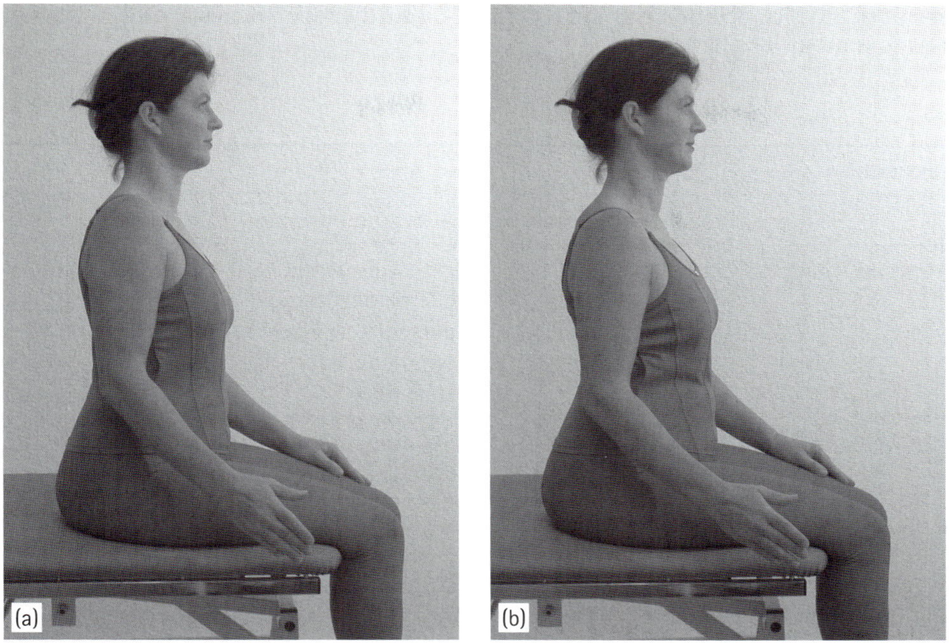

Figure 4.4a and b Area localization with symptomatic movement of the elbow into extension; differentiation between neural structures and elbow complex; provocation. **a**, Starting position. **b**, End position.

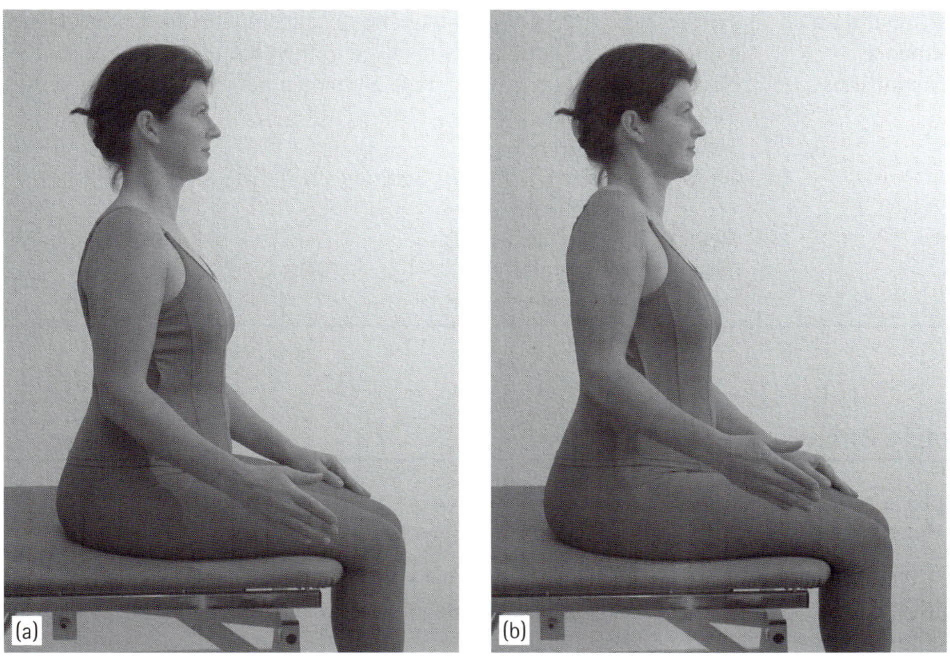

Figure 4.5a and b Area localization with symptomatic movement of the elbow into extension; differentiation between neural structures and elbow complex; alleviation. **a**, Starting position. **b**, End position.

The result of area localization has to be verified by further specific tests; otherwise the result will be open to question.

Assessment			
Goal	**Provocation of pain**	**Alleviation of pain**	**Remarks**
Starting position	Extension of the elbow to a position immediately before symptoms appear	Extension of the elbow to a position immediately after symptoms have appeared	
Test movement	Depression of the shoulder girdle	Elevation of the shoulder girdle	All other joints must not move
Explanation	The test movement produces mechanical stress on neural structures and structures associated with them	The test movement reduces mechanical stress on neural structures and structures associated with them	If the typical pain is provoked or alleviated by these manoeuvres without moving the elbow, this suggests at least an involvement of the neural structures
Additional data to support the hypothesis	Further movements of proximal and distal components to increase neural tension that are not directly involved in the painful movement History, symptom behaviour, type of complaints, 24-hour behaviour Palpation Neurodynamic tests Nerve provocation tests (e.g., Spurling's test, Tinel's sign) Nerve palpation tests Reproducibility of test results Test treatment Imaging procedures (CT, MRI)		

Example 2: Flexion

Symptom area: lateral elbow
Symptom provocation: flexion of the elbow (Fig. 4.6)

With this clinical presentation, clinical experience suggests primarily the cervical spine, the shoulder complex, the elbow complex, and the neural structures as symptom-provoking areas.

Below, examples illustrate how to differentiate between these areas. To this end, area localization is first attempted by means of active movements alone. If this is not possible, tests will be performed by means of assistive movements.

Hypothesis 1: The symptom-provoking area is the cervical spine

Differentiation: cervical spine vs. elbow complex.

The change in symptoms can be demonstrated exactly:

- provocation of pain (Fig. 4.7a and b, film 173)
- alleviation of pain (Fig. 4.8a and b, film 174).

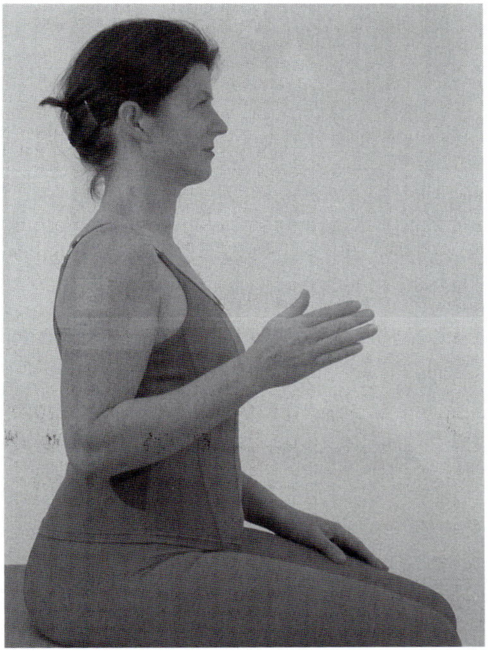

Figure 4.6 Symptom-provoking movement: movement of the elbow into flexion provokes pain in the area of the lateral elbow.

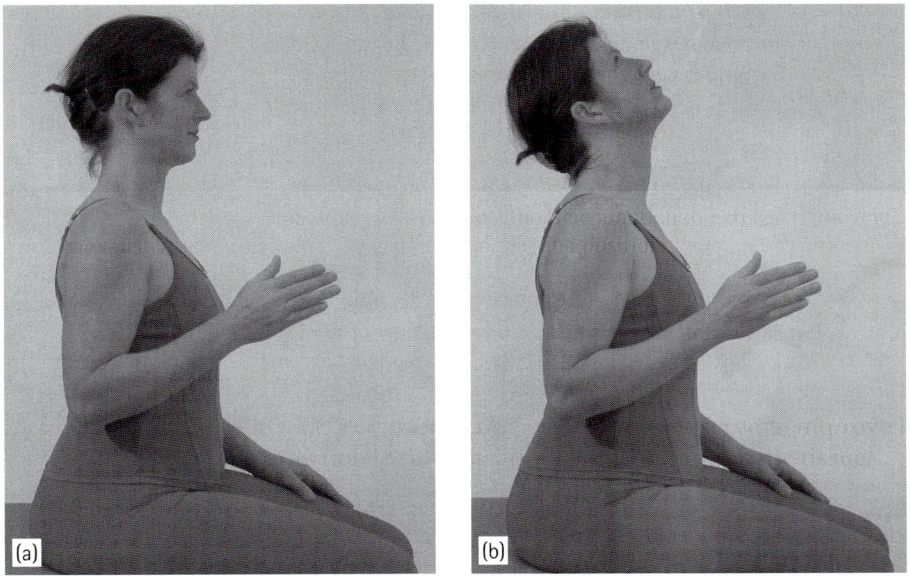

Figure 4.7a and b Area localization with symptomatic movement of the elbow into flexion; differentiation between cervical spine and elbow complex; provocation. a, Starting position. b, End position.

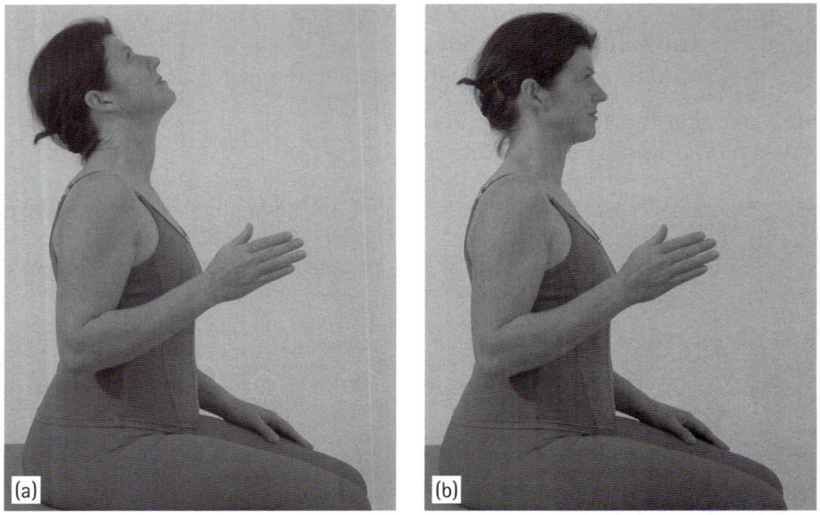

Figure 4.8a and b Area localization with symptomatic movement of the elbow into flexion; differentiation between cervical spine and elbow complex; alleviation. **a**, Starting position. **b**, End position.

The result of area localization has to be verified by further specific tests; otherwise the result will be open to question.

Assessment

Goal	Provocation of pain	Alleviation of pain	Remarks
Starting position	Flexion of the elbow to a position immediately before symptoms appear	With the cervical spine pre-positioned in extension, flexion of the elbow to a position immediately after symptoms have appeared	
Test movement	Extension of the cervical spine	Moving the cervical spine back to neutral position	Elbow remains in starting position
Explanation	If by any movement of the cervical spine (here, as an example, extension) the typical symptoms are reproduced, an isolated lesion of the elbow is doubtful	If by any movement of the cervical spine (here, as an example, moving the cervical spine back to neutral position) the typical symptoms are alleviated, an isolated lesion of the elbow is doubtful	
Additional data to support the hypothesis	General and specific mobility of cervical spine and elbow complex (potential positive findings have to be found under neural relaxation as well)		

Goal	Provocation of pain	Alleviation of pain	Remarks
	History, symptom behaviour, type of complaints, 24-hour behaviour Palpation Reproducibility of test results Test treatment Imaging procedures (CT, MRI)		

Hypothesis 2: The symptom-provoking area is the neural structures

Differentiation: neural involvement vs. elbow complex.

The change in symptoms can be demonstrated exactly:

- provocation of pain (Fig. 4.9a and b, film 175)
- alleviation of pain (Fig. 4.10a and b, film 176).

The result of area localization has to be verified by further specific tests; otherwise the result will be open to question.

Assessment			
Goal	**Provocation of pain**	**Alleviation of pain**	**Remarks**
Starting position	Flexion of the elbow to a position immediately before symptoms appear	Flexion of the elbow to a position immediately after symptoms have appeared	
Test movement	Depression of the shoulder girdle	Elevation of the shoulder girdle	All other joints must not move
Explanation	The test movement produces mechanical stress on neural structures and structures associated with them	The test movement reduces mechanical stress on neural structures and structures associated with them	If the typical pain is provoked or alleviated by these manoeuvres without moving the elbow, this suggests at least an involvement of the neural structures
Additional data to support the hypothesis	Further movements of proximal and distal components to increase neural tension that are not directly involved in the painful movement of the elbow History, symptom behaviour, type of complaints, 24-hour behaviour Palpation Neurodynamic tests Nerve provocation tests (e.g., Spurling's test, Tinel's sign) Nerve palpation tests Reproducibility of test results Test treatment Imaging procedures (CT, MRI)		

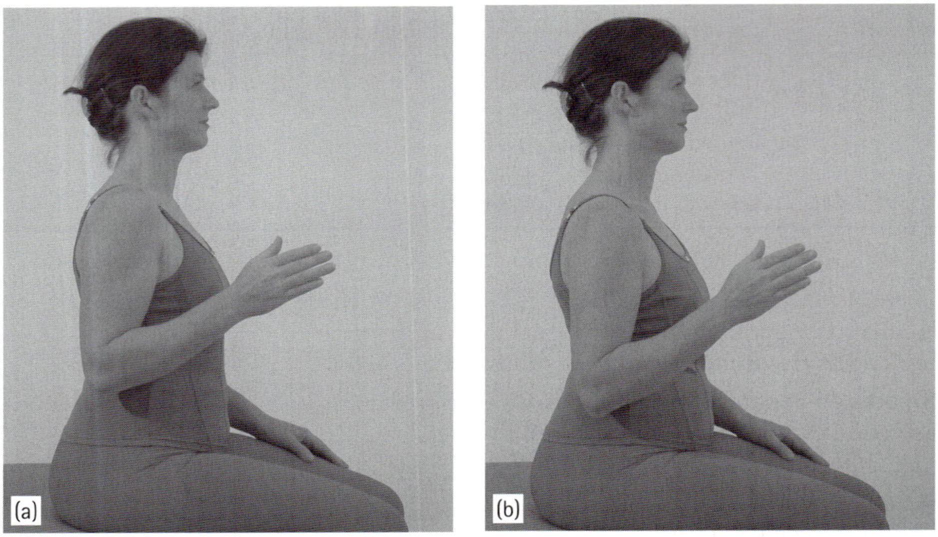

Figure 4.9a and b Area localization with symptomatic movement of the elbow into flexion; differentiation between neural structures and elbow complex; provocation. **a**, Starting position. **b**, End position.

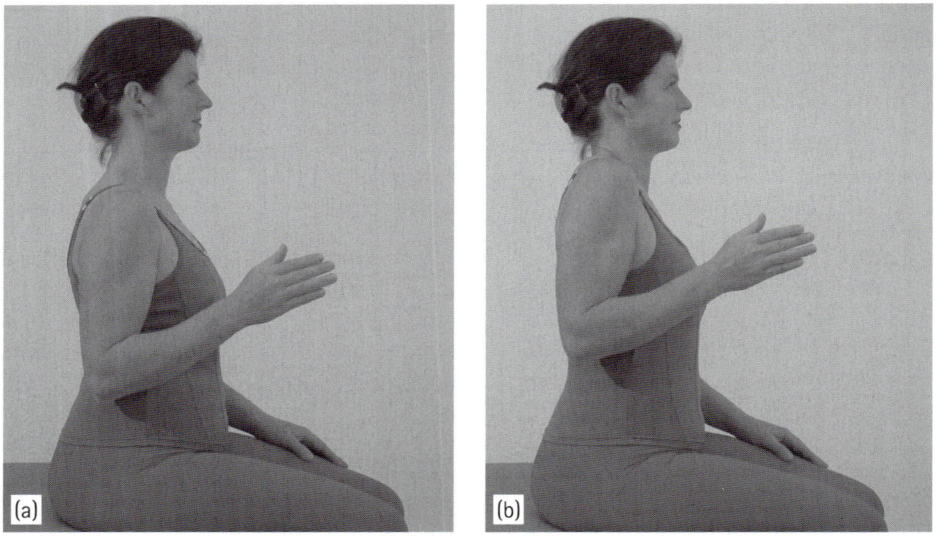

Figure 4.10a and b Area localization with symptomatic movement of the elbow into flexion; differentiation between neural structures and elbow complex; alleviation. **a**, Starting position. **b**, End position.

Example 3: Supination

Symptom area: lateral elbow
Symptom provocation: supination of the forearm (Fig. 4.11)

With this clinical presentation, clinical experience suggests primarily the cervical spine, the shoulder complex, the elbow complex, and the neural structures as symptom-provoking areas.

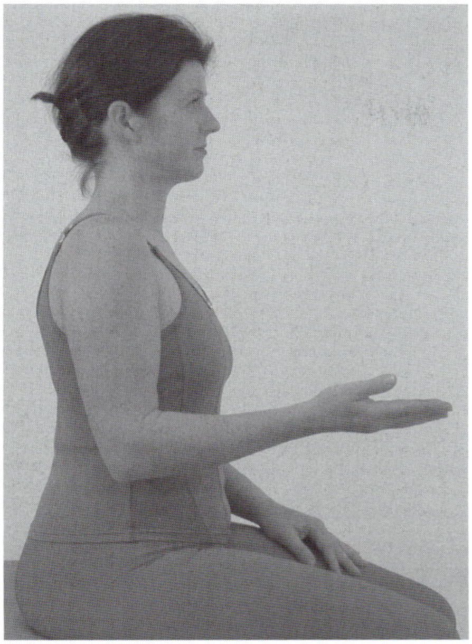

Figure 4.11 Symptom-provoking movement: movement of the elbow into supination provokes pain in the area of the lateral elbow.

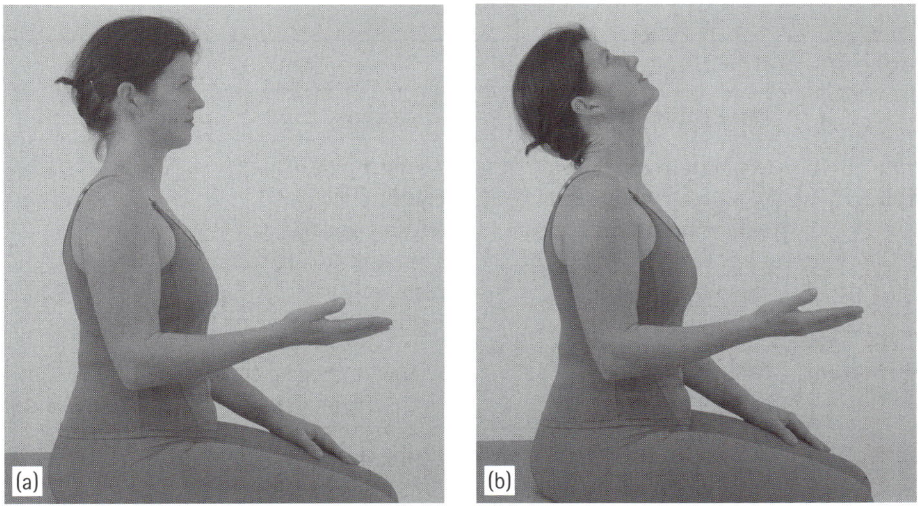

Figure 4.12a and b Area localization with symptomatic movement of the elbow into supination; differentiation between cervical spine and elbow complex; provocation. **a**, Starting position. **b**, End position.

Below, examples illustrate how to differentiate between these areas. To this end, area localization is first attempted by means of active movements alone. If this is not possible, tests will be performed by means of assistive movements.

Hypothesis 1: The symptom-provoking area is the cervical spine

Differentiation: cervical spine vs. elbow complex.

The change in symptoms can be demonstrated exactly:

- provocation of pain (Fig. 4.12a and b, film 189)
- alleviation of pain (Fig. 4.13a and b, film 190).

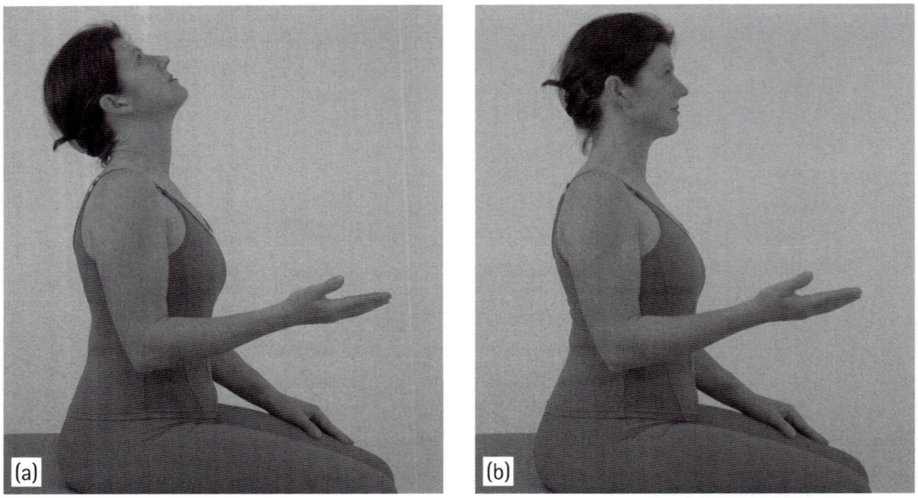

Figure 4.13a and b Area localization with symptomatic movement of the elbow into supination; differentiation between cervical spine and elbow complex; alleviation. **a**, Starting position. **b**, End position.

The result of area localization has to be verified by further specific tests; otherwise the result will be open to question.

Assessment

Goal	Provocation of pain	Alleviation of pain	Remarks
Starting position	Supination of the forearm to a position immediately before symptoms appear	With the cervical spine pre-positioned in extension, supination of the forearm to a position immediately after symptoms have appeared	
Test movement	Extension of the cervical spine	Moving the cervical spine back to neutral position	Elbow remains in starting position
Explanation	If by any movement of the cervical spine (here, as an example, extension) the typical symptoms are reproduced, an isolated lesion of the elbow is doubtful	If by any movement of the cervical spine (here, as an example, moving the cervical spine back to neutral position) the typical symptoms are alleviated, an isolated lesion of the elbow is doubtful	
Additional data to support the hypothesis	General and specific mobility of cervical spine and elbow complex (potential positive findings have to be found under neural relaxation as well) History, symptom behaviour, type of complaints, 24-hour behaviour Palpation		

Goal	Provocation of pain	Alleviation of pain	Remarks
	Reproducibility of test results Test treatment Imaging procedures (CT, MRI)		

Hypothesis 2: The symptom-provoking area is the neural structures

Differentiation: neural involvement vs. elbow complex.

The change in symptoms can be demonstrated exactly:

- provocation of pain (Fig. 4.14a and b, film 191)
- alleviation of pain (Fig. 4.15a and b, film 192).

The result of area localization has to be verified by further specific tests; otherwise the result will be open to question.

Assessment

Goal	Provocation of pain	Alleviation of pain	Remarks
Starting position	Supination of the forearm to a position immediately before symptoms appear	Supination of the forearm to a position immediately after symptoms have appeared	
Test movement	Depression of the shoulder girdle	Elevation of the shoulder girdle	All other joints must not move
Explanation	The test movement produces mechanical stress on neural structures and structures associated with them	The test movement reduces mechanical stress on neural structures and structures associated with them	If the typical pain is provoked or alleviated by these manoeuvres without moving the forearm, this suggests at least an involvement of the neural structures
Additional data to support the hypothesis	Further movements of proximal and distal components to increase neural tension that are not directly involved in the painful movement of the elbow History, symptom behaviour, type of complaints, 24-hour behaviour Palpation Neurodynamic tests Nerve provocation tests (e.g., Spurling's test, Tinel's sign) Nerve palpation tests Reproducibility of test results Test treatment Imaging procedures (CT, MRI)		

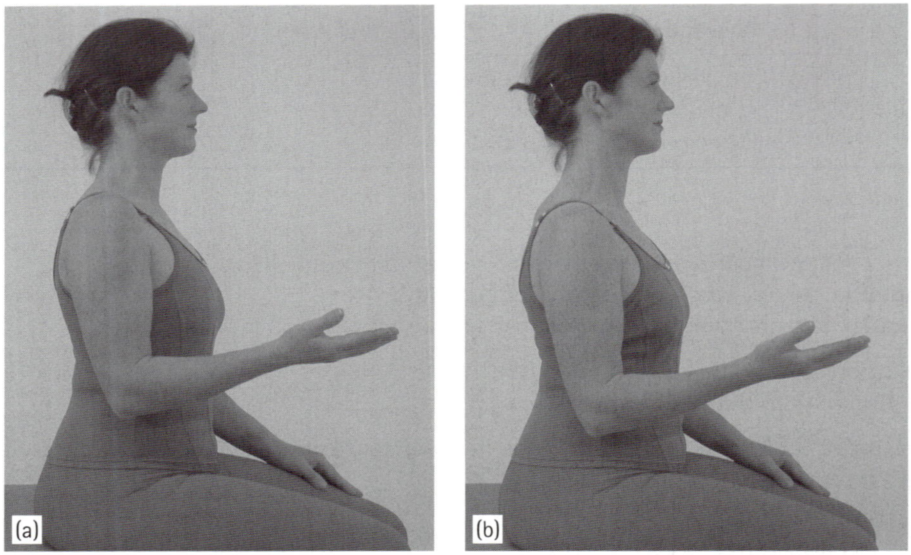

Figure 4.14a and b Area localization with symptomatic movement of the elbow into supination; differentiation between neural structures and elbow complex; provocation. **a**, Starting position. **b**, End position.

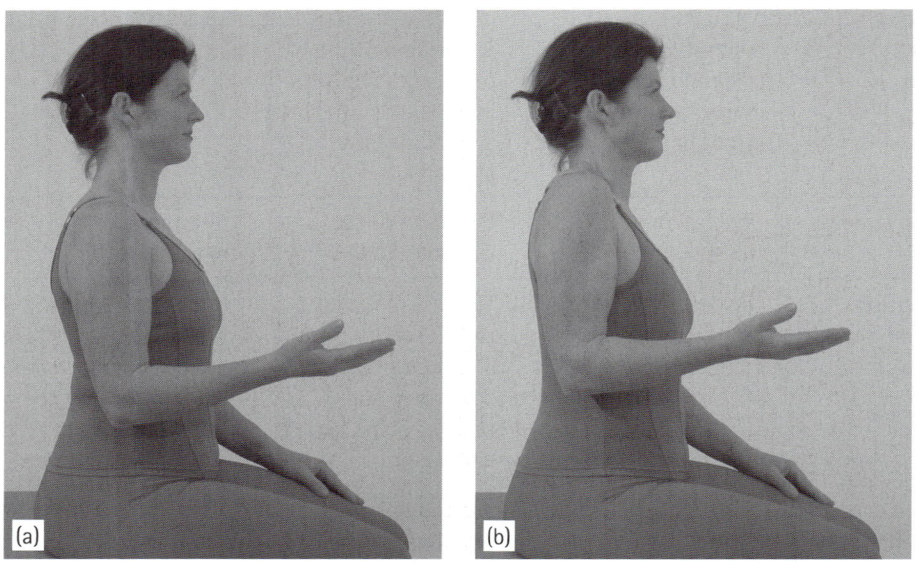

Figure 4.15a and b Area localization with symptomatic movement of the elbow into supination; differentiation between neural structures and elbow complex; alleviation. **a**, Starting position. **b**, End position.

Example 4: Pronation

Symptom area: lateral elbow
Symptom provocation: pronation of the forearm (Fig. 4.16)

With this clinical presentation, clinical experience suggests primarily the cervical spine, the shoulder complex, the elbow complex, and the neural structures as symptom-provoking areas.

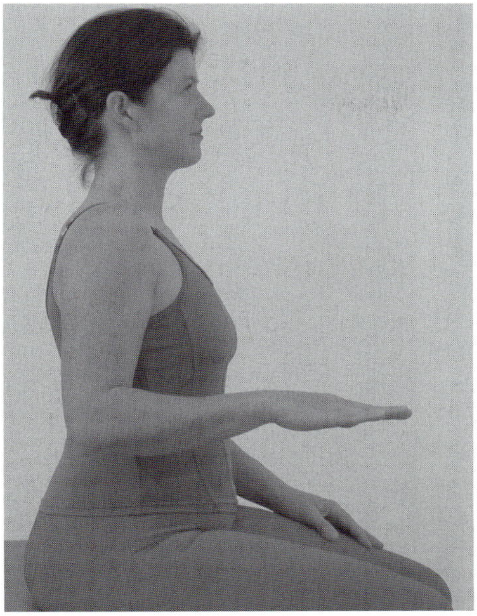

Figure 4.16 Symptom-provoking movement: movement of the elbow into pronation provokes pain in the area of the lateral elbow.

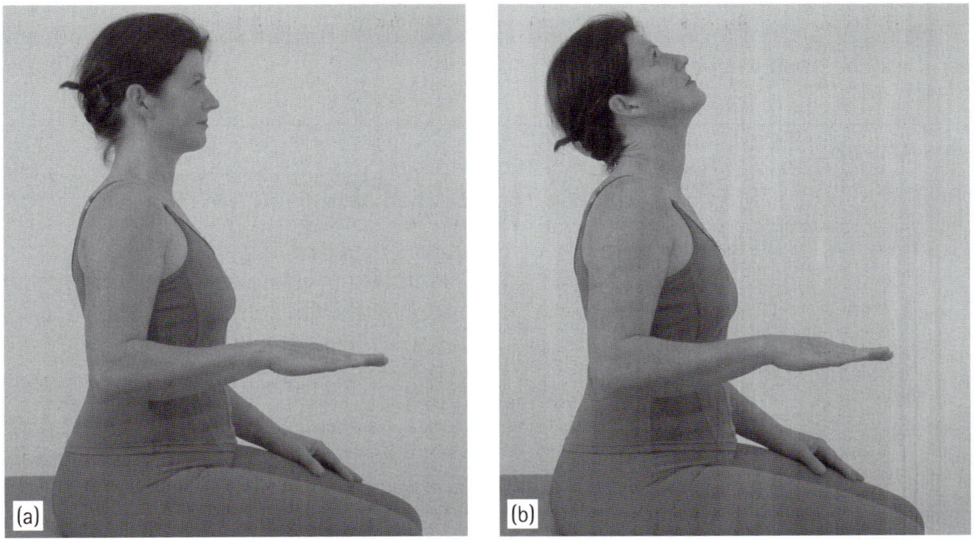

Figure 4.17a and b Area localization with symptomatic movement of the elbow into pronation; differentiation between cervical spine and elbow complex; provocation. a, Starting position. b, End position.

Below, examples illustrate how to differentiate between these areas. To this end, area localization is first attempted by means of active movements alone. If this is not possible, tests will be performed by means of assistive movements.

Hypothesis 1: The symptom-provoking area is the cervical spine

Differentiation: cervical spine vs. elbow complex.

The change in symptoms can be demonstrated exactly:

- provocation of pain (Fig. 4.17a and b, film 198)
- alleviation of pain (Fig. 4.18a and b, film 199).

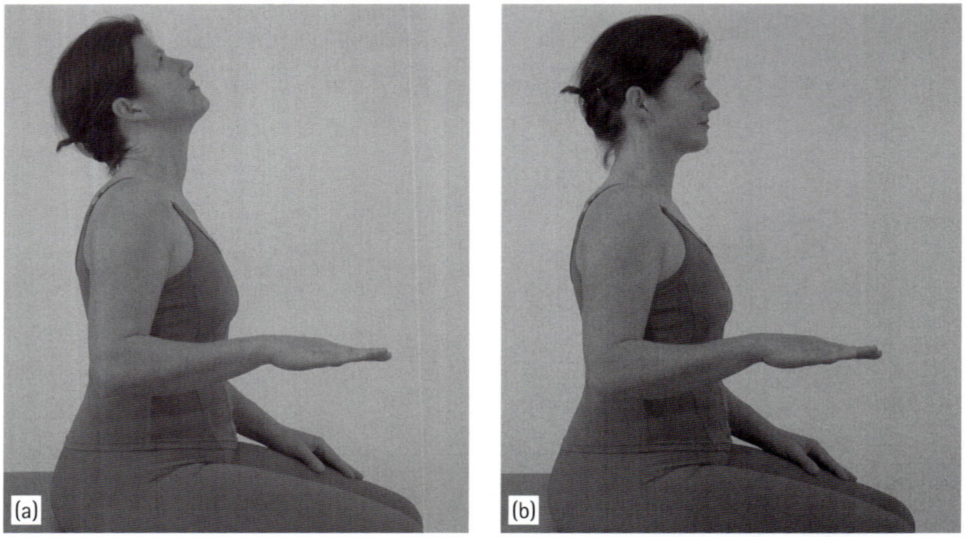

Figure 4.18a and b Area localization with symptomatic movement of the elbow into pronation; differentiation between cervical spine and elbow complex; alleviation. **a**, Starting position. **b**, End position.

The result of area localization has to be verified by further specific tests; otherwise the result will be open to question.

Assessment			
Goal	**Provocation of pain**	**Alleviation of pain**	**Remarks**
Starting position	Pronation of the forearm to a position immediately before symptoms appear	With the cervical spine pre-positioned in extension, pronation of the forearm to a position immediately after symptoms have appeared	
Test movement	Extension of the cervical spine	Moving the cervical spine back to neutral position	Elbow remains in starting position
Explanation	If by any movement of the cervical spine (here, as an example, extension) the typical symptoms are reproduced, an isolated lesion of the elbow is doubtful	If by any movement of the cervical spine (here, as an example, moving the cervical spine back to neutral position) the typical symptoms are alleviated, an isolated lesion of the elbow is doubtful	
Additional data to support	General and specific mobility of cervical spine and elbow complex (potential positive findings have to be found under neural relaxation as well)		

Goal	Provocation of pain	Alleviation of pain	Remarks
the hypothesis	History, symptom behaviour, type of complaints, 24-hour behaviour Palpation Reproducibility of test results Test treatment Imaging procedures (CT, MRI)		

Hypothesis 2: The symptom-provoking area is the neural structures
Differentiation: neural involvement vs. elbow complex.

The change in symptoms can be demonstrated exactly:

- provocation of pain (Fig. 4.19a and b, film 200)
- alleviation of pain (Fig. 4.20a and b, film 201).

The result of area localization has to be verified by further specific tests; otherwise the result will be open to question.

Assessment			
Goal	**Provocation of pain**	**Alleviation of pain**	**Remarks**
Starting position	Pronation of the forearm to a position immediately before symptoms appear	Pronation of the forearm to a position immediately after symptoms have appeared	
Test movement	Depression of the shoulder girdle	Elevation of the shoulder girdle	All other joints must not move
Explanation	The test movement produces mechanical stress on neural structures and structures associated with them	The test movement reduces mechanical stress on neural structures and structures associated with them	If the typical pain is provoked or alleviated by these manoeuvres without moving the forearm, this suggests at least an involvement of the neural structures
Additional data to support the hypothesis	Further movements of proximal and distal components to increase neural tension that are not directly involved in the painful movement of the elbow History, symptom behaviour, type of complaints, 24-hour behaviour Palpation Neurodynamic tests Nerve provocation tests (e.g., Spurling's test, Tinel's sign) Nerve palpation tests Reproducibility of test results Test treatment Imaging procedures (CT, MRI)		

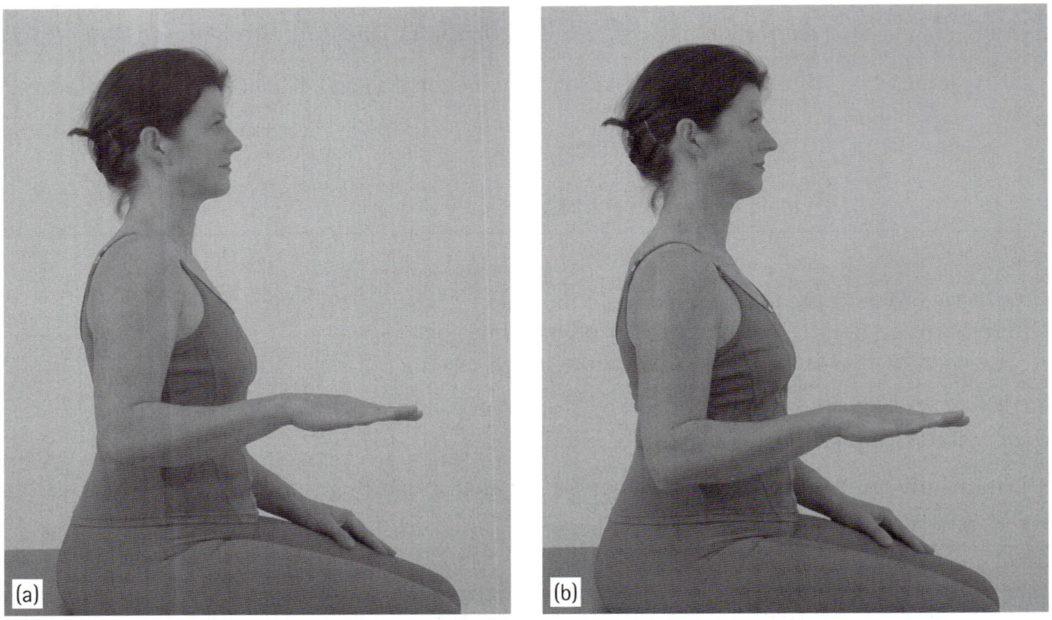

Figure 4.19a and b Area localization with symptomatic movement of the elbow into pronation; differentiation between neural structures and elbow complex; provocation. **a**, Starting position. **b**, End position.

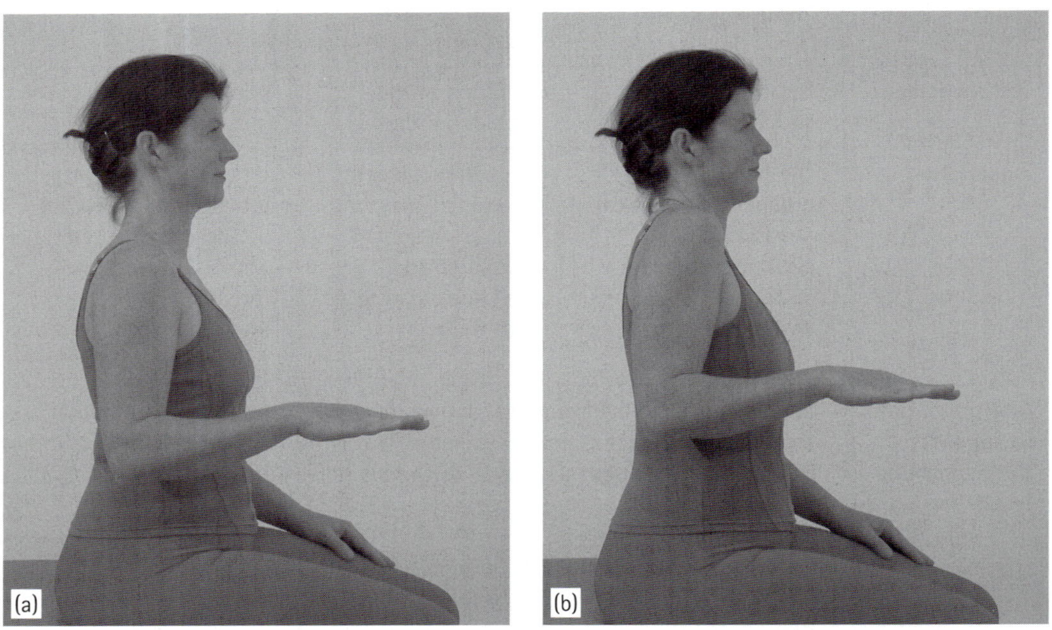

Figure 4.20a and b Area localization with symptomatic movement of the elbow into pronation; differentiation between neural structures and elbow complex; alleviation. **a**, Starting position. **b**, End position.

QUICK CHECK – SYMPTOMS, LATERAL ELBOW

If neither the area nor a symptom-provoking or symptom-reducing action is known, the quick check is used to try to load individual potential areas with specific biomechanically provocative movement combinations. The chosen movement combinations correspond with the straining and often symptom-provoking movements of the individual sections.

CERVICAL SPINE

Movement

- Extension/lateral flexion, and rotation to the opposite side (Figs 4.21 and 4.22, film 15)
- Extension/lateral flexion, and rotation to the same side (Figs 4.23 and 4.24, film 15).

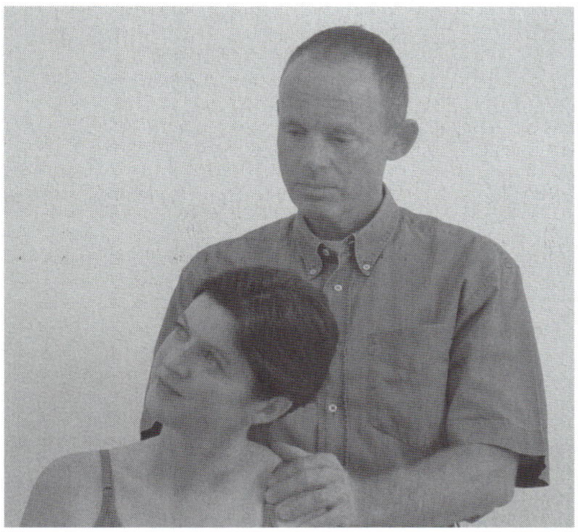

Figure 4.21 Quick check cervical spine; lateral flexion to the left with rotation to the opposite side.

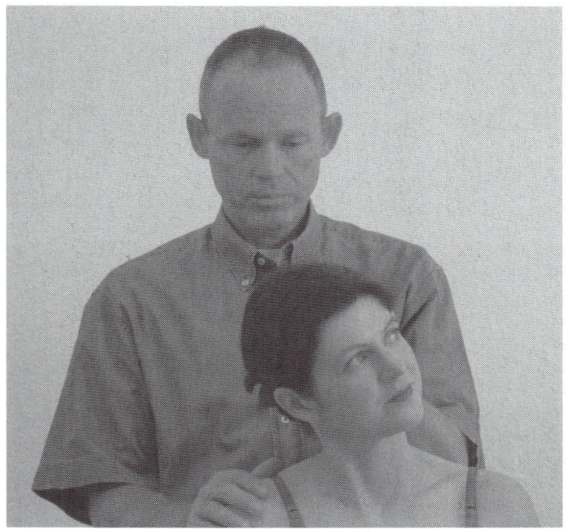

Figure 4.22 Quick check cervical spine; lateral flexion to the right with rotation to the opposite side.

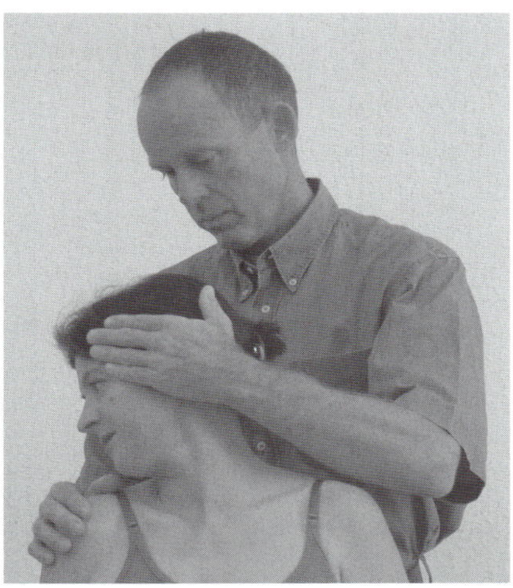

Figure 4.23 Quick check cervical spine; lateral flexion to the right with rotation to the same side.

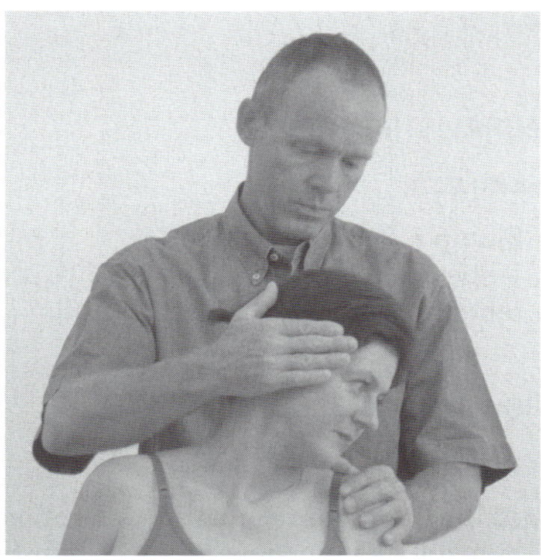

Figure 4.24 Quick check cervical spine; lateral flexion to the left with rotation to the same side.

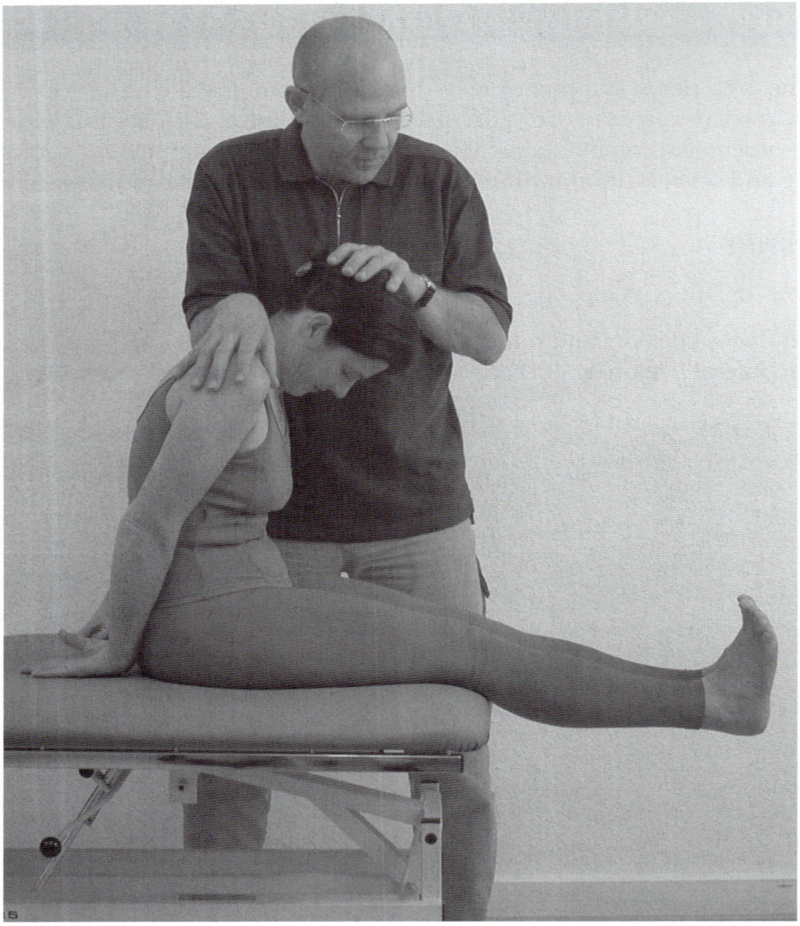

Figure 4.25 Quick check neurodynamics; slump test.

NEURAL STRUCTURES

Tension tests

- Slump test (Fig. 4.25, film 16)
- Upper limb neurodynamic test 1 (ULNT-1; Fig. 4.26, film 17)
- Straight leg raise (SLR; Fig. 4.27, film 18).

SHOULDER COMPLEX

Movement

- Abduction/internal rotation/elevation (Fig. 4.28, film 108)
- Horizontal adduction (Fig. 4.29, film 109)
- Extension/adduction/internal rotation (Fig. 4.30, film 110)
- With 90° abduction, maximum internal rotation (Fig. 4.31, film 111).

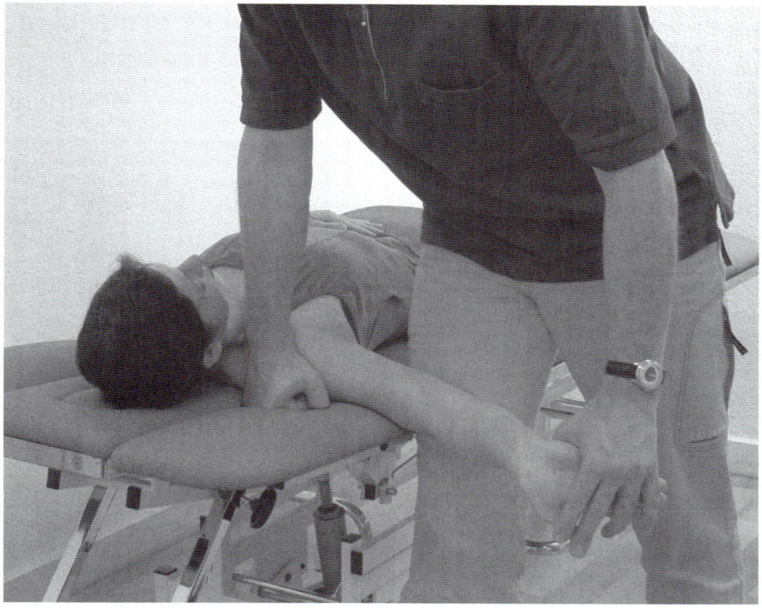

Figure 4.26 Quick check neurodynamics; upper limb tension test 1.

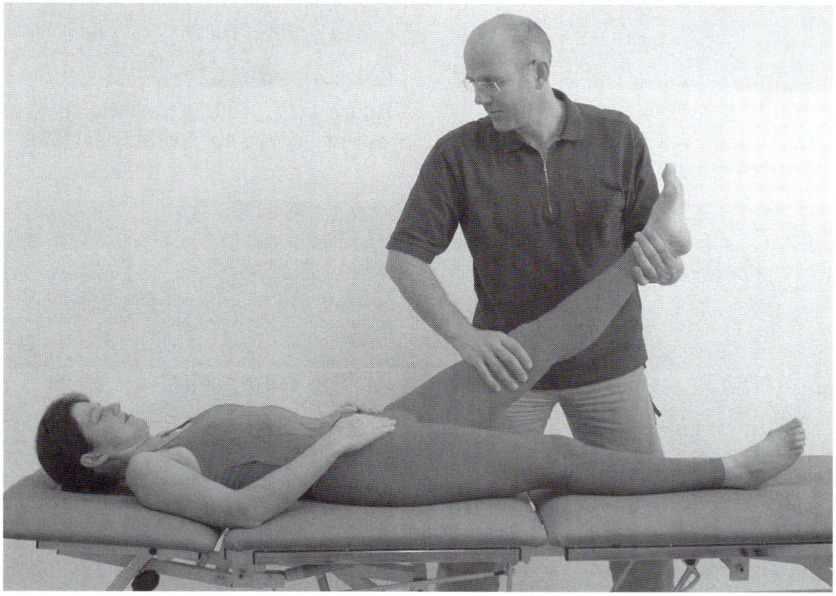

Figure 4.27 Quick check neurodynamics; straight leg raise test.

ELBOW COMPLEX

Movement

- Extension/supination (Fig. 4.32, film 249)
- Flexion/pronation (Fig. 4.33, film 250).

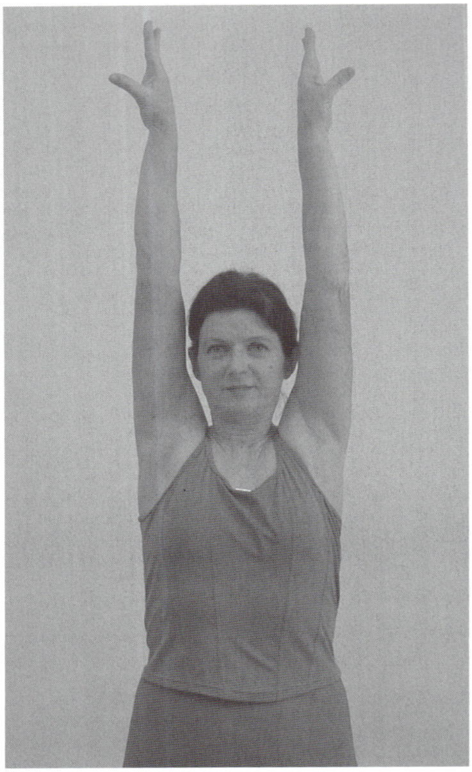

Figure 4.28 Quick check shoulder complex; movement into abduction/elevation, with previously adjusted internal rotation.

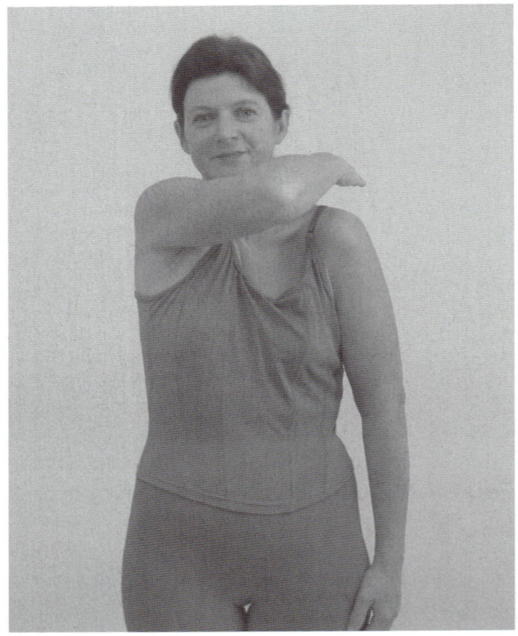

Figure 4.29 Quick check shoulder complex; movement into horizontal adduction.

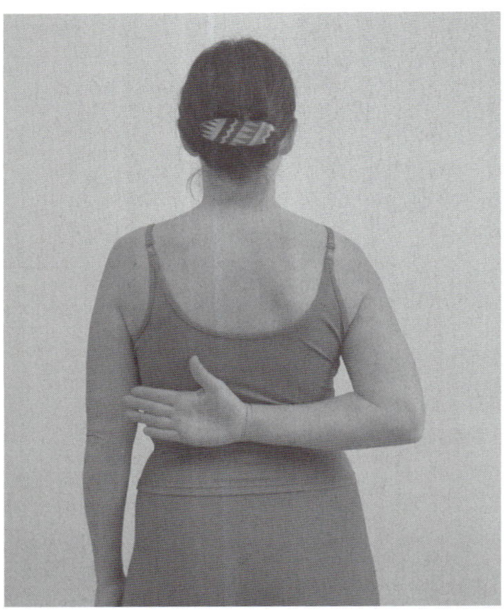

Figure 4.30 Quick check shoulder complex; movement into extension/adduction/internal rotation.

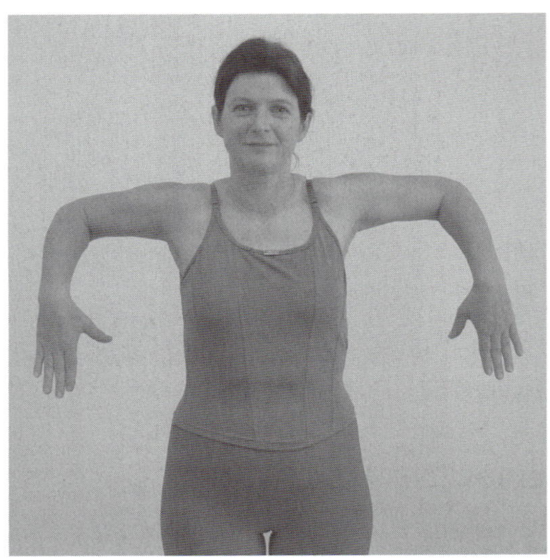

Figure 4.31 Quick check shoulder complex; movement into internal rotation, with previously adjusted abduction.

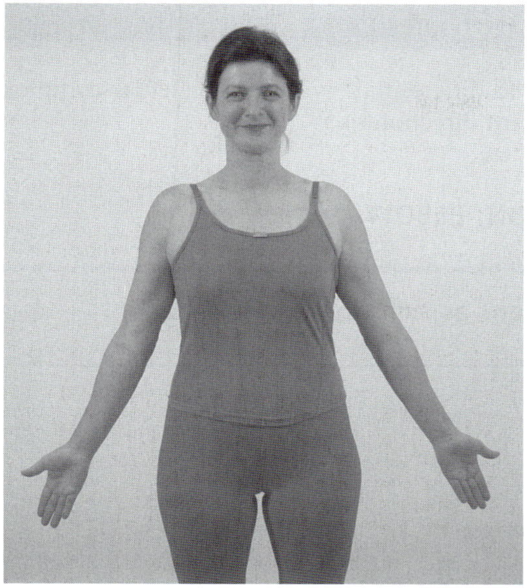

Figure 4.32 Quick check elbow complex; movement into extension, with previously adjusted supination.

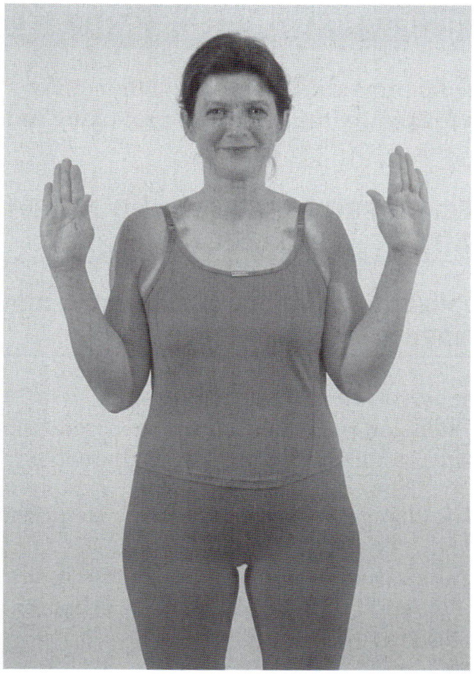

Figure 4.33 Quick check elbow complex; movement into flexion, with previously adjusted pronation.

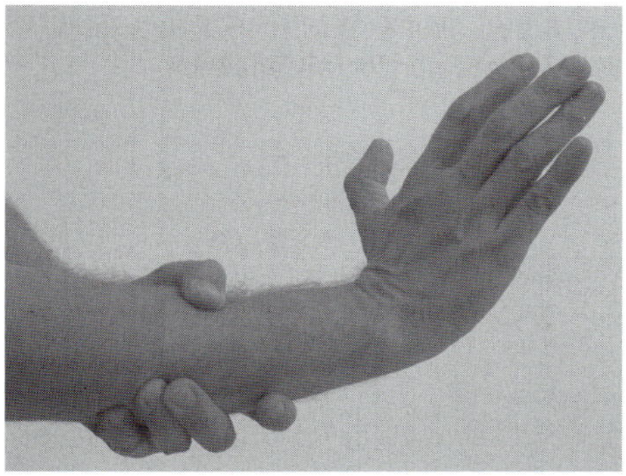

Figure 4.34 Quick check hand complex; movement into dorsal flexion and radial abduction.

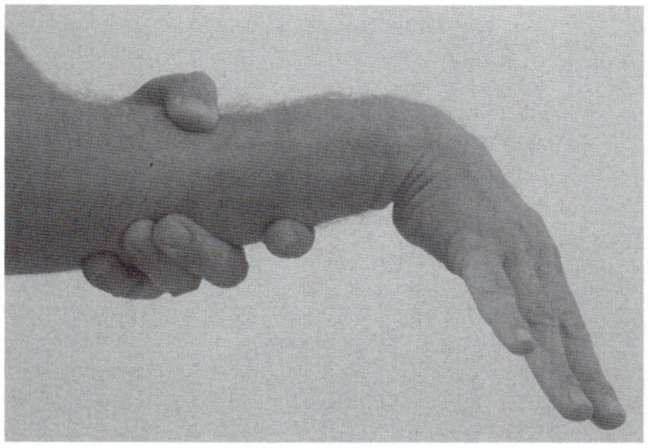

Figure 4.35 Quick check hand complex; movement into volar flexion and ulnar abduction.

HAND COMPLEX

Movement

- Dorsal flexion/radial abduction (Fig. 4.34, film 251)
- Volar flexion/ulnar abduction (Fig. 4.35, film 251).

Note: Even an area that proves negative in the quick check may possibly be symptom-provoking (another movement combination, or passive overpressure may be required).

SPECIFIC PROVOCATION AND ALLEVIATION

Specific provocation and alleviation allows one to differentiate within an articular complex and to identify the symptom-provoking movement direction(s).

SPECIFIC PROVOCATION AND ALLEVIATION, ELBOW COMPLEX – EXTENSION

Localization, humeroradial joint – movement as symptom-provoking component

Pain-provoking movement (Fig. 4.36)

- Extension provokes pain in the lateral elbow.
- Area localization hints at the elbow complex.

The change in symptoms can be demonstrated exactly:

- provocation of pain (Fig. 4.37a and b, film 134)
- alleviation of pain (Fig. 4.38a and b, film 135).

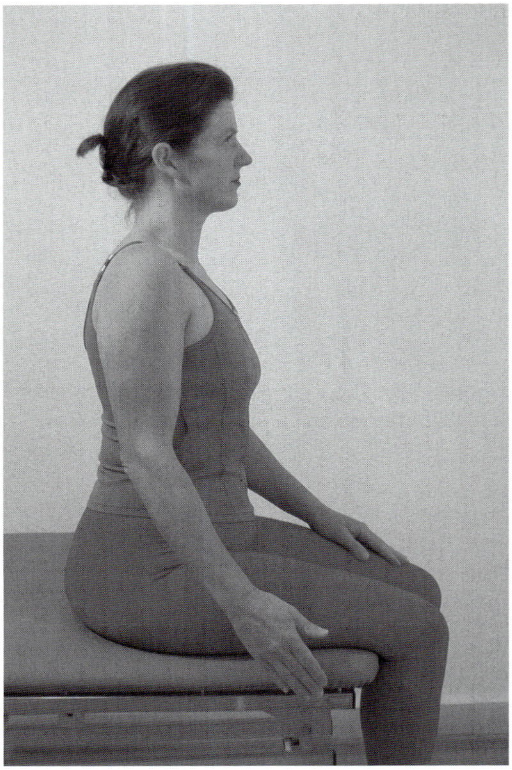

Figure 4.36 Symptom-provoking movement: movement of the elbow into extension provokes pain in the area of the lateral elbow.

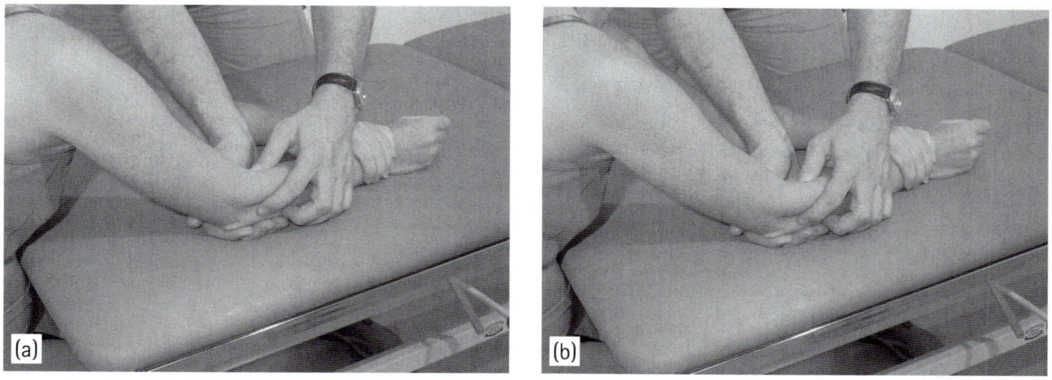

Figure 4.37a and b Specific provocation and alleviation in the area of the humeroradial joint with symptomatic movement of the elbow into extension; movement as symptom-provoking component; provocation. **a**, Starting position. **b**, End position.

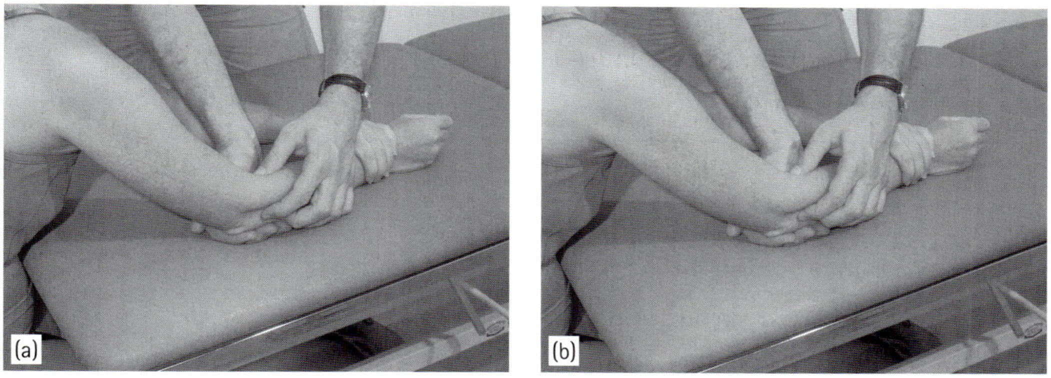

Figure 4.38a and b Specific provocation and alleviation in the area of the humeroradial joint with symptomatic movement of the elbow into extension; movement as symptom-provoking component; alleviation. **a**, Starting position. **b**, End position.

Assessment

Goal	Provocation of pain	Alleviation of pain	Remarks
Starting position	Extension to a position immediately before symptoms appear	Extension to a position immediately after symptoms have appeared	
Test movement	Radius moves in posterior direction, with fixed humerus	Radius moves in anterior direction, with fixed humerus	

Goal	Provocation of pain	Alleviation of pain	Remarks
Neural involvement	Proximal and/or distal component without change of position in the relevant area	Proximal and/or distal component without change of position in the relevant area	
Explanation	If the symptoms are provoked by movement of the radius in posterior direction, symptoms are increased by this manoeuvre, both with intra-articular and with extra-articular dysfunctions	If the symptoms are alleviated by movement of the radius in anterior direction, symptoms are reduced by this manoeuvre, both with intra-articular and with extra-articular dysfunctions	
Additional data to support the hypothesis	General and specific mobility of the elbow History, symptom behaviour, type of complaints, 24-hour behaviour Specific palpation Reproducibility of test results Test treatment Imaging procedures (CT, MRI)		

Differentiation, humeroradial joint – intra-articular vs. extra-articular (symptom provocation by an intra-articular component)

The change in symptoms can be demonstrated exactly:

- provocation of pain (Fig. 4.39a and b, film 136)
- alleviation of pain (Fig. 4.40a and b, film 137).

Assessment			
Goal	**Provocation of pain**	**Alleviation of pain**	**Remarks**
Starting position	Extension to a position immediately after symptoms have appeared	Extension to a position immediately after symptoms have appeared	Since, with pre-positioning to a position before symptoms appear, non-symptomatic parts of the affected joint may be compressed, a symptomatic position is chosen also for provocation
Test movement	Radius moves proximally, with fixed humerus	Radius moves distally, with fixed humerus	

Goal	Provocation of pain	Alleviation of pain	Remarks
Neural involvement	Proximal and/or distal component without change of position in the relevant area	Proximal and/or distal component without change of position in the relevant area	
Explanation	This manoeuvre increases intra-articular compression in pain-provoking position	This manoeuvre reduces intra-articular compression in pain-provoking position	
Additional data to support the hypothesis	General and specific mobility of the elbow History, symptom behaviour, type of complaints, 24-hour behaviour Specific palpation Reproducibility of test results Test treatment Imaging procedures (CT, MRI)		

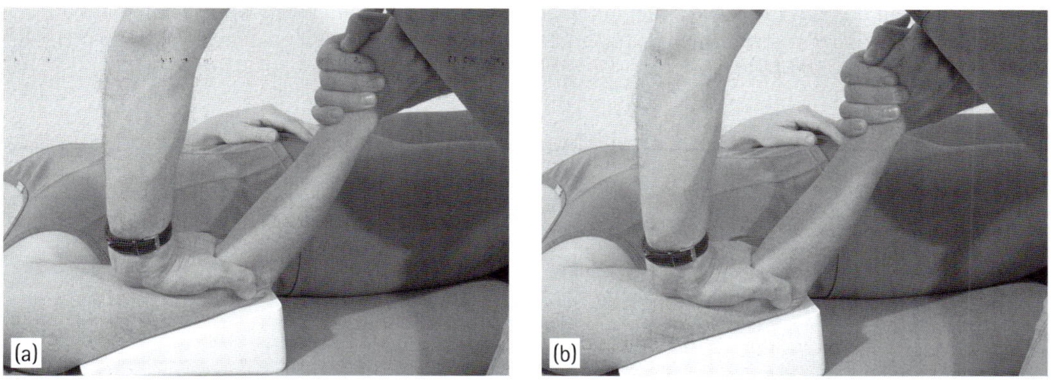

Figure 4.39a and b Specific provocation and alleviation in the area of the humeroradial joint with symptomatic movement of the elbow into extension; intra-articular mechanism as symptom-provoking component; provocation. **a**, Starting position. **b**, End position.

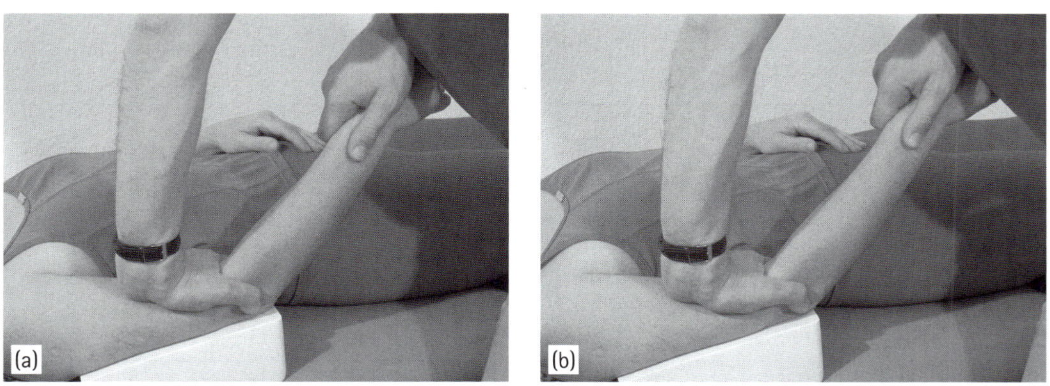

Figure 4.40a and b Specific provocation and alleviation in the area of the humeroradial joint with symptomatic movement of the elbow into extension; intra-articular mechanism as symptom-provoking component; alleviation. **a**, Starting position. **b**, End position.

Differentiation, humeroradial joint – extra-articular vs. intra-articular (symptom provocation by an extra-articular component)

The change in symptoms can be demonstrated exactly:

- provocation of pain (Fig. 4.41a and b, film 138).

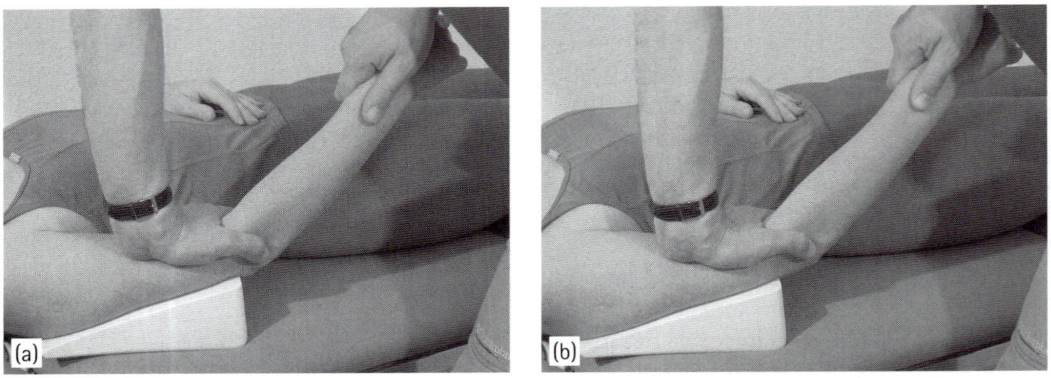

Figure 4.41a and b Specific provocation in the area of the humeroradial joint with symptomatic movement of the elbow into extension; extra-articular mechanism as symptom-provoking component. **a**, Starting position. **b**, End position.

Assessment

Goal	Provocation of pain	Alleviation of pain	Remarks
Starting position	Extension to a position immediately after symptoms have appeared	None	
Test movement	Radius moves distally, with fixed humerus	None	Usually, alleviation is not possible, as approximation of the joint surfaces seems too little for relaxation of the extra-articular structures
Neural involvement	Proximal and/or distal component without change of position in the relevant area	None	
Explanation	This manoeuvre increases the extra-articular tractive forces		
Additional data to support	General and specific mobility of the elbow History, symptom behaviour, type of complaints, 24-hour behaviour		

Goal	Provocation of pain	Alleviation of pain	Remarks
the hypothesis	Specific palpation Reproducibility of test results Test treatment Imaging procedures (CT, MRI)		

Differentiation, humero-ulnar joint – intra-articular vs. extra-articular (symptom provocation by an intra-articular component – central aspect)

The change in symptoms can be demonstrated exactly:

- provocation of pain (Fig. 4.42a and b, film 139)
- alleviation of pain (Fig. 4.43a and b, film 140).

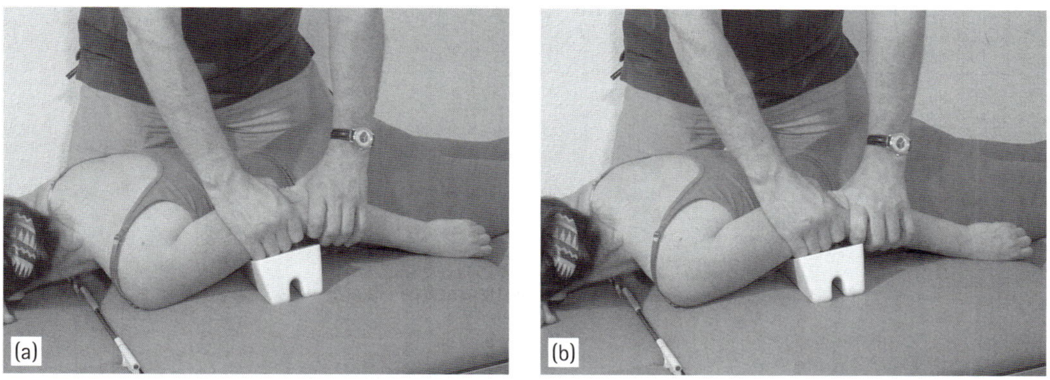

Figure 4.42a and b Specific provocation and alleviation in the area of the humero-ulnar joint with symptomatic movement of the elbow into extension; intra-articular mechanism in the central part of the joint as symptom-provoking component; provocation. **a**, Starting position. **b**, End position.

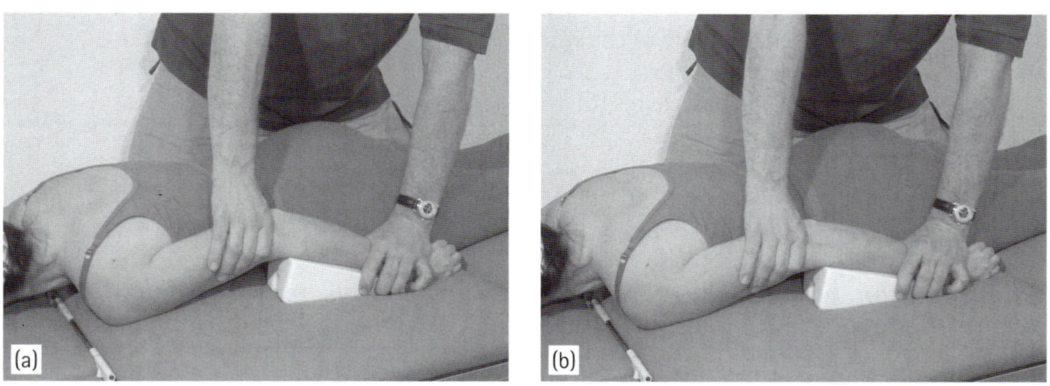

Figure 4.43a and b Specific provocation and alleviation in the area of the humero-ulnar joint with symptomatic movement of the elbow into extension; intra-articular mechanism in the central part of the joint as symptom-provoking component; alleviation. **a**, Starting position. **b**, End position.

Assessment			
Goal	**Provocation of pain**	**Alleviation of pain**	**Remarks**
Starting position	Extension to a position immediately after symptoms have appeared	Extension to a position immediately after symptoms have appeared	Since, with pre-positioning to a position before symptoms appear, non-symptomatic parts of the affected joint may be compressed, a symptomatic position is chosen also for provocation
Test movement	Compression in the humero-ulnar joint vertical to the treatment plane	Traction in the humero-ulnar joint vertical to the treatment plane	
Neural involvement	Proximal and/or distal component without change of position in the relevant area	Proximal and/or distal component without change of position in the relevant area	
Explanation	This manoeuvre increases the intra-articular compression forces in the central part of the joint	This manoeuvre reduces the intra-articular compression forces in the central part of the joint	
Additional data to support the hypothesis	General and specific mobility of the elbow History, symptom behaviour, type of complaints, 24-hour behaviour Specific palpation Reproducibility of test results Test treatment Imaging procedures (CT, MRI)		

Differentiation, humero-ulnar joint – intra-articular vs. extra-articular (symptom provocation by an intra-articular component – posterior aspect)

The change in symptoms can be demonstrated exactly:

- provocation of pain (Fig. 4.44a and b, film 141)
- alleviation of pain (Fig. 4.45a and b, film 142).

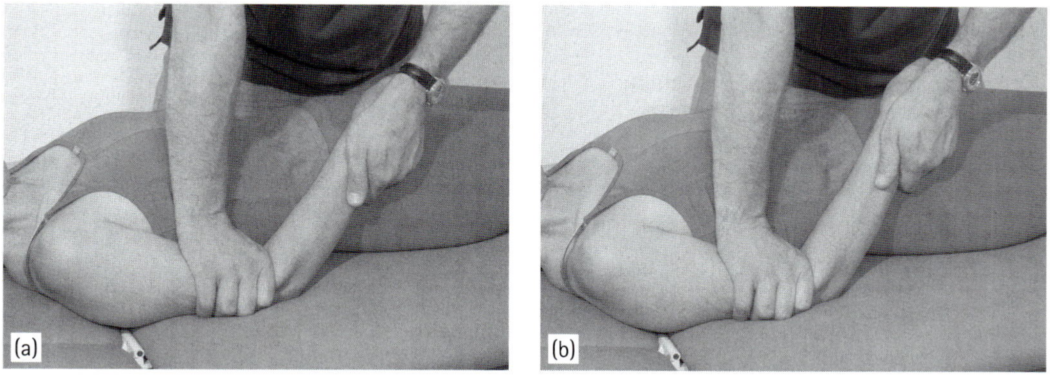

Figure 4.44a and b Specific provocation and alleviation in the area of the humero-ulnar joint with symptomatic movement of the elbow into extension; intra-articular mechanism in the posterior aspect of the joint as symptom-provoking component; provocation. **a**, Starting position. **b**, End position.

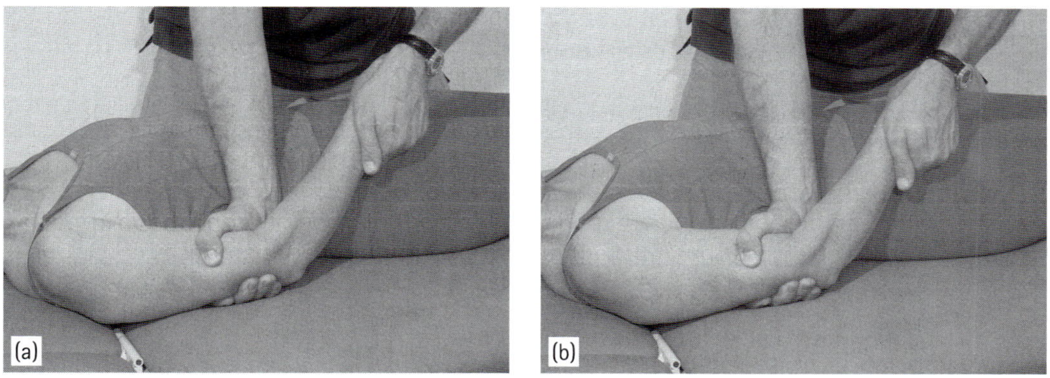

Figure 4.45a and b Specific provocation and alleviation in the area of the humero-ulnar joint with symptomatic movement of the elbow into extension; intra-articular mechanism in the posterior aspect of the joint as symptom-provoking component; alleviation. **a**, Starting position. **b**, End position.

Assessment

Goal	Provocation of pain	Alleviation of pain	Remarks
Starting position	Extension to a position immediately after symptoms have appeared	Extension to a position immediately after symptoms have appeared	Since, with pre-positioning to a position before symptoms appear, non-symptomatic parts of the affected joint may be compressed, a symptomatic position is chosen also for provocation

Goal	Provocation of pain	Alleviation of pain	Remarks
Test movement	Ulna moves distally, with fixed humerus	Ulna moves proximally, with fixed humerus	
Neural involvement	Proximal and/or distal component without change of position in the relevant area	Proximal and/or distal component without change of position in the relevant area	
Explanation	This manoeuvre increases the intra-articular compression forces in the posterior part of the joint	This manoeuvre reduces the intra-articular compression forces in the posterior part of the joint	
Additional data to support the hypothesis	General and specific mobility of the elbow History, symptom behaviour, type of complaints, 24-hour behaviour Specific palpation Reproducibility of test results Test treatment Imaging procedures (CT, MRI)		

Differentiation, humero-ulnar joint – intra-articular vs. extra-articular (symptom provocation by an intra-articular component – anterior aspect)

The change in symptoms can be demonstrated exactly:

- provocation of pain (Fig. 4.46a and b, film 143)
- alleviation of pain (Fig. 4.47a and b, film 144).

Assessment			
Goal	Provocation of pain	Alleviation of pain	Remarks
Starting position	Extension to a position immediately after symptoms have appeared	Extension to a position immediately after symptoms have appeared	Since, with pre-positioning to a position before symptoms appear, non-symptomatic parts of the affected joint may be compressed, a symptomatic position is chosen also for provocation
Test movement	Ulna moves proximally, with fixed humerus	Ulna moves distally, with fixed humerus	
Neural involvement	Proximal and/or distal component without	Proximal and/or distal component without	

Goal	Provocation of pain	Alleviation of pain	Remarks
	change of position in the relevant area	change of position in the relevant area	
Explanation	This manoeuvre increases the intra-articular compression forces in the anterior part of the joint	This manoeuvre reduces the intra-articular compression forces in the anterior part of the joint	
Additional data to support the hypothesis	General and specific mobility of the elbow History, symptom behaviour, type of complaints, 24-hour behaviour Specific palpation Reproducibility of test results Test treatment Imaging procedures (CT, MRI)		

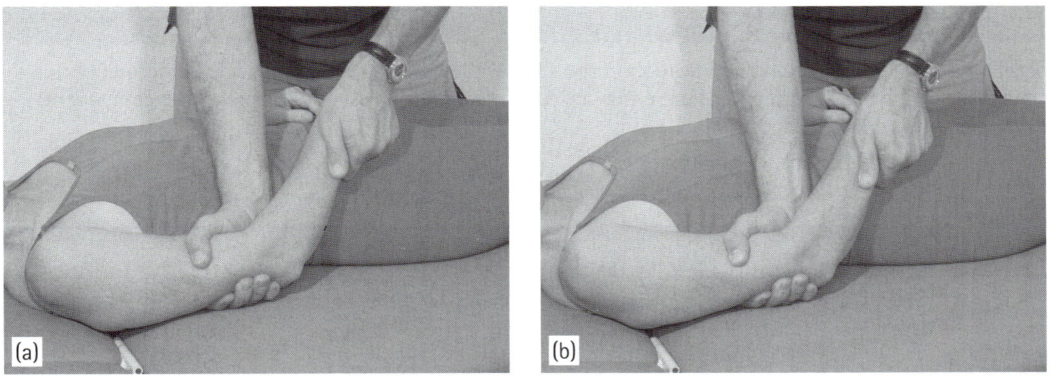

Figure 4.46a and b Specific provocation and alleviation in the area of the humero-ulnar joint with symptomatic movement of the elbow into extension; intra-articular mechanism in the anterior aspect of the joint as symptom-provoking component; provocation. **a**, Starting position. **b**, End position.

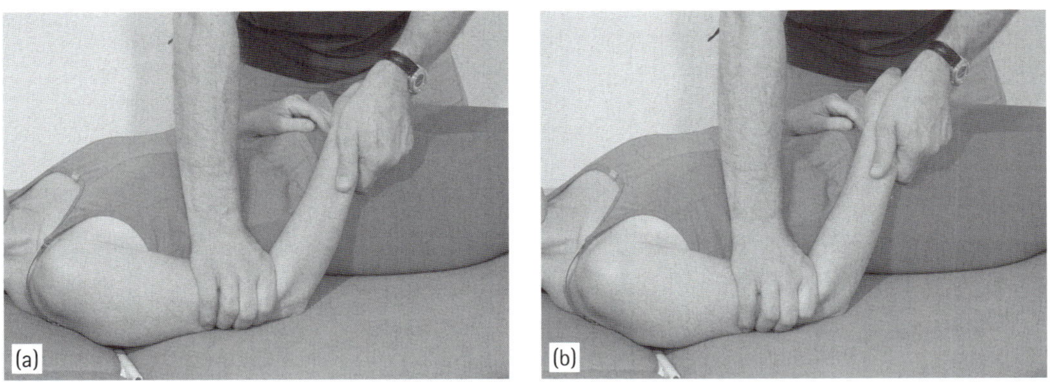

Figure 4.47a and b Specific provocation and alleviation in the area of the humero-ulnar joint with symptomatic movement of the elbow into extension; intra-articular mechanism in the anterior aspect of the joint as symptom-provoking component; alleviation. **a**, Starting position. **b**, End position.

Differentiation, humero-ulnar joint – intra-articular vs. extra-articular (symptom provocation by an extra-articular component)

The change in symptoms can be demonstrated exactly:

- provocation of pain (Fig. 4.48a and b, film 145).

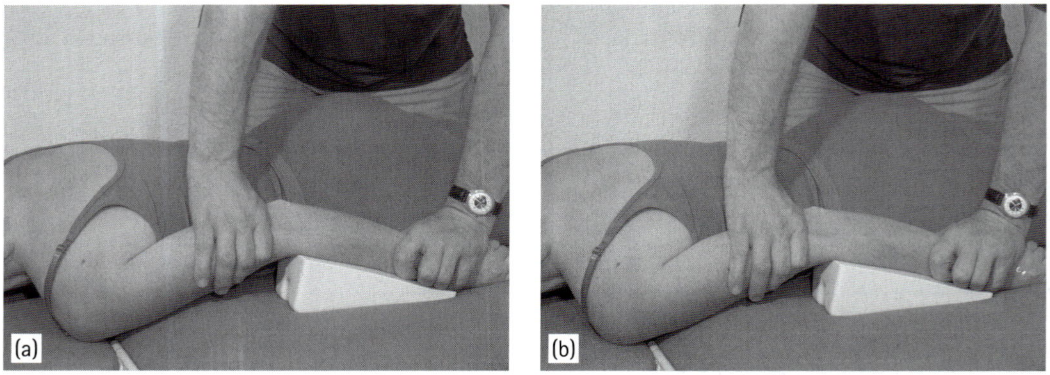

Figure 4.48a and b Specific provocation in the area of the humero-ulnar joint with symptomatic movement of the elbow into extension; extra-articular mechanism as symptom-provoking component. a, Starting position. b, End position.

Assessment

Goal	Provocation of pain	Alleviation of pain	Remarks
Starting position	Extension to a position exactly when symptoms appear	None	
Test movement	Traction in the humero-ulnar joint vertical to the treatment plane	None	Usually, alleviation is not possible, as approximation of the joint surfaces seems too little for relaxation of the extra-articular structures
Neural involvement	Proximal and/or distal component without change of position in the relevant area		
Explanation	This manoeuvre increases the extra-articular tractive forces		An extra-articular lesion is assumed when the intra-articular differentiation is negative

Goal	Provocation of pain	Alleviation of pain	Remarks
Additional data to support the hypothesis	General and specific mobility of the elbow History, symptom behaviour, type of complaints, 24-hour behaviour Specific palpation Reproducibility of test results Test treatment Imaging procedures (CT, MRI)		

SPECIFIC PROVOCATION AND ALLEVIATION, ELBOW COMPLEX – FLEXION

Localization, humeroradial joint – movement as symptom-provoking component

Pain-provoking movement (Fig. 4.49)

- Flexion provokes pain in the lateral elbow.
- Area localization hints at the elbow complex.

The change in symptoms can be demonstrated exactly:

- provocation of pain (Fig. 4.50a and b, film 177)
- alleviation of pain (Fig. 4.51a and b, film 178).

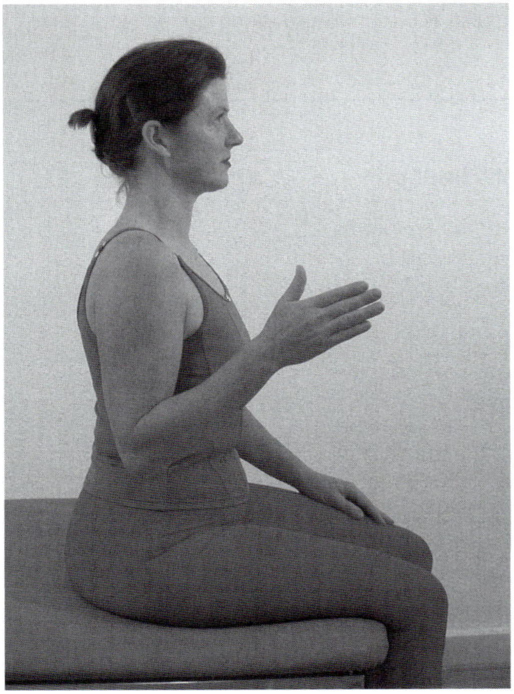

Figure 4.49 Symptom-provoking movement: movement of the elbow into flexion provokes pain in the area of the lateral elbow.

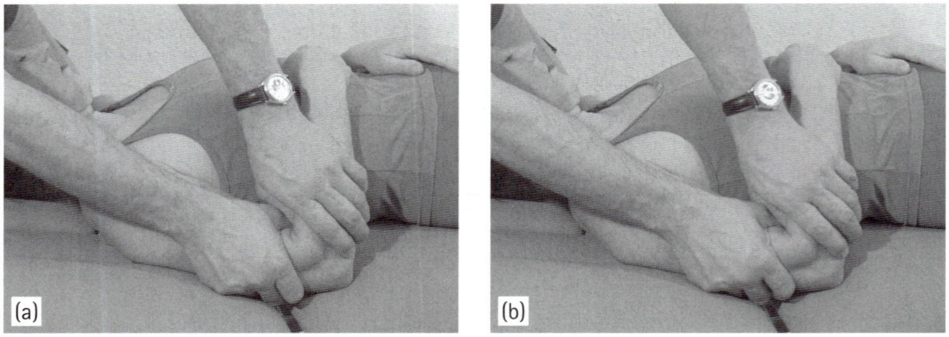

Figure 4.50a and b Specific provocation and alleviation in the area of the humeroradial joint with symptomatic movement of the elbow into flexion; movement as symptom-provoking component; provocation. **a**, Starting position. **b**, End position.

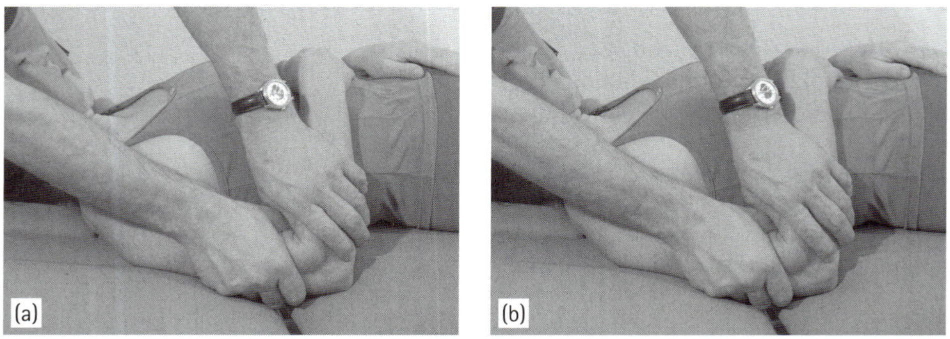

Figure 4.51a and b Specific provocation and alleviation in the area of the humeroradial joint with symptomatic movement of the elbow into flexion; movement as symptom-provoking component; alleviation. **a**, Starting position. **b**, End position.

Assessment

Goal	Provocation of pain	Alleviation of pain	Remarks
Starting position	Flexion to a position immediately before symptoms appear	Flexion to a position immediately after symptoms have appeared	
Test movement	Radius moves in anterior direction, with fixed humerus	Radius moves in posterior direction, with fixed humerus	
Neural involvement	Proximal and/or distal component without change of position in the relevant area	Proximal and/or distal component without change of position in the relevant area	
Explanation	If the symptoms are provoked by movement of the radius in anterior direction, symptoms are	If the symptoms are alleviated by movement of the radius in posterior direction, symptoms are	

Goal	Provocation of pain	Alleviation of pain	Remarks
	increased by this manoeuvre, both with intra-articular and with extra-articular dysfunctions	reduced by this manoeuvre, both with intra-articular and with extra-articular dysfunctions	
Additional data to support the hypothesis	General and specific mobility of the elbow History, symptom behaviour, type of complaints, 24-hour behaviour Specific palpation Reproducibility of test results Test treatment Imaging procedures (CT, MRI)		

Differentiation, humeroradial joint – intra-articular vs. extra-articular (symptom provocation by an intra-articular component)

The change in symptoms can be demonstrated exactly:

- provocation of pain (Fig. 4.52a and b, film 179)
- alleviation of pain (Fig. 4.53a and b, film 252).

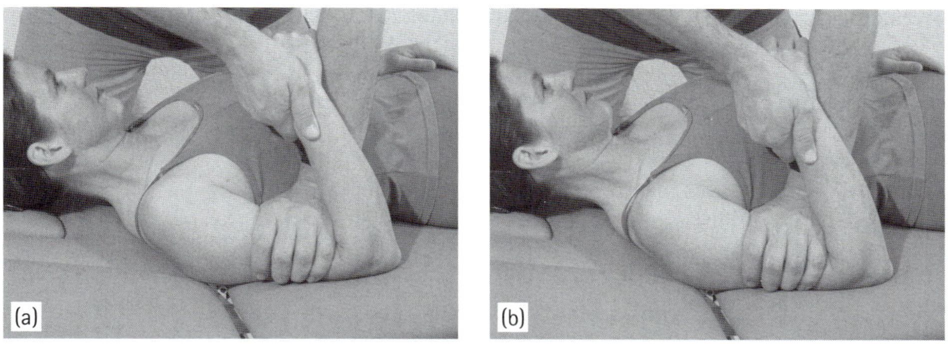

Figure 4.52a and b Specific provocation and alleviation in the area of the humeroradial joint with symptomatic movement of the elbow into flexion; intra-articular mechanism as symptom-provoking component; provocation. **a**, Starting position. **b**, End position.

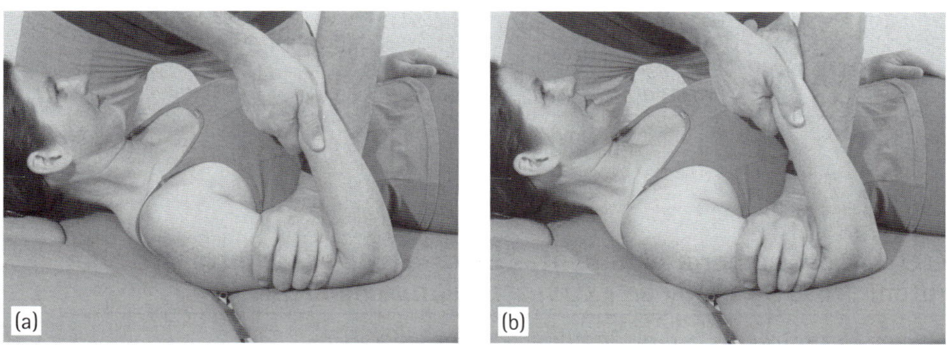

Figure 4.53a and b Specific provocation and alleviation in the area of the humeroradial joint with symptomatic movement of the elbow into flexion; intra-articular mechanism as symptom-provoking component; alleviation. **a**, Starting position. **b**, End position.

Assessment			
Goal	Provocation of pain	Alleviation of pain	Remarks
Starting position	Flexion to a position immediately after symptoms have appeared	Flexion to a position immediately after symptoms have appeared	Since, with pre-positioning to a position before symptoms appear, non-symptomatic parts of the affected joint may be compressed, a symptomatic position is chosen also for provocation
Test movement	Radius moves proximally, with fixed humerus	Radius moves distally, with fixed humerus	
Neural involvement	Proximal and/or distal component without change of position in the relevant area	Proximal and/or distal component without change of position in the relevant area	
Explanation	This manoeuvre increases the intra-articular compression in pain-provoking position	This manoeuvre reduces the intra-articular compression in pain-provoking position	
Additional data to support the hypothesis	General and specific mobility of the elbow History, symptom behaviour, type of complaints, 24-hour behaviour Specific palpation Reproducibility of test results Test treatment Imaging procedures (CT, MRI)		

Differentiation, humeroradial joint – extra-articular vs. intra-articular (symptom provocation by an extra-articular component)

The change in symptoms can be demonstrated exactly:

- provocation of pain (Fig. 4.54a and b, film 253).

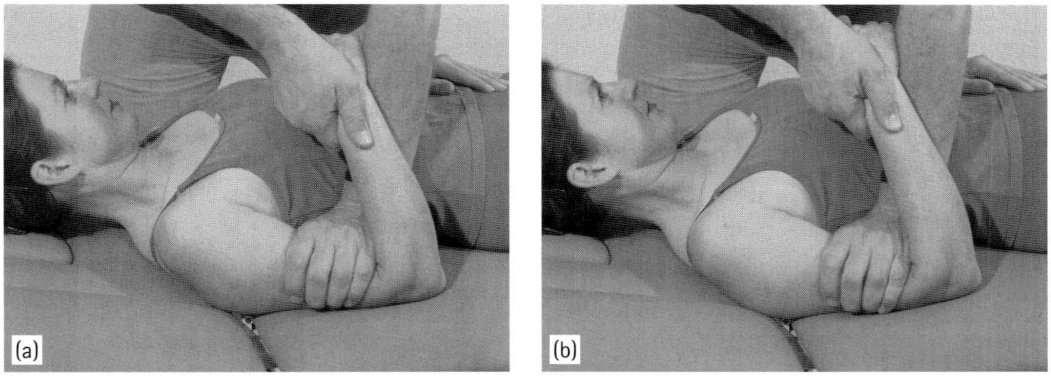

Figure 4.54a and b Specific provocation in the area of the humeroradial joint with symptomatic movement of the elbow into flexion; extra-articular mechanism as symptom-provoking component. a, Starting position. b, End position.

Assessment			
Goal	**Provocation of pain**	**Alleviation of pain**	**Remarks**
Starting position	Flexion to a position immediately after symptoms have appeared	None	
Test movement	Radius moves distally, with fixed humerus	None	Usually, alleviation is not possible, as approximation of the joint surfaces seems too little for relaxation of the extra-articular structures
Neural involvement	Proximal and/or distal component without change of position in the relevant area	None	
Explanation	This manoeuvre increases the extra-articular tractive forces		An extra-articular lesion is assumed when intra-articular differentiation is negative
Additional data to support the hypothesis	General and specific mobility of the elbow History, symptom behaviour, type of complaints, 24-hour behaviour Specific palpation Reproducibility of test results Test treatment Imaging procedures (CT, MRI)		

Differentiation, humero-ulnar joint – intra-articular vs. extra-articular (symptom provocation by an intra-articular component – central aspect)

The change in symptoms can be demonstrated exactly:

- provocation of pain (Fig. 4.55a and b, film 180)
- alleviation of pain (Fig. 4.56a and b, film 181).

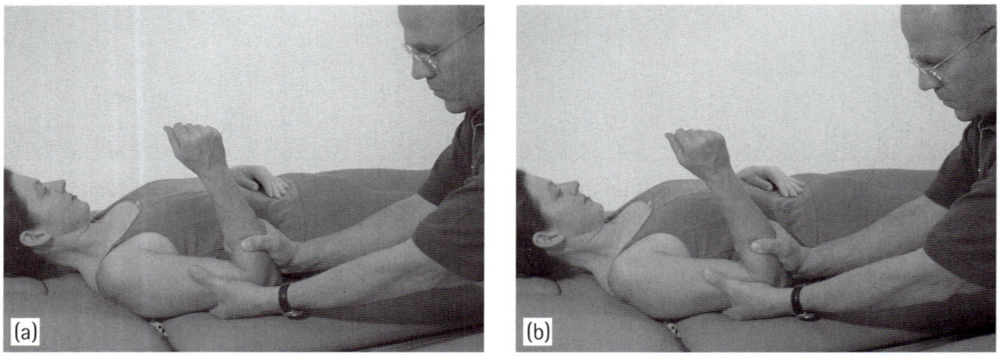

Figure 4.55a and b Specific provocation and alleviation in the area of the humero-ulnar joint with symptomatic movement of the elbow into flexion; intra-articular mechanism in the central aspect of the joint as symptom-provoking component; provocation. **a**, Starting position. **b**, End position.

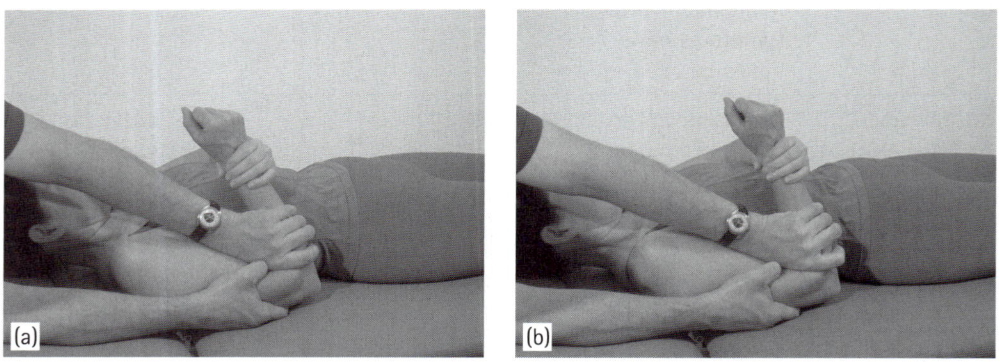

Figure 4.56a and b Specific provocation and alleviation in the area of the humero-ulnar joint with symptomatic movement of the elbow into flexion; intra-articular mechanism in the central aspect of the joint as symptom-provoking component; alleviation. **a**, Starting position. **b**, End position.

Assessment

Goal	Provocation of pain	Alleviation of pain	Remarks
Starting position	Flexion to a position immediately after symptoms have appeared	Flexion to a position immediately after symptoms have appeared	Since, with pre-positioning to a position before symptoms appear, non-symptomatic parts of the affected joint may be compressed, a symptomatic

Goal	Provocation of pain	Alleviation of pain	Remarks
			position is chosen also for provocation
Test movement	Compression in the humero-ulnar joint vertical to the treatment plane	Traction in the humero-ulnar joint vertical to the treatment plane	
Neural involvement	Proximal and/or distal component without change of position in the relevant area	Proximal and/or distal component without change of position in the relevant area	
Explanation	This manoeuvre increases the intra-articular compression forces in the central part of the joint	This manoeuvre reduces the intra-articular compression forces in the central part of the joint	
Additional data to support the hypothesis	General and specific mobility of the elbow History, symptom behaviour, type of complaints, 24-hour behaviour Specific palpation Reproducibility of test results Test treatment Imaging procedures (CT, MRI)		

Differentiation, humero-ulnar joint – intra-articular vs. extra-articular (symptom provocation by an intra-articular component – anterior aspect)

The change in symptoms can be demonstrated exactly:

- provocation of pain (Fig. 4.57a and b, film 182)
- alleviation of pain (Fig. 4.58a and b, film 183).

Assessment			
Goal	**Provocation of pain**	**Alleviation of pain**	**Remarks**
Starting position	Flexion to a position immediately after symptoms have appeared	Flexion to a position immediately after symptoms have appeared	Since, with pre-positioning to a position before symptoms appear, non-symptomatic parts of the affected joint may be compressed, a symptomatic position is chosen also for provocation
Test movement	Ulna moves proximally, with fixed humerus	Ulna moves distally, with fixed humerus	

Goal	Provocation of pain	Alleviation of pain	Remarks
Neural involvement	Proximal and/or distal component without change of position in the relevant area	Proximal and/or distal component without change of position in the relevant area	
Explanation	This manoeuvre increases the intra-articular compression forces in the anterior part of the joint	This manoeuvre reduces the intra-articular compression forces in the anterior part of the joint	
Additional data to support the hypothesis	General and specific mobility of the elbow History, symptom behaviour, type of complaints, 24-hour behaviour Specific palpation Reproducibility of test results Test treatment Imaging procedures (CT, MRI)		

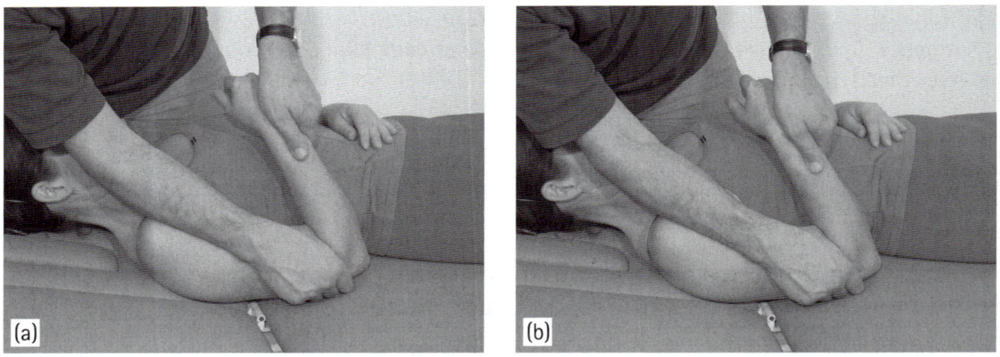

Figure 4.57a and b Specific provocation and alleviation in the area of the humero-ulnar joint with symptomatic movement of the elbow into flexion; intra-articular mechanism in the anterior aspect of the joint as symptom-provoking component; provocation. **a**, Starting position. **b**, End position.

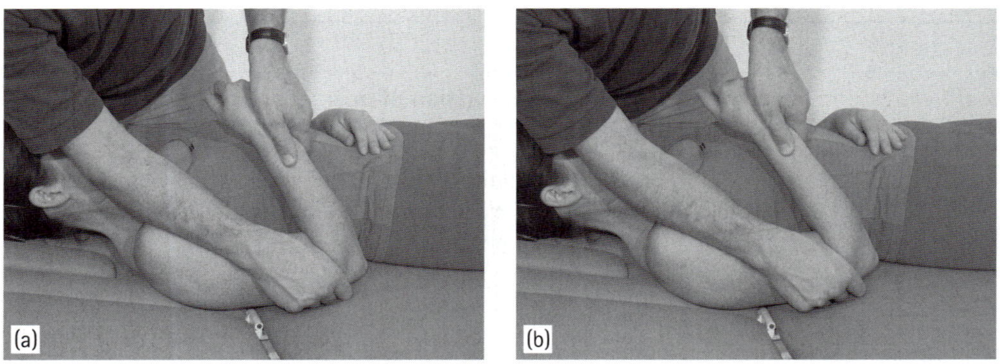

Figure 4.58a and b Specific provocation and alleviation in the area of the humero-ulnar joint with symptomatic movement of the elbow into flexion; intra-articular mechanism in the anterior aspect of the joint as symptom-provoking component; alleviation. **a**, Starting position. **b**, End position.

Differentiation, humero-ulnar joint – intra-articular vs. extra-articular (symptom provocation by an intra-articular component – posterior aspect)

The change in symptoms can be demonstrated exactly:

- provocation of pain (Fig. 4.59a and b, film 184)
- alleviation of pain (Fig. 4.60a and b, film 185).

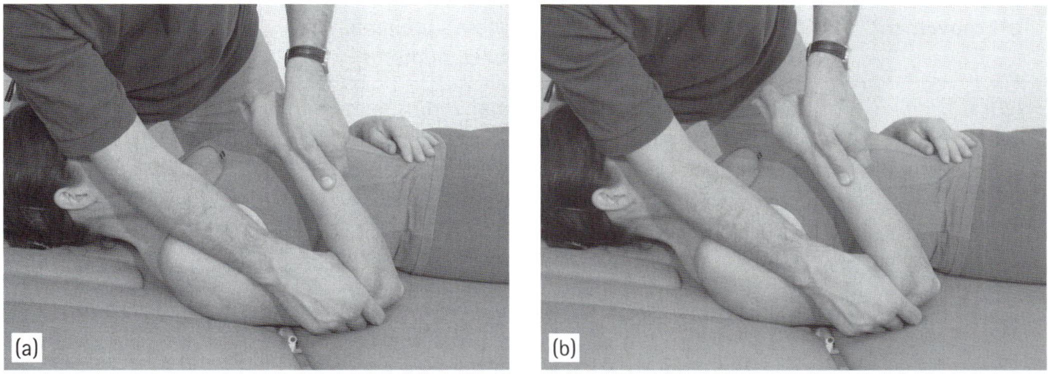

Figure 4.59a and b Specific provocation and alleviation in the area of the humero-ulnar joint with symptomatic movement of the elbow into flexion; intra-articular mechanism in the posterior aspect of the joint as symptom-provoking component; provocation. **a**, Starting position. **b**, End position.

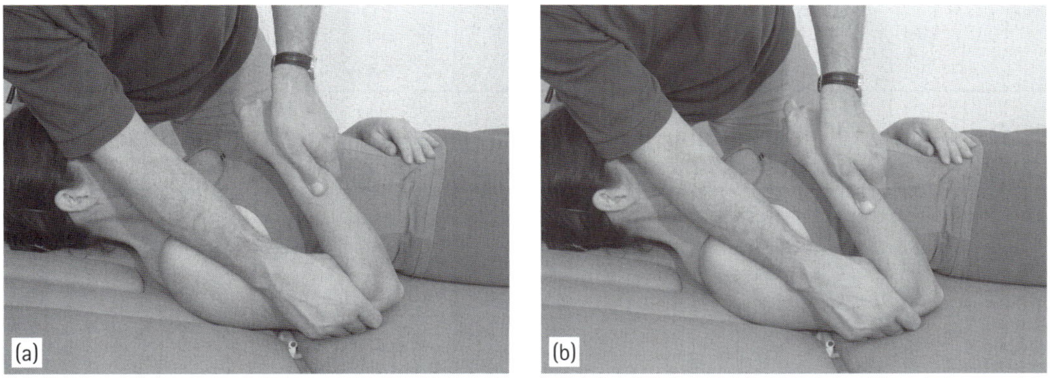

Figure 4.60a and b Specific provocation and alleviation in the area of the humero-ulnar joint with symptomatic movement of the elbow into flexion; intra-articular mechanism in the posterior aspect of the joint as symptom-provoking component; alleviation. **a**, Starting position. **b**, End position.

Assessment

Goal	Provocation of pain	Alleviation of pain	Remarks
Starting position	Flexion to a position immediately after symptoms have appeared	Flexion to a position immediately after symptoms have appeared	Since, with pre-positioning to a position before symptoms appear,

Goal	Provocation of pain	Alleviation of pain	Remarks
			non-symptomatic parts of the affected joint may be compressed, a symptomatic position is chosen also for provocation
Test movement	Ulna moves distally, with fixed humerus	Ulna moves proximally, with fixed humerus	
Neural involvement	Proximal and/or distal component without change of position in the relevant area	Proximal and/or distal component without change of position in the relevant area	
Explanation	This manoeuvre increases the intra-articular compression forces in the posterior part of the joint	This manoeuvre reduces the intra-articular compression forces in the posterior part of the joint	
Additional data to support the hypothesis	General and specific mobility of the elbow History, symptom behaviour, type of complaints, 24-hour behaviour Specific palpation Reproducibility of test results Test treatment Imaging procedures (CT, MRI)		

Differentiation humero-ulnar joint – extra-articular vs. intra-articular (symptom provocation by an extra-articular component)

The change in symptoms can be demonstrated exactly:

- provocation of pain (Fig. 4.61a and b, film 186).

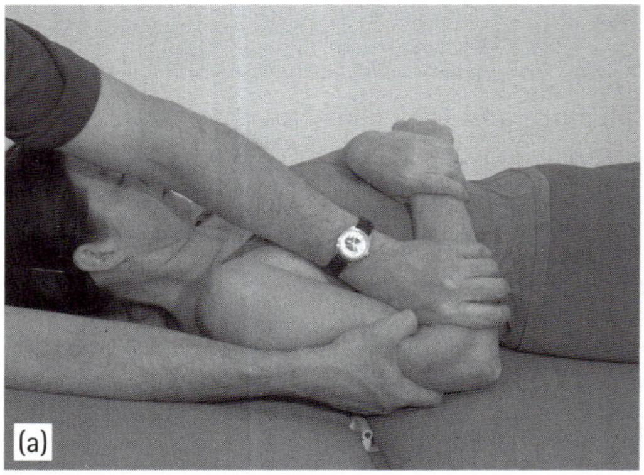

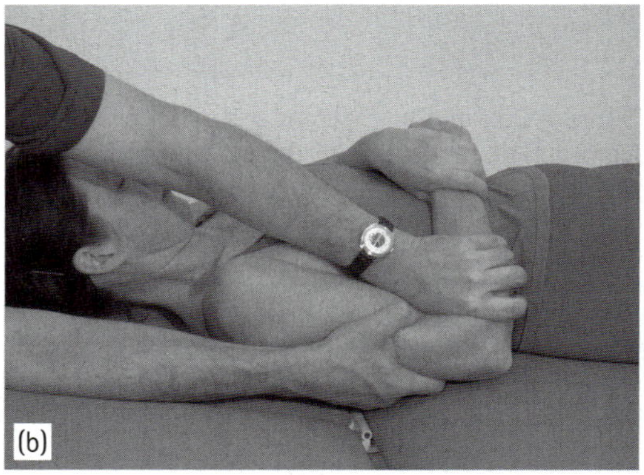

Figure 4.61a and b Specific provocation in the area of the humero-ulnar joint with symptomatic movement of the elbow into flexion; extra-articular mechanism as symptom-provoking component. a, Starting position. b, End position.

Assessment

Goal	Provocation of pain	Alleviation of pain	Remarks
Starting position	Flexion to a position exactly when symptoms appear		
Test movement	Traction in the humero-ulnar joint vertical to the treatment plane	None	Usually, alleviation is not possible, as approximation of the joint surfaces seems too little for relaxation of the extra-articular structures
Neural involvement	Proximal and/or distal component without change of position in the relevant area	None	
Explanation	This manoeuvre increases the extra-articular tractive forces	None	An extra-articular lesion is assumed when the intra-articular differentiation is negative
Additional data to support the hypothesis	General and specific mobility of the elbow History, symptom behaviour, type of complaints, 24-hour behaviour Specific palpation Reproducibility of test results Test treatment Imaging procedures (CT, MRI)		

SPECIFIC PROVOCATION AND ALLEVIATION, ELBOW COMPLEX – SUPINATION

Localization, proximal radio-ulnar joint – movement as symptom-provoking component – rolling

Pain-provoking movement (Fig. 4.62)

- Supination of the forearm provokes pain in the lateral elbow.
- Area localization hints at the elbow complex.

The change in symptoms can be demonstrated exactly:

- provocation of pain (Fig. 4.63a and b, film 193)
- alleviation of pain (Fig. 4.64a and b, film 194).

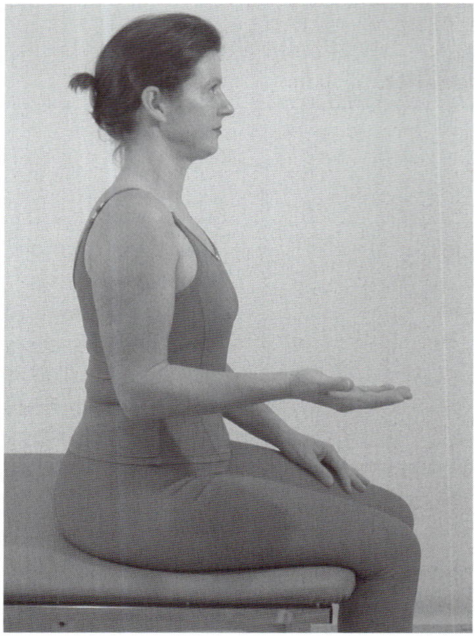

Figure 4.62 Symptom-provoking movement: movement of the elbow into supination provokes pain in the area of the lateral elbow.

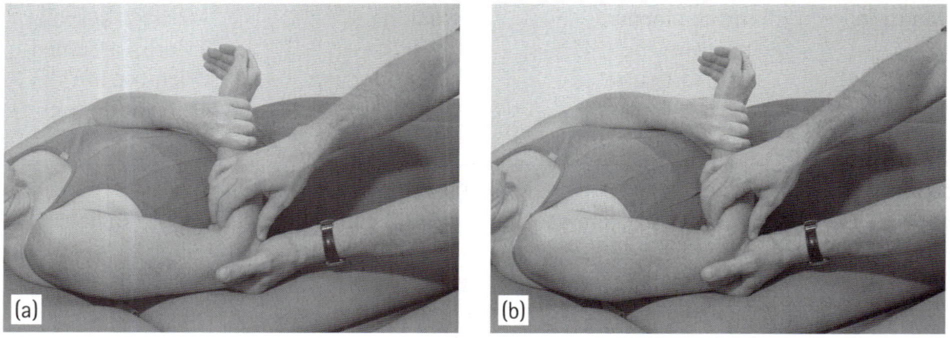

Figure 4.63a and b Specific provocation and alleviation in the area of the proximal radio-ulnar joint with symptomatic movement of the elbow into supination; rolling as symptom-provoking component; provocation. a, Starting position. b, End position.

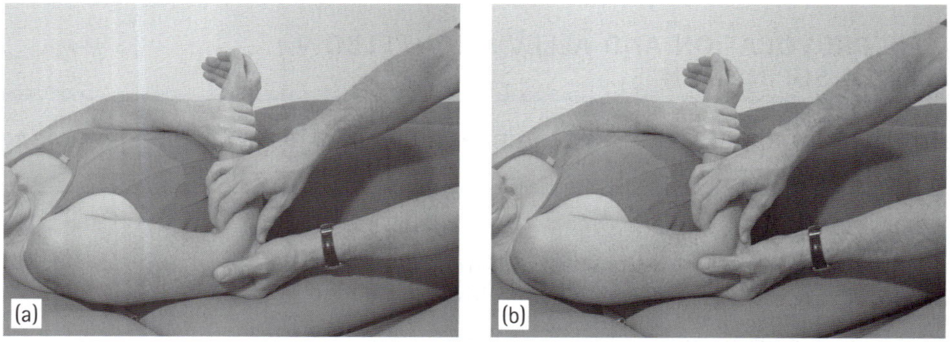

Figure 4.64a and b Specific provocation and alleviation in the area of the proximal radio-ulnar joint with symptomatic movement of the elbow into supination; rolling as symptom-provoking component; alleviation. a, Starting position. b, End position.

Assessment

Goal	Provocation of pain	Alleviation of pain	Remarks
Starting position	Supination to a position immediately before symptoms appear	Supination to a position immediately after symptoms have appeared	
Test movement	Radius moves in posterior direction	Radius moves in anterior direction	
Neural involvement	Proximal and/or distal component without change of position in the relevant area	Proximal and/or distal component without change of position in the relevant area	
Explanation	It is assumed that decentring of the radius by posterior rolling will provoke pain in sensitive structures in the posterior area	Anterior glide of the radius reduces load on pain-sensitive structures in the posterior area of the joint	
Additional data to support the hypothesis	General and specific mobility of the elbow History, symptom behaviour, type of complaints, 24-hour behaviour Specific palpation Reproducibility of test results Test treatment Imaging procedures (CT, MRI)		

Note: This example is based on the assumption that disturbed gliding of the radius in an anterior direction induces increased rolling in a posterior direction. This leads to a decentring of the radial head with simultaneous provocation of pain-sensitive structures in the posterior part of the joint.

Localization, proximal radio-ulnar joint – movement as symptom-provoking component – gliding

The change in symptoms can be demonstrated exactly:

- provocation of pain (Fig. 4.65a and b, film 195)
- alleviation of pain (Fig. 4.66a and b, film 196).

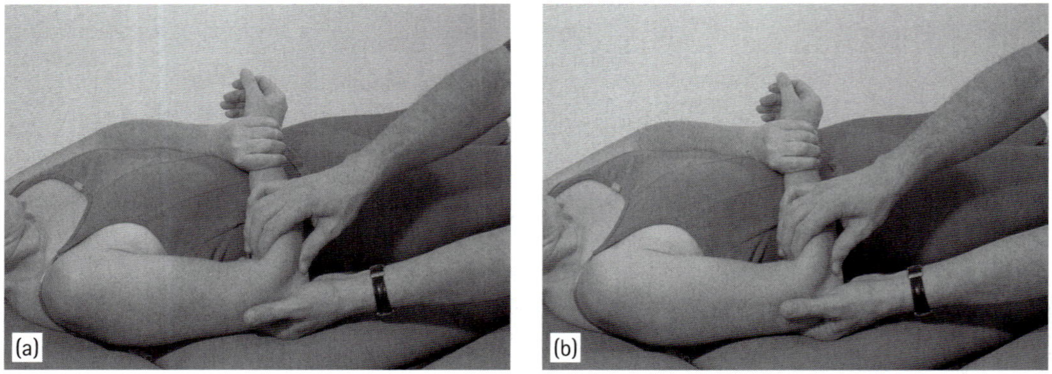

Figure 4.65a and b Specific provocation and alleviation in the area of the proximal radio-ulnar joint with symptomatic movement of the elbow into supination; gliding as symptom-provoking component; provocation. **a**, Starting position. **b**, End position.

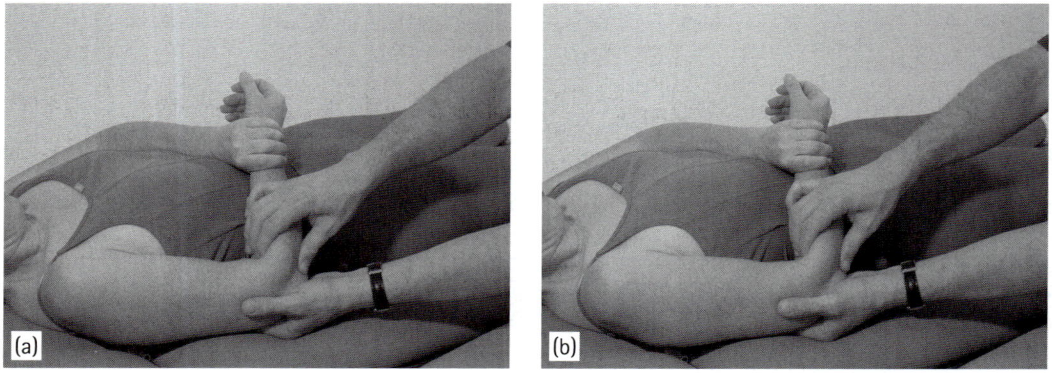

Figure 4.66a and b Specific provocation and alleviation in the area of the proximal radio-ulnar joint with symptomatic movement of the elbow into supination; gliding as symptom-provoking component; alleviation. **a**, Starting position. **b**, End position.

Assessment

Goal	Provocation of pain	Alleviation of pain	Remarks
Starting position	Supination to a position immediately before symptoms appear	Supination to a position immediately after symptoms have appeared	
Test movement	Radius moves in anterior direction	Radius moves in posterior direction	
Neural involvement	Proximal and/or distal component without change of position in the relevant area	Proximal and/or distal component without change of position in the relevant area	

Goal	Provocation of pain	Alleviation of pain	Remarks
Explanation	With this manoeuvre, pain-sensitive structures in the anterior part of the joint are provoked	With this manoeuvre, the provocation of pain-sensitive structures in the anterior part of the joint is reduced	
Additional data to support the hypothesis	General and specific mobility of the elbow History, symptom behaviour, type of complaints, 24-hour behaviour Specific palpation Reproducibility of test results Test treatment Imaging procedures (CT, MRI)		

Note: This example is based on the assumption that disturbed gliding of the radius in an anterior direction provokes pain-sensitive structures in the anterior part of the joint.

SPECIFIC PROVOCATION AND ALLEVIATION, ELBOW COMPLEX – PRONATION

Localization, proximal radio-ulnar joint – movement as symptom-provoking component – rolling

Pain-provoking movement (Fig. 4.67)

- Pronation of the forearm provokes pain in the lateral elbow.
- Area localization hints at the elbow complex.

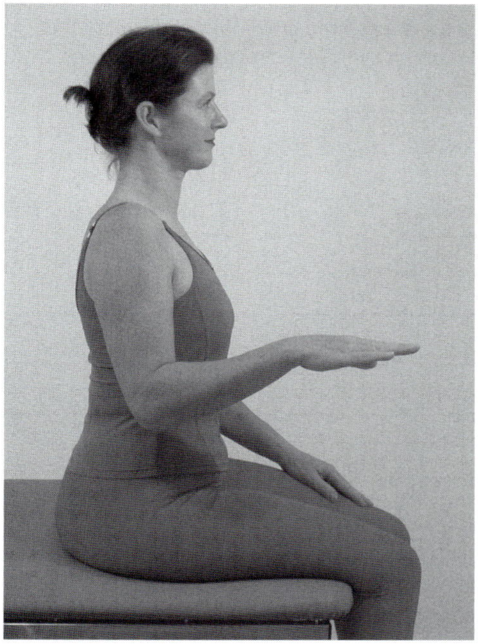

Figure 4.67 Symptom-provoking movement: movement of the elbow into pronation provokes pain in the area of the lateral elbow.

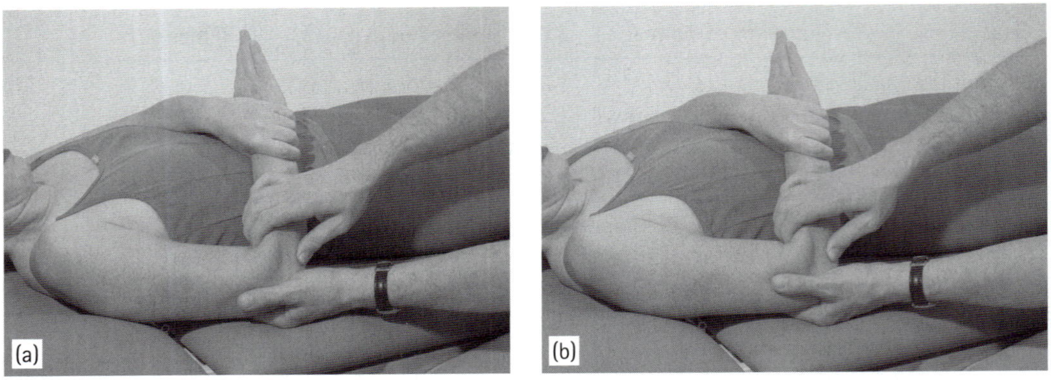

Figure 4.68a and b Specific provocation and alleviation in the area of the proximal radio-ulnar joint with symptomatic movement of the elbow into pronation; rolling as symptom-provoking component; provocation. **a**, Starting position. **b**, End position.

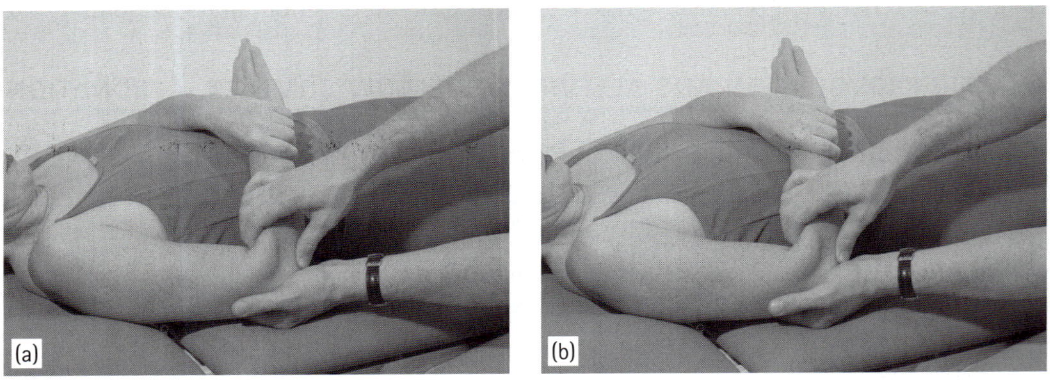

Figure 4.69a and b Specific provocation and alleviation in the area of the proximal radio-ulnar joint with symptomatic movement of the elbow into pronation; rolling as symptom-provoking component; alleviation. **a**, Starting position. **b**, End position.

The change in symptoms can be demonstrated exactly:

- provocation of pain (Fig. 4.68a and b, film 202)
- alleviation of pain (Fig. 4.69a and b, film 203).

Assessment

Goal	Provocation of pain	Alleviation of pain	Remarks
Starting position	Pronation to a position immediately before symptoms appear	Pronation to a position immediately after symptoms have appeared	
Test movement	Radius moves in anterior direction	Radius moves in posterior direction	

Goal	Provocation of pain	Alleviation of pain	Remarks
Neural involvement	Proximal and/or distal component without change of position in the relevant area	Proximal and/or distal component without change of position in the relevant area	
Explanation	It is assumed that decentring of the radius by anterior rolling provokes pain in sensitive structures in the anterior area	Posterior glide of the radius reduces load on the pain-sensitive structures in the anterior area of the joint	
Additional data to support the hypothesis	General and specific mobility of the elbow History, symptom behaviour, type of complaints, 24-hour behaviour Specific palpation Reproducibility of test results Test treatment Imaging procedures (CT, MRI)		

Note: This example is based on the assumption that disturbed gliding of the radius in a posterior direction induces increased rolling in an anterior direction. This leads to a decentring of the radial head with simultaneous provocation of pain-sensitive structures in the anterior part of the joint.

Localization, proximal radio-ulnar joint – movement as symptom-provoking component – gliding

The change in symptoms can be demonstrated exactly:

- provocation of pain (Fig. 4.70a and b, film 204)
- alleviation of pain (Fig. 4.71a and b, film 205).

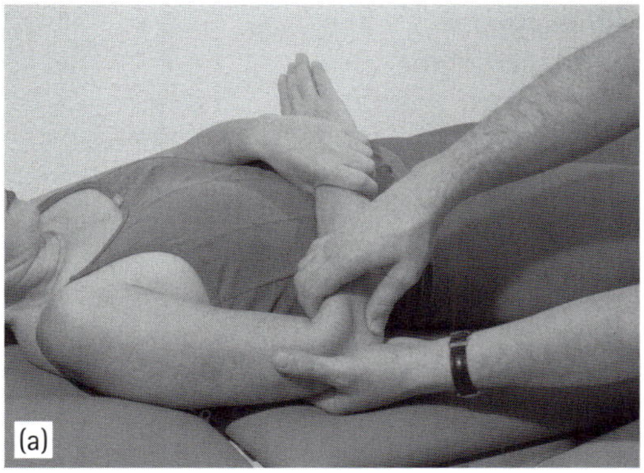

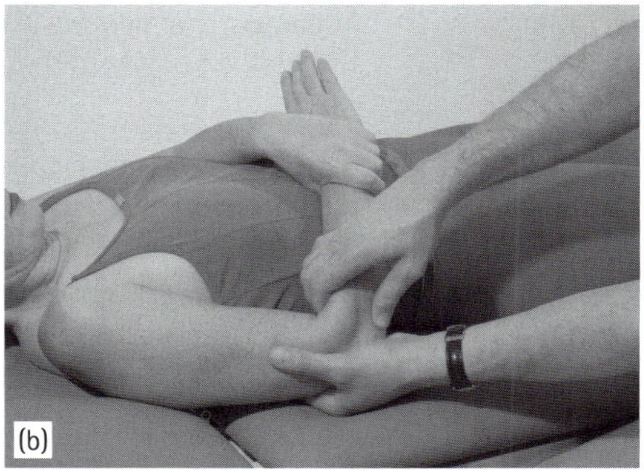

Figure 4.70a and b Specific provocation and alleviation in the area of the proximal radio-ulnar joint with symptomatic movement of the elbow into pronation; gliding as symptom-provoking component; provocation. **a**, Starting position. **b**, End position.

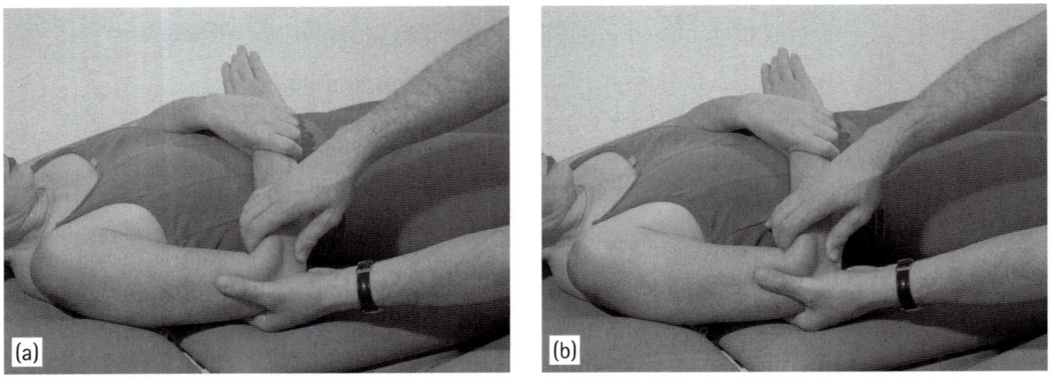

Figure 4.71a and b Specific provocation and alleviation in the area of the proximal radio-ulnar joint with symptomatic movement of the elbow into pronation; gliding as symptom-provoking component; alleviation. **a**, Starting position. **b**, End position.

Assessment

Goal	Provocation of pain	Alleviation of pain	Remarks
Starting position	Pronation to a position immediately before symptoms appear	Pronation to a position immediately after symptoms have appeared	
Test movement	Radius moves in posterior direction	Radius moves in anterior direction	
Neural involvement	Proximal and/or distal component without change of position in the relevant area	Proximal and/or distal component without change of position in the relevant area	
Explanation	With this manoeuvre, pain-sensitive structures in the posterior part of the joint are provoked	With this manoeuvre, the provocation of pain-sensitive structures in the posterior part of the joint is reduced	
Additional data to support the hypothesis	General and specific mobility of the elbow History, symptom behaviour, type of complaints, 24-hour behaviour Specific palpation Reproducibility of test results Test treatment Imaging procedures (CT, MRI)		

Note: This example is based on the assumption that disturbed gliding of the radius in a posterior direction provokes pain-sensitive structures in the posterior part of the joint.

GENERAL MOVEMENT TESTS

General movement tests identify individual anatomical movements and, in part, movement combinations in the area concerned. The individual manual therapy concepts have respective protocols at their disposal, which more or less have the same goals.

Information gained in this way is used to check or modify the relevant hypotheses developed on the basis of the anamnesis and area localization and will help in deciding how to proceed.

General question: Is there enough information available to skip general movement tests?	
No	Yes
⇓	⇓
Performance of the general movement tests	● Additional tests ● Test treatment

In view of the described clinical presentation and the results of area localization, general movement tests of the following regions seem to be useful.

Cervical spine		
	Active	Passive (assistive)
Lower cervical spine (below C2) in general	Flexion Extension Rotation (to the right and left) Lateral flexion (to the right and left)	Flexion Extension Rotation (to the right and left) Lateral flexion (to the right and left)
Shoulder complex		
	Active	Passive
Movement combination shoulder girdle and shoulder	Abduction/elevation Flexion/elevation Horizontal adduction Internal rotation in abduction of 90°	Abduction/elevation Flexion/elevation Horizontal adduction Internal rotation in abduction of 90°
Shoulder girdle	Elevation Depression Protraction Retraction	Elevation Depression Protraction Retraction

	Active	Passive
Glenohumeral joint	Flexion Extension Internal rotation External rotation Abduction Adduction	Flexion Extension Internal rotation External rotation Abduction Adduction
Elbow complex		
	Active	Passive
Elbow	Flexion Extension Pronation Supination	Flexion Extension Pronation Supination
Hand complex		
	Active	Passive
Wrist	Dorsal flexion Volar flexion Radial abduction Ulnar abduction	Dorsal flexion Volar flexion Radial abduction Ulnar abduction

TREATMENT EXAMPLE, HUMERO-ULNAR JOINT

SYMPTOMATIC MOVEMENT

Extension of the elbow is restricted as compared with the opposite side and provokes pain (VAS 2–3/10) in the lateral area of the right elbow (Fig. 4.72).

ASSESSMENTS

Area localization

Area localization hints at a provocation of symptoms by the elbow complex. There is no contraindication for movement.

Specific provocation and alleviation

Specific provocation and alleviation hints at a provocation of symptoms by movement of the humero-ulnar joint and shows an intra-articular mechanism in the posterior aspect of the joint.

Specific mobility

Specific mobility tests show hypomobility of the ulna in a posterior and ulnar direction.

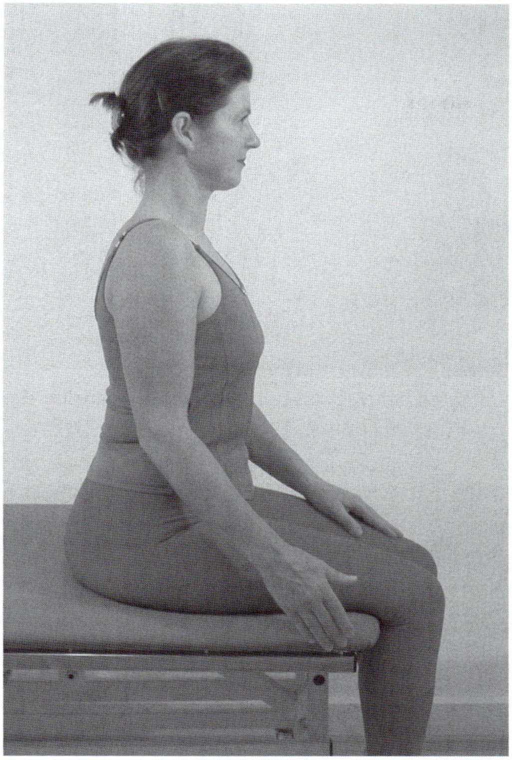

Figure 4.72 Symptom-provoking movement: movement of the elbow into extension provokes pain in the area of the lateral elbow.

Palpation

Palpation of the periarticular structures indicates a change of tissue as compared with the non-affected side. The patient's specific pain cannot be reproduced by palpation.

HYPOTHESIS

A painfully restricted extension of the humero-ulnar joint due to an intra-articular mechanism (compression) in the posterior aspect of the joint with simultaneously restricted translatory mobility in a posterior and ulnar direction is suspected (Fig. 4.72).

RELAXATION TECHNIQUES

Hold–relax techniques

MOVEMENT-DIRECTED CONTRACTION IN THE DIRECTION OPPOSING THE PAINFUL AND/OR RESTRICTED DIRECTION

Therapy technique (film 146)

- Patient's starting position: supine.
- Therapist's starting position: standing, at the patient's right side, fixation of the distal humerus as well as the shoulder (Fig. 4.73a).
- Movement: isometric flexion of the elbow while the patient tries to prevent the movement by muscle contraction (Fig. 4.73b).

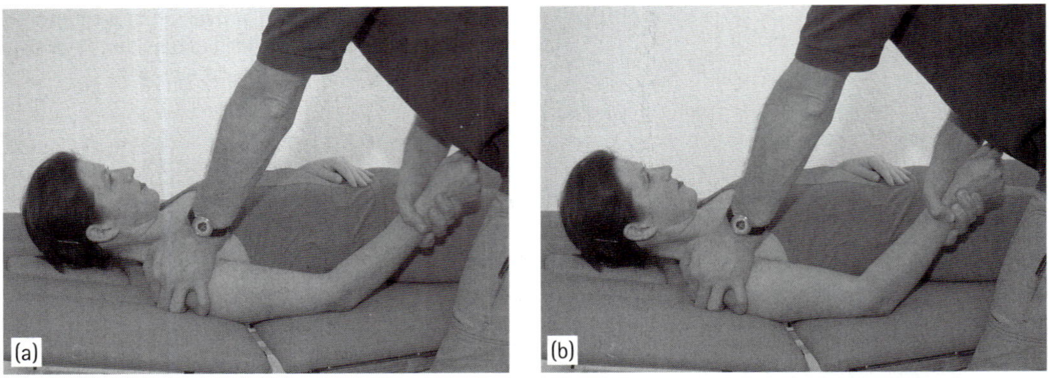

Figure 4.73a and b Hold-relax technique; movement-directed contraction in the direction opposing the painful and/or restricted direction; therapy technique. **a**, Starting position. **b**, End position.

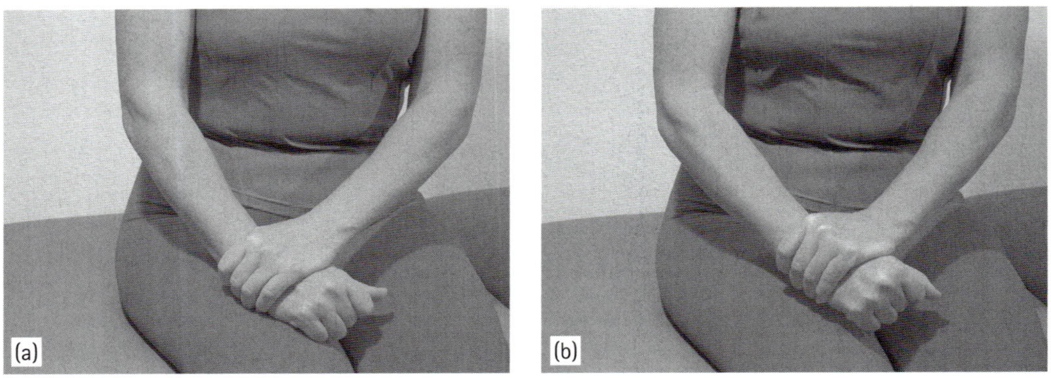

Figure 4.74a and b Hold-relax technique; movement-directed contraction in the direction opposing the painful and/or restricted direction; self-exercise. **a**, Starting position. **b**, End position.

Self-exercise (film 147)

- Patient's starting position: sitting, fixation of the distal forearm (Fig. 4.74a).
- Movement: isometric flexion of the elbow while trying to prevent the movement by muscle contraction (Fig. 4.74b).

MOVEMENT-DIRECTED CONTRACTION IN THE PAINFUL AND/OR RESTRICTED DIRECTION

Therapy technique (film 148)

- Patient's starting position: supine.
- Therapist's starting position: standing, at the patient's right side, fixation of the distal humerus as well as the shoulder (Fig. 4.75a).
- Movement: isometric extension of the elbow while the patient tries to prevent the movement by muscle contraction (Fig. 4.75b).

Self-exercise (film 149)

- Patient's starting position: sitting, fixation of the distal forearm (Fig. 4.76a).
- Movement: isometric extension of the elbow while trying to prevent the movement by muscle contraction (Fig. 4.76b).

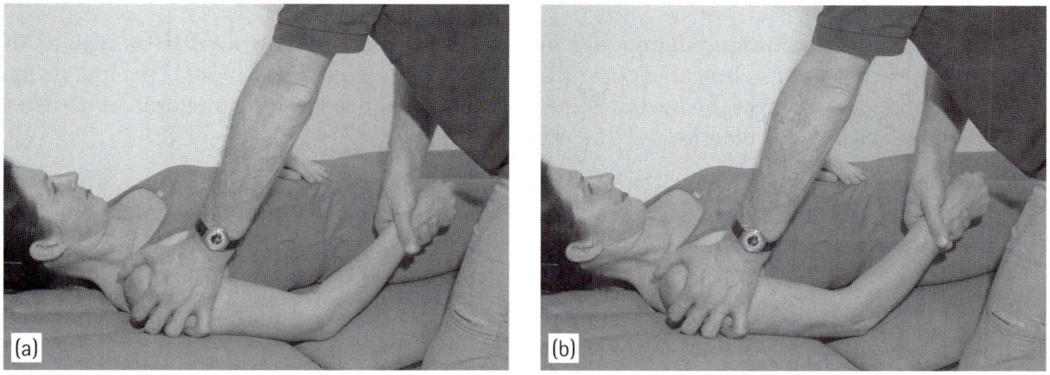

Figure 4.75a and b Hold-relax technique; movement-directed contraction in the painful and/or restricted direction; therapy technique. **a**, Starting position. **b**, End position.

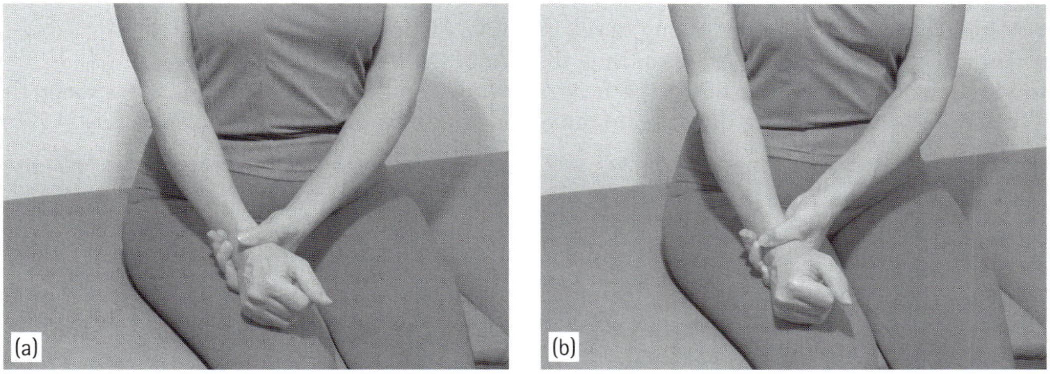

Figure 4.76a and b Hold-relax technique; movement-directed contraction in the painful and/or restricted direction; self-exercise. **a**, Starting position. **b**, End position.

Remarks (regarding hold-relax techniques)

Goal of the technique

With a painfully restricted extension of the humero-ulnar joint due to an intra-articular mechanism (compression) in the posterior area of the joint, with simultaneously restricted translatory mobility in posterior and ulnar direction, the techniques described serve to:

- reduce tonicity and improve the metabolism of the periarticular tissues
- restore pain-free function (change the input to respective centres of the central nervous system (CNS).

Performance

According to irritability or desired treatment goal, the joint to be treated is pre-positioned as necessary before treatment. As the self-exercise is performed without 'specific fixation', an uncontrolled continuation of movement has to be considered when the indication for this exercise is determined.

Dosage (regarding the affected symptomatic structure)

Both with an acute and with a chronic presentation, the contraction should always be pain-free.

Choice of technique

The selection of the technique depends, among other things, on the therapist as well as the patient, on the therapist's clinical experience, but primarily on reassessment. This means that even if all preconditions on the part of therapist and patient seem to be met, it is of no use to continue the technique if reassessment is negative.

Contributing factors

For a satisfactory solution of the patient's current problems it is important to consider the contributing factors and include them in the treatment.

The authors will, however, not go into a description of the various possibilities and their complex contexts as this would exceed the scope of the present book.

Soft tissue techniques

EXTENSORS OF FINGERS AND WRIST ORIGINATING IN THE ELBOW COMPLEX

Therapy technique (film 152)

- Patient's starting position: sitting, wrist in dorsal flexion.
- Therapist's starting position: standing, in front of the patient (Fig. 4.77a).
- Movement: passive volar flexion of the wrist, while simultaneously exerting pressure on the extensors, then releasing pressure on the muscles, and back to starting position (Fig. 4.77b).

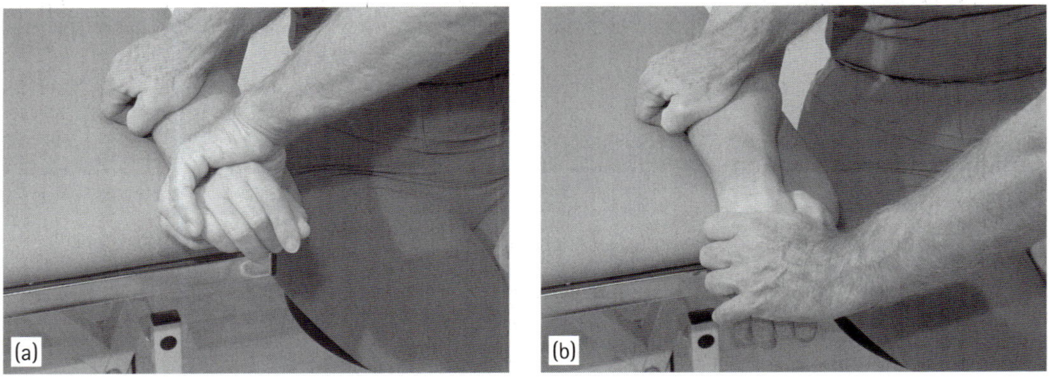

Figure 4.77a and b Soft tissue technique; wrist extensors; therapy technique. **a**, Starting position. **b**, End position.

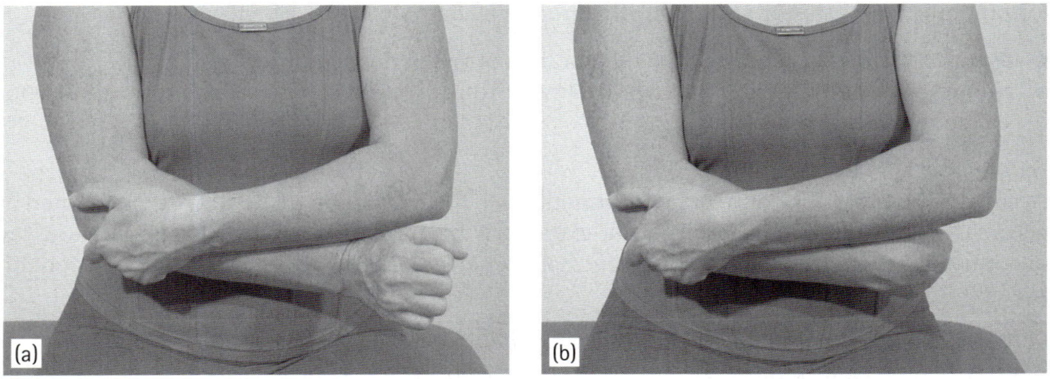

Figure 4.78a and b Soft tissue technique; wrist extensors; self-exercise. **a**, Starting position. **b**, End position.

Note: If the patient is not able to relax or if performance of the movement seems too difficult, this soft tissue technique can also be performed assistively. Application of the assistive technique leads to a simultaneous reciprocal inhibition of the treated muscles, which might facilitate relaxation.

Self-exercise (film 153)

- Patient's starting position: sitting, elbow flexed, wrist in dorsal flexion (Fig. 4.78a).
- Movement: active volar flexion in the wrist, with simultaneously exerting pressure on the extensors, then releasing the pressure on the muscles, and back to starting position (Fig. 4.78b).

FLEXORS OF FINGERS AND WRIST ORIGINATING IN THE ELBOW COMPLEX

Therapy technique (film 150)

- Patient's starting position: sitting, wrist in volar flexion.
- Therapist's starting position: standing, in front of the patient (Fig. 4.79a).
- Movement: passive dorsal flexion of the wrist, with simultaneously exerting pressure on the flexors, then releasing the pressure on the muscles, and back to starting position (Fig. 4.79b).

Note: If the patient is not able to relax or if performance of the movement seems too difficult, this soft tissue technique can also be performed assistively. Application of the assistive technique leads to a simultaneous reciprocal inhibition of the treated muscles, which might facilitate relaxation.

Self-exercise (film 151)

- Patient's starting position: sitting, elbow flexed, wrist in dorsal flexion (Fig. 4.80a).
- Movement: active dorsal flexion of the wrist, with simultaneously exerting pressure on the flexors, then releasing the pressure on the muscles, and back to starting position (Fig. 4.80b).

FLEXORS OF THE ELBOW JOINT

Therapy technique (film 154)

- Patient's starting position: side-lying, elbow flexed, forearm in supination.
- Therapist's starting position: standing, behind the patient (Fig. 4.81a).
- Movement: passive extension and pronation of the elbow, and simultaneously exerting pressure on the elbow flexors, then releasing the pressure on the muscles, and back to starting position (Fig. 4.81b).

Note: If the patient is not able to relax or if performance of the movement seems too difficult, this soft tissue technique can also be performed assistively. Application of the assistive technique leads to a simultaneous reciprocal inhibition of the treated muscles, which might facilitate relaxation.

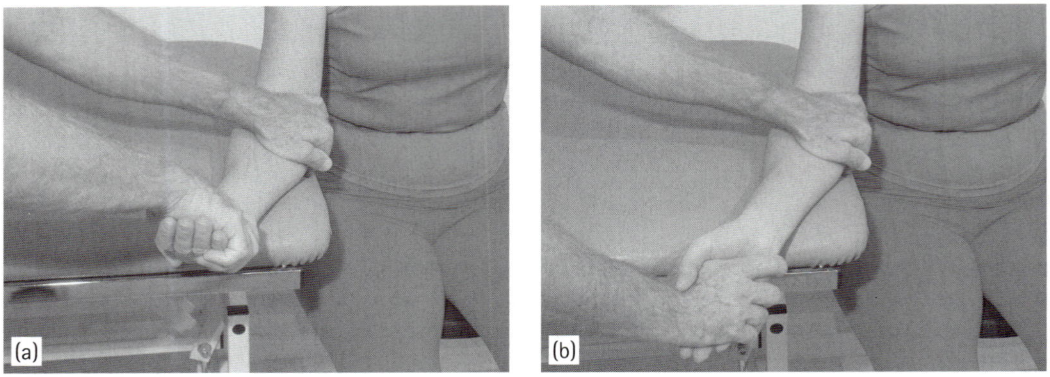

Figure 4.79a and b Soft tissue technique; wrist flexors; therapy technique. **a**, Starting position. **b**, End position.

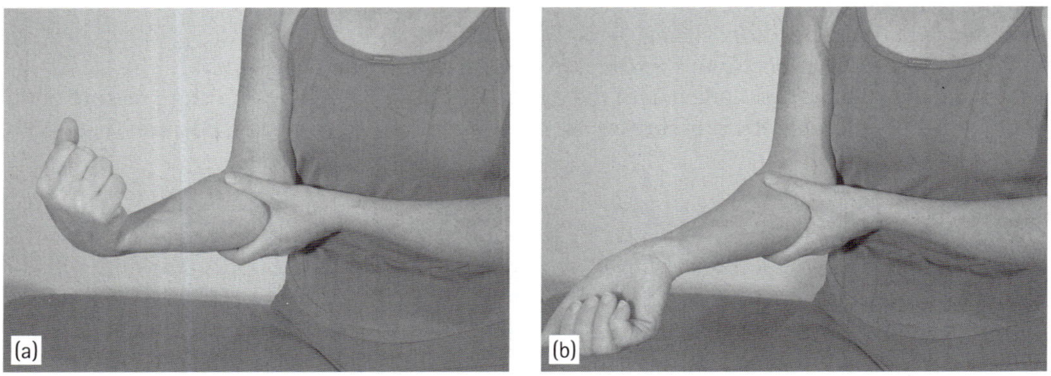

Figure 4.80a and b Soft tissue technique; wrist flexors; self-exercise. **a**, Starting position. **b**, End position.

Self-exercise (film 155)

- Patient's starting position: sitting, elbow flexed, forearm in supination (Fig. 4.82a).
- Movement: active extension of the elbow, and simultaneously exerting pressure on the elbow flexors, then releasing the pressure on the muscles, and back to starting position (Fig. 4.82b).

Remarks (regarding soft tissue techniques)

Goal of the technique

With a painfully restricted extension of the humero-ulnar joint due to an intra-articular mechanism (compression) in the posterior area of the joint, with simultaneously restricted translatory mobility in posterior and ulnar direction, the techniques described serve to:

- reduce tonicity and improve the metabolism of the treated soft tissues
- restore pain-free function (change the input to respective centres of the CNS).

Performance

Treatment is done in the pain-free range of movement.

Dosage (regarding the affected symptomatic structure)

Both with an acute and with a chronic presentation, application of this technique should always be pain-free.

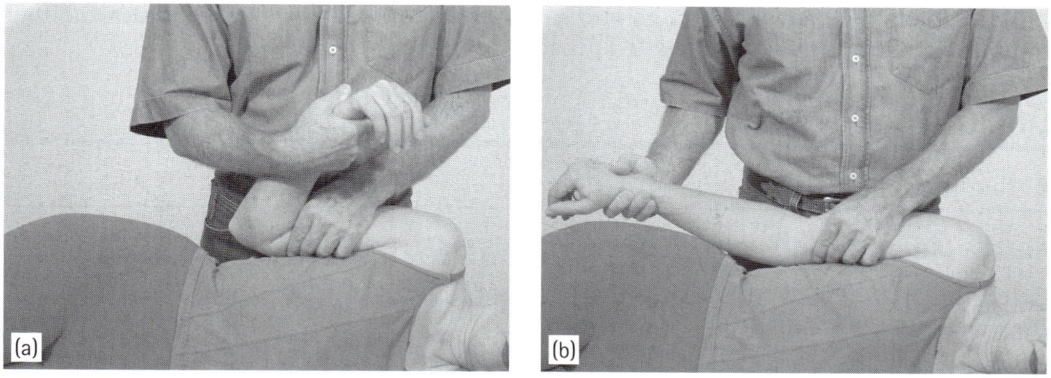

Figure 4.81a and b Soft tissue technique; flexors of the elbow; therapy technique. a, Starting position. b, End position.

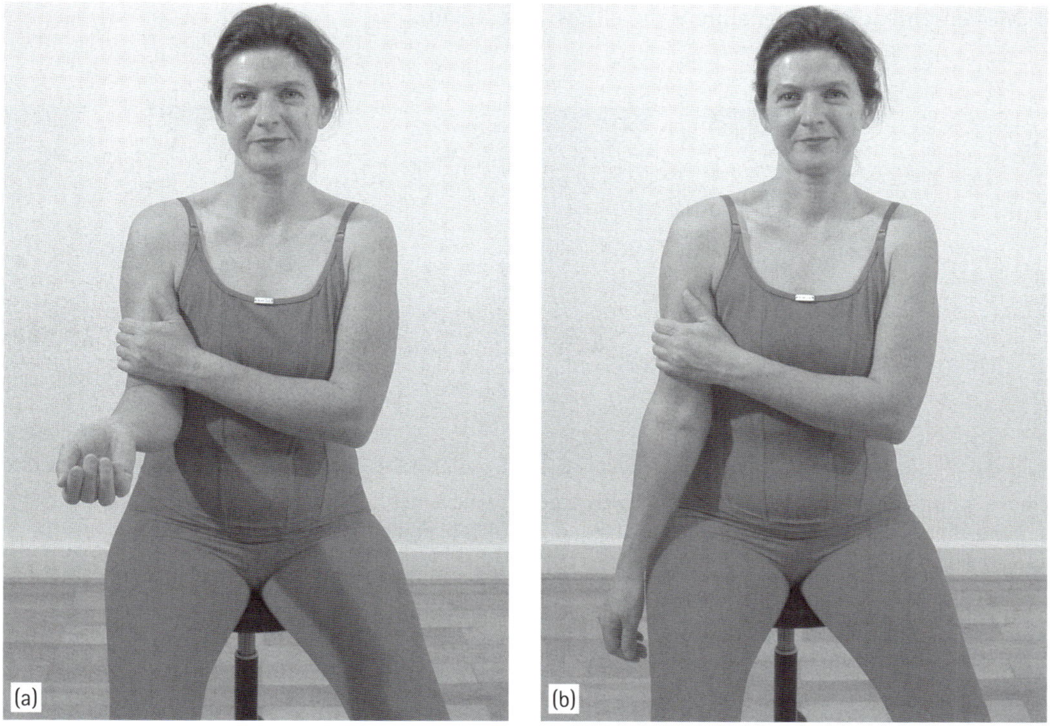

Figure 4.82a and b Soft tissue technique; flexors of the elbow; self-exercise. a, Starting position. b, End position.

Choice of technique

The selection of the technique depends, among other things, on the therapist as well as the patient, on the therapist's clinical experience, but primarily on reassessment. This means that even if all preconditions on the part of therapist and patient seem to be met, it is of no use to continue the technique if reassessment is negative.

Contributing factors

For a satisfactory solution of the patient's current problems it is important to consider the contributing factors and include them in the treatment.

The authors will, however, not go into a description of the various possibilities and their complex contexts as this would exceed the scope of the present book.

MOBILIZATION TECHNIQUES

Active procedures

ACTIVE MOBILIZATION PLUS ACCESSORY MOVEMENT

Extension of the elbow with posterior glide of the ulna

Therapy technique (film 156)

- Patient's starting position: supine.
- Therapist's starting position: standing, at the patient's right side, fixation of the distal humerus on a wedge or sandbag, the olecranon has to be free, contact with the right hand at the ulna, proximal of the ulnar head, pushing the ulna in a proximal direction (Fig. 4.83a).
- Movement: active extension of the elbow (Fig. 4.83b).

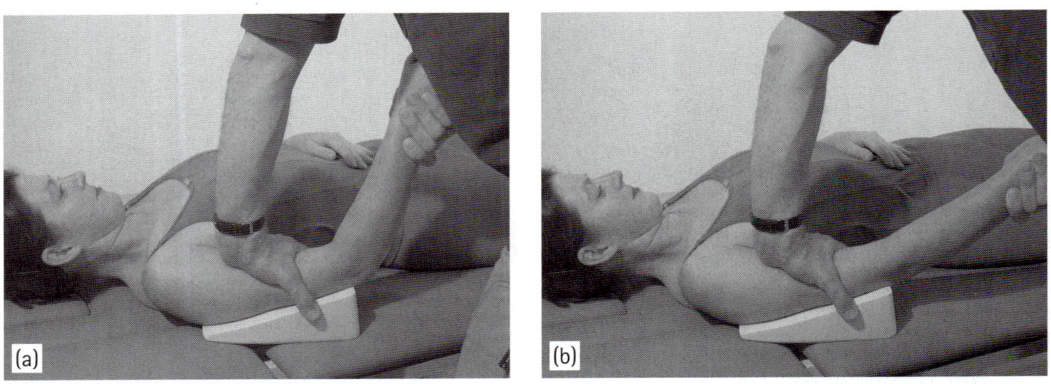

Figure 4.83a and b Active mobilization with accessory movement; extension with posterior glide in the humero-ulnar joint; therapy technique. **a**, Starting position. **b**, End position.

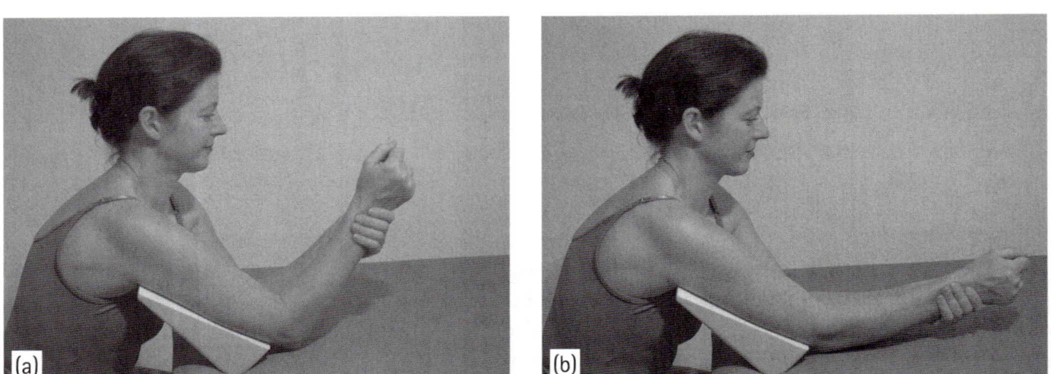

Figure 4.84a and b Active mobilization with accessory movement; extension with posterior glide in the humero-ulnar joint; self-exercise. **a**, Starting position. **b**, End position.

Self-exercise (film 157)

- Patient's starting position: sitting, at the end of the plinth, the humerus fixed by a wedge (the olecranon has to be free) on the plinth, with simultaneous push of the ulna in a proximal direction (Fig. 4.84a).
- Movement: extension of the elbow (Fig. 4.84b).

EXTENSION OF THE ELBOW WITH ULNAR GLIDE OF THE ULNA

Therapy technique (film 158)

- Patient's starting position: supine.
- Therapist's starting position: standing, at the patient's right side, fixation of the humerus with the right hand, contact with the left hand from the radial side against the proximal forearm, and simultaneous push of the forearm in an ulnar direction (Fig. 4.85a).
- Movement: active extension of the elbow (Fig. 4.85b).

Self-exercise (film 159)

- Patient's starting position: sitting, fixation of the humerus with a belt, and simultaneous pull of the ulna in an ulnar direction with the other hand (Fig. 4.86a).
- Movement: extension of the elbow, and moving forearm back into starting position (Fig. 4.86b).

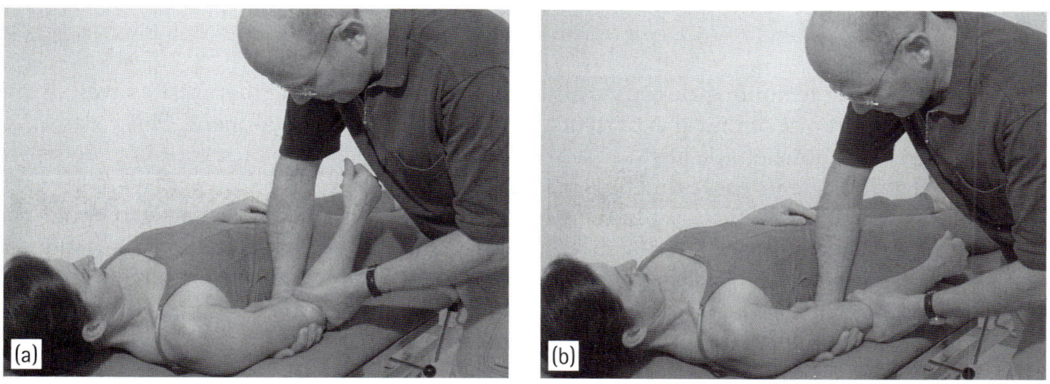

Figure 4.85a and b Active mobilization with accessory movement; extension with ulnar glide in the humero-ulnar joint; therapy technique. **a**, Starting position. **b**, End position.

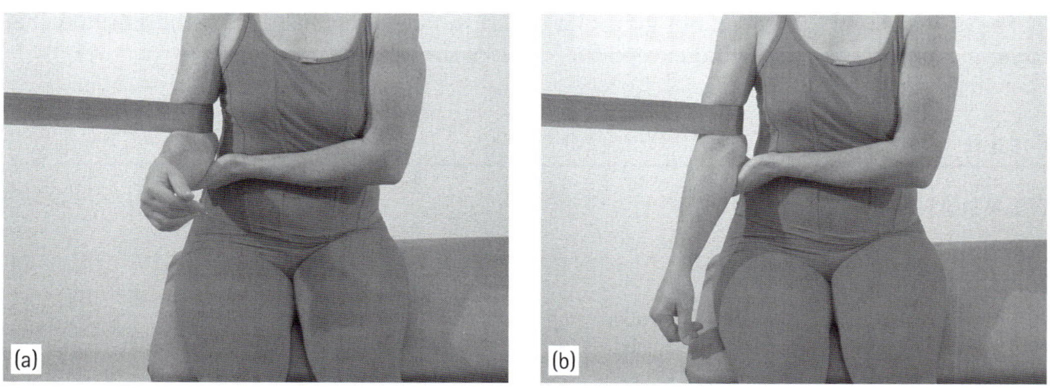

Figure 4.86a and b Active mobilization with accessory movement; extension with ulnar glide in the humero-ulnar joint; self-exercise. **a**, Starting position. **b**, End position.

Remarks (regarding active mobilization plus accessory movement)

Goal of the technique

With a painfully restricted extension of the humero-ulnar joint due to an intra-articular mechanism (compression) in the posterior area of the joint, with simultaneously restricted translatory mobility in posterior and ulnar direction, these techniques serve to:

- reduce tonicity and improve the metabolism of the affected tissues
- restore pain-free function (change the input to respective centres of the CNS).

Performance

Extension of the elbow with ulnar glide of the ulna.

Due to the great anatomical variability and the individual pathology, the ulnar push may have to be slightly modified in direction in some cases, so as to maintain ulnar glide during the movement into extension.

Dosage (regarding the affected structure)

Both with an acute (predominantly peripheral pain mechanisms) and with a chronic presentation (predominantly central pain mechanisms), these techniques should not provoke the patient's symptoms. Their dosage is determined by the course of healing and/or the expected training state of the tissue, as well as by reassessment.

Choice of technique

The selection of the technique depends, among other things, on the therapist as well as the patient, on the therapist's clinical experience, but primarily on reassessment. This means that even if all preconditions on the part of therapist and patient seem to be met, it is of no use to continue the technique if reassessment is negative.

If the ulnar push does not result in the desired success, it may be necessary to change the direction of push (e.g., in a radial direction). Here, again, reassessment serves to test the current hypothesis. If reassessment shows improvement although the chosen direction of the accessory movement cannot be explained on the basis of our current biomechanical understanding, the respective treatment is applied nevertheless!

Contributing factors

For a satisfactory solution of the patient's current problems it is important to consider the contributing factors and include them in the treatment.

The authors will, however, not go into a description of the various possibilities and their complex contexts as this would exceed the scope of the present book.

Passive procedures

TRANSLATORY MOVEMENTS

Traction

Therapy technique (film 162)

- Patient's starting position: prone.
- Therapist's starting position: standing, at the patient's right side, fixation of the ulna on a wedge or sandbag (Fig. 4.87a).
- Movement: traction in the humero-ulnar joint by pushing the humerus in an anterior direction (Fig. 4.87b).

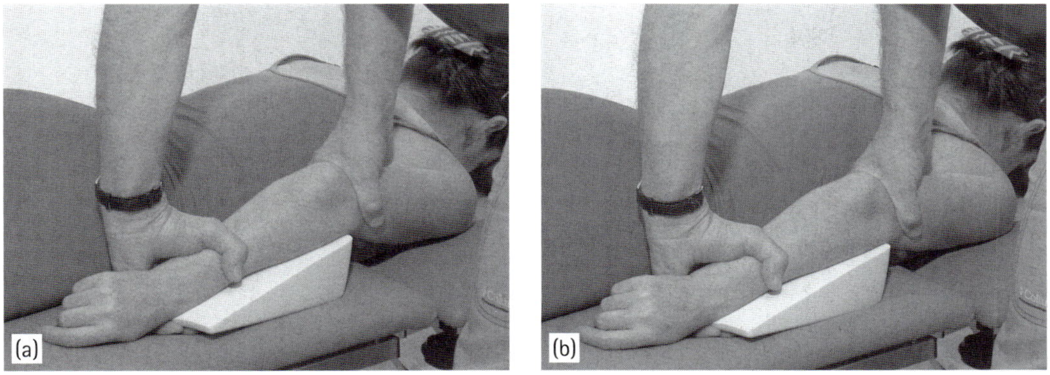

Figure 4.87a and b Passive mobilization; translatory movement; traction in the humero-ulnar joint; therapy technique. a, Starting position. b, End position.

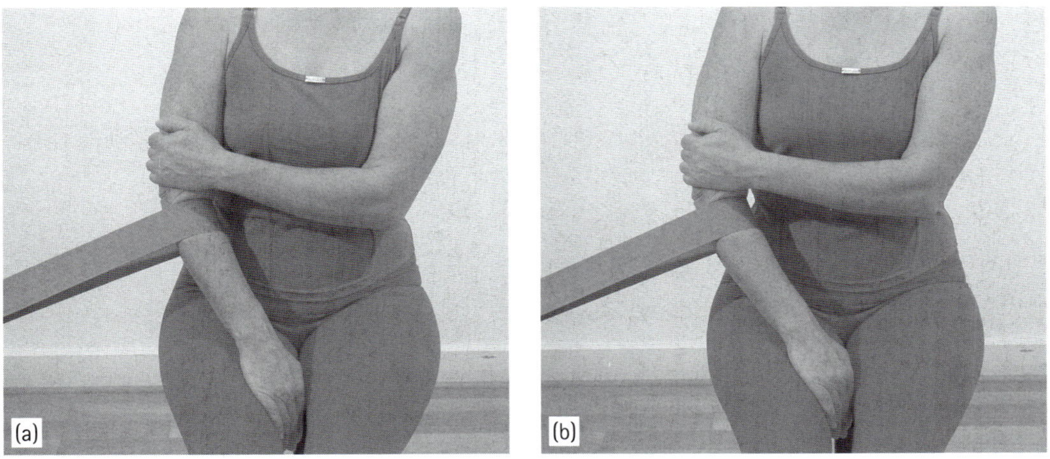

Figure 4.88a and b Passive mobilization; translatory movement; traction in the humero-ulnar joint; self-exercise. a, Starting position. b, End position.

Self-exercise (film 163)

- Patient's starting position: sitting, fixation of the forearm by a belt and by the patient's legs (Fig. 4.88a).
- Movement: traction in the humero-ulnar joint by pushing the humerus in an anterior direction (Fig. 4.88b).

Posterior glide

Therapy technique (film 164)

- Patient's starting position: supine, the elbow pre-positioned in submaximal extension, and the humerus supported on a wedge or sandbag.
- Therapist's starting position: standing, at the patient's right side, stabilization of the distal humerus with the left hand, the olecranon not in contact with the wedge, contact with the right hand in the distal area of the ulna (Fig. 4.89a).
- Movement: push of the ulna in a proximal direction (posterior glide) (Fig. 4.89b).

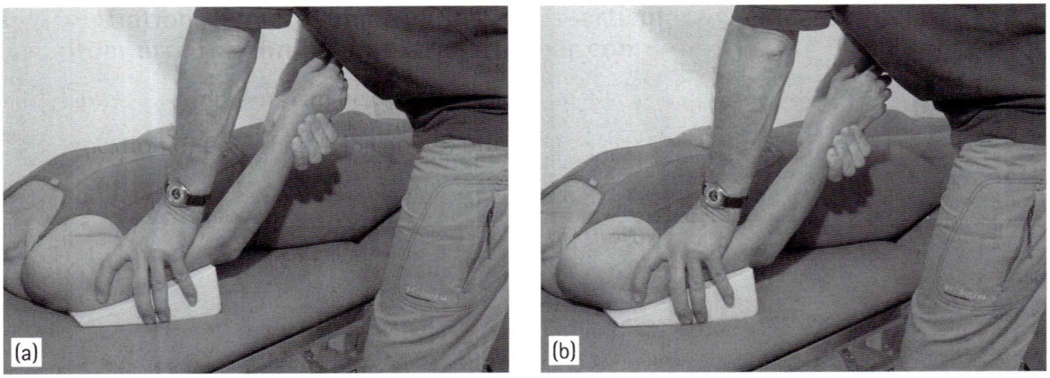

Figure 4.89a and b Passive mobilization; translatory movement; posterior glide in the humero-ulnar joint; therapy technique. a, Starting position. b, End position.

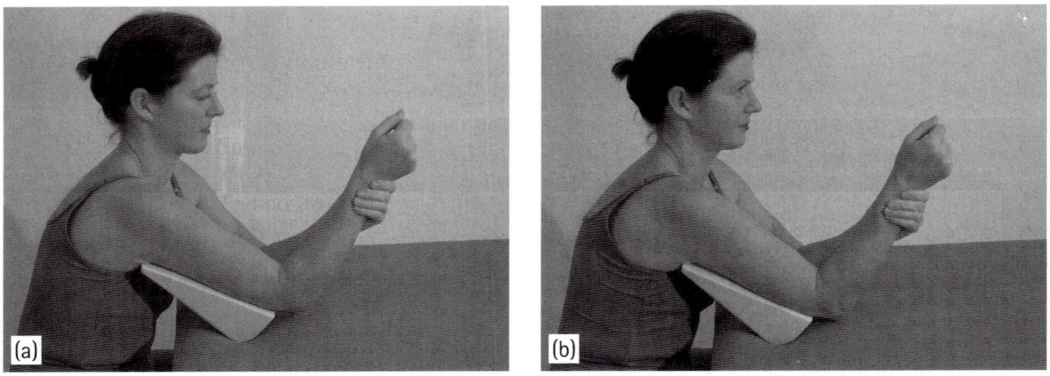

Figure 4.90a and b Passive mobilization; translatory movement; posterior glide in the humero-ulnar joint; self-exercise. a, Starting position. b, End position.

Self-exercise (film 165)

- Patient's starting position: sitting, fixation of the humerus on a wedge, the olecranon has to be free, elbow in submaximal extension (Fig. 4.90a).
- Movement: contact at the distal end of the ulna, and push of the ulna in a proximal direction (posterior glide) (Fig. 4.90b).

Ulnar glide

Therapy technique (film 168)

- Patient's starting position: lying on the right side, elbow in submaximal extension.
- Therapist's starting position: standing, at the patient's right side, fixation of the forearm radially with a wedge, just distally of the humeroradial joint cavity (Fig. 4.91a).
- Movement: push of the humerus in direction of the radial epicondyle of the humerus (Fig. 4.91b).

Self-exercise (film 169)

- Patient's starting position: sitting, fixation of the pronated forearm by a belt and the patient's legs (Fig. 4.92a).
- Movement: ulnar glide by push of the humerus in direction of the radial epicondyle of the humerus (Fig. 4.92b).

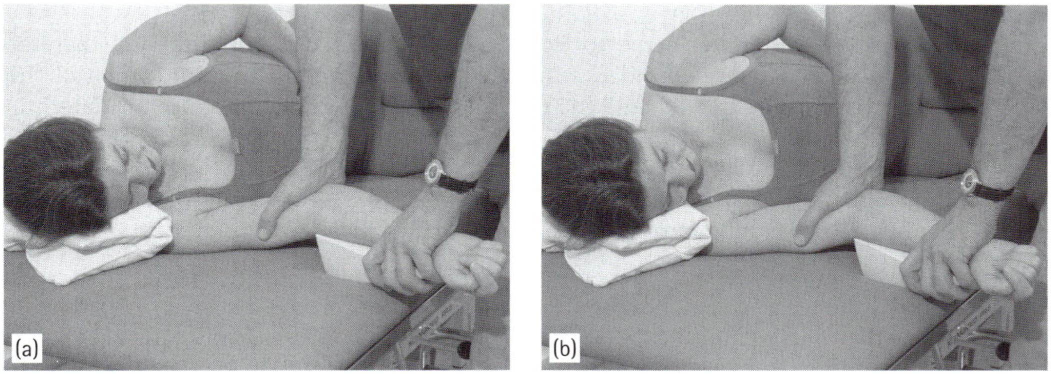

Figure 4.91a and b Passive mobilization; translatory movement; ulnar glide in the humero-ulnar joint; therapy technique. **a**, Starting position. **b**, End position.

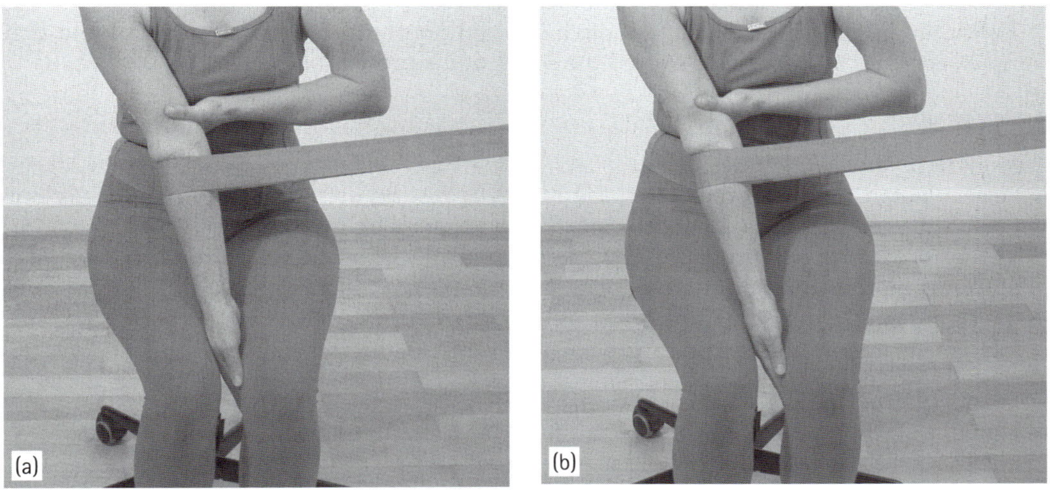

Figure 4.92a and b Passive mobilization; translatory movement; ulnar glide in the humero-ulnar joint; self-exercise. **a**, Starting position. **b**, End position.

Remarks (regarding translatory movements)

Goal of the technique

With a painfully restricted extension of the humero-ulnar joint due to an intra-articular mechanism (compression) in the posterior aspect of the joint, with simultaneously restricted translatory mobility in a posterior and ulnar direction, the described techniques serve to improve mobility by mobilization of non-symptom-provoking tissues.

Performance

Movement of the humerus in a radial direction with fixed forearm results in an ulnar glide in the humero-ulnar joint. Taking the oblique joint surface of the humero-ulnar joint into account, it is often necessary to modify the push in a proximal direction with respect to the ulna.

Dosage

Here, the described techniques serve to treat a non-symptomatic structure, and therefore dosage is not determined by wound healing. Rather, the expected training state (loading capacity) of the tissue to be treated, and the patient's personal expectations are the determining factors.

If there is any doubt, treatment is always started with very low force, and further increase is made conditional on reassessment. Thus, in treatment of the non-symptomatic structure, pain is not always the limiting factor for the dosage of a particular technique.

Choice of technique

The selection of the technique depends, among other things, on the therapist as well as the patient, on the therapist's clinical experience, but primarily on reassessment. This means that even if all preconditions on the part of therapist and patient seem to be met, it is of no use to continue the technique if reassessment is negative.

Contributing factors

For a satisfactory solution of the patient's current problems it is important to consider the contributing factors and include them in the treatment.

The authors will, however, not go into a description of the various possibilities and their complex contexts as this would exceed the scope of the present book.

Anterior glide

Therapy technique (film 166)

- Patient's starting position: supine, the humerus resting on a wedge or sandbag, elbow pre-positioned in submaximal extension.
- Therapist's starting position: standing, at the patient's right side, stabilization of the distal humerus by the left hand, with patient's olecranon not touching the plinth, contact with the right hand in the distal area of the ulna (Fig. 4.93a).
- Movement: intermittent traction at the ulna in an anterior direction (anterior glide) (Fig. 4.93b).

Self-exercise (film 167)

- Patient's starting position: sitting, fixation of the forearm on the thigh, elbow in submaximal extension (Fig. 4.94a).
- Movement: intermittent traction of the ulna in an anterior direction by repositioning the upper arm. With fixed ulna, this produces an anterior glide of the ulna (Fig. 4.94b).

Remarks

Goal of the technique

With a painfully restricted extension of the humero-ulnar joint due to an intra-articular mechanism (compression) in the posterior aspect of the joint, with simultaneously restricted translatory mobility in a posterior and ulnar direction, the described techniques serve to restore normal function of the symptomatic tissue by graduated application of the symptom-provoking stimulus (here: compression) in the symptomatic area of the joint.

Performance

The frequency of application of the technique depends on reassessment.

Dosage (regarding the affected structure)

Acute presentation (predominantly peripheral mechanisms): The described technique is applied in the first phase of wound healing (inflammation/proliferation phase). Consequently, it has to be performed without provoking pain.

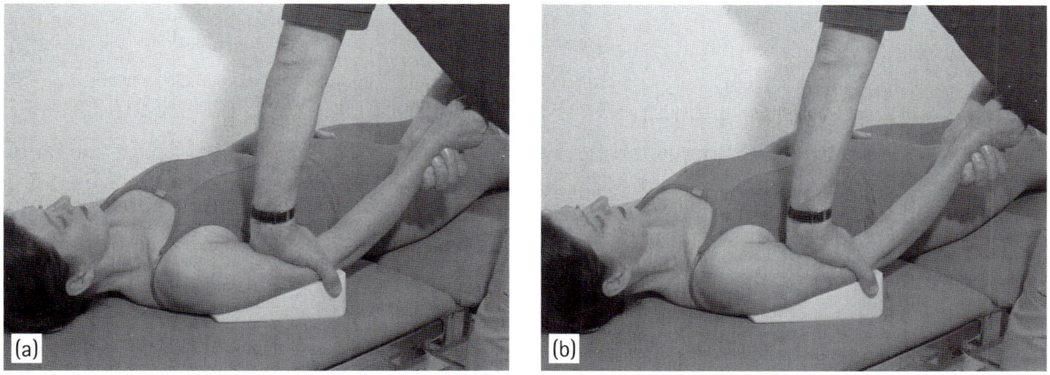

Figure 4.93a and b Passive mobilization; translatory movement; anterior glide in the humero-ulnar joint; therapy technique. **a**, Starting position. **b**, End position.

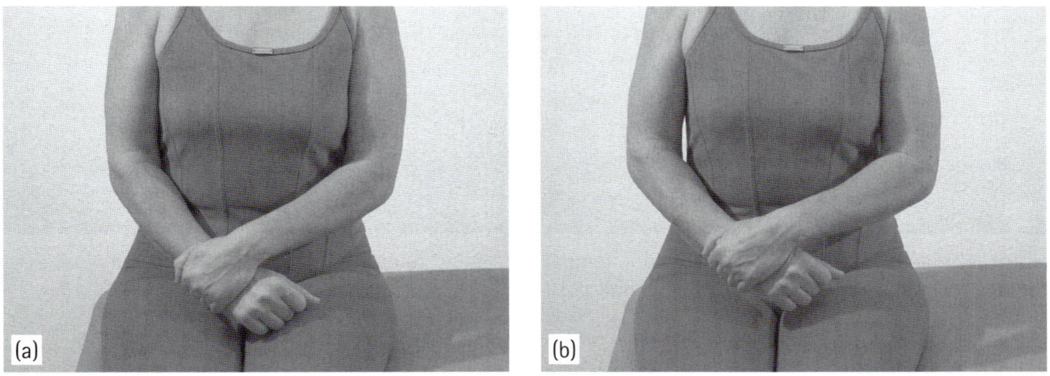

Figure 4.94a and b Passive mobilization; translatory movement; anterior glide in the humero-ulnar joint; self-exercise. **a**, Starting position. **b**, End position.

In the course of further healing (end of the proliferation/remodelling phase), in addition to functional stimulation of the affected tissue, angular movements with simultaneous compression are applied. Based on clinical experience, only the range of movement with free joint play is used.

With self-exercise at a more advanced state of healing, dosage of the compression component is determined by the amount of contraction of the periarticular muscles (e.g., co-contraction of the wrist flexors and wrist extensors with simultaneous movement in the elbow).

Choice of technique

The selection of the technique depends, among other things, on the therapist as well as the patient, on the therapist's clinical experience, but primarily on reassessment. This means that even if all preconditions on the part of therapist and patient seem to be met, it is of no use to continue the technique if reassessment is negative.

Contributing factors

For a satisfactory solution of the patient's current problems it is important to consider the contributing factors and include them in the treatment.

The authors will, however, not go into a description of the various possibilities and their complex contexts as this would exceed the scope of the present book.

ANGULAR MOVEMENTS

Ulnar gapping

Therapy technique (film 170)

- Patient's starting position: supine.
- Therapist's starting position: standing, at the patient's right side, contact over the elbow with the left hand from the radial side, and simultaneously fixing the forearm adjusted in pronation with the right hand, elbow adjusted in submaximal extension (Fig. 4.95a).
- Movement: ulnar gapping by pushing the left hand in the direction of the ulnar epicondyle of the humerus (Fig. 4.95b).

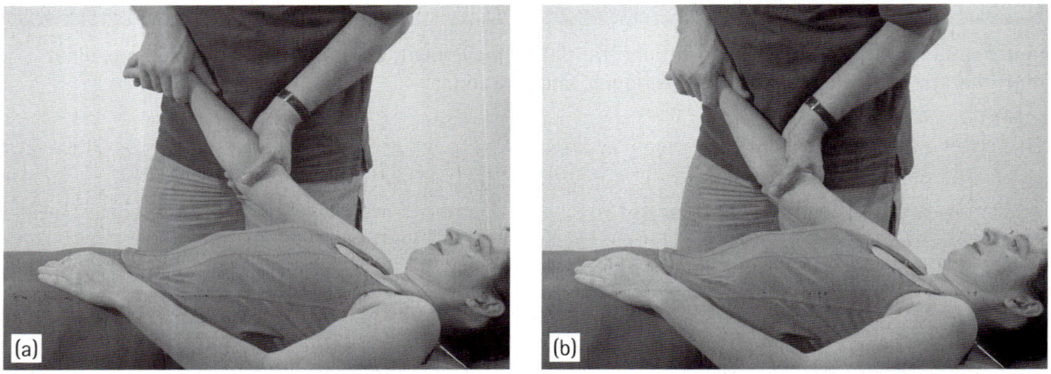

Figure 4.95a and b Passive mobilization; angular movement; ulnar gapping in the elbow complex; therapy technique. **a**, Starting position. **b**, End position.

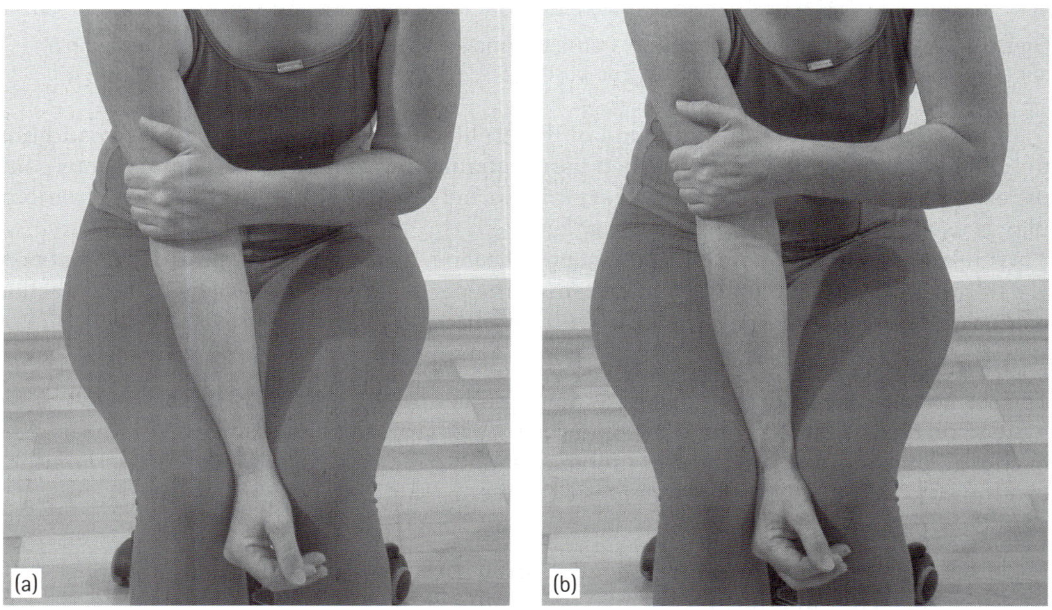

Figure 4.96a and b Passive mobilization; angular movement; ulnar gapping in the elbow complex; self-exercise. **a**, Starting position. **b**, End position.

Self-exercise (film 171)

- Patient's starting position: sitting, grasping the front edge of the seat with the right hand, further fixation by entrapping the distal forearm between the knees, external rotation of the right shoulder joint to adjust the forearm in pronation, contact over the elbow with the left hand from the radial side, the right elbow adjusted in submaximal extension (Fig. 4.96a).
- Movement: ulnar gapping by pulling the left hand in the direction of the ulnar epicondyle of the humerus (Fig. 4.96b).

Remarks (regarding angular movements)

Goal of the technique

With a painfully restricted extension of the humero-ulnar joint due to an intra-articular mechanism (compression) in the posterior area of the joint, with simultaneously restricted translatory mobility in a posterior and ulnar direction, the described techniques serve to improve mobility by mobilization of non-symptom-provoking tissues.

Performance

To achieve ulnar gapping and no extension or flexion by the push transversally across the joint, it is essential to determine the direction first by palpation of the radial and ulnar epicondyles. During ulnar gapping, the patient may feel some pulling sensation on the ulnar side of the joint, but the typical pain with extension must not appear.

Dosage (regarding the affected structure)

Here, the described technique serves to treat a non-symptomatic structure, and therefore dosage is not determined by wound healing. Rather, the expected training state (loading capacity) of the tissue to be treated, and the patient's personal expectations are the determining factors.

If there is any doubt, treatment is always started with very low force, and further increase is made conditional on reassessment. Thus, in treatment of the non-symptomatic structure, pain is not always the limiting factor for the dosage of a particular technique.

Choice of technique

The selection of the technique depends, among other things, on the therapist as well as the patient, on the therapist's clinical experience, but primarily on reassessment. This means that even if all preconditions on the part of therapist and patient seem to be met, it is of no use to continue the technique if reassessment is negative.

Contributing factors

For a satisfactory solution of the patient's current problems it is essential to consider the contributing factors and include them in the treatment.

The authors will, however, not go into a description of the various possibilities and their complex contexts as this would exceed the scope of the present book.

Chapter 5

Radial distal forearm

CHAPTER CONTENTS

AREA LOCALIZATION

IDENTIFICATION OF THE POTENTIALLY AFFECTED AREA BY DEMONSTRATION OF A SYMPTOMATIC FUNCTIONAL MOVEMENT/POSITION

Based on the information gained from the anamnesis so far, the therapist tries to ascertain more details about potentially affected sections. This is done by means of area localization, which represents the beginning of the physical examination. Information gained in this way is used to check or modify the relevant hypotheses developed on the basis of the anamnesis and will determine how to proceed.

Area localization is explained by means of examples. In both examples, the patient feels pain in the area of the radial distal forearm. Based on clinical experience and known clinical patterns, primarily the following sections are considered as potential sources of the current complaints:

- cervical spine
- elbow complex
- hand complex
- neural structures.

General question: Is there enough information available to skip area localization?	
No	Yes
⇓	⇓
Performance of area localization	• General movement tests • Additional tests • Test treatment

Example 1: Volar flexion

Symptom area: radial distal forearm
Symptom provocation: volar flexion of the wrist (Fig. 5.1)

With this clinical presentation, the underlying theoretical model and clinical experience suggest primarily the cervical spine, the hand complex, the elbow complex, and the neural structures as potential symptom-provoking areas.

Below, examples illustrate how to differentiate between these areas. To this end, area localization is first attempted by means of active movements alone. If this is not possible, tests will be performed by means of assistive movements.

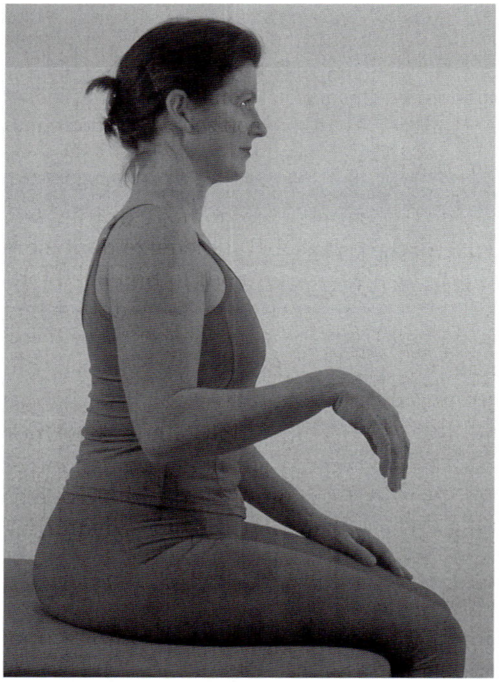

Figure 5.1 Symptom-provoking movement: movement of the hand into volar flexion provokes symptoms in the area of the distal lateral forearm.

Hypothesis 1: The symptom-provoking area is the cervical spine
Differentiation: cervical spine vs. hand complex.

The change in symptoms can be demonstrated exactly:

- provocation of pain (Fig. 5.2a and b, film 208)
- alleviation of pain (Fig. 5.3a and b, film 209).

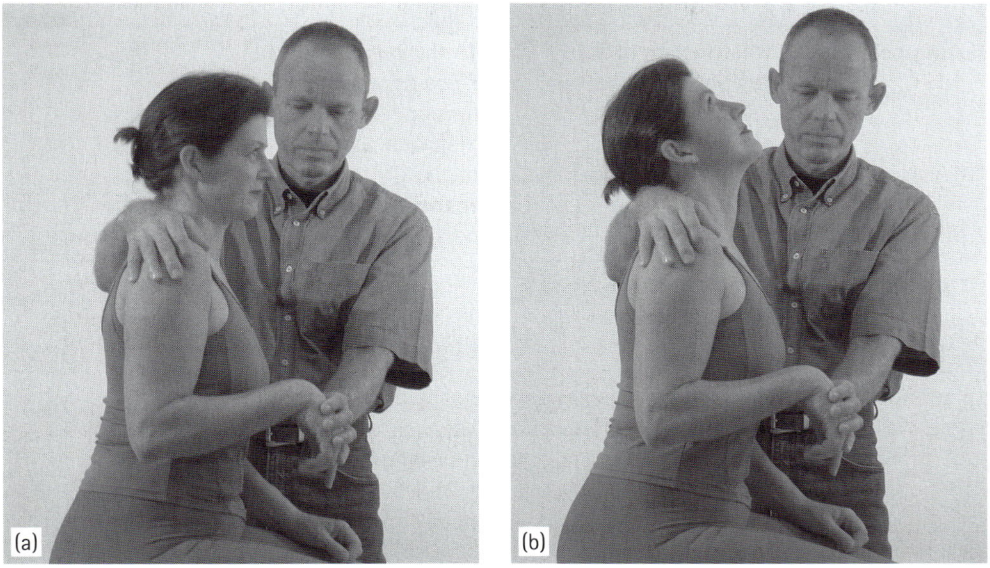

Figure 5.2a and b Area localization with symptomatic volar flexion of the wrist; differentiation between cervical spine and hand complex; provocation. **a**, Starting position. **b**, End position.

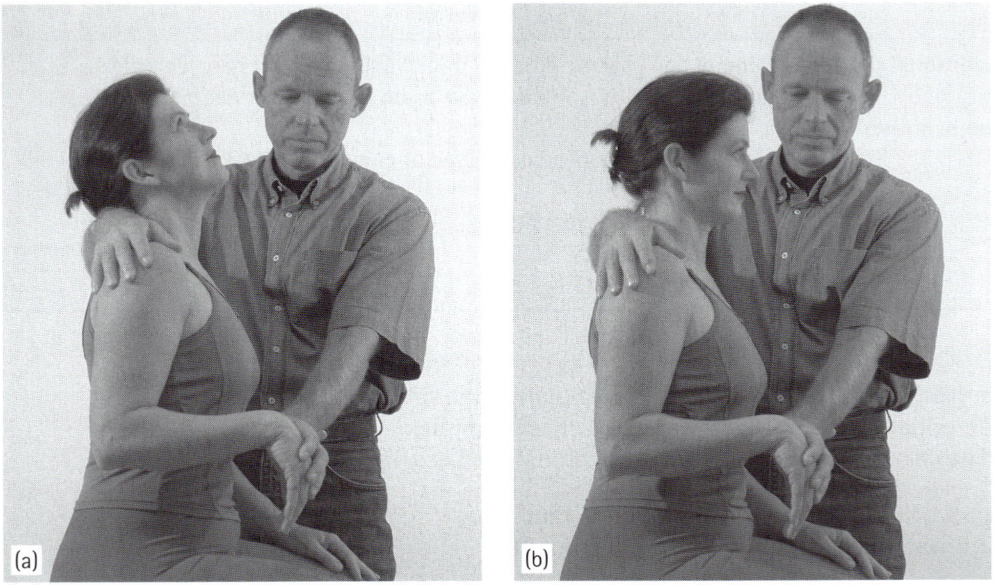

Figure 5.3a and b Area localization with symptomatic volar flexion of the wrist; differentiation between cervical spine and hand complex; alleviation. **a**, Starting position. **b**, End position.

The result of area localization has to be verified by further specific tests; otherwise the result will be open to question.

Assessment

Goal	Provocation of pain	Alleviation of pain	Remarks
Starting position	Volar flexion to a position immediately before symptoms appear	With the cervical spine pre-positioned in extension, volar flexion to a position immediately after symptoms have appeared	
Test movement	Extension of the cervical spine	Moving the cervical spine back to neutral position	Hand remains in starting position
Explanation	If by any movement of the cervical spine (here, as an example, extension) the typical symptoms are reproduced, an isolated lesion of the hand complex is doubtful	If by any movement of the cervical spine (here, as an example, moving the cervical spine back to neutral position) the typical symptoms are alleviated, an isolated lesion of the hand complex is doubtful	
Additional data to support the hypothesis	General and specific mobility of cervical spine and hand complex (potential positive findings have to be found under neural relaxation as well) History, symptom behaviour, type of complaints, 24-hour behaviour Palpation Reproducibility of test results Test treatment Imaging procedures (CT, MRI)		

Hypothesis 2: The symptom-provoking area is the neural structures

Differentiation: neural involvement vs. hand complex.

The change in symptoms can be demonstrated exactly:

- provocation of pain (Fig. 5.4a and b, film 210)
- alleviation of pain (Fig. 5.5a and b, film 211).

The result of area localization has to be verified by further specific tests; otherwise the result will be open to question.

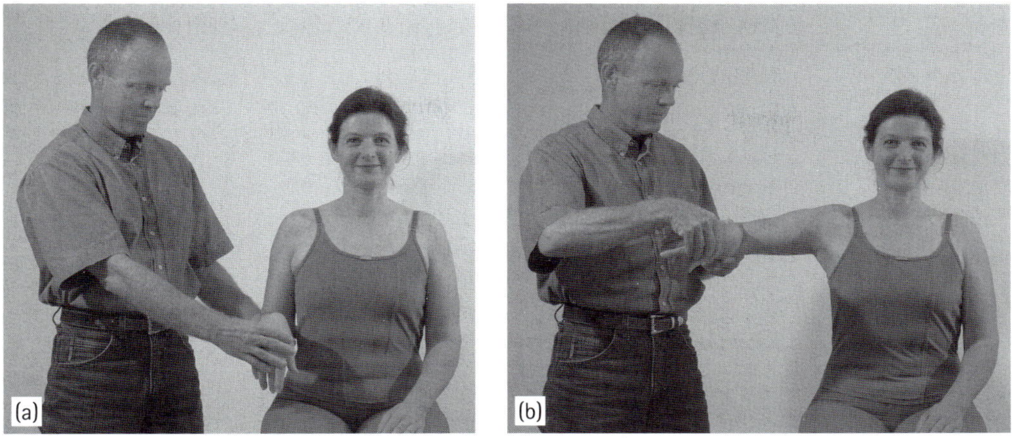

Figure 5.4a and b Area localization with symptomatic volar flexion of the wrist; differentiation between neural structures and hand complex; provocation. **a**, Starting position. **b**, End position.

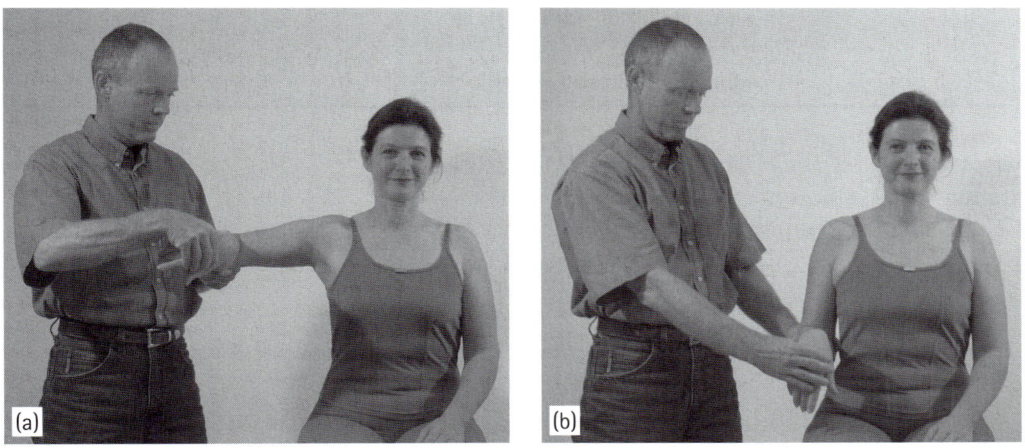

Figure 5.5a and b Area localization with symptomatic volar flexion of the wrist; differentiation between neural structures and hand complex; alleviation. **a**, Starting position. **b**, End position.

Assessment

Goal	Provocation of pain	Alleviation of pain	Remarks
Starting position	Volar flexion to a position immediately before symptoms appear	Volar flexion to a position immediately after symptoms have appeared, with the glenohumeral joint adjusted in abduction before	

Goal	Provocation of pain	Alleviation of pain	Remarks
Test movement	Abduction of the glenohumeral joint	Adduction of the glenohumeral joint	All other joints have to remain immobile
Explanation	Abduction of the glenohumeral joint produces mechanical stress on the neural structures and the structures associated with them	Adduction of the glenohumeral joint reduces mechanical stress on the neural structures and the structures associated with them	
Additional data to support the hypothesis	Further movements of proximal and/or distal components to increase neural tension not involved in dorsal flexion of the wrist History, symptom behaviour, type of complaints, 24-hour behaviour Neurodynamic tests Nerve provocation tests (Spurling's test) Nerve palpation Reproducibility of test results Test treatment Imaging procedures (CT, MRI)		

Hypothesis 3: The symptom-provoking area is the elbow complex

Differentiation: elbow complex vs. hand complex.

The change in symptoms can be demonstrated exactly:

- provocation of pain (Fig. 5.6a and b, film 212)
- alleviation of pain (Fig. 5.7a and b, film 213).

The result of area localization has to be verified by further specific tests; otherwise the result will be open to question.

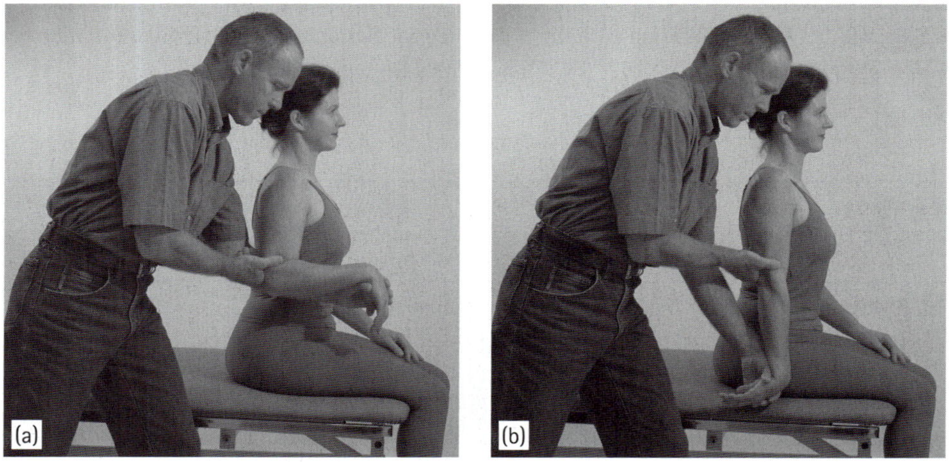

Figure 5.6a and b Area localization with symptomatic volar flexion of the wrist; differentiation between elbow complex and hand complex; provocation. **a**, Starting position. **b**, End position.

Assessment			
Goal	**Provocation of pain**	**Alleviation of pain**	**Remarks**
Starting position	Volar flexion to a position immediately before symptoms appear	With the elbow pre-positioned in extension, volar flexion to a position immediately after symptoms have appeared	
Test movement	Extension of the elbow	Flexion of the elbow	Hand remains in starting position
Explanation	If, with elbow adjusted in flexion and wrist adjusted in volar flexion shortly before P1, pain is provoked by extension of the elbow, this suggests that there is probably no isolated lesion of the wrist itself	If, with elbow adjusted in extension and wrist adjusted in volar flexion shortly before P1, pain is alleviated by flexion of the elbow, this suggests that there is probably no isolated lesion of the wrist	
Additional data to support the hypothesis	General and specific mobility of elbow complex and hand complex History, symptom behaviour, type of complaints, 24-hour behaviour Palpation Reproducibility of test results Test treatment Imaging procedures (CT, MRI)		

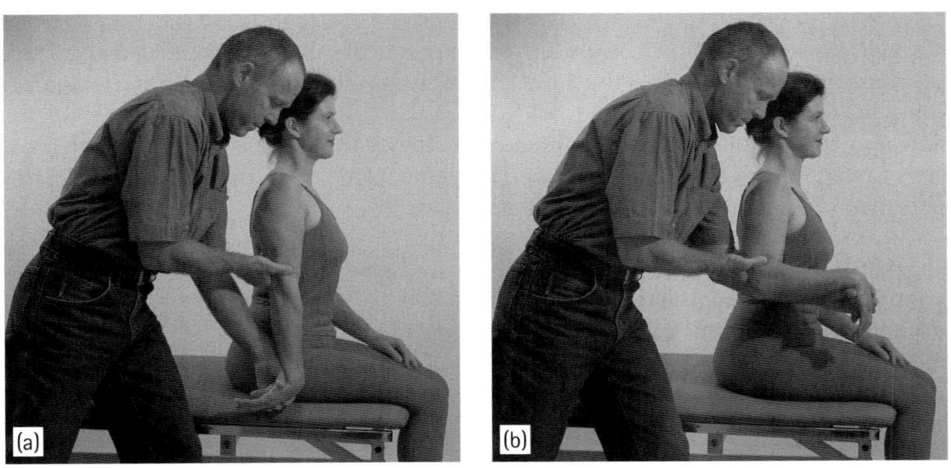

Figure 5.7a and b Area localization with symptomatic volar flexion of the wrist; differentiation between elbow complex and hand complex; alleviation. **a**, Starting position. **b**, End position.

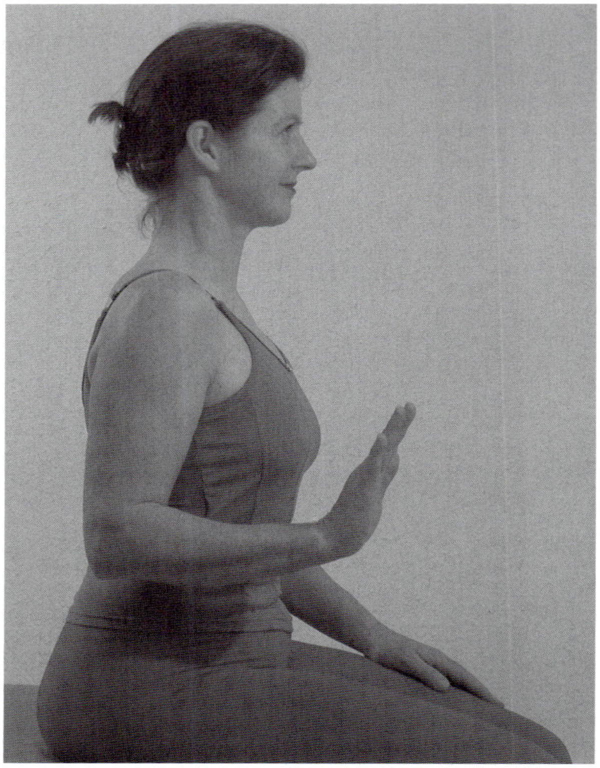

Figure 5.8 Symptom-provoking movement: movement of the hand into dorsal flexion provokes symptoms in the area of the distal lateral forearm.

Example 2: Dorsal flexion

Symptom area: radial distal forearm
Symptom provocation: dorsal flexion of the wrist (Fig. 5.8)

With this clinical presentation, the underlying theoretical model and clinical experience suggest primarily the cervical spine, the hand complex, the elbow complex, and the neural structures as symptom-provoking areas.

Below, examples illustrate how to differentiate between these areas. To this end, area localization is first attempted by means of active movements alone. If this is not possible, tests will be performed by means of assistive movements.

Hypothesis 1: The symptom-provoking area is the cervical spine
Differentiation: cervical spine vs. hand complex.

The change in symptoms can be demonstrated exactly:

- provocation of pain (Fig. 5.9a and b, film 220)
- alleviation of pain (Fig. 5.10a and b, film 221).

The result of area localization has to be verified by further specific tests; otherwise the result will be open to question.

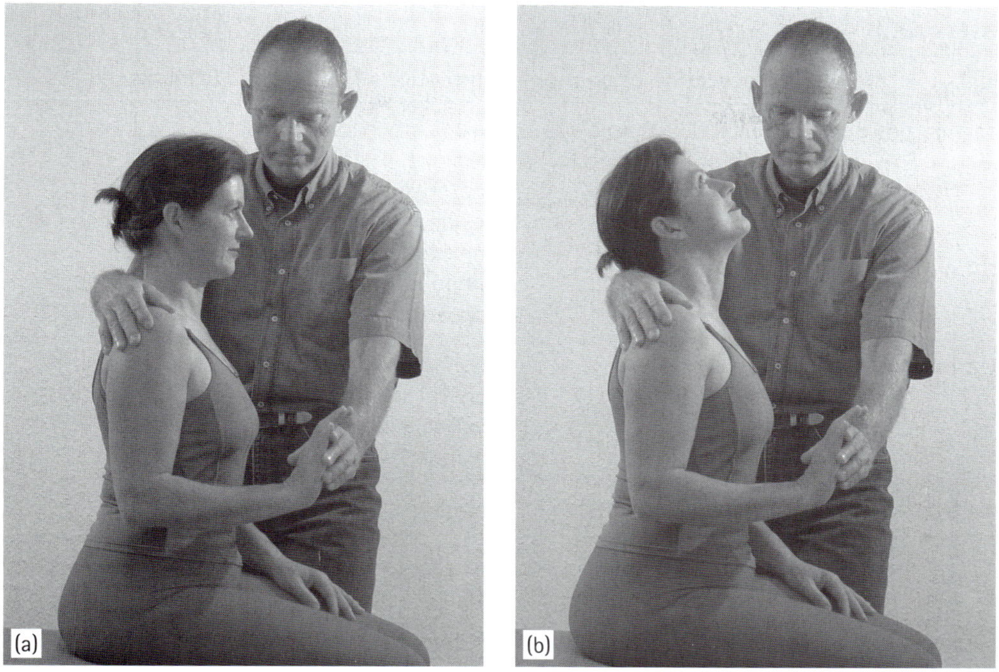

Figure 5.9a and b Area localization with symptomatic dorsal flexion of the wrist; differentiation between cervical spine and hand complex; provocation. **a**, Starting position. **b**, End position.

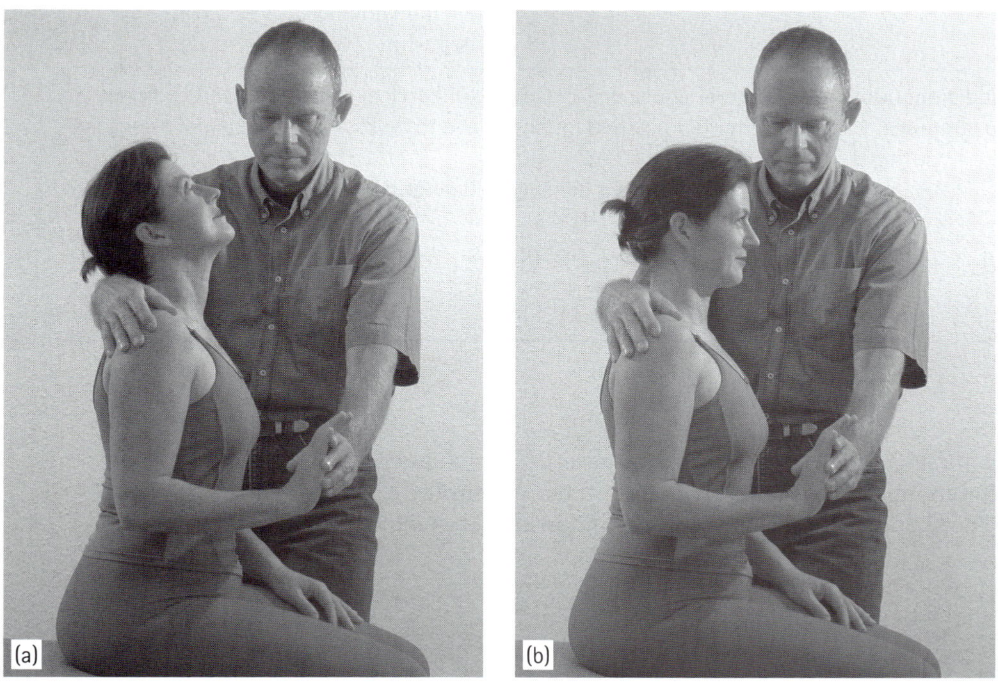

Figure 5.10a and b Area localization with symptomatic dorsal flexion of the wrist; differentiation between cervical spine and hand complex; alleviation. **a**, Starting position. **b**, End position.

Assessment			
Goal	**Provocation of pain**	**Alleviation of pain**	**Remarks**
Starting position	Dorsal flexion to a position immediately before symptoms appear	With the cervical spine pre-positioned in extension, dorsal flexion to a position immediately after symptoms have appeared	
Test movement	Extension of the cervical spine	Moving the cervical spine back to neutral position	Hand remains in starting position
Explanation	If by any movement of the cervical spine (here, as an example, extension) the typical symptoms are reproduced, an isolated lesion of the hand complex is doubtful	If by any movement of the cervical spine (here, as an example, moving the cervical spine back to neutral position) the typical symptoms are alleviated, an isolated lesion of the hand complex is doubtful	
Additional data to support the hypothesis	General and specific mobility of cervical spine and hand complex (potential positive findings have to be found under neural relaxation as well) History, symptom behaviour, type of complaints, 24-hour behaviour Palpation Reproducibility of test results Test treatment Imaging procedures (CT, MRI)		

Hypothesis 2: The symptom-provoking area is the neural structures
Differentiation: neural involvement vs. hand complex.

The change in symptoms can be demonstrated exactly:

- provocation of pain (Fig. 5.11a and b, film 222)
- alleviation of pain (Fig. 5.12a and b, film 223).

The result of area localization has to be verified by further specific tests; otherwise the result will be open to question.

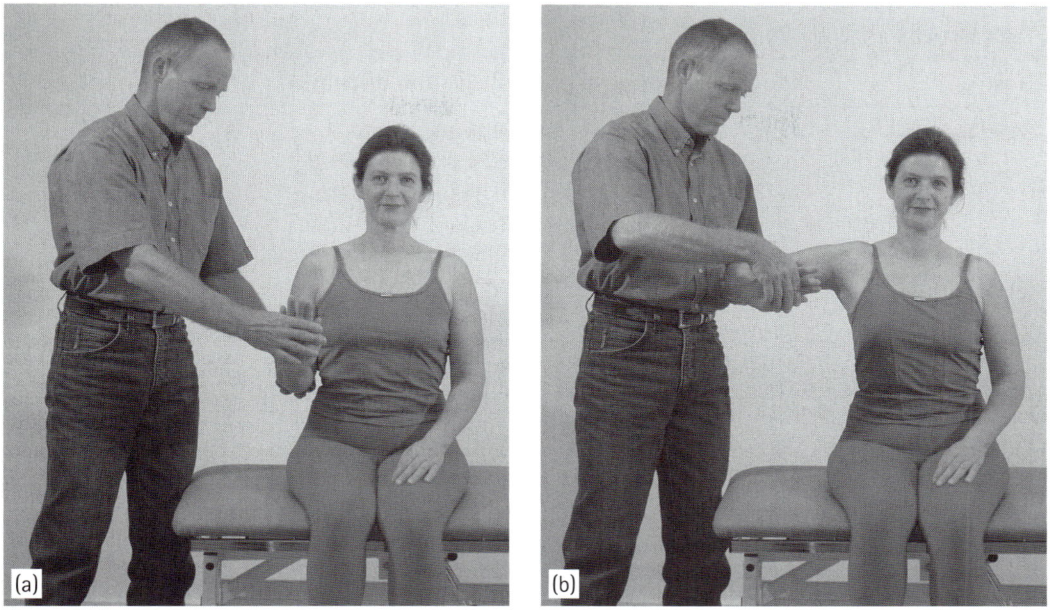

Figure 5.11a and b Area localization with symptomatic dorsal flexion of the wrist; differentiation between neural structures and hand complex; provocation. **a**, Starting position. **b**, End position.

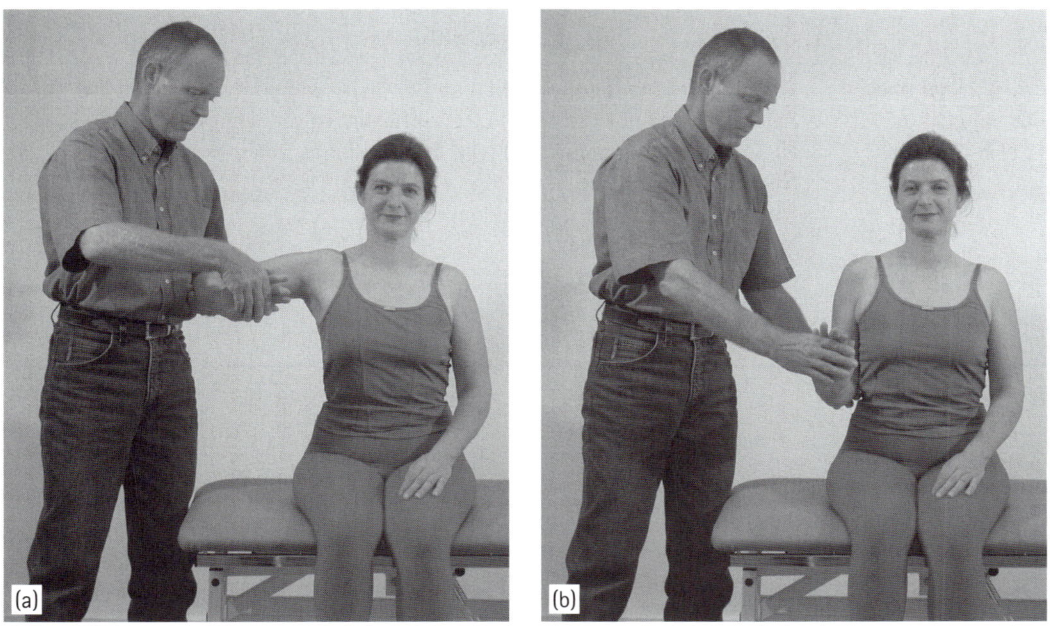

Figure 5.12a and b Area localization with symptomatic dorsal flexion of the wrist; differentiation between neural structures and hand complex; alleviation. **a**, Starting position. **b**, End position.

Assessment			
Goal	**Provocation of pain**	**Alleviation of pain**	**Remarks**
Starting position	Dorsal flexion to a position immediately before symptoms appear	With the glenohumeral joint pre-positioned in abduction, dorsal flexion to a position immediately after symptoms have appeared	
Test movement	Abduction of the glenohumeral joint	Adduction of the glenohumeral joint	All other joints have to remain immobile
Explanation	Abduction of the glenohumeral joint produces mechanical stress on the brachial plexus and the structures associated with it. If the patient's symptoms can be provoked by these manoeuvres, an isolated lesion of the hand complex is doubtful	Adduction of the glenohumeral joint reduces mechanical stress on the brachial plexus and the structures associated with it. If the patient's symptoms can be alleviated by these manoeuvres, an isolated lesion of the hand complex is doubtful	
Additional data to support the hypothesis	Further movements of proximal and/or distal components to increase neural tension not involved in dorsal flexion of the wrist History, symptom behaviour, type of complaints, 24-hour behaviour Neurodynamic tests Nerve provocation tests (Spurling's test) Nerve palpation Reproducibility of test results Test treatment Imaging procedures (CT, MRI)s		

Hypothesis 3: The symptom-provoking area is the elbow complex
Differentiation: elbow complex vs. hand complex.

The change in symptoms can be demonstrated exactly:

- provocation of pain (Fig. 5.13a and b, film 224)
- alleviation of pain (Fig. 5.14a and b, film 225).

The result of area localization has to be verified by further specific tests; otherwise the result will be open to question.

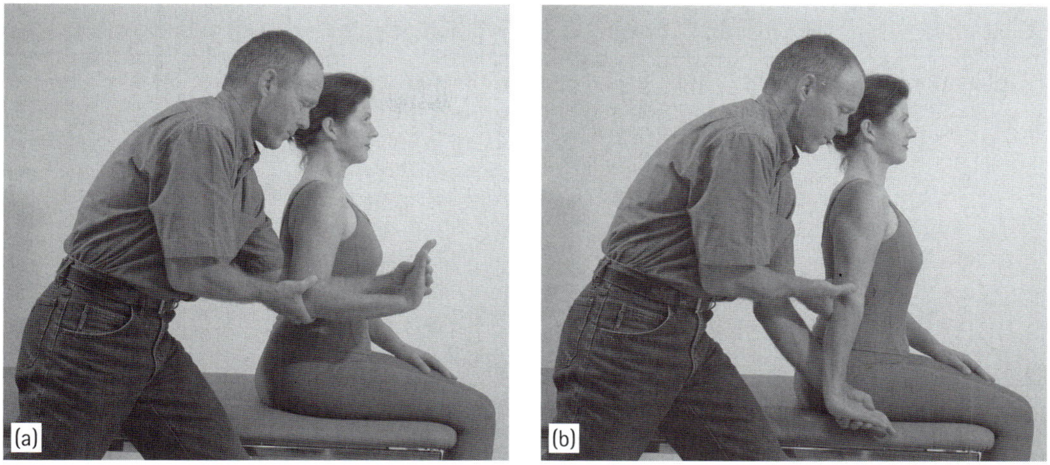

Figure 5.13a and b Area localization with symptomatic dorsal flexion of the wrist; differentiation between elbow complex and hand complex; provocation. **a**, Starting position. **b**, End position.

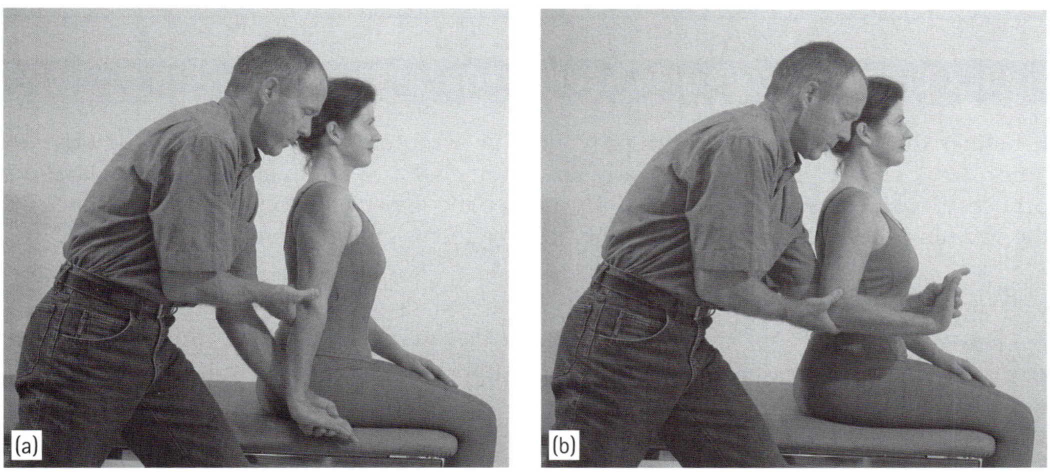

Figure 5.14a and b Area localization with symptomatic dorsal flexion of the wrist; differentiation between elbow complex and hand complex; alleviation. **a**, Starting position. **b**, End position.

Assessment

Goal	Provocation of pain	Alleviation of pain	Remarks
Starting position	Dorsal flexion to a position immediately before symptoms appear	Dorsal flexion to a position immediately after symptoms have appeared	
Test movement	Extension of the elbow	Flexion of the elbow	Hand remains in starting position

Goal	Provocation of pain	Alleviation of pain	Remarks
Explanation	If, with flexed elbow and the hand adjusted in volar flexion shortly before P1, extension of the elbow provokes pain, this means that an isolated lesion of the wrist itself is improbable	If, with extended elbow and the hand adjusted in volar flexion shortly after P1, flexion of the elbow alleviates pain, this means that an isolated lesion of the wrist itself is improbable	
Additional data to support the hypothesis	General and specific mobility of elbow complex and hand complex History, symptom behaviour, type of complaints, 24-hour behaviour Palpation Reproducibility of test results Test treatment Imaging procedures (CT, MRI)		

QUICK CHECK – SYMPTOMS, RADIAL FOREARM

If neither the area nor a symptom-provoking or symptom-reducing action is known, the quick check is used to try to load individual potential areas with specific biomechanically provocative movement combinations. The chosen movement combinations correspond with the straining and often symptom-provoking movements of the individual sections.

CERVICAL SPINE (film 15)

Movement

- Extension/lateral flexion, and rotation to the opposite side (Figs 5.15 and 5.16)
- Extension/lateral flexion, and rotation to the same side (Figs 5.17 and 5.18).

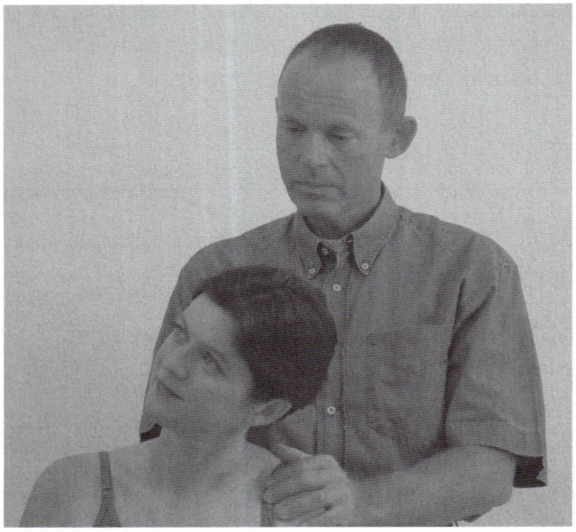

Figure 5.15 Quick check cervical spine; lateral flexion to the left with rotation to the opposite side.

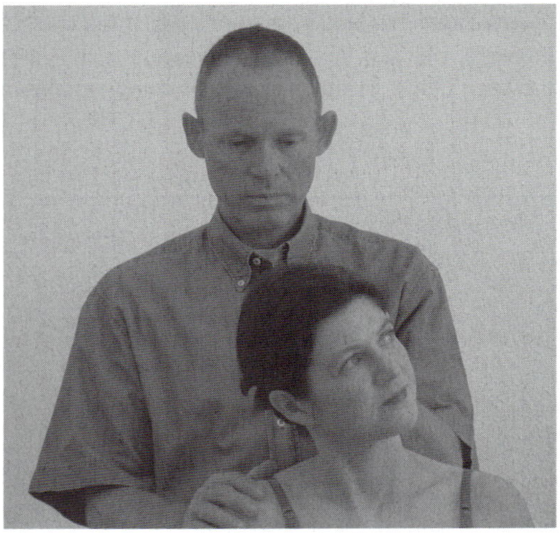

Figure 5.16 Quick check cervical spine; lateral flexion to the right with rotation to the opposite side.

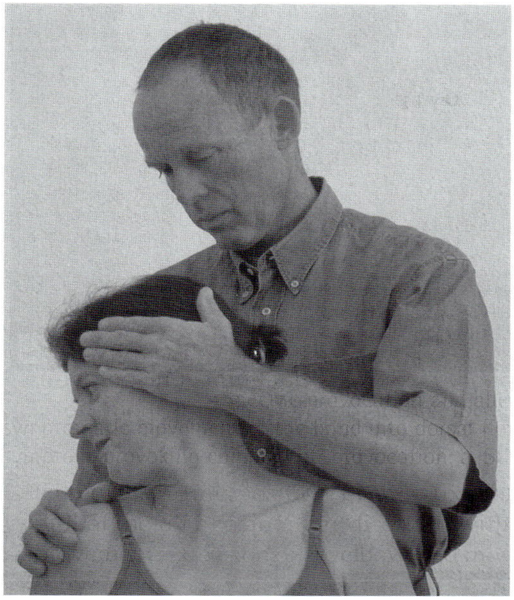

Figure 5.17 Quick check cervical spine; lateral flexion to the right with rotation to the same side.

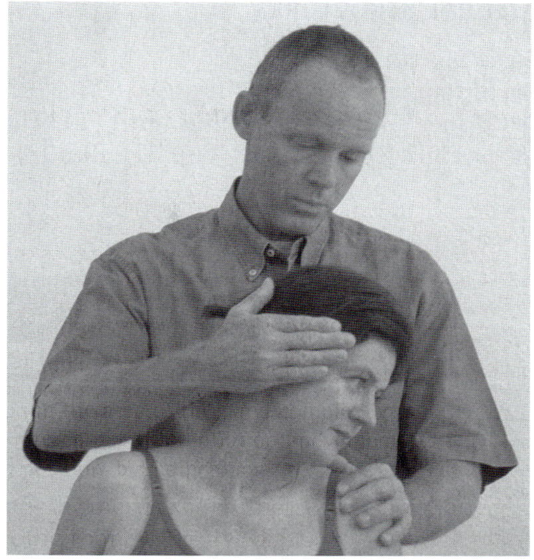

Figure 5.18 Quick check cervical spine; lateral flexion to the left with rotation to the same side.

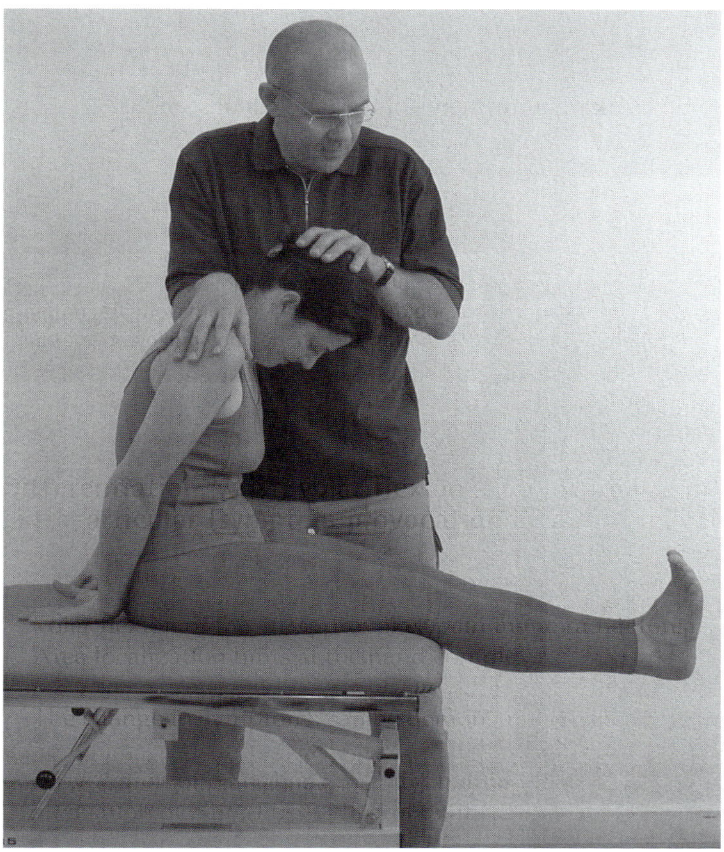

Figure 5.19 Quick check neurodynamics; slump test.

NEURAL STRUCTURES

Tension tests

- Slump test (Fig. 5.19, film 16)
- Upper limb neurodynamic test 1 (ULNT-1; Fig. 5.20, film 17)
- Straight leg raise (SLR; Fig. 5.21, film 18).

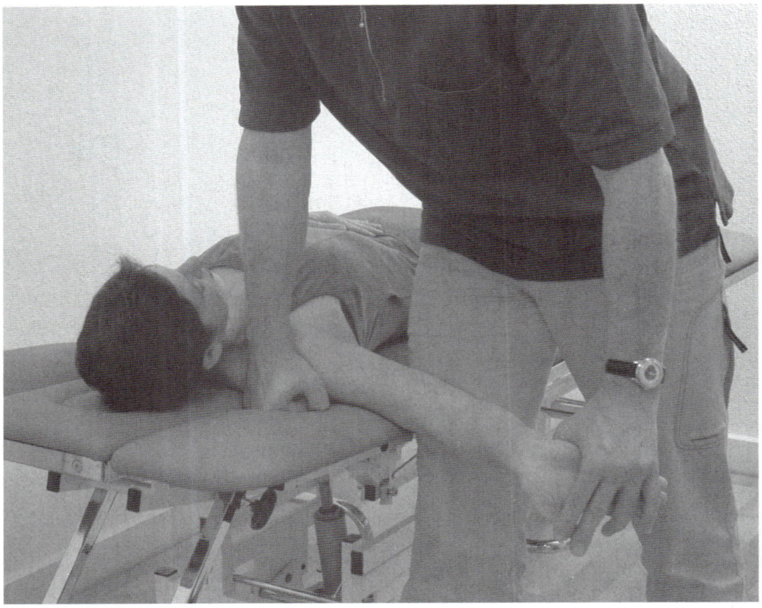

Figure 5.20 Quick check neurodynamics; upper limb tension test 1 (ULNT-1).

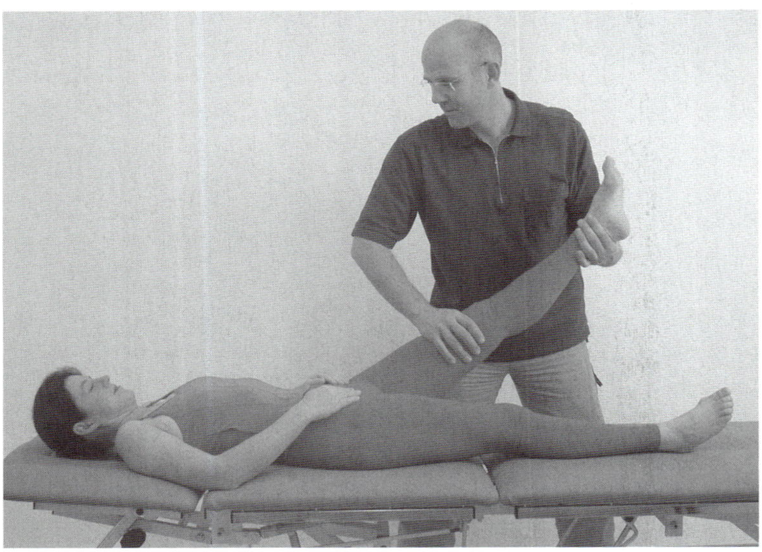

Figure 5.21 Quick check neurodynamics; straight leg raise test (SLR).

ELBOW COMPLEX

Movement

- Extension/supination (Fig. 5.22, film 249)
- Flexion/pronation (Fig. 5.23, film 250).

HAND COMPLEX (film 251)

Movement

- Dorsal flexion/radial abduction (Fig. 5.24)
- Volar flexion/ulnar abduction (Fig. 5.25).

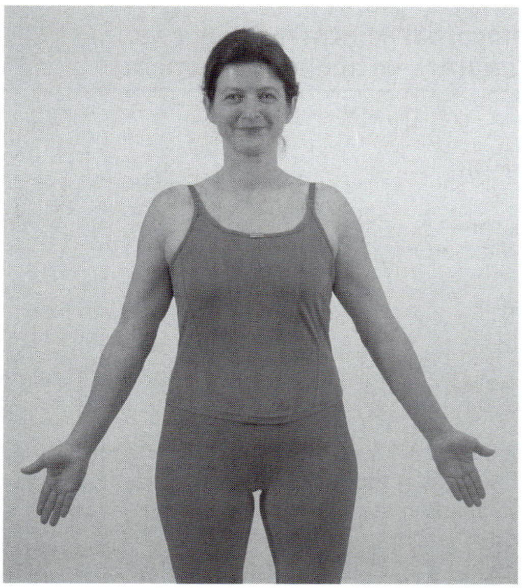

Figure 5.22 Quick check elbow complex; movement into extension, with previously adjusted supination.

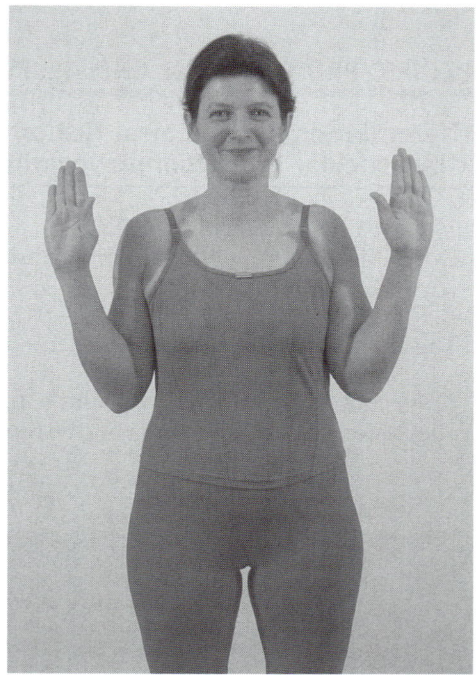

Figure 5.23 Quick check elbow complex; movement into flexion, with previously adjusted pronation.

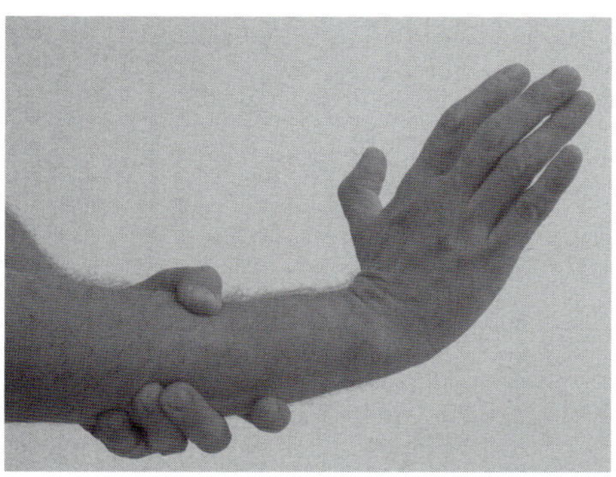

Figure 5.24 Quick check hand complex; movement into dorsal flexion and radial abduction.

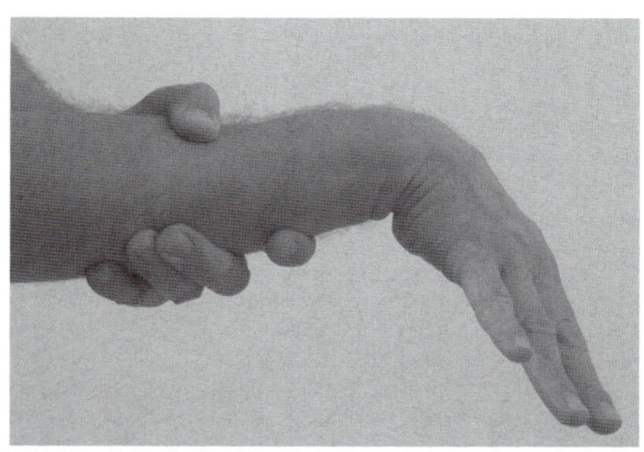

Figure 5.25 Quick check hand complex; movement into volar flexion and ulnar abduction.

Note: Even an area that proves negative in the quick check may possibly be symptom-provoking (another movement combination, or passive overpressure may be required).

SPECIFIC PROVOCATION AND ALLEVIATION

Specific provocation and alleviation allows one to differentiate within an articular complex and to identify the symptom-provoking movement direction(s).

SPECIFIC PROVOCATION AND ALLEVIATION, HAND COMPLEX

Differentiation, wrist, dorsal flexion – radiocarpal – intra-articular vs. extra-articular (symptom provocation by an intra-articular component)

Pain-provoking movement (Fig. 5.26)

- Dorsal flexion provokes pain in the radial forearm.
- Area localization hints at the hand complex.

The change in symptoms can be demonstrated exactly:

- provocation of pain (Fig. 5.27a and b, film 226)
- alleviation of pain (Fig. 5.28a and b, film 227).

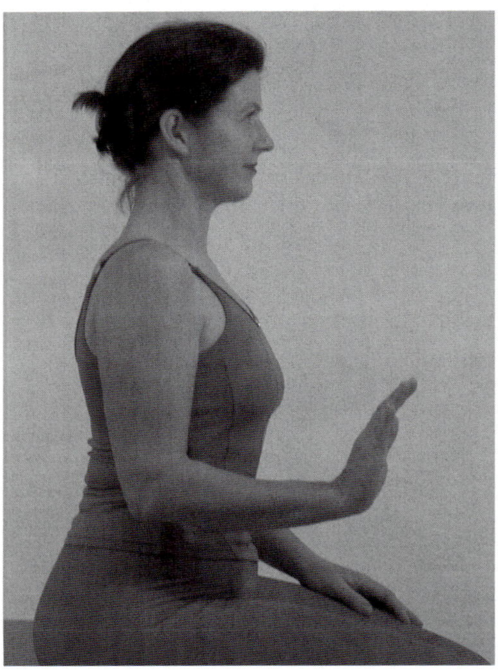

Figure 5.26 Symptom-provoking movement: movement of the hand into dorsal flexion provokes symptoms in the area of the distal lateral forearm.

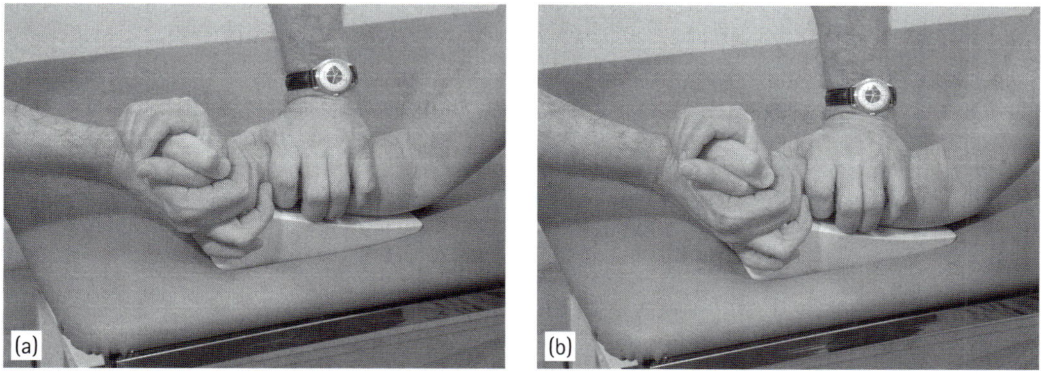

Figure 5.27a and b Specific provocation and alleviation in the area of the hand complex with symptomatic movement of the hand into dorsal flexion, intra-articular mechanism as symptom-provoking component; provocation. **a**, Starting position. **b**, End position.

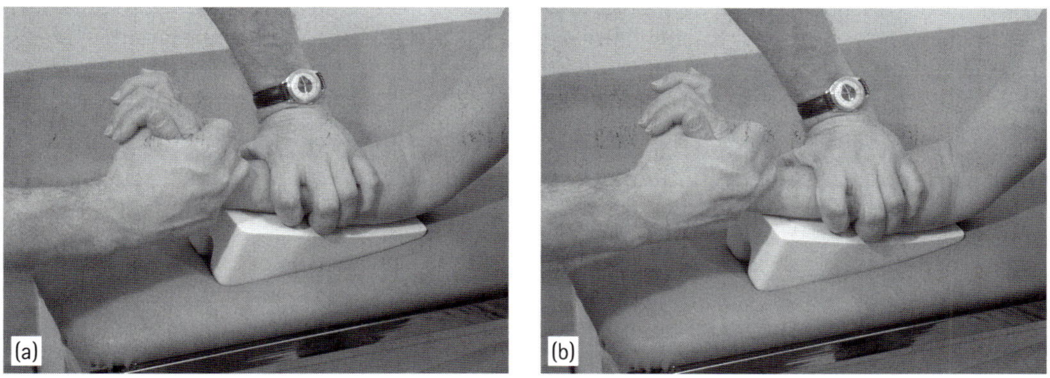

Figure 5.28a and b Specific provocation and alleviation in the area of the hand complex with symptomatic movement of the hand into dorsal flexion, intra-articular mechanism as symptom-provoking component; alleviation. **a**, Starting position. **b**, End position.

Assessment

Goal	Provocation of pain	Alleviation of pain	Remarks
Starting position	Dorsal flexion to a position immediately after symptoms have appeared	Dorsal flexion to a position immediately after symptoms have appeared	The starting position for pain provocation must not be symptom-free, since in a symptom-free position symptomatic tissue might possibly not be compressed, and thus the patient's symptoms cannot be reproduced

Goal	Provocation of pain	Alleviation of pain	Remarks
Test movement	Compression of the carpus, with fixed radius	Traction of the carpus, with fixed radius	
Neural involvement	Proximal component without change of position in the relevant area	Proximal component without change of position in the relevant area	
Explanation	This manoeuvre increases the intra-articular compression in pain-provoking position	This manoeuvre reduces the intra-articular compression in pain-provoking position	
Additional data to support the hypothesis	General and specific mobility of the hand complex History, symptom behaviour, type of complaints, 24-hour behaviour Specific palpation Reproducibility of test results Test treatment Imaging procedures (CT, MRI)		

Differentiation, wrist, dorsal flexion – radiocarpal – extra-articular vs. intra-articular (symptom provocation by an extra-articular component)

The change in symptoms can be demonstrated exactly:

- provocation of pain (Fig. 5.29a and b, film 228).

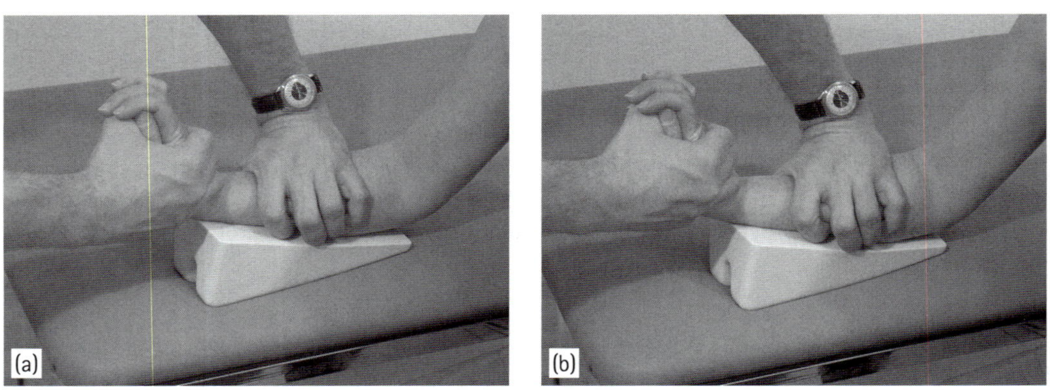

Figure 5.29a and b Specific provocation in the area of the hand complex with symptomatic movement of the hand into dorsal flexion, extra-articular mechanism as symptom-provoking component. **a**, Starting position. **b**, End position.

Assessment			
Goal	**Provocation of pain**	**Alleviation of pain**	**Remarks**
Starting position	Dorsal flexion to a position immediately before symptoms appear		
Test movement	Traction of the carpus, with fixed radius		It is questionable whether, by compression of the joint, the extra-articular structures can be sufficiently relaxed to alleviate symptoms. Therefore, alleviation is not described here
Neural involvement	Proximal component without change of position in the relevant area		
Explanation	This manoeuvre increases the pull on the extra-articular structures		
Additional data to support the hypothesis	General and specific mobility of the hand complex History, symptom behaviour, type of complaints, 24-hour behaviour Specific palpation Reproducibility of test results Test treatment Imaging procedures (CT, MRI)		

Differentiation, wrist, dorsal flexion – intercarpal – radiocarpal

The change in symptoms can be demonstrated exactly:

- provocation of pain (Fig. 5.30a and b, film 229)
- alleviation of pain (Fig. 5.31a and b, film 230).

Assessment			
Goal	**Provocation of pain**	**Alleviation of pain**	**Remarks**
Starting position	Dorsal flexion to a position immediately	Dorsal flexion to a position immediately	

Goal	Provocation of pain	Alleviation of pain	Remarks
	before symptoms appear	after symptoms have appeared	
Test movement	● Trapezium bones in dorsal direction with fixed scaphoid bone ● Scaphoid bone in volar direction with fixed radius ● Lunar bone in volar direction with fixed radius and ulna ● Capitate bone in volar direction with fixed lunar bone	● Trapezium bones in volar direction with fixed scaphoid bone ● Scaphoid bone in dorsal direction with fixed radius ● Lunar bone in dorsal direction with fixed radius and ulna ● Capitate bone in dorsal direction with fixed lunar bone	
Neural involvement	Proximal component without change of position in the relevant area (here, e.g., depression of the shoulder girdle)	Proximal component without change of position in the relevant area (here, e.g., elevation of the shoulder girdle)	
Explanation	If the patient's symptoms can be provoked by the described movements of the individual carpal bones, this hints at symptomatic tissue in the tested area	If the patient's symptoms can be alleviated by the described movements of the individual carpal bones, this hints at symptomatic tissue in the tested area	
Additional data to support the hypothesis	General and specific mobility of the hand complex History, symptom behaviour, type of complaints, 24-hour behaviour Specific palpation Reproducibility of test results Test treatment Imaging procedures (CT, MRI)		

Note: If the pain-provoking component is the rolling component with decentring effect, the push for provocation or alleviation must, with convex joint partners, go in the same direction of the hand movement. Based on pain localization, symptom provocation by the intercarpal bones of the ulnar column seems less probable and therefore is not described here. To check the hypothesis of symptom provocation by the ulnar column, the respective bones will have to be tested according to the same principles.

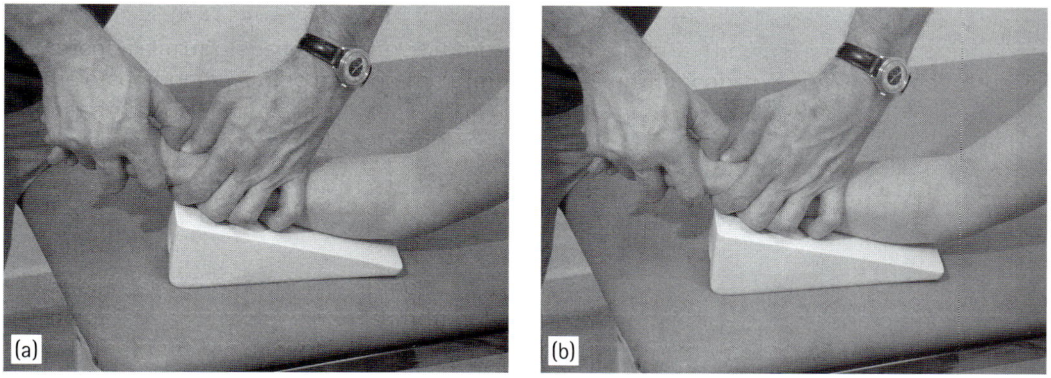

Figure 5.30a and b Specific provocation and alleviation in the area of the hand complex with symptomatic movement of the hand into dorsal flexion; intercarpal differentiation; movement as symptom-provoking component; provocation. **a**, Starting position. **b**, End position.

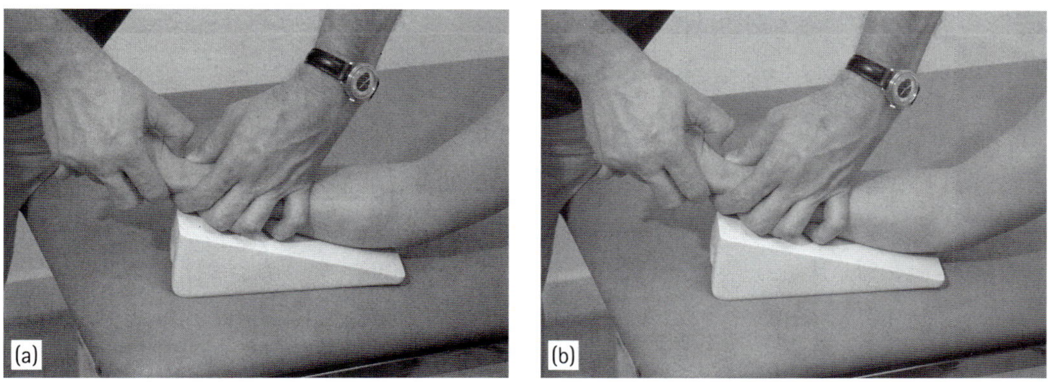

Figure 5.31a and b Specific provocation and alleviation in the area of the hand complex with symptomatic movement of the hand into dorsal flexion; intercarpal differentiation; movement as symptom-provoking component; alleviation. **a**, Starting position. **b**, End position.

Differentiation, wrist, volar flexion – radiocarpal – intra-articular vs. extra-articular (symptom provocation by an intra-articular component)

Pain-provoking movement (Fig. 5.32)

- Volar flexion of the wrist provokes pain in the radial forearm.
- Area localization hints at the hand complex.

The change in symptoms can be demonstrated exactly:

- provocation of pain (Fig. 5.33a and b, film 214)
- alleviation of pain (Fig. 5.34a and b, film 215).

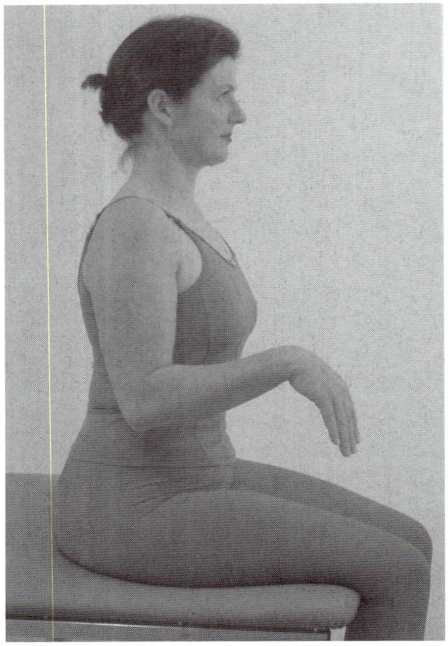

Figure 5.32 Symptom-provoking movement: movement of the hand into volar flexion provokes symptoms in the area of the distal lateral forearm.

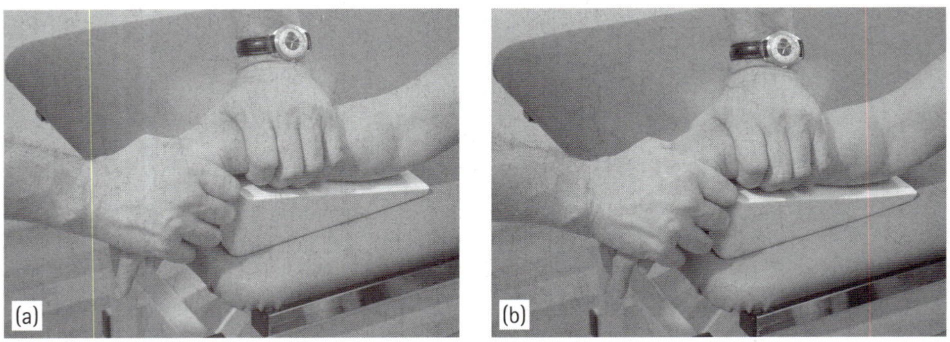

Figure 5.33a and b Specific provocation and alleviation in the area of the hand complex with symptomatic movement of the hand into volar flexion, intra-articular mechanism as symptom-provoking component; provocation. **a**, Starting position. **b**, End position.

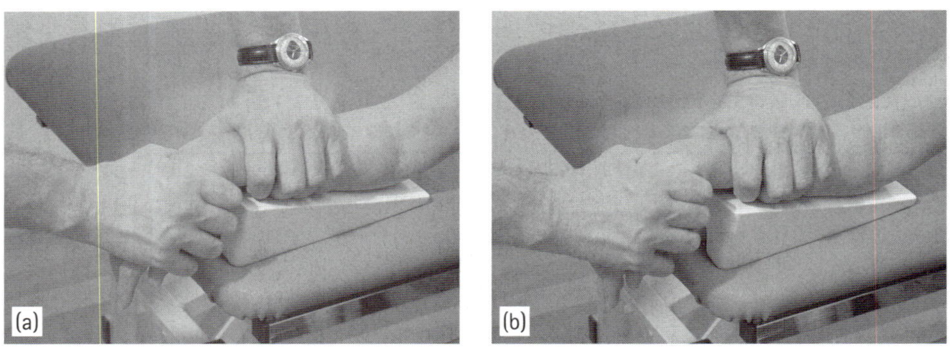

Figure 5.34a and b Specific provocation and alleviation in the area of the hand complex with symptomatic movement of the hand into volar flexion, intra-articular mechanism as symptom-provoking component; alleviation. **a**, Starting position. **b**, End position.

Assessment			
Goal	**Provocation of pain**	**Alleviation of pain**	**Remarks**
Starting position	Volar flexion to a position immediately after symptoms have appeared	Volar flexion to a position immediately after symptoms have appeared	The starting position for pain provocation must not be symptom-free, since in a symptom-free position symptomatic tissue might possibly not be compressed, and thus the patient's symptoms cannot be reproduced
Test movement	Compression of the carpus, with fixed radius	Traction of the carpus, with fixed radius	
Neural involvement	Proximal component without change of position in the relevant area	Proximal component without change of position in the relevant area	
Explanation	This manoeuvre increases the intra-articular compression in pain-provoking position	This manoeuvre reduces the intra-articular compression in pain-provoking position	
Additional data to support the hypothesis	General and specific mobility of the hand complex History, symptom behaviour, type of complaints, 24-hour behaviour Specific palpation Reproducibility of test results Test treatment Imaging procedures (CT, MRI)		

Differentiation, wrist, volar flexion – radiocarpal – extra-articular vs. intra-articular (symptom provocation by an extra-articular component)

The change in symptoms can be demonstrated exactly:

- provocation of pain (Fig. 5.35a and b, film 216).

Assessment			
Goal	**Provocation of pain**	**Alleviation of pain**	**Remarks**
Starting position	Volar flexion to a position immediately		

Goal	Provocation of pain	Alleviation of pain	Remarks
	before symptoms appear		
Test movement	Traction of the carpus, with fixed radius		It is questionable whether, by compression of the joint, the extra-articular structures can be sufficiently relaxed to alleviate symptoms. Therefore, alleviation is not described here
Neural involvement	Proximal component without change of position in the relevant area		
Explanation	This manoeuvre increases the pull on the extra-articular structures		
Additional data to support the hypothesis	General and specific mobility of the hand complex History, symptom behaviour, type of complaints, 24-hour behaviour Specific palpation Reproducibility of test results Test treatment Imaging procedures (CT, MRI)		

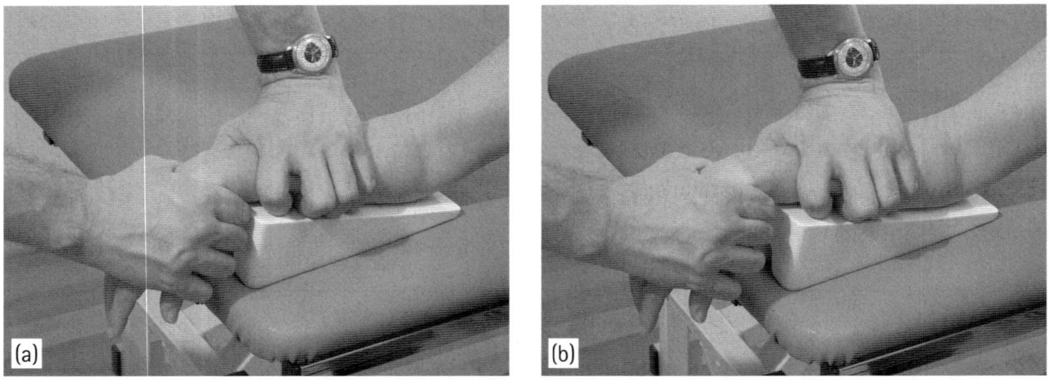

Figure 5.35a and b Specific provocation in the area of the hand complex with symptomatic movement of the hand into volar flexion, extra-articular mechanism as symptom-provoking component. **a**, Starting position. **b**, End position.

Differentiation, wrist, volar flexion – intercarpal – radiocarpal

The change in symptoms can be demonstrated exactly:

- provocation of pain (Fig. 5.36a and b, film 217)
- alleviation of pain (Fig. 5.37a and b, film 218).

Assessment			
Goal	**Provocation of pain**	**Alleviation of pain**	**Remarks**
Starting position	Volar flexion to a position immediately before symptoms appear	Volar flexion to a position immediately after symptoms have appeared	
Test movement	• Trapezium bones in volar direction with fixed scaphoid bone • Scaphoid bone in dorsal direction with fixed radius • Lunar bone in dorsal direction with fixed radius and ulna • Capitate bone in dorsal direction with fixed lunar bone	• Trapezium bones in dorsal direction with fixed scaphoid bone • Scaphoid bone in volar direction with fixed radius • Lunar bone in volar direction with fixed radius and ulna • Capitate bone in volar direction with fixed lunar bone	
Neural involvement	Proximal component without change of position in the relevant area (here, e.g., depression of the shoulder girdle)	Proximal component without change of position in the relevant area (here, e.g., elevation of the shoulder girdle)	
Explanation	If the patient's symptoms can be provoked by the described movements of the individual carpal bones, this hints at symptomatic tissue in the tested area	If the patient's symptoms can be alleviated by the described movements of the individual carpal bones, this hints at symptomatic tissue in the tested area	

Goal	Provocation of pain	Alleviation of pain	Remarks
Additional data to support the hypothesis	General and specific mobility of the hand complex History, symptom behaviour, type of complaints, 24-hour behaviour Specific palpation Reproducibility of test results Test treatment Imaging procedures (CT, MRI)		

Note: If the pain-provoking component is the rolling component with decentring effect, the push for provocation or alleviation must, with convex joint partners, go in the opposite direction of the hand movement. Based on pain localization, symptom provocation by the intercarpal bones of the ulnar column seems less probable and therefore is not described here. To check the hypothesis of symptom provocation by the ulnar column, the respective bones will have to be tested according to the same principles.

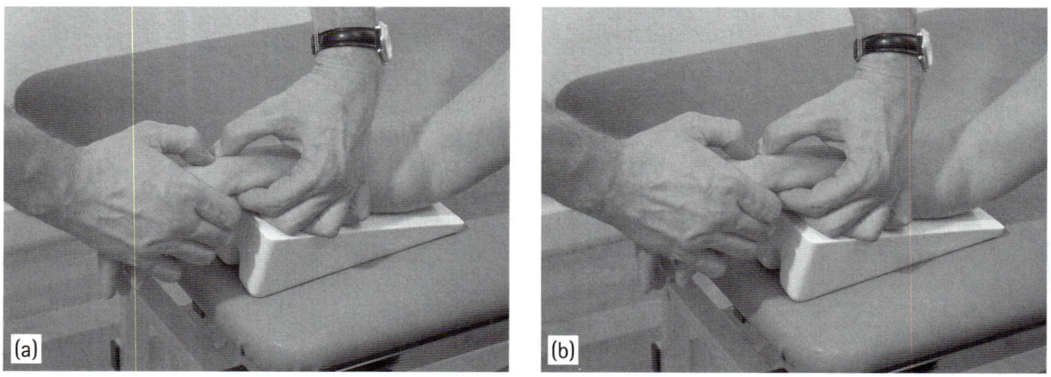

Figure 5.36a and b Specific provocation and alleviation in the area of the hand complex with symptomatic movement of the hand into volar flexion; intercarpal differentiation; movement as symptom-provoking component; provocation. **a**, Starting position. **b**, End position.

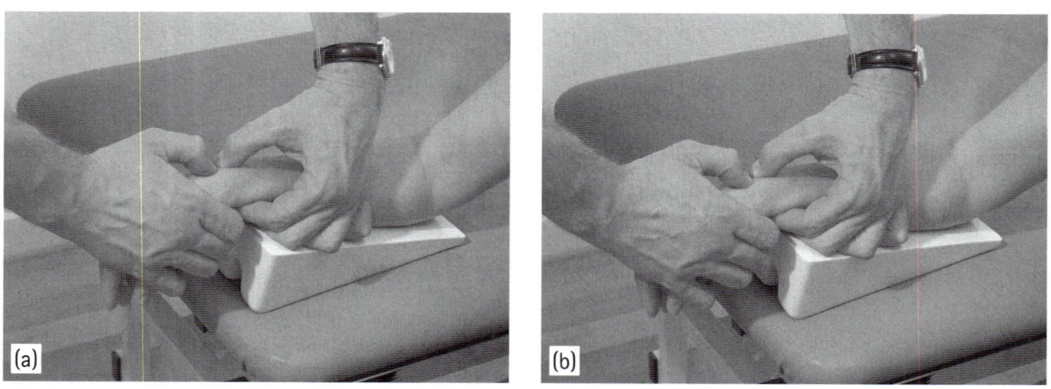

Figure 5.37a and b Specific provocation and alleviation in the area of the hand complex with symptomatic movement of the hand into volar flexion; intercarpal differentiation; movement as symptom-provoking component; alleviation. **a**, Starting position. **b**, End position.

GENERAL MOVEMENT TESTS

General movement tests identify anatomical individual movements and, in part, movement combinations in the area concerned. The individual manual therapy concepts have respective protocols at their disposal, which more or less have the same goals.

Information gained in this way is useful for checking or modifying the relevant hypotheses developed on the basis of anamnesis and area localization and will help in deciding how to proceed.

General question: Is there enough information available to skip general movement tests?	
No	Yes
⇓	⇓
Performance of the general movement tests	• Additional tests • Test treatment

In view of the described clinical presentation and the results of area localization, general movement tests of the following regions seem to be useful.

Cervical spine		
	Active	**Passive (assistive)**
Lower cervical spine (below C2) in general	Flexion Extension Rotation (to the right and left) Lateral flexion (to the right and left)	Flexion Extension Rotation (to the right and left) Lateral flexion (to the right and left)
Elbow complex		
	Active	**Passive**
Elbow	Flexion Extension Pronation Supination	Flexion Extension Pronation Supination
Hand complex		
	Active	**Passive**
Wrist	Dorsal flexion Volar flexion Radial abduction Ulnar abduction	Dorsal flexion Volar flexion Radial abduction Ulnar abduction

TREATMENT EXAMPLE, SCAPHOID BONE

SYMPTOMATIC MOVEMENT

Dorsal flexion of the wrist is restricted by 20% as compared with the opposite side and, in end-range positions, provokes pain (VAS 3/10) in the area of the distal forearm, right side.

ASSESSMENTS

Area localization

Area localization hints at a provocation of symptoms by the hand complex. There is no contraindication for movement (negative imaging procedures).

Specific provocation and alleviation

- Specific provocation and alleviation hints at a provocation of symptoms by movement of the scaphoid bone in a volar direction.
- In a symptomatic position, distraction reduces the symptoms, while compression increases them.

Specific mobility

Specific mobility tests show hypomobility of the scaphoid bone in a volar direction.

Palpation

Palpation indicates a painful change in tissue over the scaphoid bone.

HYPOTHESIS

Painfully restricted movement of the scaphoid bone in dorsal flexion. Symptom provocation by an intra-articular component (Fig. 5.38).

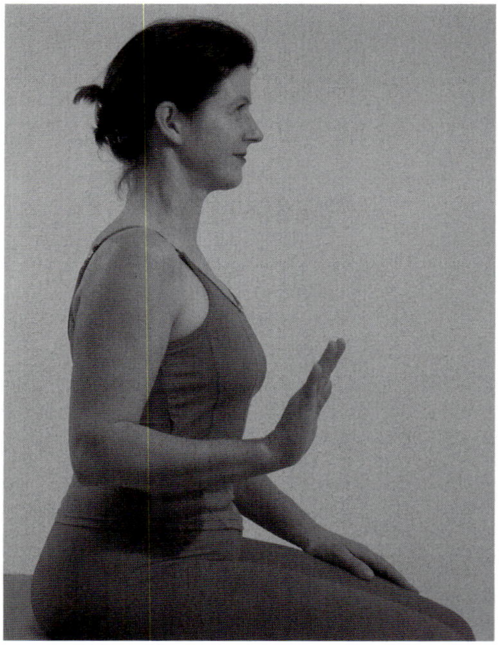

Figure 5.38 Symptom-provoking movement: movement of the hand into dorsal flexion provokes symptoms in the area of the distal lateral forearm.

MOBILIZATION TECHNIQUES

Active procedures

ACTIVE MOBILIZATION PLUS ACCESSORY MOVEMENT

Dorsal flexion of the wrist with volar glide of the scaphoid bone (film 231)

Therapy technique

- Patient's starting position: sitting, the forearm rests on the treatment wedge.
- Therapist's starting position: standing, at the patient's side, fixation of the radius on the treatment wedge, contact with the scaphoid bone (Fig. 5.39a).
- Movement: push of the scaphoid bone in a volar direction followed by active dorsal flexion of the wrist (Fig. 5.39b).

Self-exercise (film 232)

- Patient's starting position: sitting, contact with the scaphoid bone with the thumb from dorsal, with the index finger on the radius from volar (Fig. 5.40a).
- Movement: pressing thumb and index together, then active movement into dorsal flexion, and moving the wrist back to the starting position (Fig. 5.40b).

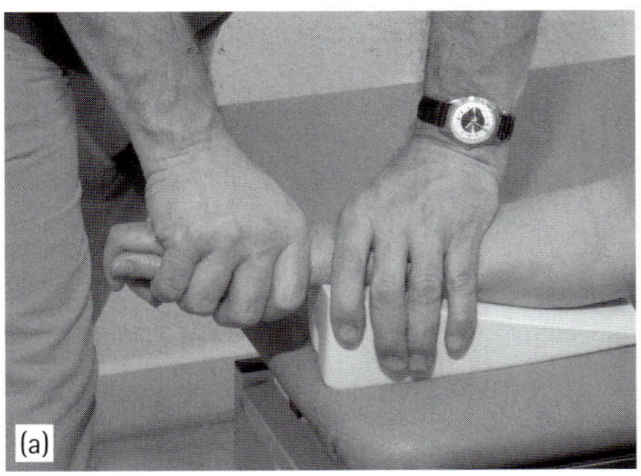
(a)

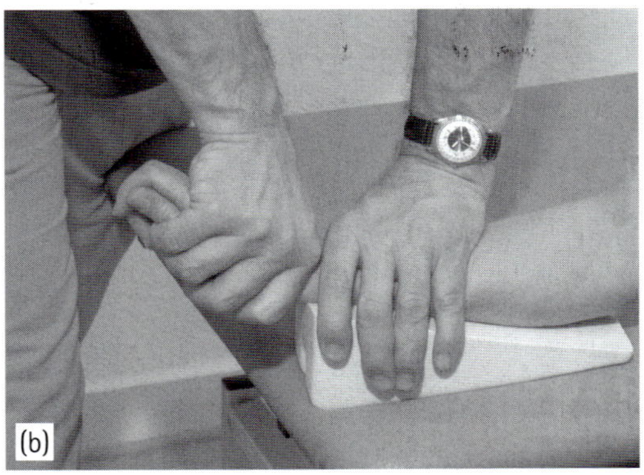
(b)

Figure 5.39a and b Active mobilization with accessory movement; dorsal flexion with volar glide; therapy technique. **a**, Starting position. **b**, End position.

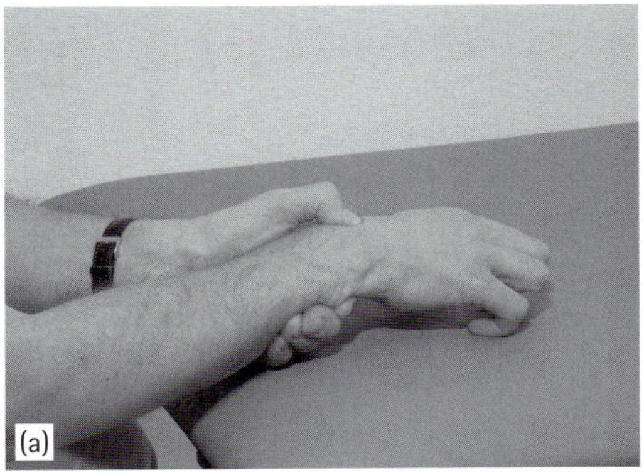
(a)

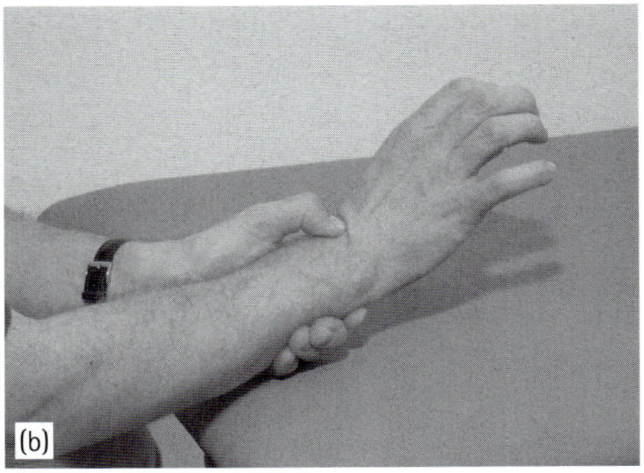
(b)

Figure 40a and b Active mobilization with accessory movement; dorsal flexion with volar glide; self-exercise. **a**, Starting position. **b**, End position.

Dorsal flexion of the wrist with ulnar glide of the scaphoid bone (film 235)

Therapy technique

- Patient's starting position: sitting, the forearm rests on the treatment wedge.
- Therapist's starting position: standing, at the patient's side, fixation of the forearm and grasping the proximal row of carpal bones from the ulnar side (Fig. 5.41a).
- Movement: gliding of the wrist in an ulnar direction, followed by active movement into dorsal flexion, and moving the wrist back to the starting position (Fig. 5.41b).

Self-exercise (film 236)

- Patient's starting position: sitting, the left hand siezes the wrist from the volar side, the thumb rests on the scaphoid bone from the radial side, the second and third fingers rest on the ulna from the ulnar side (Fig. 5.42a).
- Movement: pressing the thumb and second and third fingers together, then active movement into dorsal flexion, and moving the wrist back to the starting position (Fig. 5.42b).

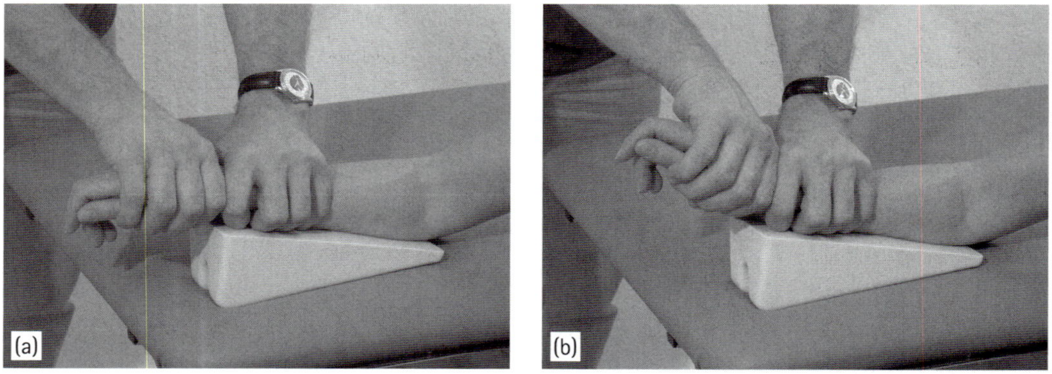

Figure 5.41a and b Active mobilization with accessory movement; dorsal flexion with ulnar glide; therapy technique. **a**, Starting position. **b**, End position.

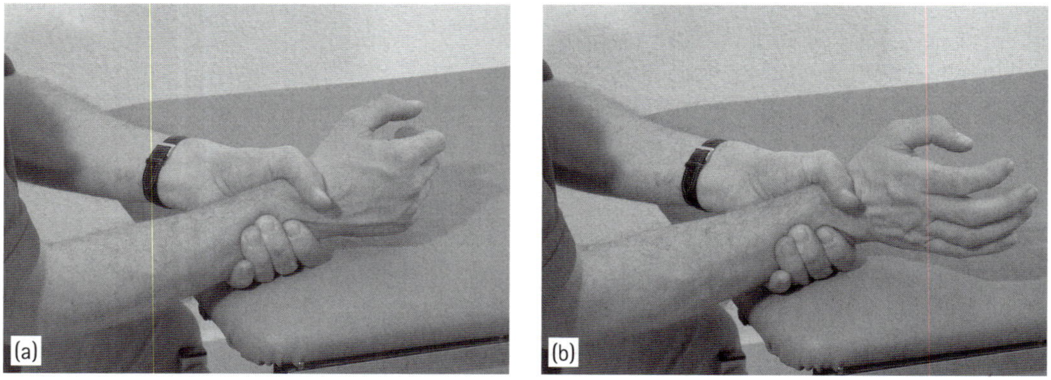

Figure 5.42a and b Active mobilization with accessory movement; dorsal flexion with ulnar glide; self-exercise. **a**, Starting position. **b**, End position.

Remarks (regarding active mobilization plus accessory movement)

Goal of the technique

With a painfully restricted dorsal flexion of the right wrist with simultaneous hypomobility of the scaphoid bone in a volar and ulnar direction, these techniques serve to:

- reduce tonicity and improve the metabolism of the affected tissues
- restore pain-free function (change the input to respective centres of the central nervous system (CNS)).

Performance

With active mobilization with volar or ulnar glide, the push is performed parallel to the treatment plane (distal joint surface of the radius).

Dosage (regarding the affected symptomatic structure)

Both with an acute (predominantly peripheral pain mechanisms) and with a chronic presentation (predominantly central pain mechanisms), these techniques should not provoke the patient's symptoms. The dosage is determined by the expected training state of the tissue as well as by reassessment.

Choice of technique

The selection of the technique depends, among other things, on the therapist as well as the patient, on the therapist's clinical experience, but primarily on reassessment. This means that even if all preconditions on the part of therapist and patient seem to be met, it is of no use to continue the technique if reassessment is negative.

Contributing factors

For a satisfactory solution of the patient's current problems it is important to consider the contributing factors and include them in the treatment.

The authors will, however, not go into a description of the various possibilities and their complex contexts as this would exceed the scope of the present book.

Passive procedures

TRANSLATORY MOVEMENTS

Traction (movement from distal, film 247)

Therapy technique

- Patient's starting position: sitting, forearm stabilized by a belt and supported on a wedge, the wrist in submaximal dorsal flexion.
- Therapist's starting position: standing, in front of the patient (Fig. 5.43a).
- Movement: traction in the radiocarpal joint (Fig. 5.43b).

Self-exercise (film 248)

- Patient's starting position: standing, the wrist in submaximal dorsal flexion, stabilized by the other hand (Fig. 5.44a).
- Movement: traction in the radiocarpal joint by elevation of the shoulder girdle (Fig. 5.44b).

Remarks

Goal of the technique

With a painfully restricted dorsal flexion of the right wrist by an intra-articular mechanism, the described technique serves to improve the mobility of non-symptom-provoking tissues.

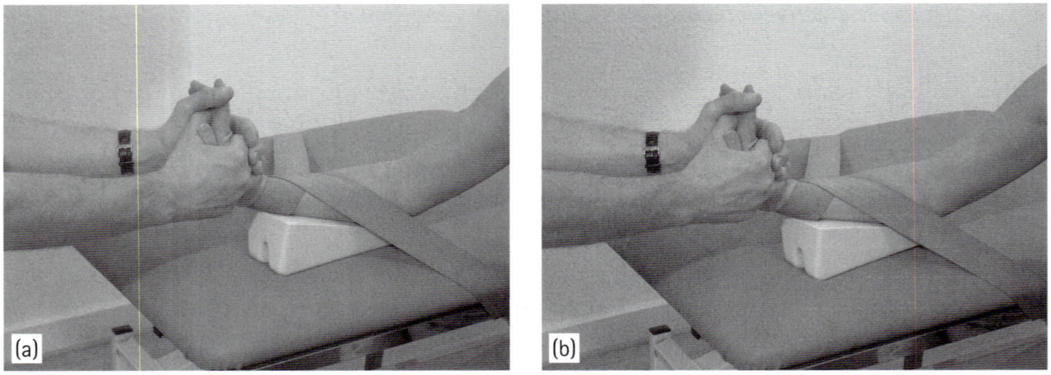

Figure 5.43a and b Passive mobilization; translatory movements; traction; therapy technique. a, Starting position. b, End position.

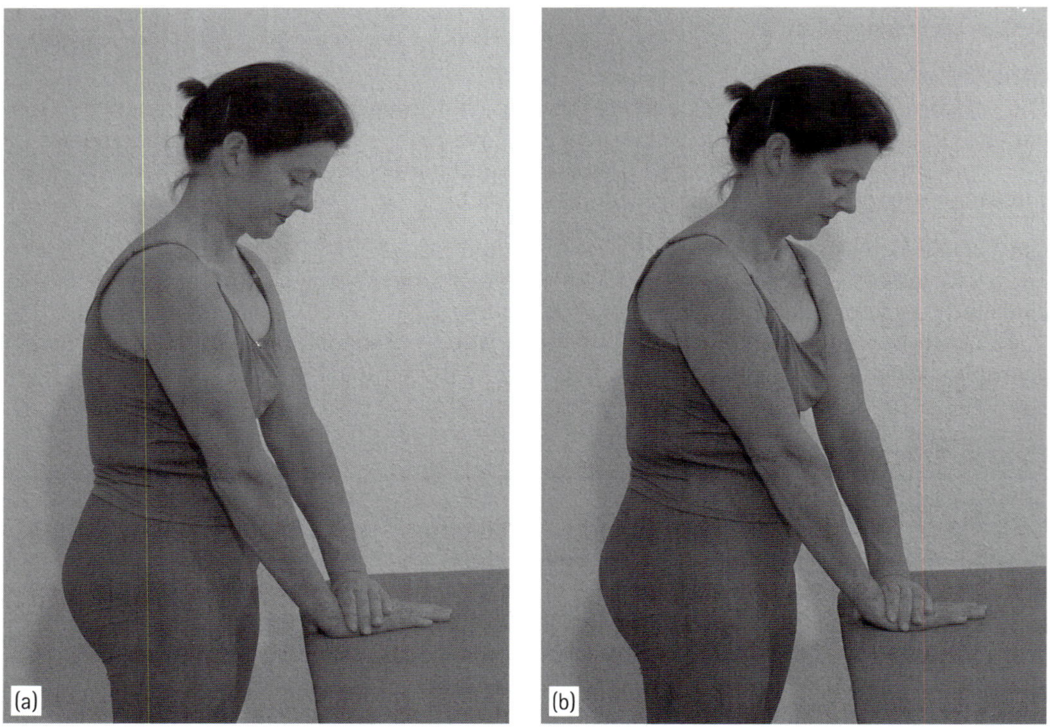

Figure 5.44a and b Passive mobilization; translatory movements; traction; self-exercise. a, Starting position. b, End position.

Performance

Traction is done vertical to the treatment plane, independently of the pre-positioned of the wrist.

Dosage

Here, the described technique serves to treat a non-symptomatic structure, and therefore dosage is not determined by wound healing. Rather, the expected training state (loading capacity) of the tissue to be treated, and the patient's personal expectations are the determining factors.

If there is any doubt, treatment is always started with very low force, and further increase is made conditional on reassessment. Thus, in treatment of the non-symptomatic structure, pain is not always the limiting factor for the dosage of a particular technique.

Choice of technique

The selection of the technique depends, among other things, on the therapist as well as the patient, on the therapist's clinical experience, but primarily on reassessment. This means that even if all preconditions on the part of therapist and patient seem to be met, it is of no use to continue the technique if reassessment is negative.

Contributing factors

For a satisfactory solution of the patient's current problems it is important to consider the contributing factors and include them in the treatment.

The authors will, however, not go into a description of the various possibilities and their complex contexts as this would exceed the scope of the present book.

Volar glide – movement via scaphoid bone (film 239)

Therapy technique

- Patient's starting position: sitting, the forearm supported on a wedge, contact with the scaphoid bone, the wrist pre-positioned in submaximal dorsal flexion.
- Therapist's starting position: standing, in front of the patient (Fig. 5.45a).
- Movement: volar glide of the scaphoid bone in relation to the stabilized radius (Fig. 5.45b).

Self-exercise (film 240)

- Patient's starting position: sitting, the forearm supported on a wedge, contact with the scaphoid bone, pre-positioning of the wrist in submaximal dorsal flexion (Fig. 5.46a).
- Movement: volar glide of the scaphoid bone in relation to the stabilized radius (Fig. 5.46b).

Volar glide – movement via radius (film 241)

Therapy technique

- Patient's starting position: sitting, the hand supported on a wedge, which fixes the scaphoid bone (from dorsal), pre-positioning of the wrist in submaximal dorsal flexion, contact with the radius from the volar side.
- Therapist's starting position: standing, in front of the patient (Fig. 5.47a).
- Movement: dorsal glide of the radius in relation to the fixed scaphoid bone (Fig. 5.47b).

Remarks (regarding volar glide)

Goals of the technique

With a painfully restricted dorsal flexion of the right wrist with simultaneous hypomobility of the scaphoid bone in volar and ulnar direction, these techniques serve to improve mobility by mobilization of symptomatic tissues.

Performance

The joint to be treated is pre-positioned first according to irritability or the desired treatment goal. By the 'specific fixation' of this technique, an uncontrolled continuation of movement is prevented as far as possible. This should be considered when the indication for this technique is determined.

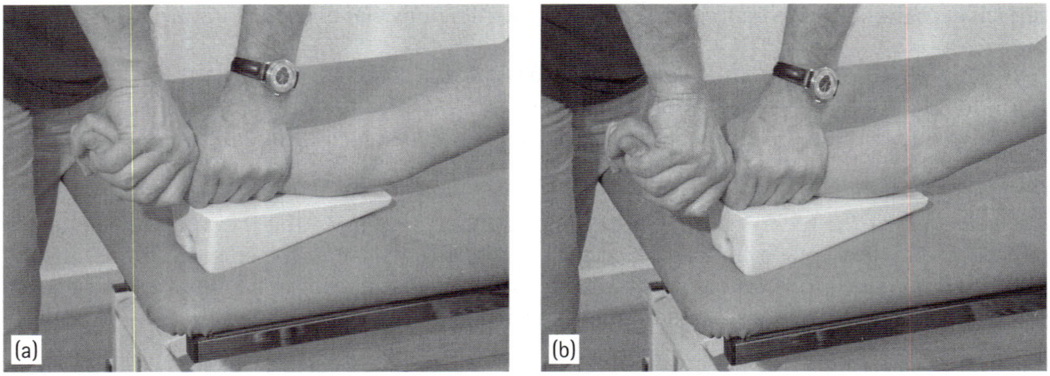

Figure 5.45a and b Passive mobilization; translatory movements; volar glide of the scaphoid bone; therapy technique. a, Starting position. b, End position.

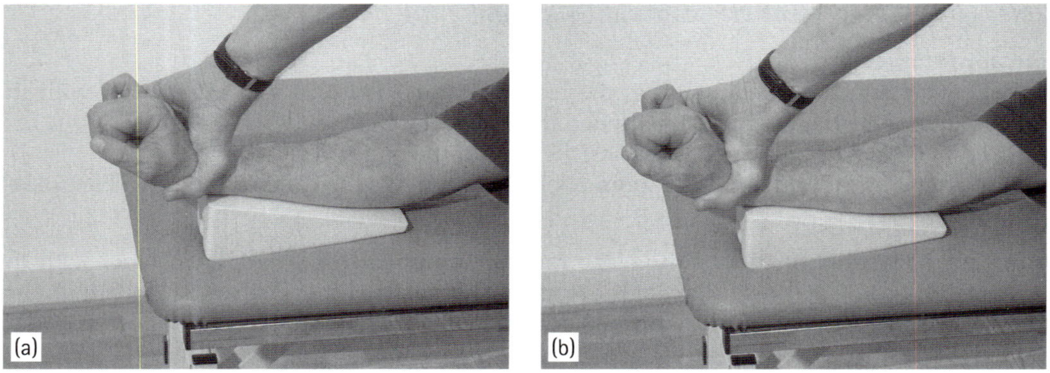

Figure 5.46a and b Passive mobilization; translatory movements; volar glide of the scaphoid bone; self-exercise. a, Starting position. b, End position.

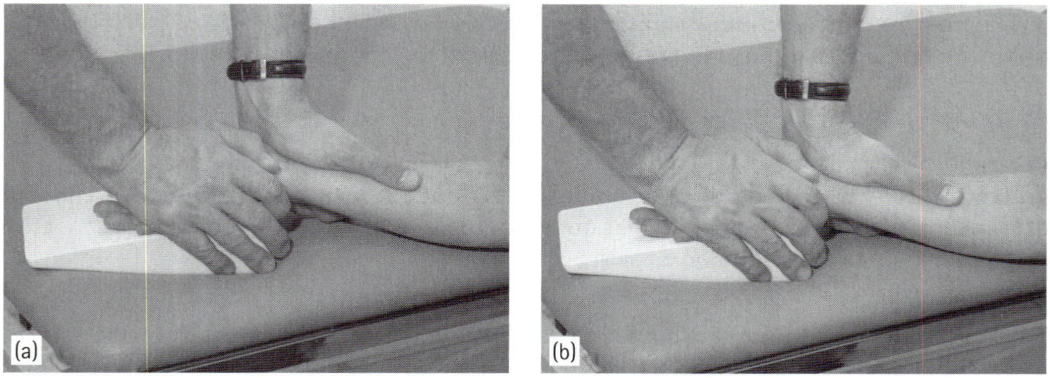

Figure 5.47a and b Passive mobilization; translatory movements; volar glide of the scaphoid bone via radius; therapy technique. a, Starting position. b, End position.

Dosage (regarding the affected structure)

Acute presentation (predominantly peripheral pain mechanisms)			
Phase	Limitation of movement due to pain and resistance	Concept	Movement grade
Inflammation phase	No pain	Kaltenborn–Evjenth	Up to the beginning of II
	No resistance	Maitland	Up to II
Proliferation phase	Up to P1	Kaltenborn–Evjenth	Up to the 1st third of II
	Slowly progressing up to low resistance	Maitland	III^{-}
Remodelling/ organization phase	Slowly progressing up to maximum resistance	Kaltenborn–Evjenth	Up to III
	(Note: duration of turnover!)	Maitland	Up to IV^{++} or III^{++}

Note: The chances of a disturbed (delayed) course of healing and the consequences for the loading capacity of the tissue (e.g., diabetes, old age, partial or general immobilization) have to be considered.

Chronic presentation (predominantly central pain mechanisms): Since here it is assumed that pain no longer represents a protection mechanism, the therapist has to consider the expected training state of the treated tissue as well as the patient's personal expectations. If there is any doubt, treatment is always started with very low force, with progression made conditional on reassessment. Hence with a chronic presentation, pain is not always the limiting factor with regard to treatment dosage.

Choice of technique

The selection of the technique depends, among other things, on the therapist as well as the patient, on the therapist's clinical experience, but primarily on reassessment. This means that even if all preconditions on the part of therapist and patient seem to be met, it is of no use to continue the technique if reassessment is negative.

Contributing factors

For a satisfactory solution of the patient's current problems it is important to consider the contributing factors and include them in the treatment.

The authors will, however, not go into a description of the various possibilities and their complex contexts as this would exceed the scope of the present book.

Chapter 6

Thoracolumbar junction

CHAPTER CONTENTS

AREA LOCALIZATION

IDENTIFICATION OF THE POTENTIALLY AFFECTED AREA BY DEMONSTRATION OF A SYMPTOMATIC FUNCTIONAL MOVEMENT/POSITION

Based on the information gained from the anamnesis so far, the therapist tries to ascertain more details about potentially affected sections. This is done by means of area localization, which represents the beginning of the physical examination. Information gained in this way is used to check or modify the relevant hypotheses developed on the basis of the anamnesis and will determine further progress.

Area localization is explained by means of examples. In all three examples, the patient feels pain in the area of the thoracolumbar junction, on the right side. Based on clinical experience and known clinical patterns, primarily the following areas are considered as potential sources of the current complaints:

- thoracic spine/lumbar spine
- ribs
- neural structures.

General question: Is there enough information available to bypass area localization?	
No	Yes
⇓	⇓
Performance of area localization	• General movement tests • Additional tests • Test treatment

Example 1: Flexion

Symptom area: thoracolumbar junction, right side
Symptom provocation: flexion of the spine (Fig. 6.1)

With this presentation, clinical experience suggests primarily the thoracic spine/lumbar spine, the ribs, and the neural structures as symptom-provoking areas.

Below, examples illustrate how to differentiate between these areas. To this end, the therapist performs area localization by means of active movements alone. If this is not possible, tests will be performed by means of assistive movements.

Hypothesis 1: The symptom-provoking area is the neural structures

Differentiation: neural involvement vs. thoracic spine/lumbar spine.

The change in symptoms can be demonstrated exactly:

- provocation of pain (Fig. 6.2a and b, film 1)
- alleviation of pain (Fig. 6.3a and b, film 2).

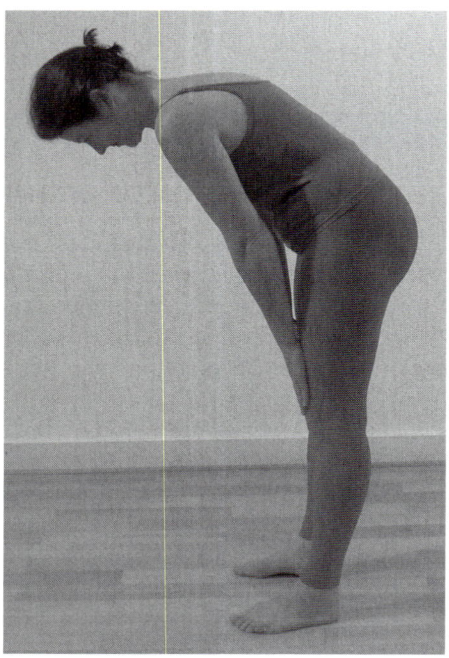

Figure 6.1 Symptom-provoking movement: flexion of the spine provokes pain at the thoracolumbar junction, right side.

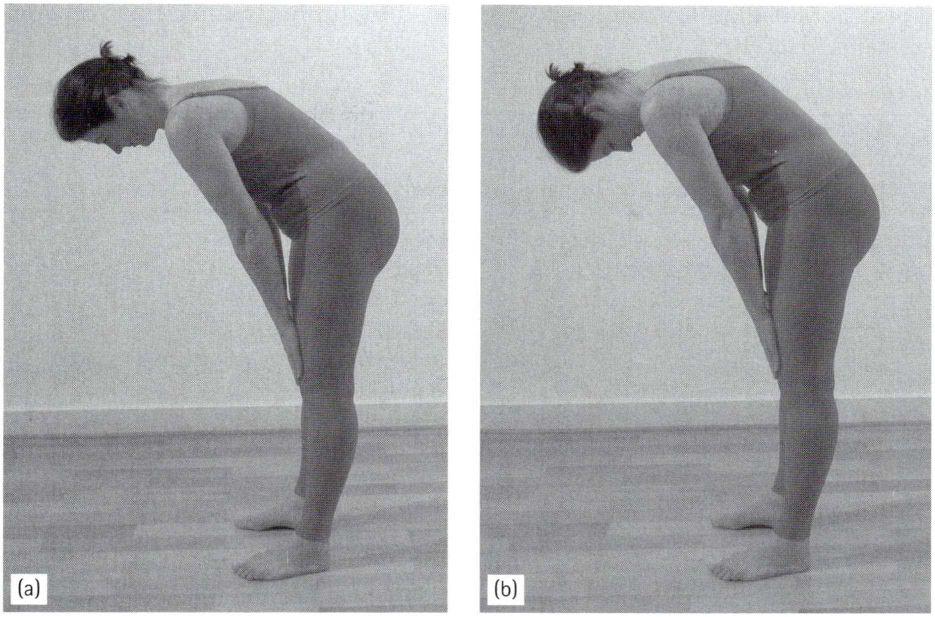

Figure 6.2a and b Area localization with symptomatic movement of the thoracolumbar junction into flexion; differentiation between neural structures and thoracic spine/lumbar spine; provocation. a, Starting position. b, End position.

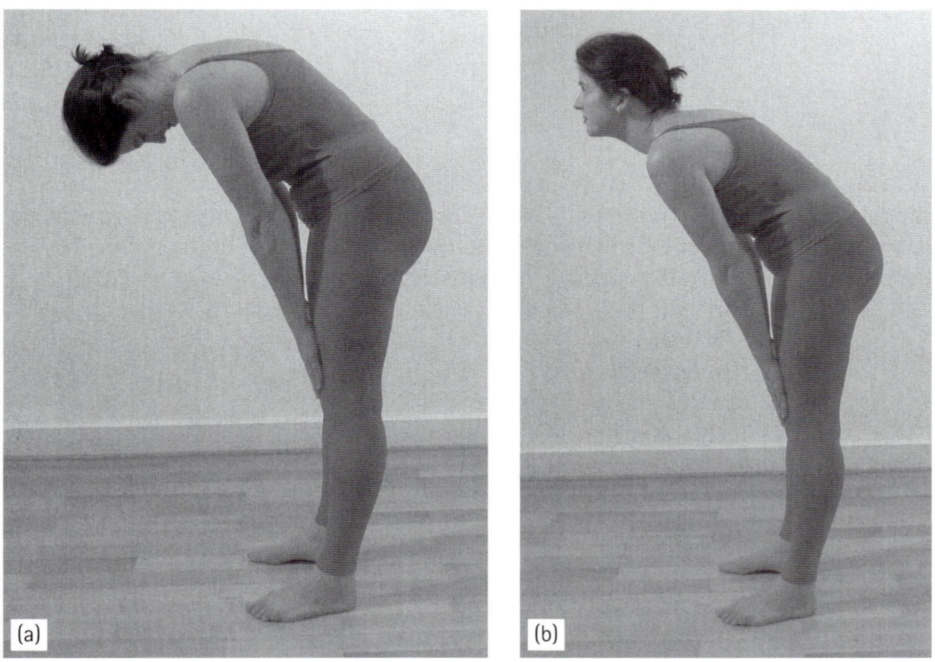

Figure 6.3a and b Area localization with symptomatic movement of the thoracolumbar junction into flexion; differentiation between neural structures and thoracic spine/lumbar spine; alleviation. a, Starting position. b, End position.

The result of area localization has to be verified by further specific tests; otherwise the result remains in doubt.

Assessment			
Goal	**Provocation of pain**	**Alleviation of pain**	**Remarks**
Starting position	Flexion of the spine to a position immediately before symptoms appear	With the cervical spine pre-positioned in flexion, flexion of the spine to a position immediately after symptoms have appeared	
Test movement	Flexion of the cervical spine	Extension of the cervical spine	
Explanation	The test movement increases tension in the neural structures	The test movement reduces tension in the neural structures	If by movements of the cervical spine (as an example: flexion for provocation and extension for alleviation) the patient's typical pain is changed, this suggests at least an involvement of the neural structures
Additional data to support the hypothesis	Further movements of proximal or distal components to increase neural tension which are not directly involved in flexion of the spine General and specific mobility of the affected area History (e.g., symptom behaviour, type of complaints, 24-hour behaviour) Palpation Neurodynamic tests Reproducibility of test results Test treatment Imaging procedures (CT, MRI)		

Hypothesis 2: The symptom-provoking area is the ribs
Differentiation: ribs vs. thoracic spine/lumbar spine.

The change in symptoms can be demonstrated exactly:

- provocation of pain (Fig. 6.4a and b, film 3)
- alleviation of pain (Fig. 6.5a and b, film 4).

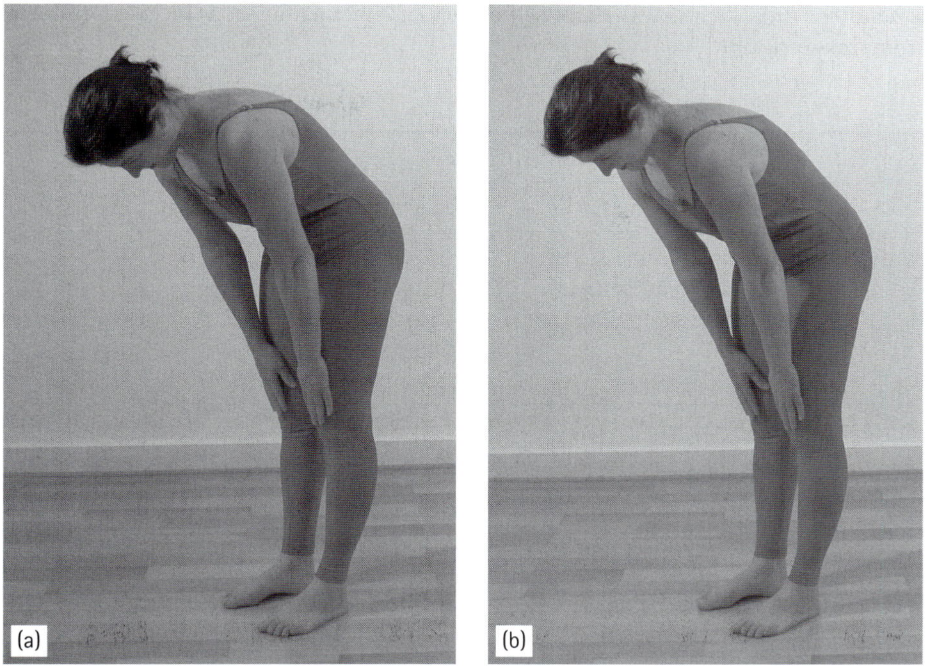

Figure 6.4a and b Area localization with symptomatic movement of the thoracolumbar junction into flexion; differentiation between ribs and thoracic spine/lumbar spine; provocation. **a**, Starting position. **b**, End position.

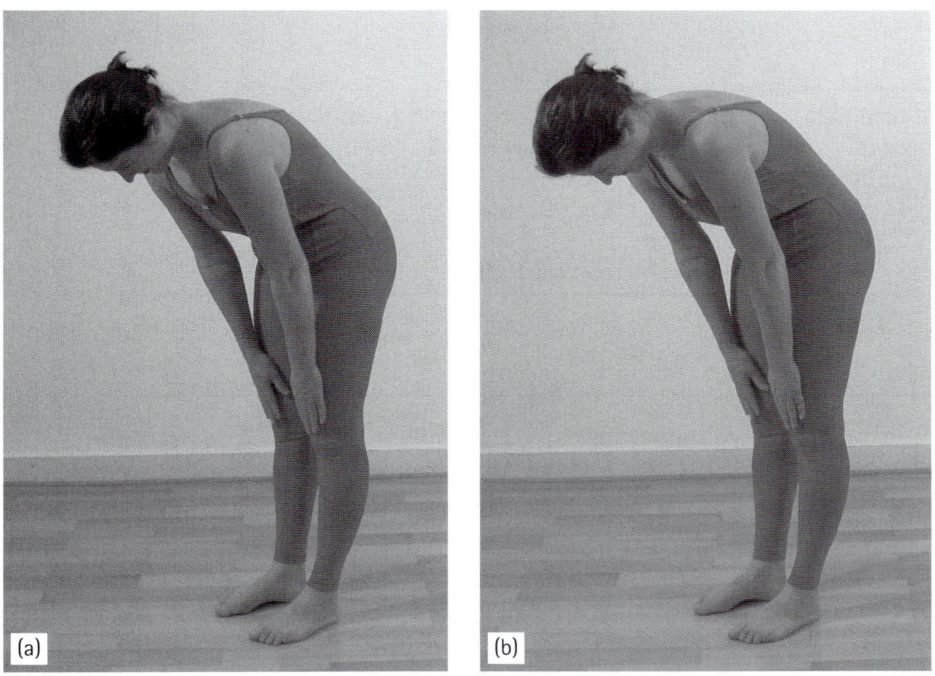

Figure 6.5a and b Area localization with symptomatic movement of the thoracolumbar junction into flexion; differentiation between ribs and thoracic spine/lumbar spine; alleviation. **a**, Starting position. **b**, End position.

The result of area localization has to be verified by further specific tests; otherwise the result remains in doubt.

Assessment			
Goal	**Provocation of pain**	**Alleviation of pain**	**Remarks**
Starting position	Flexion of the spine to a position immediately before symptoms appear	Flexion of the spine to a position immediately after symptoms have appeared	
Test movement	Inspiration	Expiration	Position of the spine must not change during test movement
Explanation	The test movement moves predominantly the ribs. Hence the rib movement during inspiration may be regarded as the symptom-provoking mechanism	The test movement moves predominantly the ribs. Hence the rib movement during expiration may be regarded as the symptom-reducing mechanism	In the authors' experience, inspiration is mostly provoking, expiration is mostly alleviating, when rib joints are involved. Due to the complexity of the movement apparatus, however, the reverse mechanism is also possible
Additional data to support the hypothesis	General and specific mobility of ribs and thoracic spine History (e.g., symptom behaviour, type of complaints, 24-hour behaviour) Palpation Reproducibility of test results Test treatment Imaging procedures (CT, MRI)		

Example 2: Extension

Symptom area: thoracolumbar junction, right side
Symptom provocation: extension of the spine (Fig. 6.6)

With this presentation, clinical experience suggests primarily the thoracic spine/lumbar spine, the ribs, and the neural structures as symptom-provoking areas.

Below, examples illustrate how to differentiate between these areas. To this end, the therapist performs area localization by means of active movements alone. If this is not possible, tests will be performed by means of assistive movements.

Hypothesis 1: The symptom-provoking area is the neural structures

Differentiation: neural involvement vs. thoracic spine/lumbar spine.

The change in symptoms can be demonstrated exactly:

- provocation of pain (Fig. 6.7a and b, film 5)
- alleviation of pain (Fig. 6.8a and b, film 6).

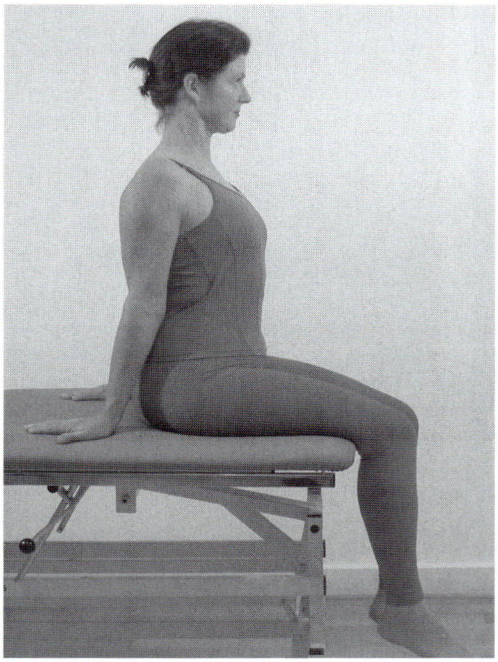

Figure 6.6 Symptom-provoking movement: extension of the spine provokes pain at the thoracolumbar junction, right side.

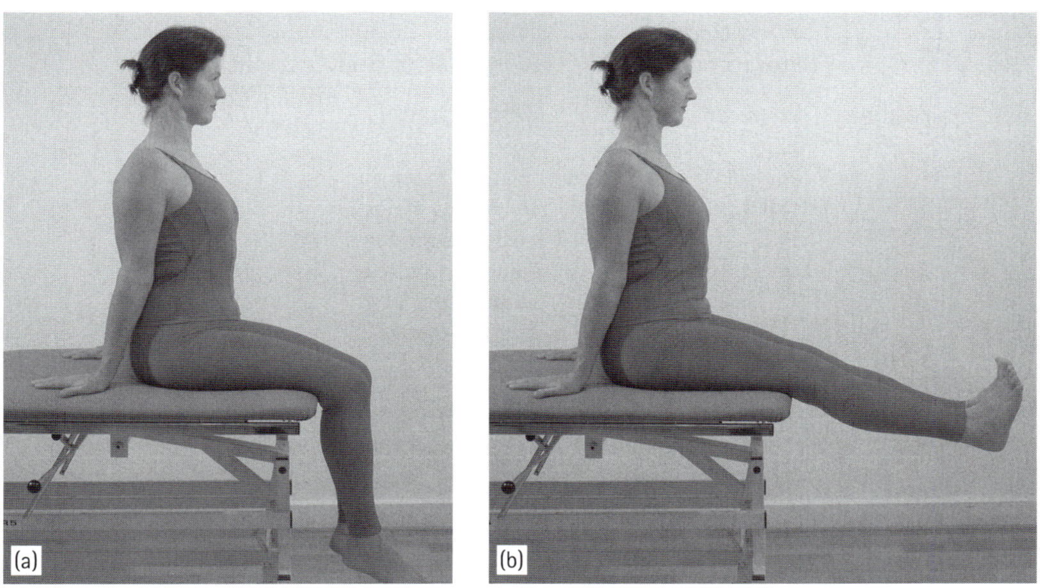

Figure 6.7a and b Area localization with symptomatic movement of the thoracolumbar junction into extension; differentiation between neural structures and thoracic spine/lumbar spine; provocation. a, Starting position. b, End position.

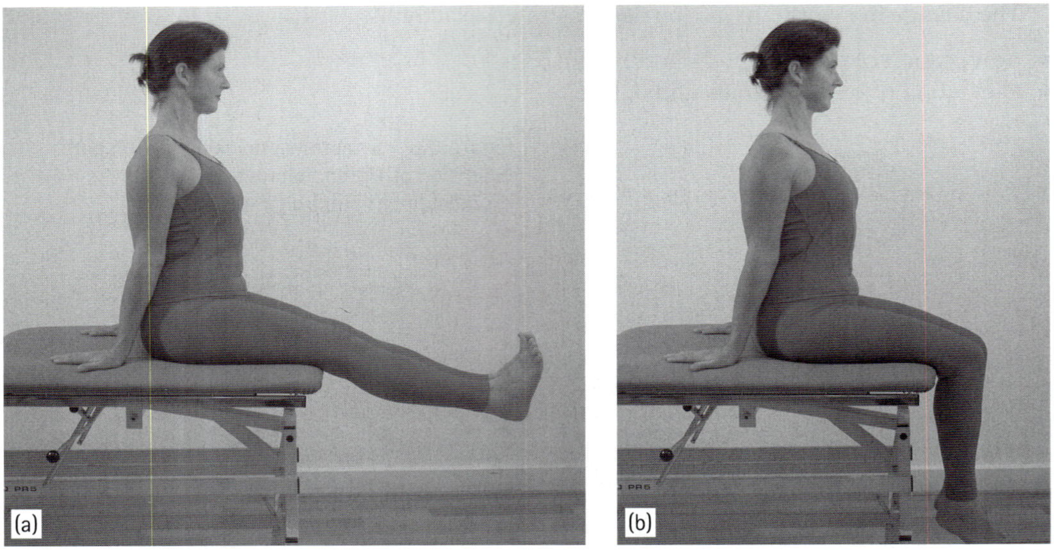

Figure 6.8a and b Area localization with symptomatic movement of the thoracolumbar junction into extension; differentiation between neural structures and thoracic spine/lumbar spine; alleviation. a, Starting position. b, End position.

The result of area localization has to be verified by further specific tests; otherwise the result remains in doubt.

Assessment			
Goal	**Provocation of pain**	**Alleviation of pain**	**Remarks**
Starting position	Extension of the spine to a position immediately before symptoms appear	With the knees pre-positioned in bilateral extension and the ankles in dorsal flexion, extension of the spine to a position immediately after symptoms have appeared	
Test movement	Bilateral extension of the knees and dorsal flexion of the upper ankles in sitting	Bilateral flexion of the knees reduces the tension in the neural structures produced by the starting position	
Explanation	The test movement increases tension in the neural structures	The test movement reduces tension in the neural structures	If the typical pain is provoked or alleviated by these manoeuvres,

Goal	Provocation of pain	Alleviation of pain	Remarks
			this suggests at least an involvement of the neural structures
Additional data to support the hypothesis	Further movements of proximal and distal components to increase neural tension which are not directly involved in flexion of the spine General and specific mobility of the affected area History (e.g., symptom behaviour, type of complaints, 24-hour behaviour) Palpation Neurodynamic tests Nerve provocation tests (e.g., bow string sign) Reproducibility of test results Test treatment Imaging procedures (CT, MRI)		

Hypothesis 2: The symptom-provoking area is the ribs

Differentiation: ribs vs. thoracic spine/lumbar spine.

The change in symptoms can be demonstrated exactly:

- provocation of pain (Fig. 6.9a and b, film 7)
- alleviation of pain (Fig. 6.10a and b, film 8).

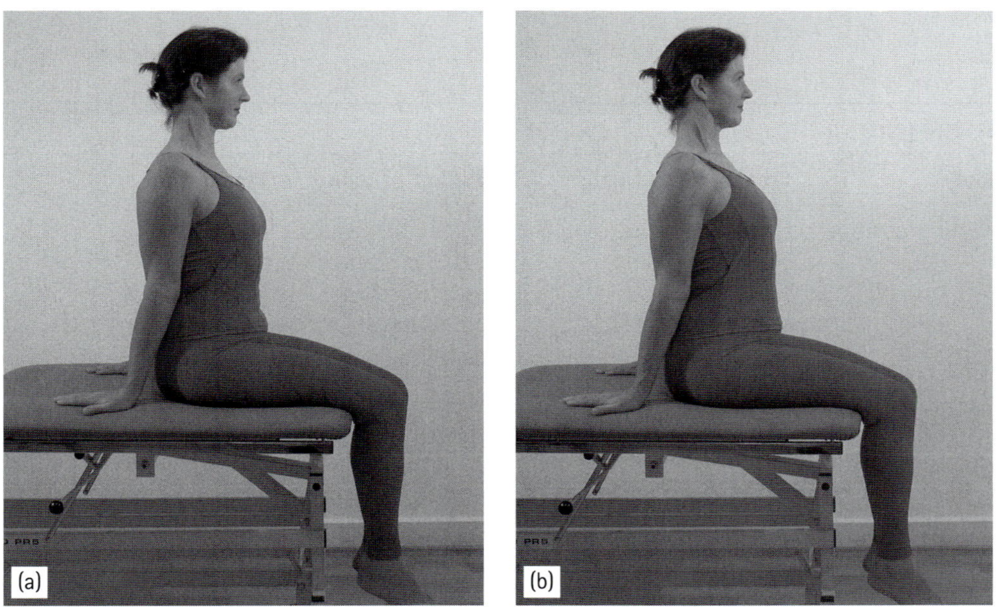

Figure 6.9a and b Area localization with symptomatic movement of the thoracolumbar junction into extension; differentiation between ribs and thoracic spine/lumbar spine; provocation. **a**, Starting position. **b**, End position.

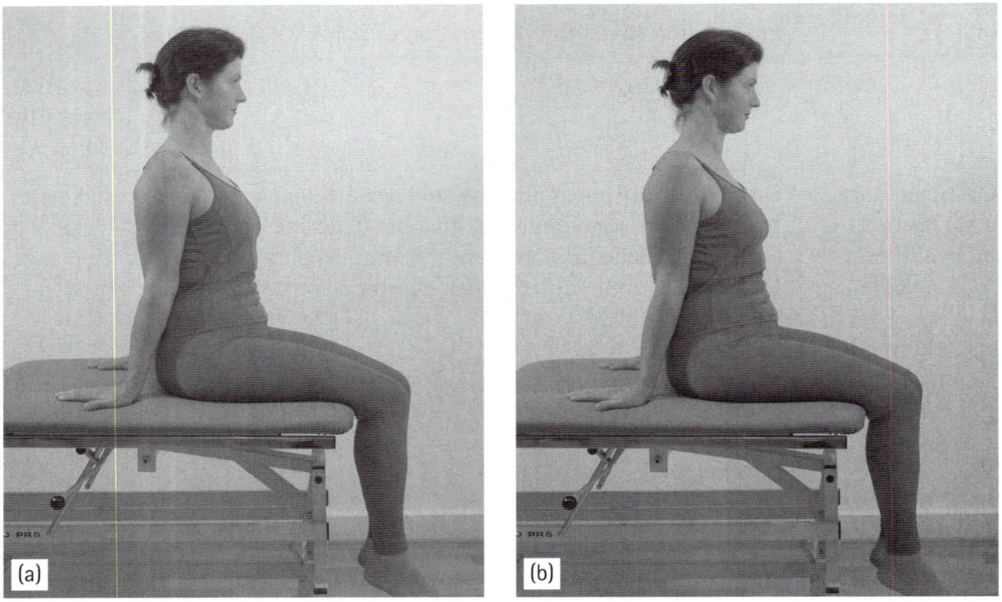

Figure 6.10a and b Area localization with symptomatic movement of the thoracolumbar junction into extension; differentiation between ribs and thoracic spine/lumbar spine; alleviation. **a**, Starting position. **b**, End position.

The result of area localization has to be verified by further specific tests; otherwise the result remains in doubt.

Assessment

Goal	Provocation of pain	Alleviation of pain	Remarks
Starting position	Extension of the spine to a position immediately before symptoms appear	Extension of the spine to a position immediately after symptoms have appeared	
Test movement	Inspiration	Expiration	Position of the spine must not change during test movement
Explanation	The test movement moves predominantly the ribs. Hence the rib movement during inspiration may be regarded as the	The test movement moves predominantly the ribs. Hence the rib movement during expiration may be regarded as the	In the authors' experience, inspiration is mostly provoking, expiration is mostly alleviating, when rib joints are involved. Due

Goal	Provocation of pain	Alleviation of pain	Remarks
	symptom-provoking mechanism	symptom-reducing mechanism	to the complexity of the movement apparatus, however, the reverse mechanism is also possible
Additional data to support the hypothesis	General and specific mobility of ribs and thoracic spine History (e.g., symptom behaviour, type of complaints, 24-hour behaviour) Palpation Reproducibility of test results Test treatment Imaging procedures (CT, MRI)		

Example 3: Rotation

Symptom area: thoracolumbar junction, right side
Symptom provocation: rotation of the spine (Fig. 6.11)

With this presentation, clinical experience suggests primarily the thoracic spine/lumbar spine, the ribs, and the neural structures as symptom-provoking areas.

Below, examples illustrate how to differentiate between these areas. To this end, the therapist performs area localization by means of active movements alone. If this is not possible, tests will be performed by means of assistive movements.

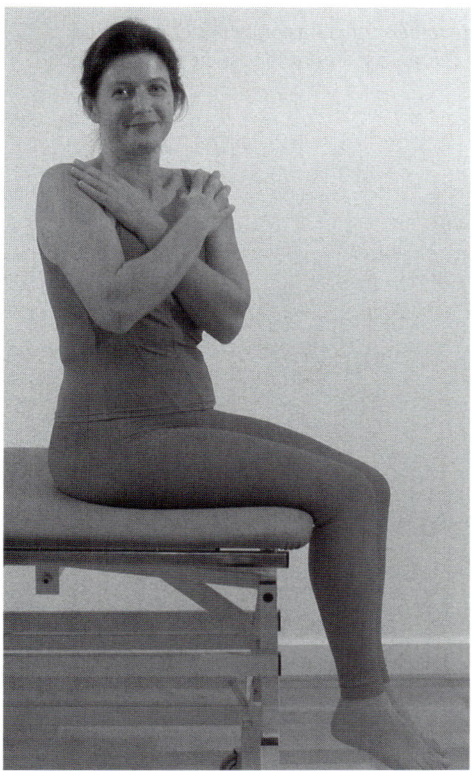

Figure 6.11 Symptom-provoking movement: rotation of the spine provokes pain at the thoracolumbar junction, right side.

Hypothesis 1: The symptom-provoking area is the neural structures

Differentiation: neural involvement vs. thoracic spine/lumbar spine.

The change in symptoms can be demonstrated exactly:

- provocation of pain (Fig. 6.12a and b, film 9)
- alleviation of pain (Fig. 6.13a and b, film 10).

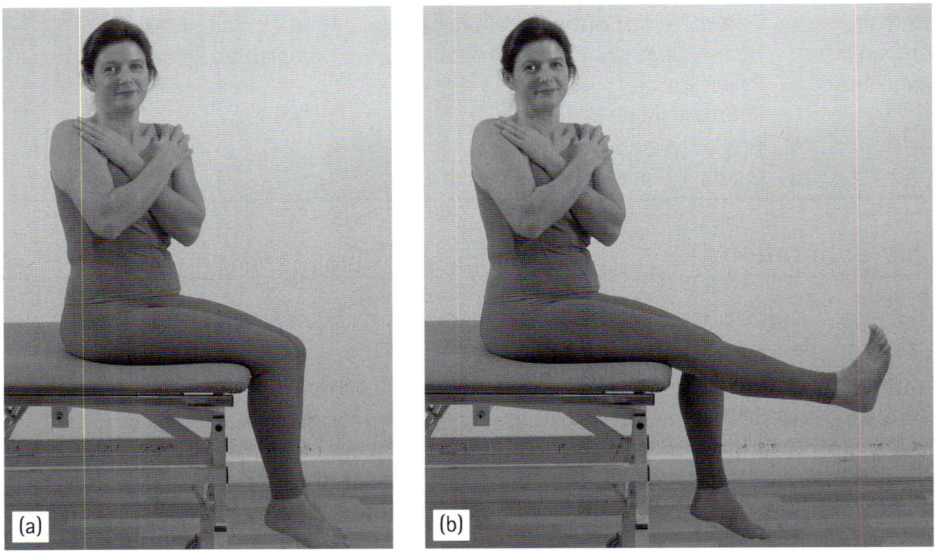

Figure 6.12a and b Area localization with symptomatic movement of the thoracolumbar junction into rotation; differentiation between neural structures and thoracic spine/lumbar spine; provocation. **a**, Starting position. **b**, End position.

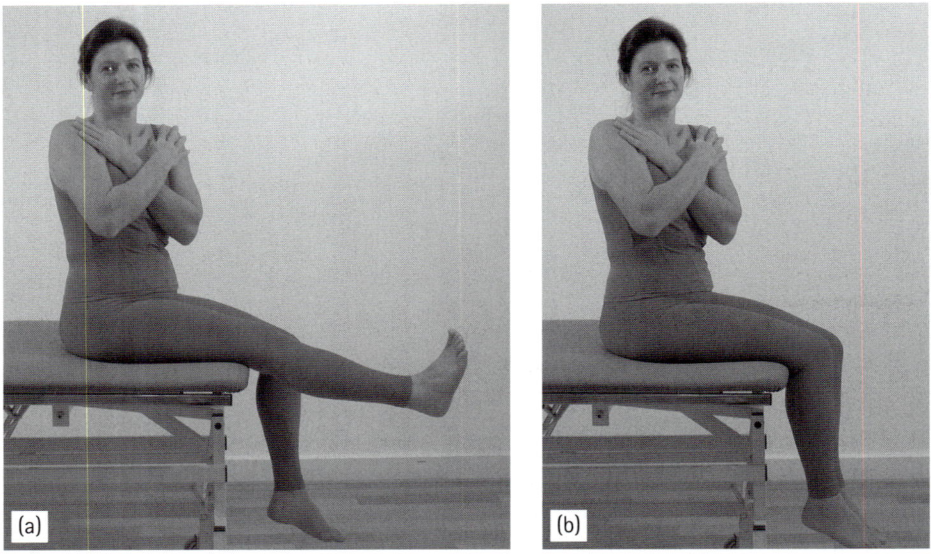

Figure 6.13a and b Area localization with symptomatic movement of the thoracolumbar junction into rotation; differentiation between neural structures and thoracic spine/lumbar spine; alleviation. **a**, Starting position. **b**, End position.

The result of area localization has to be verified by further specific tests; otherwise the result remains in doubt.

Assessment			
Goal	**Provocation of pain**	**Alleviation of pain**	**Remarks**
Starting position	Rotation of the spine to a position immediately before symptoms appear	With the right knee pre-positioned in extension and the right ankle in dorsal flexion, rotation of the spine to the right, to a position immediately after symptoms have appeared	
Test movement	Unilateral extension of the knee and dorsal flexion of the ipsilateral ankle, in sitting	Flexion of the right knee, which reduces the tension in the neural structures produced by the starting position	
Explanation	The test movement increases tension in the neural structures	The test movement reduces tension in the neural structures	If the typical pain is provoked or alleviated by these manoeuvres, this suggests at least an involvement of the neural structures
Additional data to support the hypothesis	Further movements of proximal and distal components to increase neural tension which are not directly involved in flexion of the spine General and specific mobility of the affected area History (e.g., symptom behaviour, type of complaints, 24-hour behaviour) Palpation Neurodynamic tests Nerve provocation tests (e.g., bow string sign) Reproducibility of test results Test treatment Imaging procedures (CT, MRI)		

Hypothesis 2: The symptom-provoking area is the ribs
Differentiation: ribs vs. thoracic spine/lumbar spine.

The change in symptoms can be demonstrated exactly:

- provocation of pain (Fig. 6.14a and b, film 11)
- alleviation of pain (Fig. 6.15a and b, film 12).

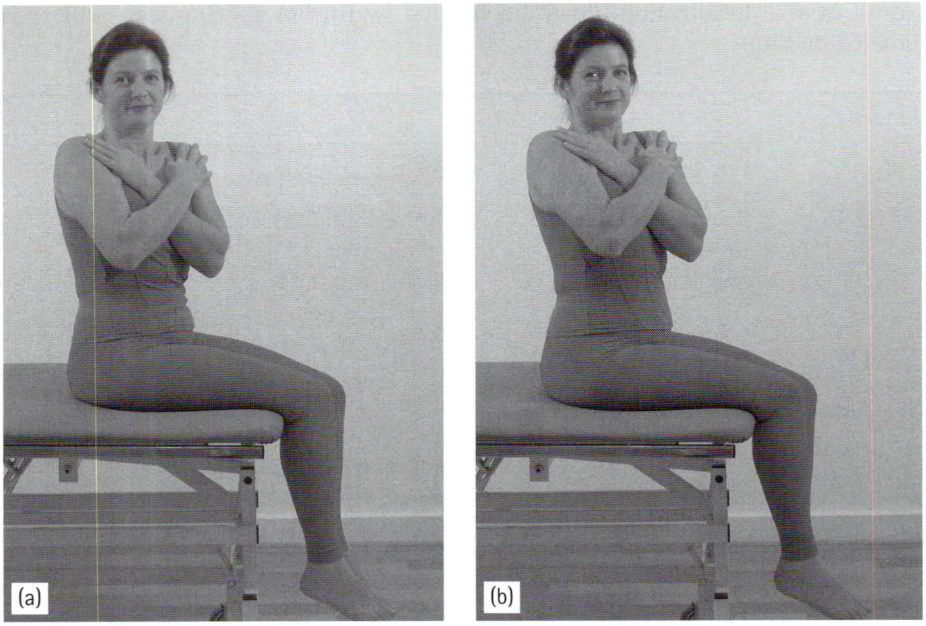

Figure 6.14a and b Area localization with symptomatic movement of the thoracolumbar junction into rotation; differentiation between ribs and thoracic spine/lumbar spine; provocation. **a**, Starting position. **b**, End position.

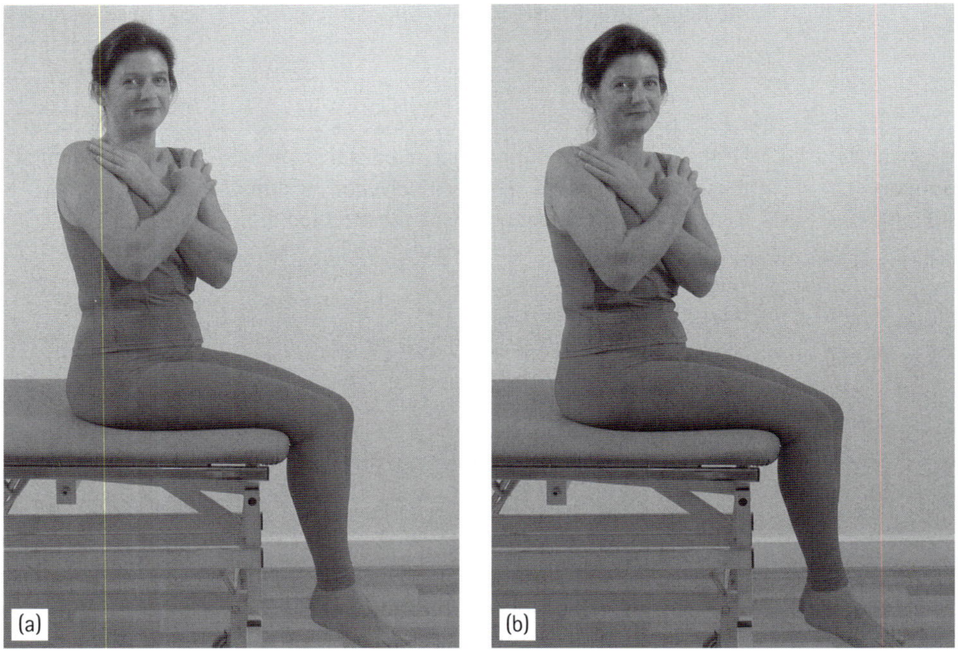

Figure 6.15a and b Area localization with symptomatic movement of the thoracolumbar junction into rotation; differentiation between ribs and thoracic spine/lumbar spine; alleviation. **a**, Starting position. **b**, End position.

The result of area localization has to be verified by further specific tests; otherwise the result remains in doubt.

Assessment			
Goal	**Provocation of pain**	**Alleviation of pain**	**Remarks**
Starting position	Rotation of the spine to a position immediately before symptoms appear	Inspiration, then rotation of the spine to a position immediately after symptoms have appeared	
Test movement	Inspiration	Expiration	Position of the spine must not change during test movement
Explanation	The test movement moves predominantly the ribs. Hence the rib movement during inspiration may be regarded as the symptom-provoking mechanism	The test movement moves predominantly the ribs. Hence the rib movement during expiration may be regarded as the symptom-reducing mechanism	In the authors' experience, inspiration is mostly provoking, expiration is mostly alleviating, when rib joints are involved. Due to the complexity of the movement apparatus, however, the reverse mechanism is also possible
Additional data to support the hypothesis	General and specific mobility of ribs and thoracic spine History (e.g., symptom behaviour, type of complaints, 24-hour behaviour) Palpation Reproducibility of test results Test treatment Imaging procedures (CT, MRI)		

QUICK CHECK – SYMPTOMS, THORACOLUMBAR JUNCTION

If neither the area nor a symptom-provoking or symptom-reducing action is known, the quick check is used to try to load individual potential areas with specific biomechanically provocative movement combinations. The chosen movement combinations correspond with the straining and often symptom-provoking movements of the individual sections.

THORACIC SPINE/LUMBAR SPINE

Movement (film 226)

- Extension/lateral flexion to the right, and rotation to the same as well as to the opposite side, with overpressure (Fig. 6.16a and b)
- Extension/lateral flexion to the left, and rotation to the same as well as to the opposite side, with overpressure (Fig. 6.17a and b).

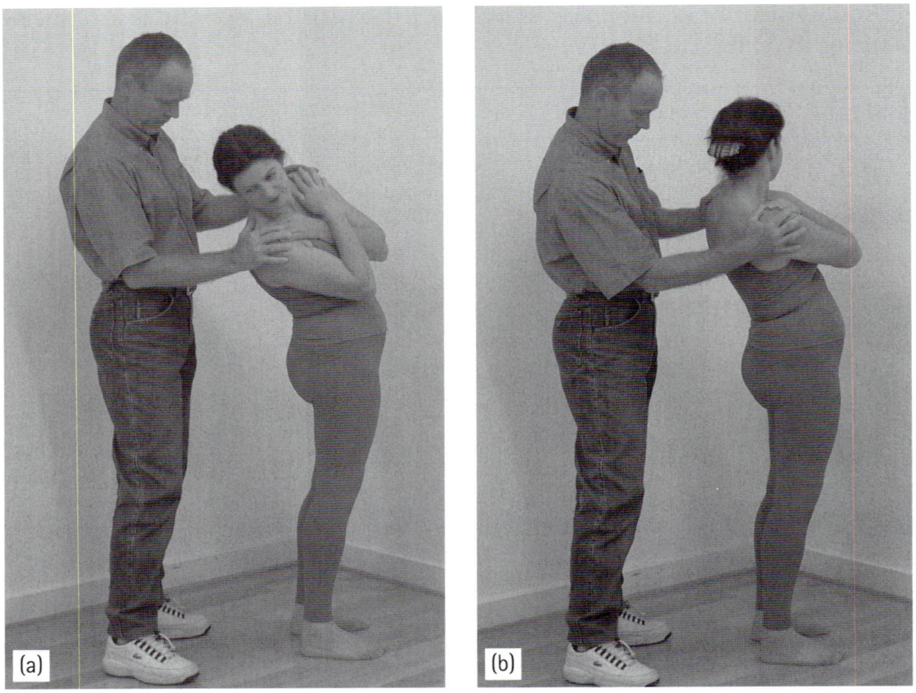

Figure 6.16a and b Quick check of the thoracic/lumbar spine; extension; lateral flexion to the right. a, Rotation to the same side. b, Rotation to the opposite side.

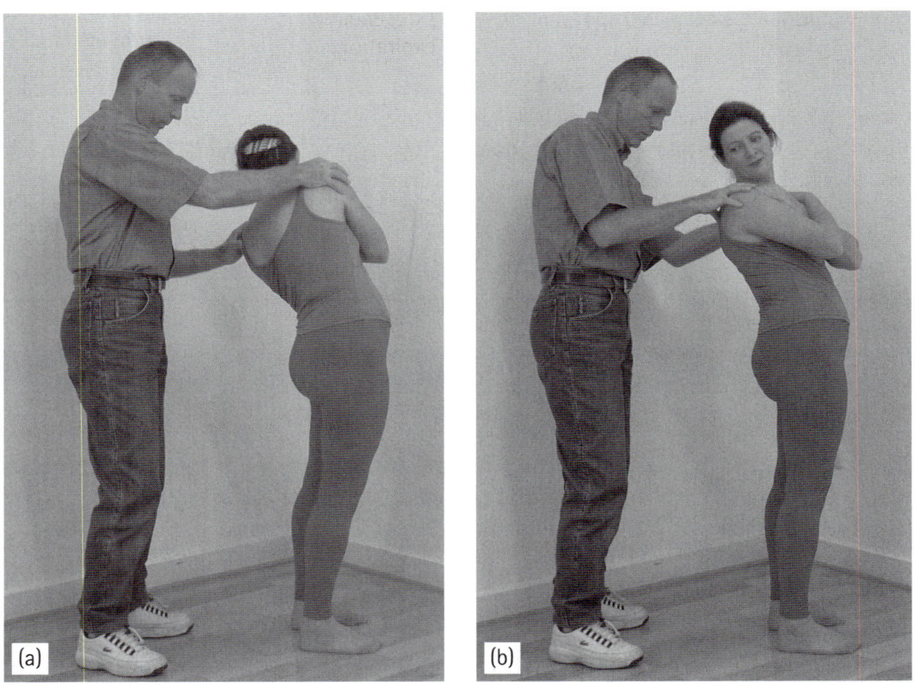

Figure 6.17a and b Quick check of the thoracic/lumbar spine; extension; lateral flexion to the left. a, Rotation to the same side. b, Rotation to the opposite side.

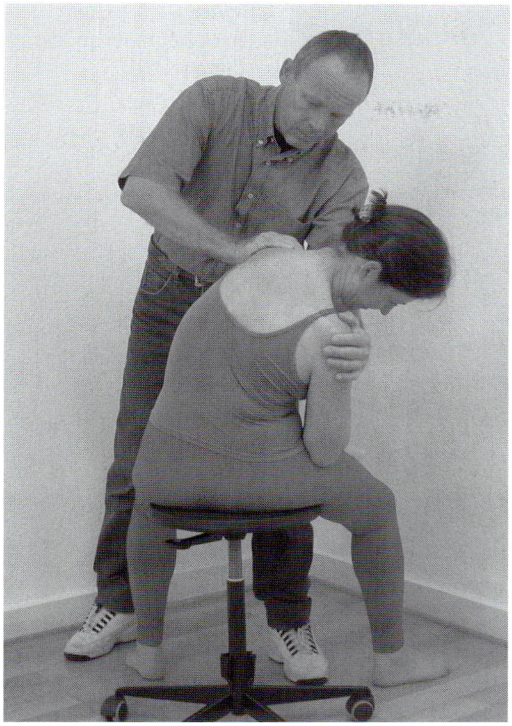

Figure 6.18 Quick check ribs; flexion, sidebending and rotation to the same side, plus inspiration.

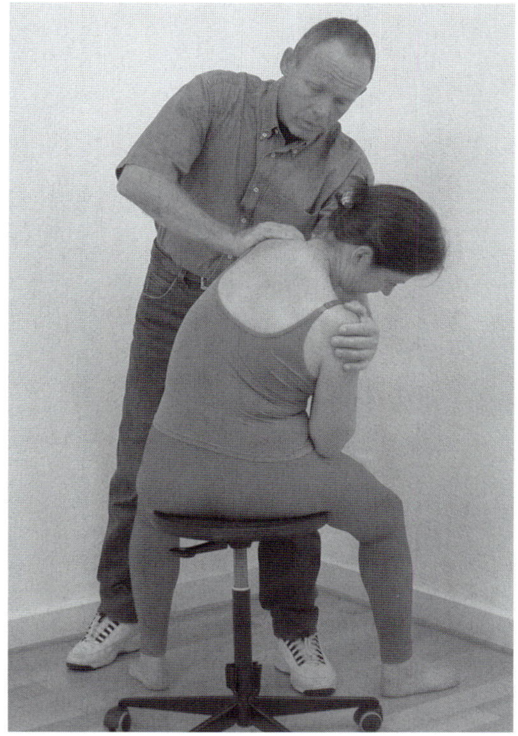

Figure 6.19 Quick check ribs; extension, sidebending and rotation to the same side, plus expiration.

RIBS

Movement (film 227)

- Maximum inspiration and expiration from neutral position
- Flexion, lateral flexion and rotation to the same side, plus inspiration (Fig. 6.18)
- Extension, lateral flexion and rotation to the same side, plus expiration (Fig. 6.19).

NEURAL STRUCTURES

Tension tests

- Slump test (Fig. 6.20, film 616)
- SLR (Fig. 6.21, film 618).

Note: Even an area that proves negative in the quick check may possibly be symptom-provoking (another movement combination, or passive overpressure may be required).

SPECIFIC PROVOCATION AND ALLEVIATION

Specific provocation and alleviation allows one to differentiate within an articular complex and to identify the symptom-provoking movement direction(s).

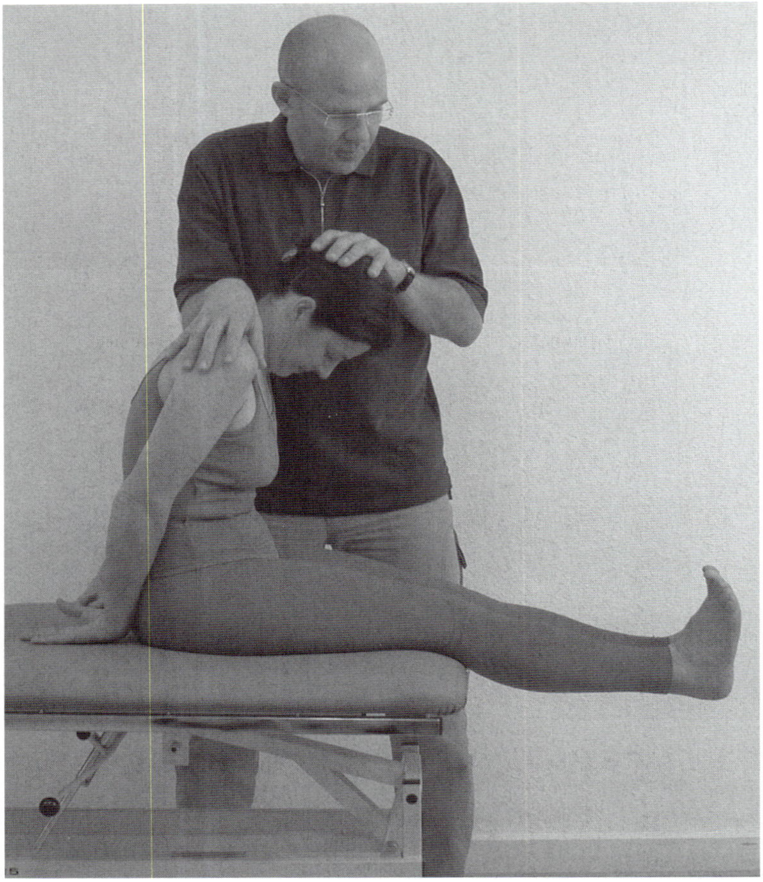

Figure 6.20 Quick check neurodynamics; slump test.

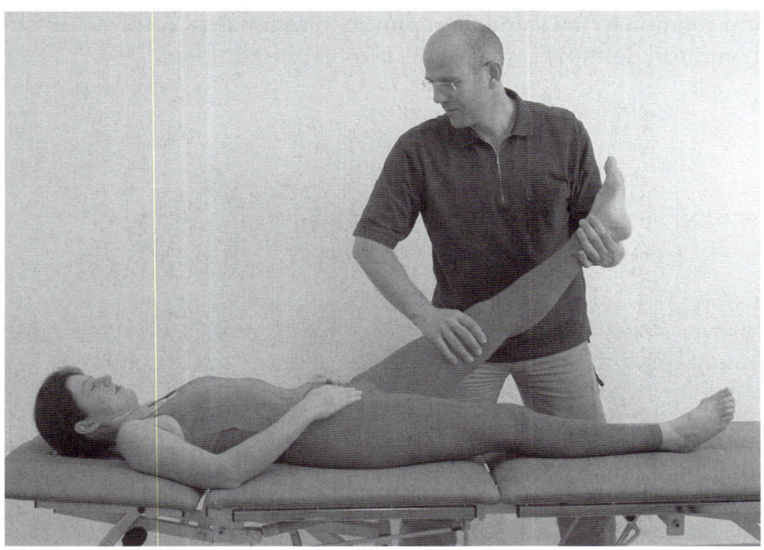

Figure 6.21 Quick check neurodynamics; straight leg raise (SLR) test.

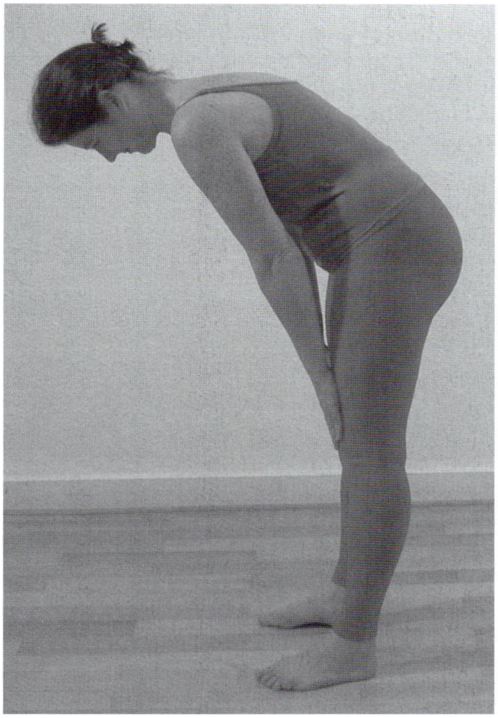

Figure 6.22 Symptom-provoking movement: flexion of the spine provokes pain at the thoracolumbar junction, right side.

SPECIFIC PROVOCATION AND ALLEVIATION, THORACOLUMBAR JUNCTION

Localization, thoracolumbar junction – flexion

Pain-provoking movement (Fig. 6.22)

- Flexion of the spine provokes pain at the thoracolumbar junction, right side.
- Area localization hints at the thoracolumbar junction.

The change in symptoms can be demonstrated exactly:

- provocation of pain (Fig. 6.23a and b, film 13)
- alleviation of pain (Fig. 6.24a and b, film 14).

Assessment			
Goal	Provocation of pain	Alleviation of pain	Remarks
Starting position	Flexion of the spine to a position immediately before symptoms appear, slight propping up on the plinth	Flexion of the spine to a position immediately after symptoms have appeared, slight propping up on the plinth	Trunk remains in starting position

Goal	Provocation of pain	Alleviation of pain	Remarks
Test movement	Pushing the vertebra via lamina or spinous process in ventrocranial direction; the movement has to be started caudally (L2–T8)	Pushing the vertebra via lamina or spinous process in ventrocranial direction; the movement has to be started cranially (T9–L3)	
Neural involvement	Proximal and/or distal component without change of position in the relevant area	Proximal and/or distal component without change of position in the relevant area	
Explanation	The symptoms are provoked when the cranial vertebra in the segment is moved (flexion in the affected segment)	The symptoms are alleviated when the caudal vertebra in the segment is moved (extension in the affected segment)	
Additional data to support the hypothesis	General and specific mobility of the thoracolumbar junction History (e.g., symptom behaviour, type of complaints, 24-hour behaviour) Specific palpation Neurodynamic tests (if specific provocation and alleviation indicate neural involvement) Reproducibility of test results Test treatment Imaging procedures (CT, MRI)		

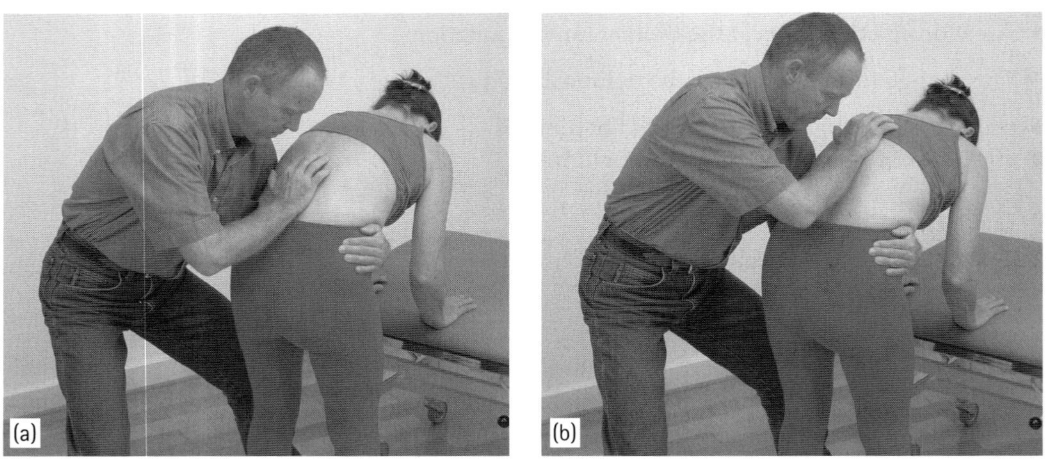

Figure 6.23a and b Specific provocation and alleviation in the area of the thoracolumbar junction with symptomatic flexion of the spine; localization of the symptomatic segment; provocation. **a**, Test start. **b**, Test end.

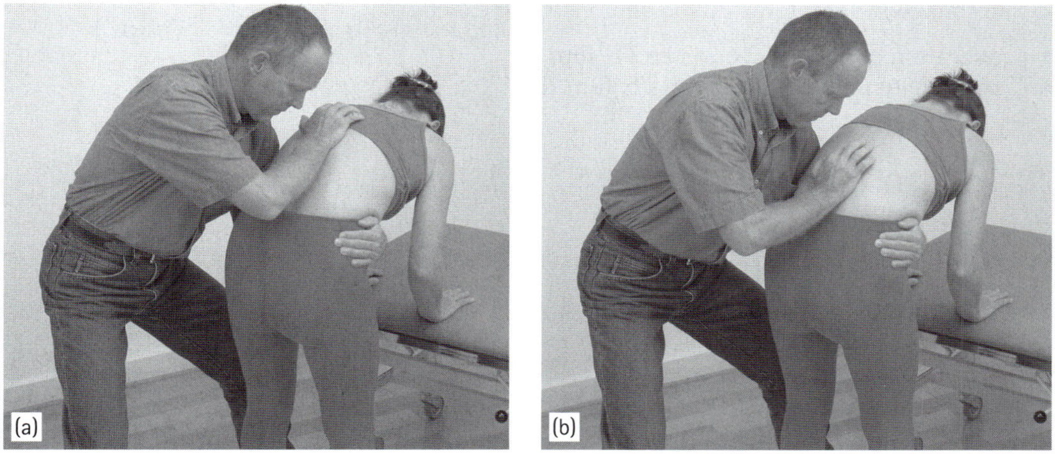

Figure 6.24a and b Specific provocation and alleviation in the area of the thoracolumbar junction with symptomatic flexion of the spine; localization of the symptomatic segment; alleviation. **a**, Test start. **b**, Test end.

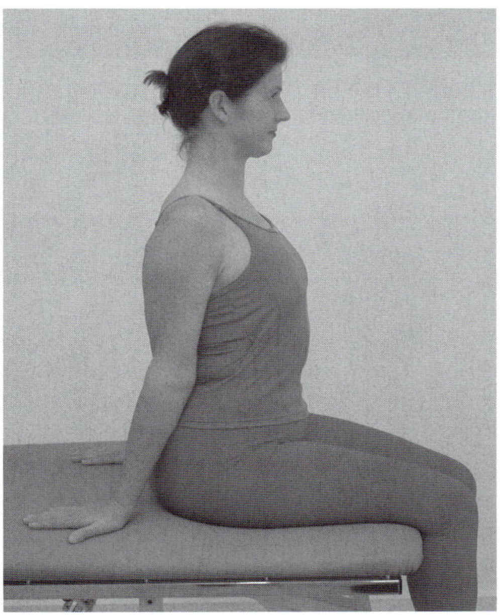

Figure 6.25 Symptom-provoking movement: extension of the spine provokes pain at the thoracolumbar junction, right side.

Localization, thoracolumbar junction – extension

Pain-provoking movement (Fig. 6.25)

- Extension of the spine provokes pain at the thoracolumbar junction, right side.
- Area localization hints at the thoracolumbar junction.

The change in symptoms can be demonstrated exactly:

- provocation of pain (Fig. 6.26a and b, film 15)
- alleviation of pain (Fig. 6.27a and b, film 16).

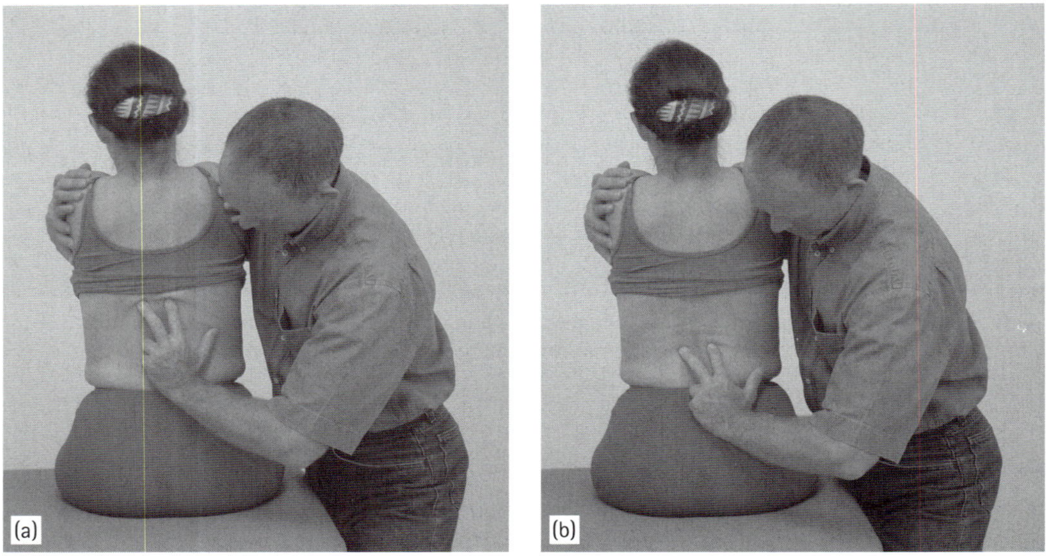

Figure 6.26a and b Specific provocation and alleviation in the area of the thoracolumbar junction with symptomatic extension of the spine; localization of the symptomatic segment; provocation. **a**, Test start. **b**, Test end.

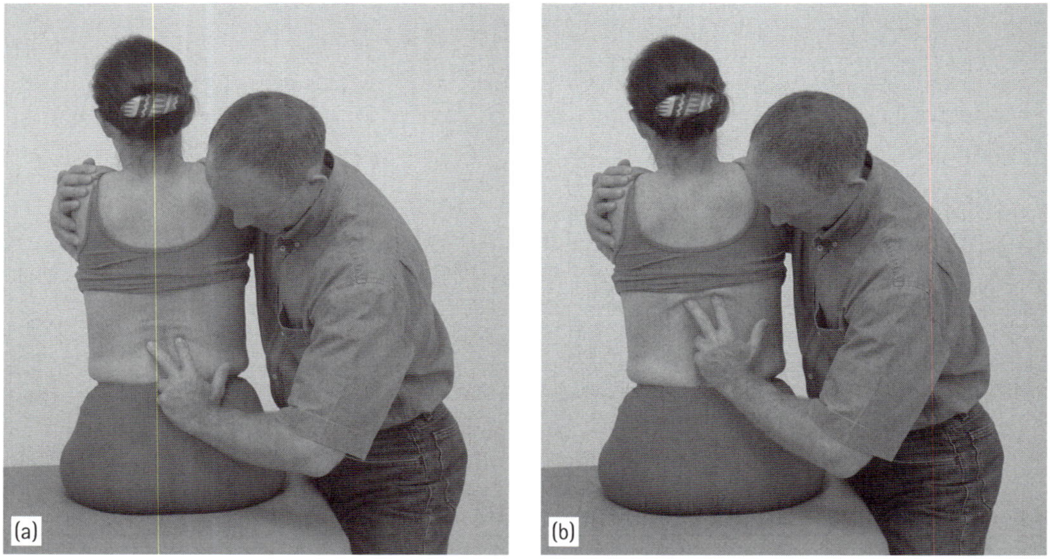

Figure 6.27a and b Specific provocation and alleviation in the area of the thoracolumbar junction with symptomatic extension of the spine; localization of the symptomatic segment; alleviation. **a**, Test start. **b**, Test end.

Assessment			
Goal	Provocation of pain	Alleviation of pain	Remarks
Starting position	Extension of the spine to a position immediately before symptoms appear	Extension of the spine to a position immediately after symptoms have appeared	Trunk remains in starting position
Test movement	Pushing the vertebra via the lamina in ventrocranial direction; the movement has to be started cranially (T9–L3)	Pushing the vertebra via the lamina in ventrocranial direction; the movement has to be started caudally (L2–T8)	
Neural involvement	Proximal and/or distal component without change of position in the relevant area	Proximal and/or distal component without change of position in the relevant area	
Explanation	The symptoms are provoked when the caudal vertebra in the segment is moved (extension in the affected segment)	The symptoms are alleviated when the cranial vertebra in the segment is moved (flexion in the affected segment)	
Additional data to support the hypothesis	General and specific mobility of the thoracolumbar junction History (e.g., symptom behaviour, type of complaints, 24-hour behaviour) Specific palpation Neurodynamic tests (if specific provocation and alleviation indicate neural involvement) Reproducibility of test results Test treatment Imaging procedures (CT, MRI)		

Localization, thoracolumbar junction – rotation

Pain-provoking movement (Fig. 6.28)

- Rotation of the spine to the right provokes pain at the thoracolumbar junction.
- Area localization hints at the thoracolumbar junction.

The change in symptoms can be demonstrated exactly:

- provocation of pain (Fig. 6.29a and b, film 17)
- alleviation of pain (Fig. 6.30a and b, film 18).

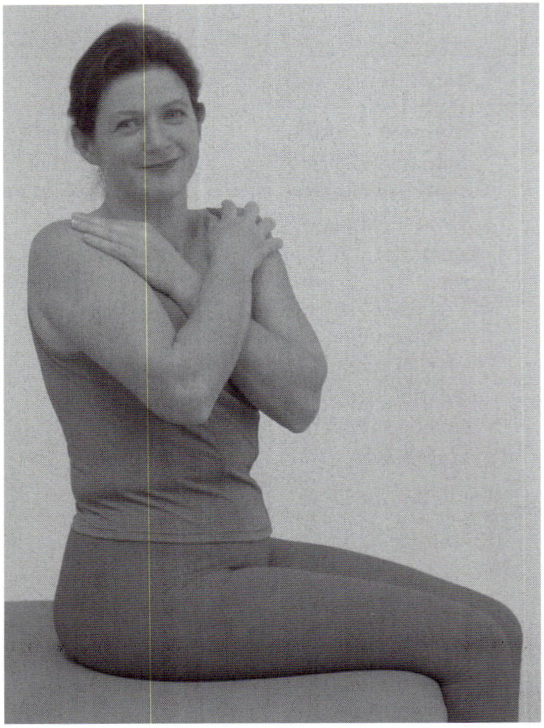

Figure 6.28 Symptom-provoking movement: rotation of the spine provokes pain at the thoracolumbar junction, right side.

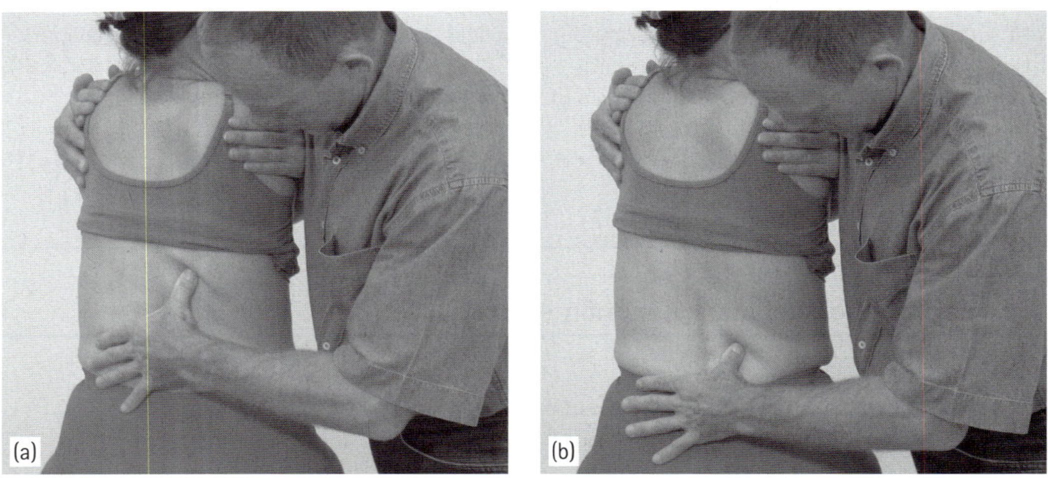

Figure 6.29a and b Specific provocation and alleviation in the area of the thoracolumbar junction with symptomatic rotation of the spine; localization of the symptomatic segment; provocation. **a**, Test start. **b**, Test end.

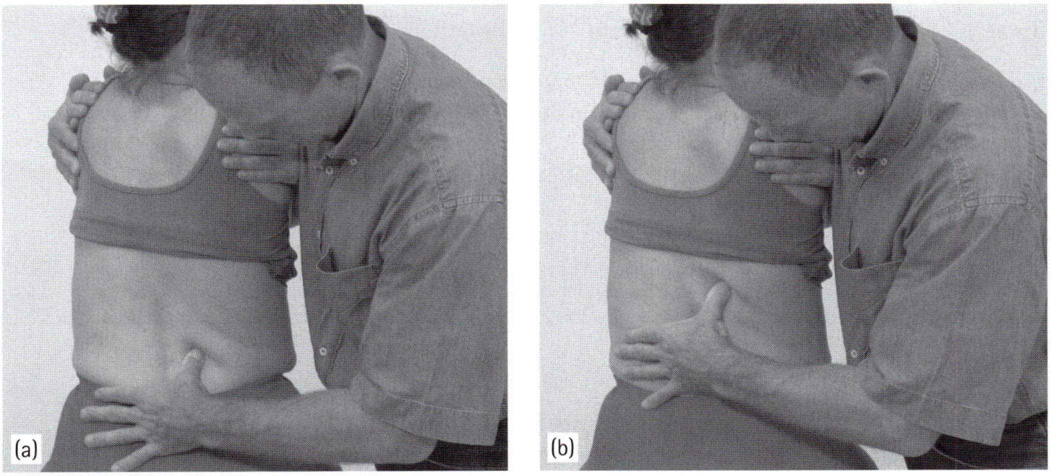

Figure 6.30a and b Specific provocation and alleviation in the area of the upper thoracolumbar junction with symptomatic rotation of the spine; localization of the symptomatic segment; alleviation. **a**, Test start. **b**, Test end.

Assessment

Goal	Provocation of pain	Alleviation of pain	Remarks
Starting position	Turning the spine to the right to a position immediately before symptoms appear	Turning the spine to the right to a position immediately after symptoms have appeared	Trunk remains in starting position
Test movement	Pushing the vertebra via right transverse process into rotation to the left; the movement has to be started cranially (T9–L3)	Pushing the vertebra via right transverse process to the left; the movement has to be started caudally (L2–T8)	If differentiation is done via pushing the vertebra into rotation to the right, provocation has to start caudally, alleviation cranially
Neural involvement	Proximal and/or distal component without change of position in the relevant area	Proximal and/or distal component without change of position in the relevant area	
Explanation	The symptoms are provoked when the caudal vertebra in the segment is moved (rotation to the right in the affected segment)	The symptoms are alleviated when the cranial vertebra in the segment is moved (rotation to the left in the affected segment)	

Goal	Provocation of pain	Alleviation of pain	Remarks
Additional data to support the hypothesis	General and specific mobility of the thoracolumbar junction History (e.g., symptom behaviour, type of complaints, 24-hour behaviour) Specific palpation Neurodynamic tests (if specific provocation and alleviation indicate neural involvement) Reproducibility of test results Test treatment Imaging procedures (CT, MRI)		

Differentiation between vertebral and costal joints within the affected segment at the thoracolumbar junction – rotation

Pain-provoking movement

Specific provocation and alleviation of symptomatic rotation to the right hints at segment T10.

The change in symptoms can be demonstrated exactly:

- provocation of pain (Fig. 6.31a and b, film 19)
- alleviation of pain (Fig. 6.32a and b, film 20).

Assessment

Goal	Provocation of pain	Alleviation of pain	Remarks
Starting position	Turning the spine to the right to a position immediately before symptoms appear	Turning the spine to the right to a position immediately after symptoms have appeared	Trunk remains in starting position
Test movement	Pushing the costal angle of the corresponding rib in ventral direction	Push from ventral against the corresponding rib	
Neural involvement	Proximal and/or distal component without change of position in the relevant area	Proximal and/or distal component without change of position in the relevant area	
Explanation	If, in this way, symptoms are provoked, the vertebra is not the cause, since it is	If, in this way, symptoms are alleviated, the vertebra is not the cause, since it is	

Goal	Provocation of pain	Alleviation of pain	Remarks
	rotated to the left in this manoeuvre	rotated to the right in this manoeuvre	
Additional data to support the hypothesis	General and specific mobility of the thoracolumbar junction and the ribs History (e.g., symptom behaviour, type of complaints, 24-hour behaviour) Specific palpation Neurodynamic tests (if specific provocation and alleviation indicate neural involvement) Reproducibility of test results Test treatment Imaging procedures (CT, MRI)		

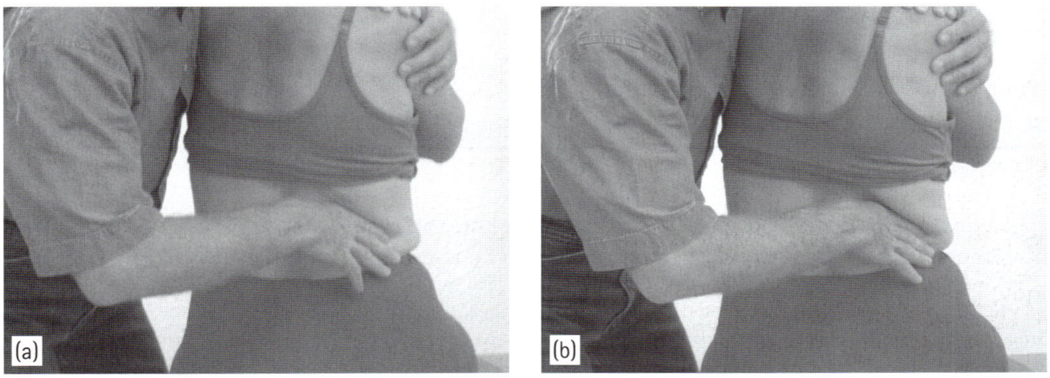

Figure 6.31a and b Specific provocation and alleviation in the area of the thoracolumbar junction with symptomatic rotation of the spine; differentiation between costal and vertebral joints (T10); provocation. **a**, Test start. **b**, Test end.

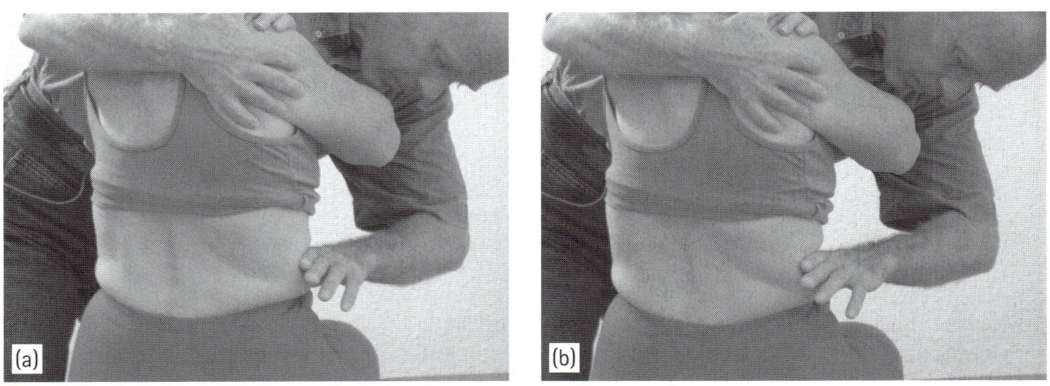

Figure 6.32a and b Specific provocation and alleviation in the area of the thoracolumbar junction with symptomatic rotation of the spine; differentiation between costal and vertebral joints (T10); alleviation. **a**, Test start. **b**, Test end.

GENERAL MOVEMENT TESTS

General movement tests identify, quantity, and qualify individual anatomical movements and, in part, movement combinations in the area concerned. The individual manual therapy concepts have respective protocols at their disposal, which more or less have the same goals.

Information gained in this way is used for checking or modifying the relevant hypotheses developed on the basis of anamnesis and area localization and will contribute to determining how to proceed.

General question: Is there enough information available to bypass general movement tests?	
No	Yes
⇓	⇓
Performance of the general movement tests	• Additional tests • Test treatment

In view of the described clinical presentation and the results of area localization, general movement tests in the following regions seem to be useful.

Thoracic spine and ribs		
	Active	**Passive**
Thoracic spine in general	Flexion	Flexion
	Extension	Extension
	Rotation (to the right and left) Lateral flexion (to the right and left)	Rotation (to the right and left) Lateral flexion (to the right and left)
Ribs in general	Inspiration Expiration	
Movement combinations thoracic spine and ribs in general	Symptomatic movements of the thoracic spine plus inspiration and expiration	Symptomatic movements of the thoracic spine plus inspiration and expiration

Lumbar spine		
	Active	Passive
Lumbar spine in general	Flexion Extension Rotation (to the right and left) Lateral flexion (to the right and left)	Flexion Extension Rotation (to the right and left) Lateral flexion (to the right and left)
Movement combinations lumbar spine in general	Symptomatic movements of the lumbar spine	Symptomatic movements of the lumbar spine

TREATMENT EXAMPLE, THORACOLUMBAR JUNCTION

SYMPTOMATIC MOVEMENT

Rotation of the spine to the right provokes pain (VAS 3/10) at the thoracolumbar junction, right side.

ASSESSMENTS

Area localization

Area localization hints at the thoracolumbar junction. There is no contraindication for movement.

Symptomatic movement combinations

Although the patient described symptoms occurring with rotation to the right, it turned out that with the spine pre-positioned in extension and lateral flexion to the right, rotation to the right (non-coupled movement) was markedly restricted. Thus in movement examination, a clearly greater rotation to the left was found with extension and lateral flexion to the left than was found with rotation to the right with extension and lateral flexion to the right. Moreover, the patient's typical symptoms could be reproduced much more markedly with this non-coupled movement combination than with coupled rotation to the right (VAS 5/10).

Coupled/non-coupled movements for thoracic spine and lumbar spine			
Movement	Plus lateral flexion	Plus rotation	Type of movement combination
Flexion	Right	Right Left	Coupled Non-coupled
	Left	Right Left	Non-coupled Coupled
Extension	Right	Right Left	Non-coupled Coupled
	Left	Right Left	Coupled Non-coupled

The concept of coupled/non-coupled movements of the spine (Zahnd 1998) describes only certain movement combinations. It has to be noted that, with a few exceptions, the movement combinations referred to as coupled occur involuntarily and allow the greatest rotation ranges (Pearcy 1984, Panjabi 1992a,b, Zahnd and Baumgartner 2000).

Occasionally, this concept can be used clinically. The arthrokinematics of the conceptual movements, however, remains hidden to the examiner. With morphological changes as well as with movement dysfunctions of the spine, a deviation from the described concept is to be expected rather frequently.

Specific provocation and alleviation

Specific provocation and alleviation hints at a provocation of symptoms by movement of T12 into rotation to the right.

Specific mobility

Specific mobility tests show hypomobility of T12 in rotation to the right. In particular, rotation to the right with extension, together with lateral flexion to the right, is heavily hypomobile at T12 as compared with neighbouring segments.

Palpation

Palpation indicates increased tension and slightly increased tenderness of the thoracolumbar paravertebral muscles at the right side as compared with the opposite side.

HYPOTHESIS

A painful movement restriction of T12 with extension, lateral flexion, and rotation to the right is suspected (Fig. 6.33).

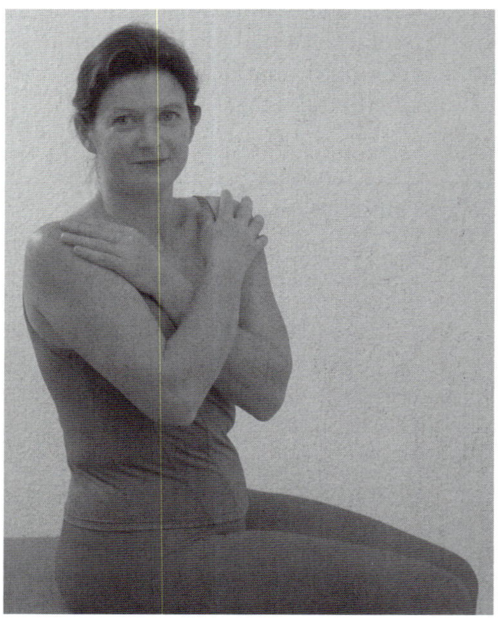

Figure 6.33 Symptom-provoking movement: rotation of the spine provokes pain at the thoracolumbar junction, right side.

RELAXATION TECHNIQUES

Hold–relax techniques

MOVEMENT-DIRECTED CONTRACTION IN THE DIRECTION OPPOSING THE PAINFUL AND/OR RESTRICTED DIRECTION

Therapy technique (film 21)

Patient's starting position:

- sitting on the plinth (Fig. 6.34a)
- the left pelvis is supported by a wedge (lateral flexion of the lumbar spine to the left), feet resting on a stool, arms folded in front of the chest
- the plinth is lowered to the point where the lumbar spine is pre-positioned in flexion at L1
- lateral flexion to the left is further increased from the cranial side.

Therapist's starting position:

- standing, at the patient's right side
- fixing patient's thorax by grasping his or her shoulder girdle from anterior.

Movement:

- adjusting the thoracic spine in lateral flexion to the right, extension and rotation to the right up to the segment to be treated (T12, Fig. 6.34b)
- in this position, the therapist tries to rotate further to the right, while the patient tries to prevent this movement by muscle contraction.

Note: Although the patient's functional demonstration had been simple rotation of the trunk to the right, the check of specific movement combinations revealed the greatest restriction when the spine was pre-positioned in extension and lateral flexion to the right. With the same movement combination, the patient's typical symptoms could be reproduced.

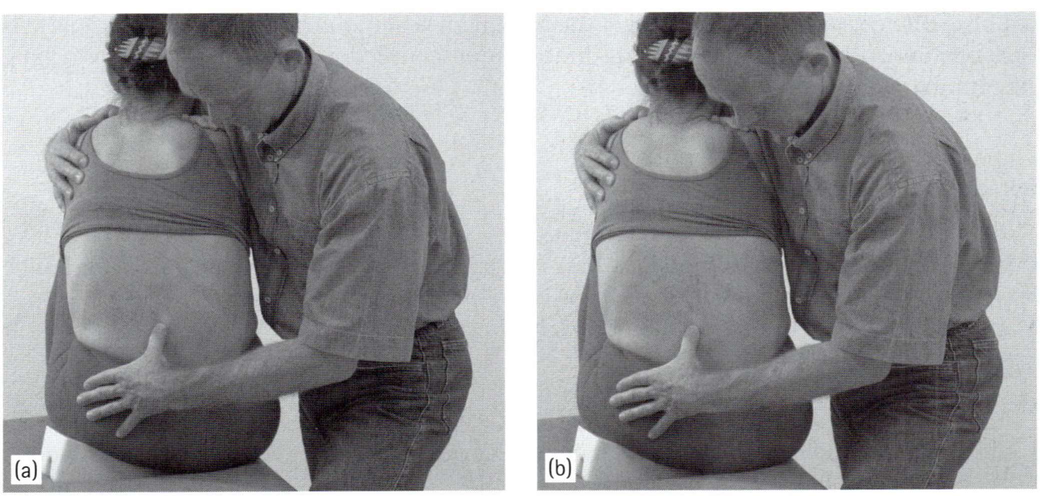

Figure 6.34a and b Hold–relax technique; movement-directed contraction in the direction opposing the painful and/or restricted direction; therapy technique. **a**, Starting position. **b**, End position.

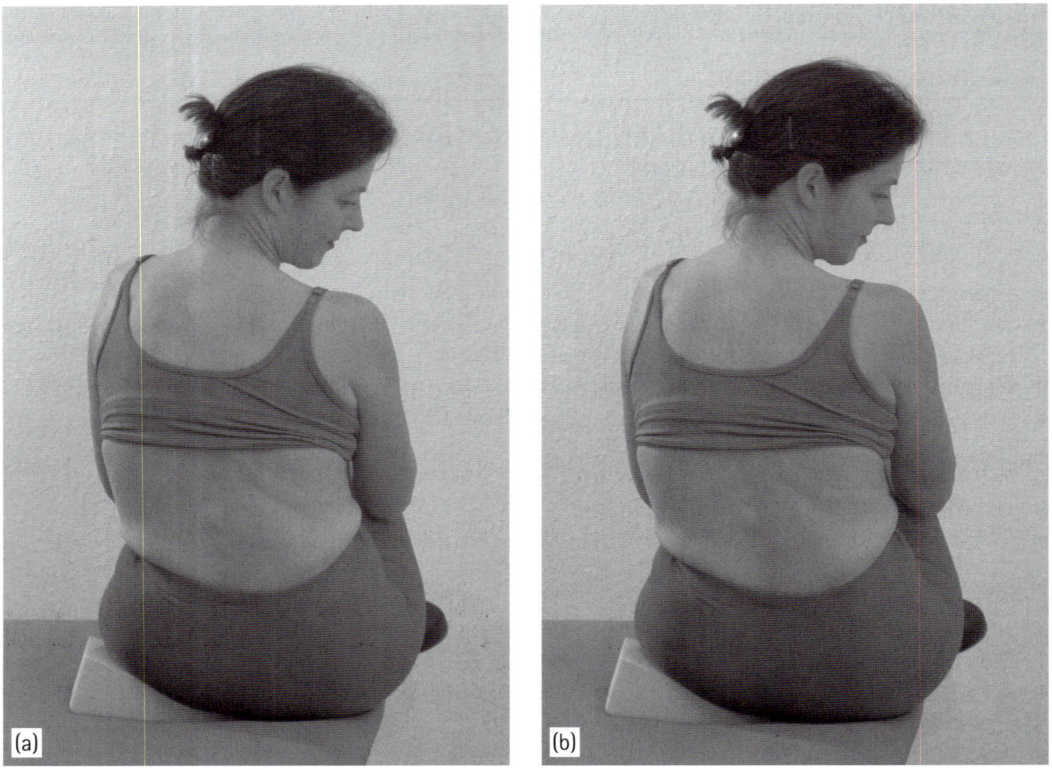

Figure 6.35a and b Hold-relax technique; movement-directed contraction in the direction opposing the painful and/or restricted direction; self-exercise. **a**, Starting position. **b**, End position.

Note (continued): For this reason, the presented technique is performed additionally in extension and lateral flexion to the right. To prevent co-rotation of the lumbar spine as far as possible, i.e. to be able to localize the treatment technique better, the lumbar spine is pre-positioned in flexion with this technique (non-coupled movement pattern → locking the lumbar spine).

Self-exercise (film 22)

Patient's starting position:

- sitting on the plinth, the left pelvis supported by a wedge, feet resting on a stool and pulled close to the body until the lumbar spine is pre-positioned in flexion at L1 (Fig. 6.35a)
- the left hand is placed on the lateral right thigh, the right hand grasps the left wrist for reinforcement.

Movement:

- the thoracic spine is pre-positioned in lateral flexion to the right, extension, and rotation to the right (Fig. 6.35b)
- in this position, the patient tries to rotate to the left, while trying to oppose this movement with hands on the thigh.

MOVEMENT-DIRECTED CONTRACTION IN THE PAINFUL AND/OR RESTRICTED DIRECTION

Therapy technique (film 23)

Patient's starting position:

- sitting on the plinth, the left pelvis is supported by a wedge (lateral flexion of the lumbar spine to the left), feet resting on a stool, arms folded in front of the chest (Fig. 6.36a)
- the plinth is lowered to the point where the lumbar spine is pre-positioned in flexion at L1
- lateral flexion to the left is still increased from cranial.

Therapist's starting position:

- standing, at the patient's right side
- fixing patient's thorax by grasping his or her shoulder girdle from anterior.

Movement:

- adjusting the thoracic spine in lateral flexion to the right, extension, and rotation to the right up to the segment to be treated (T12, Fig. 6.36b)
- in this position, the therapist tries to rotate to the left, while the patient tries to prevent this movement by muscle contraction.

> ***Note:*** Although the patient's functional demonstration had been simple rotation of the trunk to the right, the check of specific movement combinations showed the greatest restriction when the spine was pre-positioned in extension and lateral flexion to the right. With the same movement combination, the patient's typical symptoms could be reproduced.
>
> For this reason, the presented technique is performed additionally in extension and lateral flexion to the right. To prevent co-rotation of the lumbar spine as far as possible, i.e. to be able to localize the treatment technique better, the lumbar spine is pre-positioned in flexion with this technique (non-coupled movement pattern → locking the lumbar spine).

Self-exercise (film 24)

Patient's starting position:

- sitting on the plinth, the left pelvis supported by a wedge (lateral flexion to the left), feet resting on a stool and pulled close to the body so that the lumbar spine is pre-positioned in flexion at L1 (Fig. 6.37a)
- the left hand is placed on the medial right thigh, the right hand grasps the left wrist for reinforcement.

Movement:

- adjusting the thoracic spine in extension, lateral flexion to the right, and rotation to the right (Fig. 6.37b)
- in this position, the patient tries to rotate to the right, while trying to oppose this movement with hands on the thigh.

Remarks

Goals of the technique

Reduction of the tonicity and improvement of the metabolism of the periarticular tissue involved in a painfully restricted rotation to the right of T12.

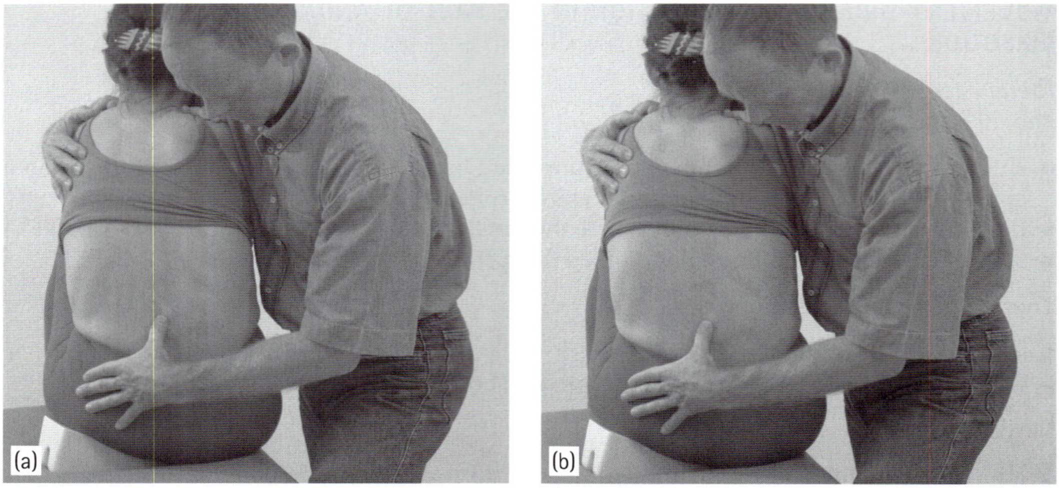

Figure 6.36a and b Hold–relax technique; movement-directed contraction in the painful and/or restricted direction; therapy technique. a, Starting position. b, End position.

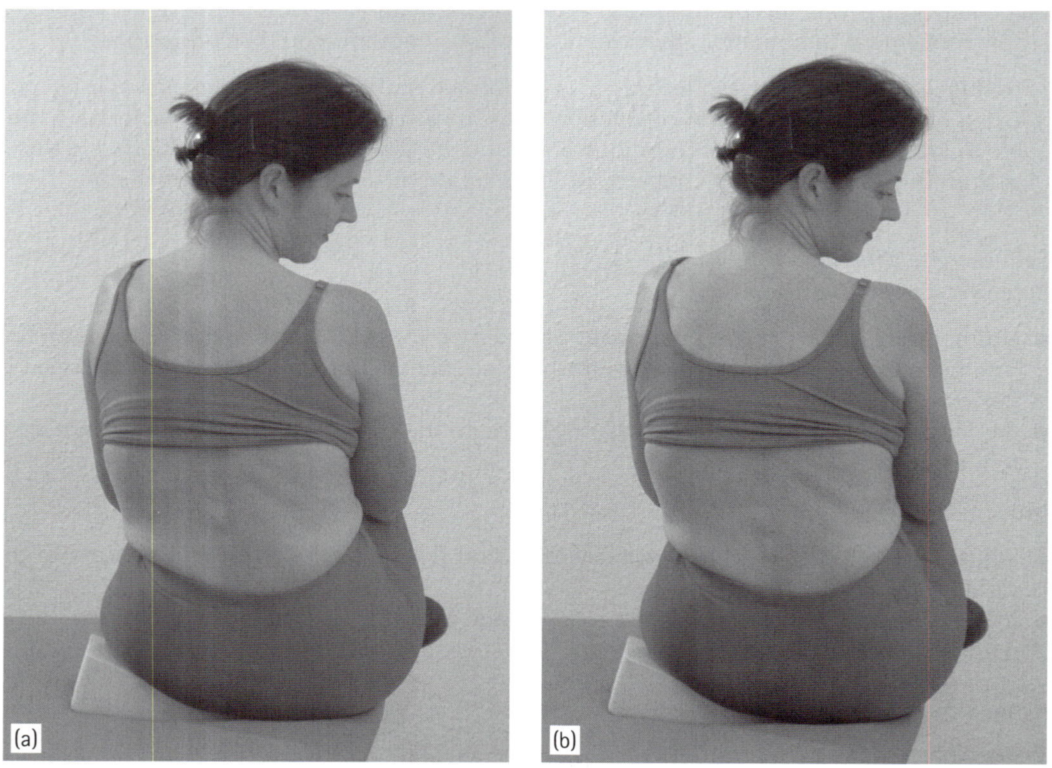

Figure 6.37a and b Hold–relax technique; movement-directed contraction in the painful and/or restricted direction; self-exercise. a, Starting position. b, End position.

Performance

Depending on irritability or the desired treatment goal, the joint to be treated is pre-positioned as necessary before treatment. As the self-exercise is performed without 'specific fixation', transferred movement has to be considered when the indication for the exercise is determined.

Dosage (regarding the affected symptomatic structure)

Neither with adjustment nor with contraction must the patient's typical symptoms be reproduced.

Choice of technique

The selection of the technique depends, among other things, on the therapist as well as the patient, on the therapist's clinical experience, but primarily on reassessment. This means that even if all preconditions on the part of therapist and patient seem to be fulfilled, it is of no use to continue the technique if reassessment is negative.

Contributing factors

For a satisfactory solution of the patient's current problems it is important to consider the contributing factors and include them in the treatment.

The authors will, however, not go into a description of the various possibilities and their complex contexts as this would exceed the scope of the present book.

Soft tissue techniques

Possible soft tissue techniques for the thoracolumbar junction are described in Chapters 7 and 8.

MOBILIZATION TECHNIQUES

Active procedures

ACTIVE MOBILIZATION

Extension and rotation of T12 to the right, in prone position (film 25)

Therapy technique

Patient's starting position:

- prone, thoracic spine and lumbar spine laterally flexed to the right, head rotated to the right, left arm resting beside the body, right hand propping up at shoulder level (Fig. 6.38a)
- if the lateral flexion to the right pre-positioned from cranial goes too far in the caudal direction, into the lumbar spine, it can be repositioned into neutral position via the legs.

Therapist's starting position:

- standing, at the patient's left side
- contact with the ulnar edge of the left hand (reinforced by the right hand) on the costal process of L1.

Movement:

- rotation of the thoracic spine to the right by having the patient push with his or her right arm, while the therapist gives resistance to this movement with the ulnar edge of left hand (reinforced by right hand) on L1 (Fig. 6.38b).

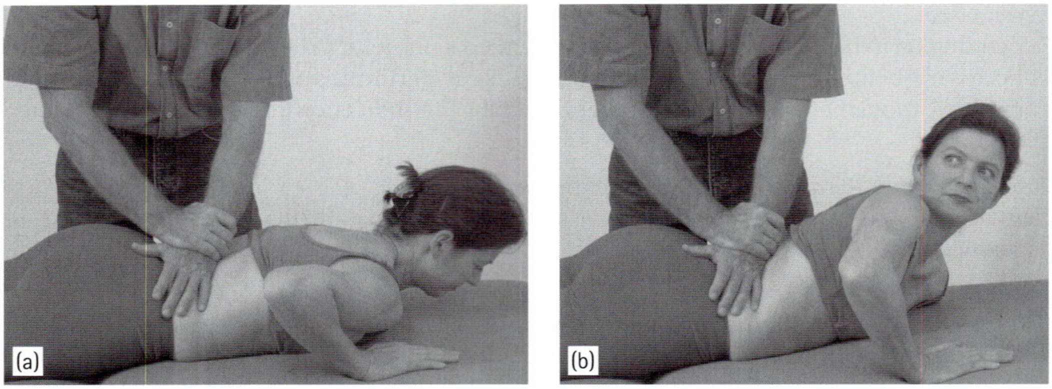

Figure 6.38a and b Active mobilization; extension and rotation to the right (T12); therapy technique. a, Starting position. b, End position.

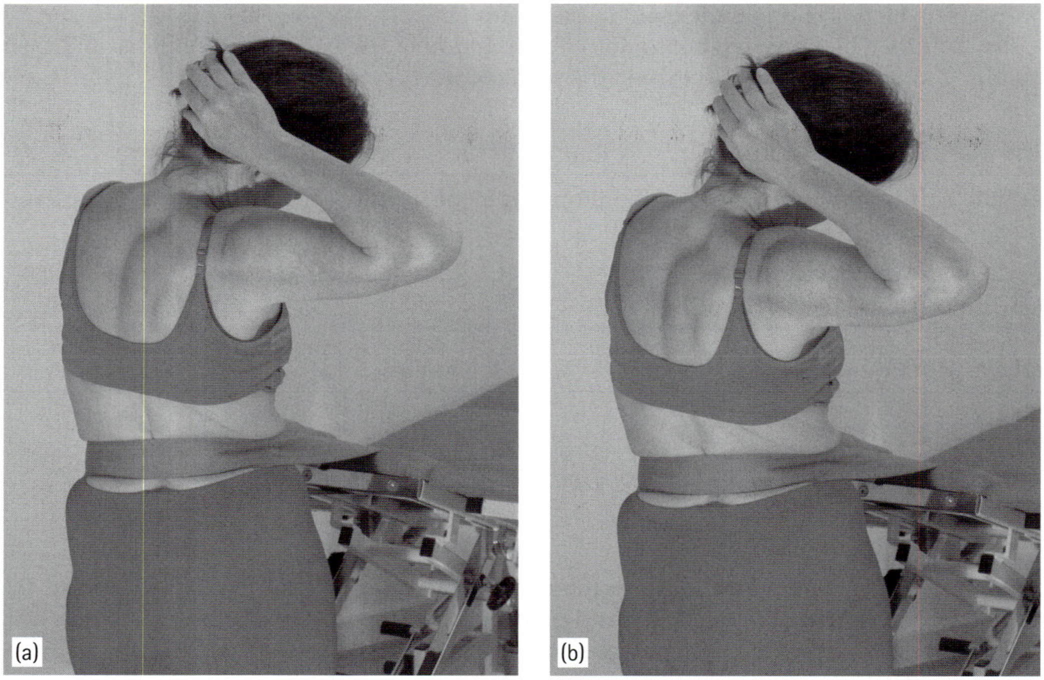

Figure 6.39a and b Active mobilization; extension and rotation to the right (T12); self-exercise. a, Starting position. b, End position.

Self-exercise (film 26)

Patient's starting position:

- standing, a belt surrounds the patient from dorsal, at level L1, and is fixed at some firm object (Fig. 6.39a)
- thoracic spine and lumbar spine are pre-positioned in extension and lateral flexion to the right.

Movement:

- leaning backwards against the belt for fixation (Fig. 6.39b)
- then movement into rotation to the right and lateral flexion to the right.

Passive procedures

ACCESSORY MOVEMENTS

Unilateral push in posterior-anterior direction

Therapy technique (film 27)

Patient's starting position:

- prone (Fig. 6.40a).

Therapist's starting position:

- standing, at the patient's left side
- hypothenar of the therapist's right hand is placed on the patient's right costal process of L1.

Movement:

- unilateral push on the costal process of L1 from posterior to anterior, right side (Fig. 6.40b).

Self-exercise (film 28)

Patient's starting position:

- sitting on a chair (Fig. 6.41a)
- a tennis ball is placed between right costal process of L1 and back of the chair
- arms are placed on the thighs.

Movement:

- increasing the pressure on the ball by pushing off with the feet against the floor and pushing the trunk backwards against the ball (Fig. 6.41b); this produces a unilateral pressure in posterior-anterior direction on L1 at the right side
- releasing pressure, and back to starting position.

ANGULAR MOVEMENTS

Extension and rotation of T12 to the right, in prone position

Therapy technique (film 29)

Patient's starting position:

- prone, head rotated to the right, arms placed beside the body (Fig. 6.42a)
- the thoracic spine is pre-positioned in extension, lateral flexion and rotation to the right, from cranial downwards up to the symptomatic segment (T12)
- the position is supported by a firm cushion.

Therapist's starting position:

- standing, at the patient's left side
- therapist's right hand is placed with its ulnar edge on patient's costal process of L1.

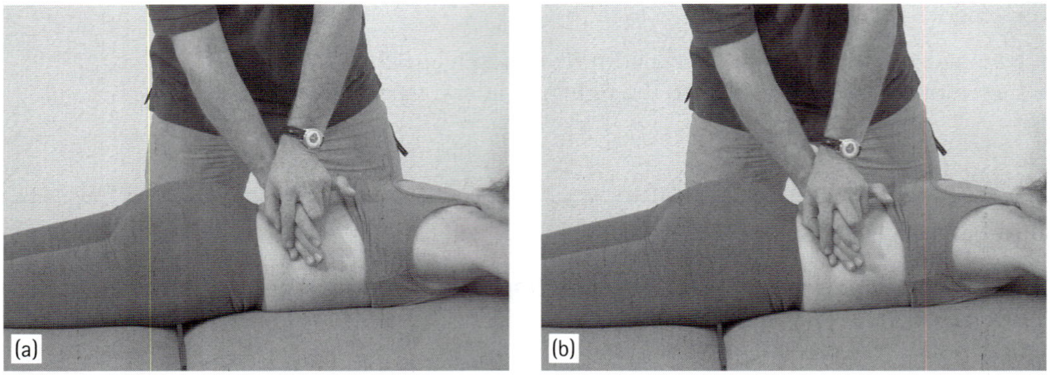

Figure 6.40a and b Accessory movement; unilateral push in posterior-anterior direction (L1); therapy technique. a, Starting position. b, End position.

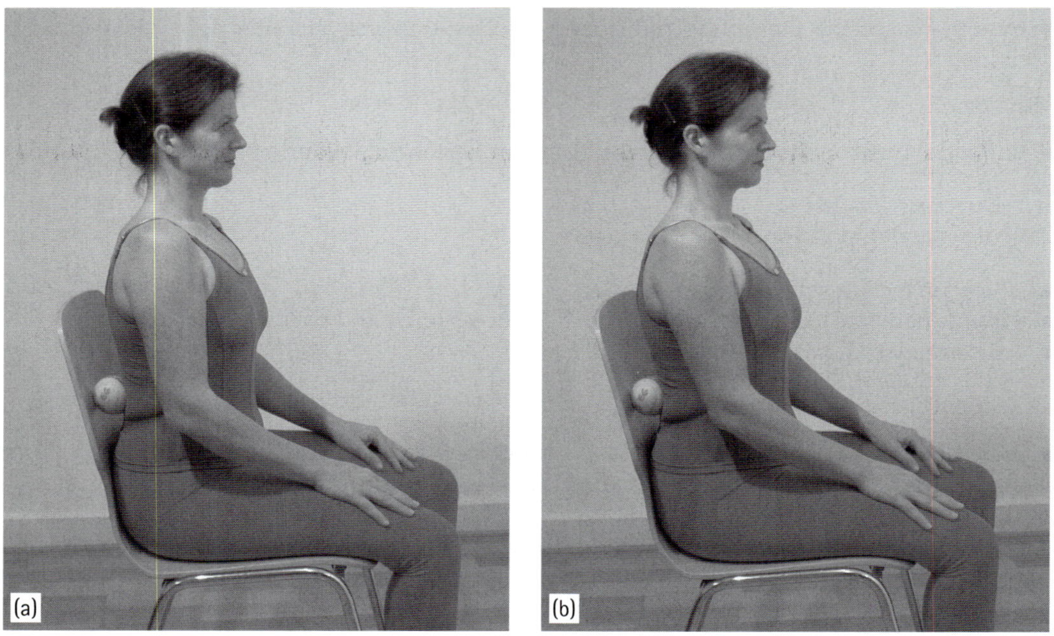

Figure 6.41a and b Accessory movement; unilateral push in posterior-anterior direction (L1); self-exercise. a, Starting position. b, End position.

Movement:

- push with the right hand on the costal process of L1 in a ventrocranial direction (Fig. 6.42b).

Self-exercise (film 26)

See self-exercise for active mobilization into extension and rotation to the right (Fig. 6.39).

For reasons of simplicity, in this situation the same exercise is chosen for self-exercise as with active mobilization.

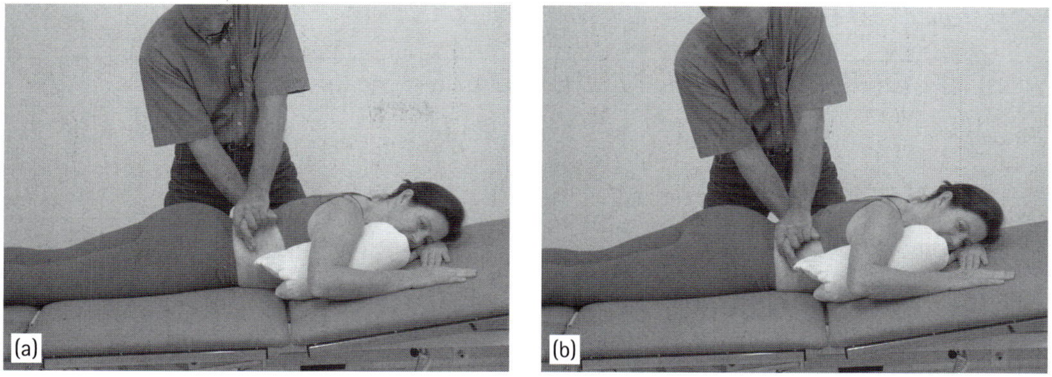

Figure 6.42a and b Passive angular movement; extension and rotation to the right (T12); therapy technique. a, Starting position. b, End position.

Note:
Regarding the technique:
For mobilization, the segment to be treated is pre-positioned in rotation to the right, extension, and lateral flexion to the right (non-coupled movement). The underlying goal is mobilization of the functionally most restricted as well as most painful movement (see explanation in assessment at the beginning of this chapter).

If, however, the technique aims at reaching the largest possible movement range, lateral flexion to the right has to end in segment T11 (non-coupled movement → locking up to T11), and segment T12 has to be pre-positioned in lateral flexion to the left (coupled movement).

Regarding self-exercise:
Although the therapy technique is performed in prone and by movement of the caudal vertebra in the segment, the self-exercise is, for reasons of simplicity, done in standing, and movement is performed from cranial, as with active mobilization.

Remarks (regarding treatment of a symptomatic structure/direction)

Goals of the technique

With a painfully restricted rotation to the right of T12, these techniques serve to:

- reduce tonicity and improve the metabolism of the affected tissues
- restore normal function of symptomatic tissue by application of the symptom-provoking stimulus dosed according to the current load tolerance.
- restore symptom-free function by changing the input to the respective centres of the central nervous system.

Performance

Depending on irritability or desired treatment goal, the joint to be treated is pre-positioned as necessary first. Due to the specific fixation with all of these techniques except *unilateral push in posterior–anterior direction*, transferred movement is prevented as far as possible. This should possibly be considered when the indication for this technique is determined.

Dosage (regarding the affected symptomatic structure)

Acute presentation (predominantly peripheral pain mechanisms)			
Phase	Limitation of movement due to pain and resistance	Concept	Movement grade
Inflammation phase	No pain	Kaltenborn-Evjenth	Up to the beginning of II
	No resistance	Maitland	Up to II
Proliferation phase	Up to P1, slowly progressing up to low resistance	Kaltenborn-Evjenth	Up to the 1st third of II
		Maitland	Up to III^{-}
Remodelling/ organization phase	Slowly progressing up to maximum resistance	Kaltenborn-Evjenth	Up to III
	(Note: duration of turnover!)	Maitland	Up to IV^{++} or III^{++}

Note: The chances of a disturbed (delayed) course of healing and the consequences for the loading capacity of the tissue (e.g., diabetes, old age, partial or general immobilization) have to be considered.

Chronic presentation (predominantly central pain mechanisms): Since here it is assumed that pain no longer represents a protection mechanism, the therapist has to consider the expected training state of the treated tissue as well as the patient's personal expectations. If there is any doubt, treatment is always started with very low force, with progression made conditional on reassessment. Hence with a chronic presentation, pain is not always the limiting factor regarding dosage of treatment.

Choice of technique

The selection of the technique depends, among other things, on the therapist as well as the patient, on the therapist's clinical experience, but primarily on reassessment. This means that even if all preconditions on the part of therapist and patient seem to be fulfilled, it is of no use to continue the technique if reassessment is negative.

Contributing factors

For a satisfactory solution of the patient's current problems it is important to consider the contributing factors and include them in the treatment.

The authors will, however, not go into a description of the various possibilities and their complex contexts as this would exceed the scope of the present book.

Chapter 7

Lumbosacral junction

CHAPTER CONTENTS

AREA LOCALIZATION

IDENTIFICATION OF THE POTENTIALLY AFFECTED AREA BY DEMONSTRATION OF A SYMPTOMATIC FUNCTIONAL MOVEMENT/POSITION

Based on the information gained from the anamnesis so far, the therapist ascertains more details about potentially affected sections. This is done by means of area localization, which represents the beginning of the physical examination. Information gained in this way is used to check or modify the relevant hypotheses developed on the basis of the anamnesis and will determine further proceedings.

Area localization is explained by means of two examples. In both, the patient feels central pain in the area of the lumbosacral junction, on the right side. On the basis of clinical experience and known clinical patterns of this presentation (Fortin et al. 1994a,b), primarily the following areas are considered as potential sources of the current complaints:

- lumbar spine
- neural structures.

General question: Is there enough information available to skip area localization?	
No	Yes
⇓	⇓
Performance of area localization	• General movement tests • Additional tests • Test treatment

Example 1: Flexion

Symptom area: lumbosacral junction
Symptom provocation: flexion of the spine (Fig. 7.1)

With this presentation, clinical experience suggests primarily the lumbar spine and the neural structures as symptom-provoking areas.

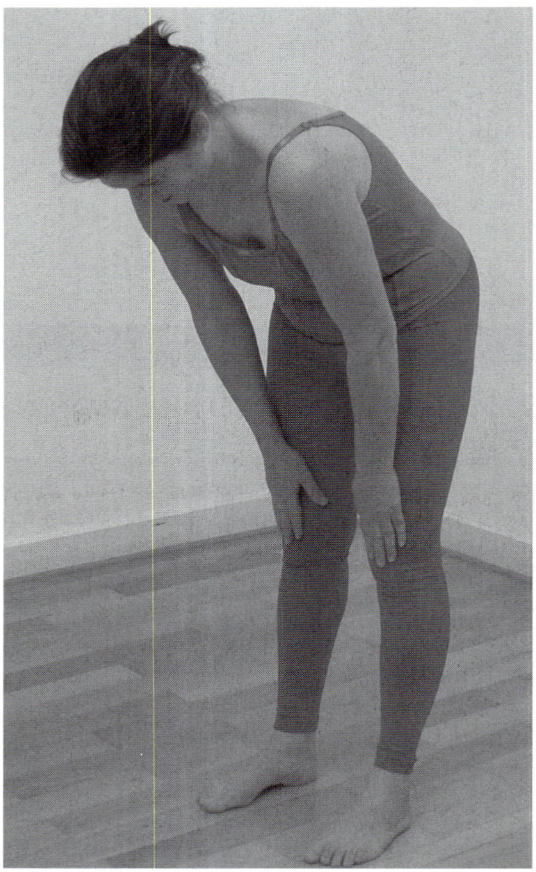

Figure 7.1 Symptom-provoking movement: flexion of the spine provokes pain at the lumbosacral junction.

Below, examples illustrate how to differentiate between these areas. To this end, the therapist performs area localization by means of active movements alone. If this is not possible, tests will be performed by means of assistive movements.

Hypothesis 1: The symptom-provoking area is the neural structures

Differentiation: neural involvement vs. lumbar spine.

The change in symptoms can be demonstrated exactly:

- provocation of pain (Fig. 7.2a and b, film 30)
- alleviation of pain (Fig. 7.3a and b, film 31).

The result of area localization should be verified by further specific tests; otherwise the result remains in doubt.

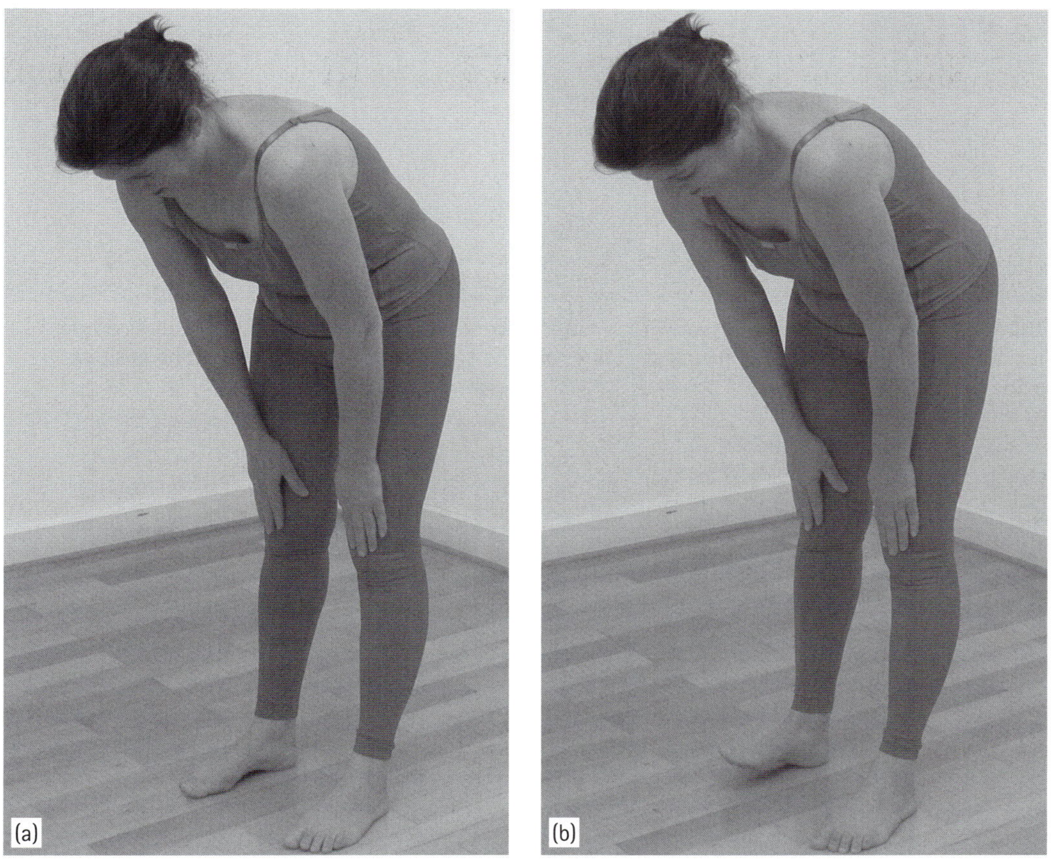

Figure 7.2a and b Area localization with symptomatic movement of the lumbosacral junction into flexion; differentiation between neural structures and lumbar spine; provocation. **a**, Starting position. **b**, End position.

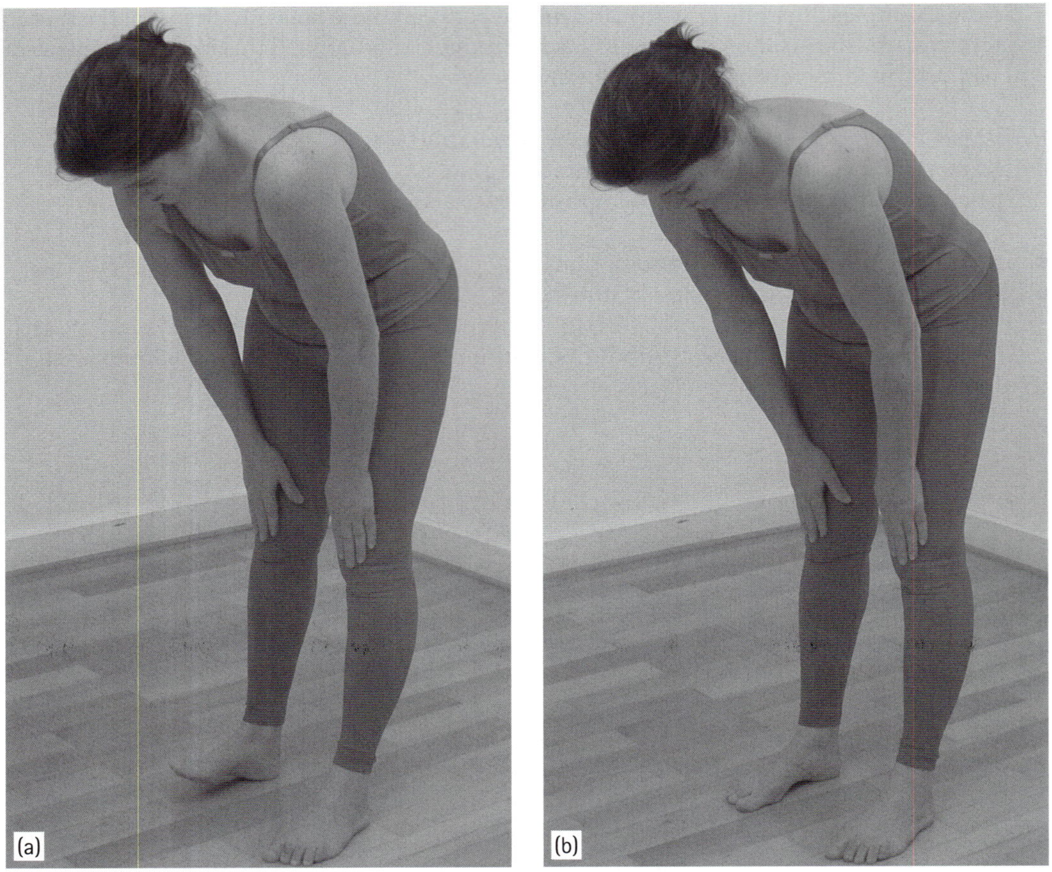

Figure 7.3a and b Area localization with symptomatic movement of the lumbosacral junction into flexion; differentiation between neural structures and lumbar spine; alleviation. **a**, Starting position. **b**, End position.

Assessment			
Goal	**Provocation of pain**	**Alleviation of pain**	**Remarks**
Starting position	Flexion of the spine to a position immediately before symptoms appear	With the foot pre-positioned in dorsal flexion, flexion of the spine to a position immediately after symptoms have appeared	
Test movement	Dorsal flexion of the feet (individually)	Plantar flexion of the foot	

Goal	Provocation of pain	Alleviation of pain	Remarks
Explanation	The test movement increases tension in the neural structures	The test movement reduces tension in the neural structures. For alleviation, that foot is chosen via which symptoms could be provoked before	If by movements of the feet the patient's typical pain is changed, this suggests at least an involvement of the neural structures
Additional data to support the hypothesis	Further movements of proximal or distal components to increase neural tension which are not directly involved in flexion of the spine General and specific mobility of the affected area History (e.g., symptom behaviour, type of complaints, 24-hour behaviour) Palpation Neurodynamic tests Nerve provocation tests (e.g., bow string sign) Reproducibility of test results Test treatment Imaging procedures (CT, MRI)		

Example 2: Extension

Symptom area: lumbosacral junction
Symptom provocation: extension of the spine (Fig. 7.4)

With this presentation, clinical experience suggests primarily the lumbar spine and the neural structures as symptom-provoking areas.

Below, examples illustrate how to differentiate between these areas. To this end, the therapist performs area localization by means of active movements alone. If this is not possible, tests will be performed by means of assistive movements.

Hypothesis 1: The symptom-provoking area is the neural structures

Differentiation: neural involvement vs. lumbar spine.

The change in symptoms can be demonstrated exactly:

- provocation of pain (Fig. 7.5a and b, film 32)
- alleviation of pain (Fig. 7.6a and b, film 33).

The result of area localization should be verified by further specific tests; otherwise the result remains in doubt.

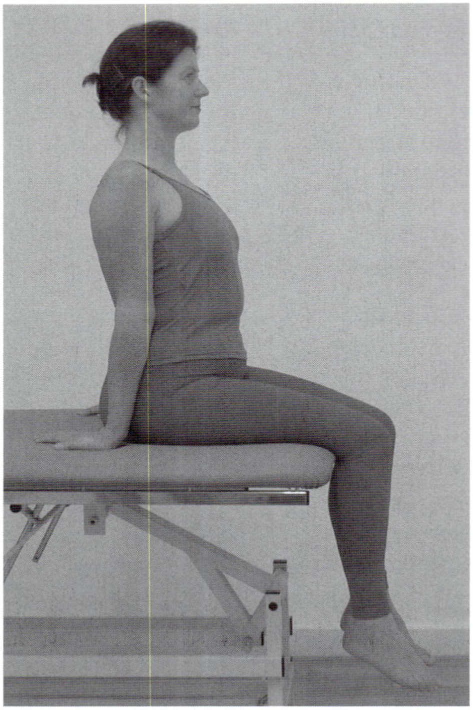

Figure 7.4 Symptom-provoking movement: extension of the spine provokes pain at the lumbosacral junction.

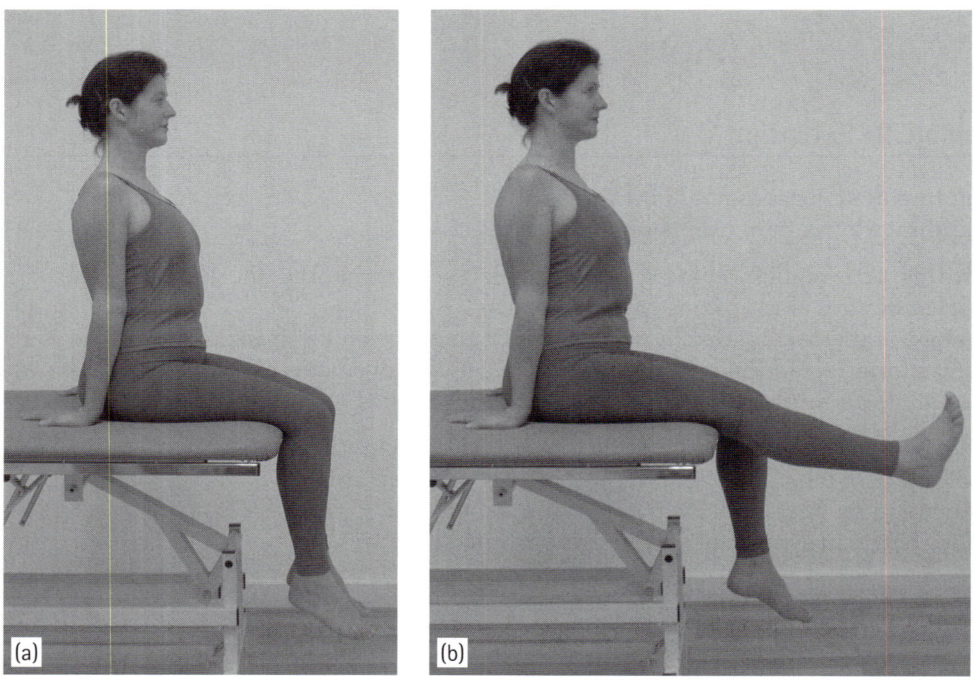

Figure 7.5a and b Area localization with symptomatic movement of the lumbosacral junction into extension; differentiation between neural structures and lumbar spine; provocation. **a**, Starting position. **b**, End position.

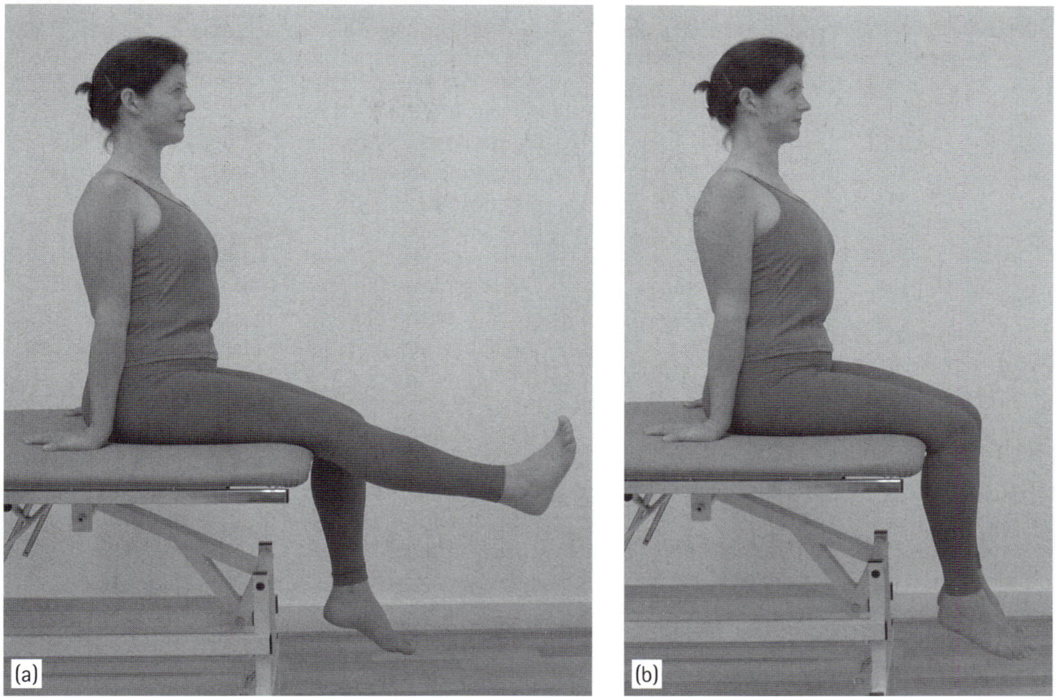

Figure 7.6a and b Area localization with symptomatic movement of the lumbosacral junction into extension; differentiation between neural structures and lumbar spine; alleviation. a, Starting position. b, End position.

Assessment

Goal	Provocation of pain	Alleviation of pain	Remarks
Starting position	Extension of the spine to a position immediately before symptoms appear	With the right knee pre-positioned in extension and the right ankle in dorsal flexion, extension of the spine to a position immediately after symptoms have appeared	
Test movement	Extension of the knees and dorsal flexion of the ankles (individually), in sitting	Flexion of the right knee reduces the tension on the neural structures produced by the starting	Here, increase and reduction of neural tension via the right leg is demonstrated as an example. It may

Goal	Provocation of pain	Alleviation of pain	Remarks
		position. For alleviation, the right leg is chosen, since symptoms could be produced before via that leg	equally be necessary to change neural tension via the left leg or via both legs
Explanation	The test movement increases tension in the neural structures	The test movement reduces tension in the neural structures	If the typical pain is provoked or alleviated by these manoeuvres, this suggests at least an involvement of the neural structures
Additional data to support the hypothesis	Further movements of proximal and distal components to increase neural tension which are not directly involved in flexion of the spine General and specific mobility of the affected area History (e.g., symptom behaviour, type of complaints, 24-hour behaviour) Palpation Neurodynamic tests Nerve provocation tests (e.g., bow string sign) Reproducibility of test results Test treatment Imaging procedures (CT, MRI)		

QUICK CHECK – SYMPTOMS, LUMBOSACRAL JUNCTION

If neither the area nor a symptom-provoking or symptom-reducing action is known, the quick check is used to try to load individual potential areas with specific biomechanically provocative movement combinations. The chosen movement combinations correspond with the straining and often symptom-provoking movements of the individual sections.

LUMBAR SPINE

Movement (film 226)

- Extension/lateral flexion to the right, and rotation to the same as well as to the opposite side, with overpressure (Fig. 7.7a and b)
- Extension/lateral flexion to the left, and rotation to the same as well as to the opposite side, with overpressure (Fig. 7.8a and b).

NEURAL STRUCTURES

Tension tests

- Slump test (Fig. 7.9, film 616)
- Straight leg raise (SLR; Fig. 7.10, film 618).

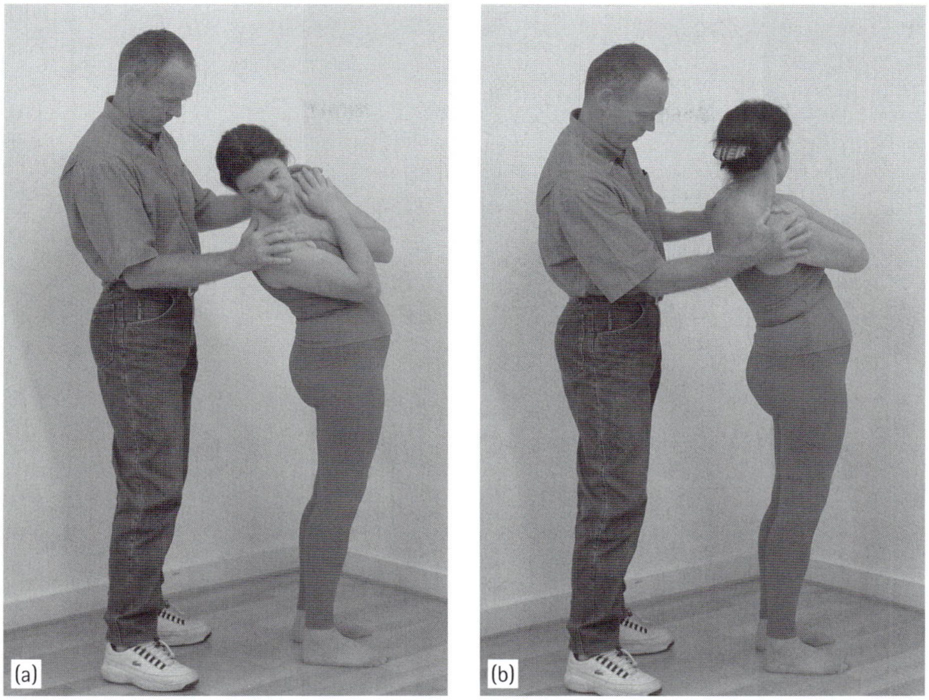

Figure 7.7a and b Quick check lumbar spine; extension, lateral flexion to the right. **a**, Rotation to the same side. **b**, Rotation to the opposite side.

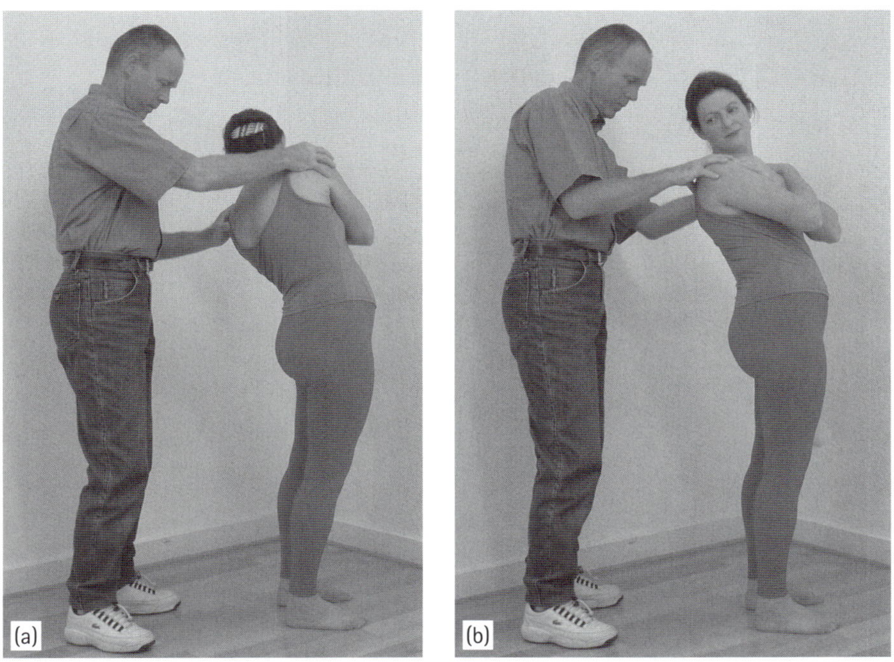

Figure 7.8a and b Quick check lumbar spine; extension, lateral flexion to the left. **a**, Rotation to the same side. **b**, Rotation to the opposite side.

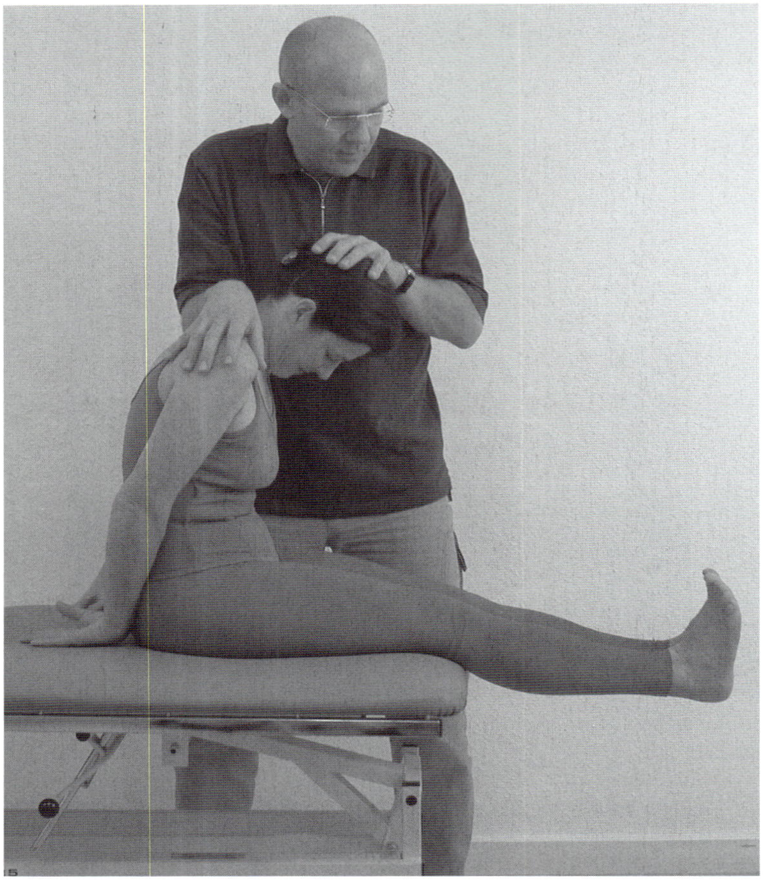

Figure 7.9 Quick check neurodynamics; slump test.

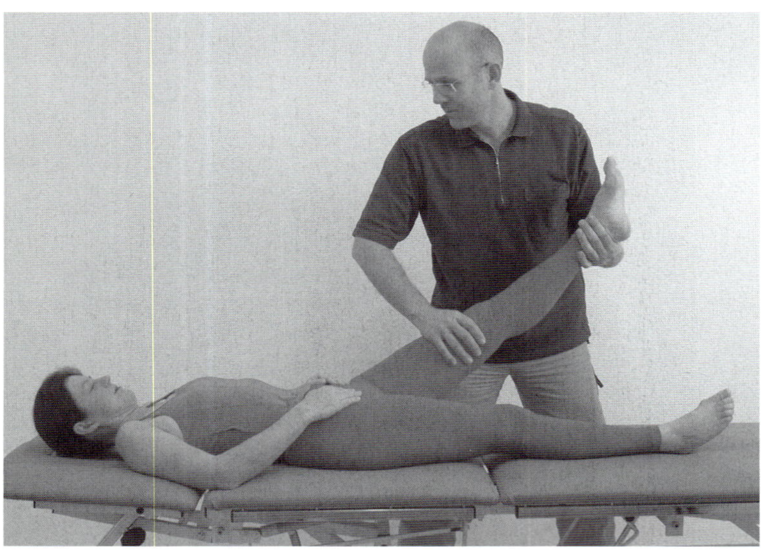

Figure 7.10 Quick check neurodynamics; straight leg raise (SLR) test.

Note: Even an area that proves negative in the quick check may possibly be symptom-provoking (another movement combination, or passive overpressure may be required).

SPECIFIC PROVOCATION AND ALLEVIATION

Specific provocation and alleviation allows one to differentiate within an articular complex and to identify the symptom-provoking movement direction(s).

SPECIFIC PROVOCATION AND ALLEVIATION, LUMBOSACRAL JUNCTION

The patient feels central pain in the area of the lumbosacral junction. On the basis of clinical experience and known clinical patterns of this presentation (Fortin et al. 1994a,b), specific provocation and alleviation is limited to the lumbar spine. If the source of symptoms cannot be localized despite careful performance of differentiation tests, alternatives should be considered. Even if such alternatives seem to be unfounded with our present knowledge, other hypotheses (e.g., sacroiliac joint) have nevertheless to be checked carefully.

Localization, lumbosacral junction – flexion

Pain-provoking movement (Fig. 7.11)

- Flexion of the spine provokes pain at the lumbosacral junction.
- Area localization hints at the lumbosacral junction.

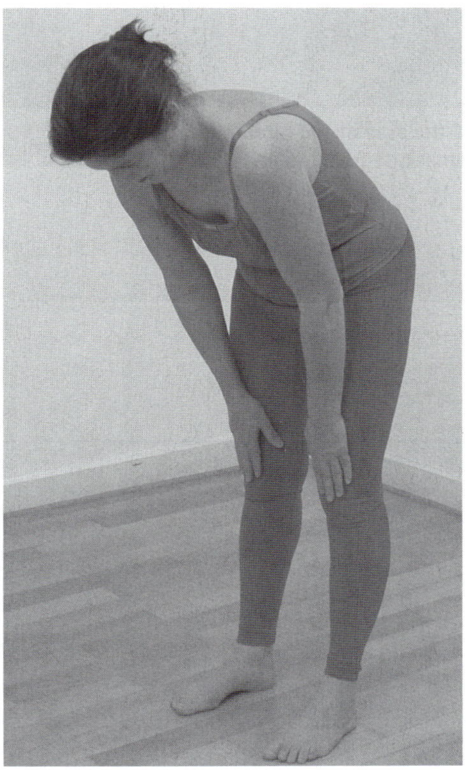

Figure 7.11 Symptom-provoking movement: flexion of the spine provokes pain at the lumbosacral junction.

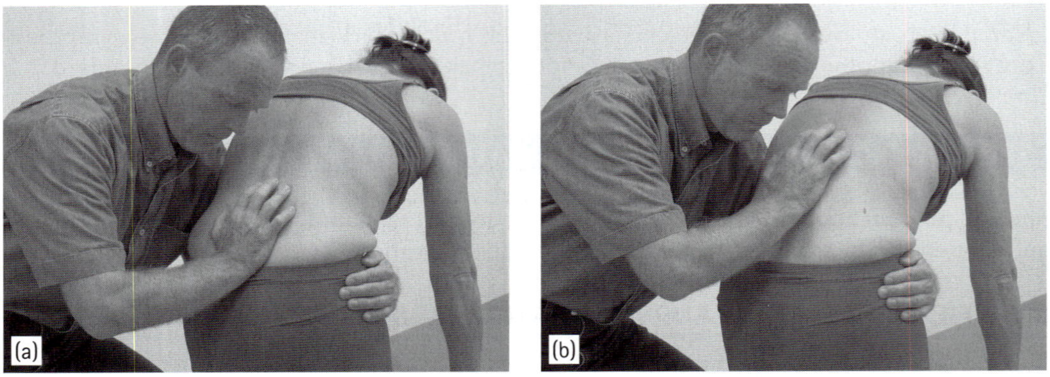

Figure 7.12a and b Specific provocation and alleviation in the area of the lumbosacral junction with symptomatic flexion of the spine; localization of the symptomatic segment; provocation. **a**, Test start. **b**, Test end.

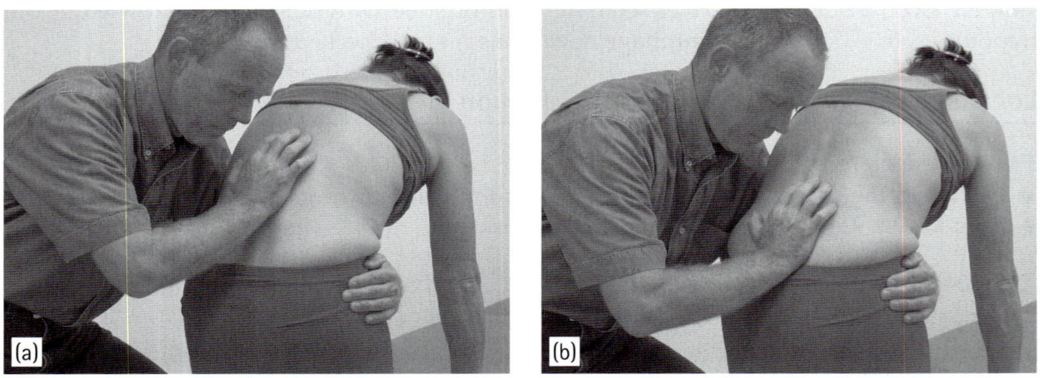

Figure 7.13a and b Specific provocation and alleviation in the area of the lumbosacral junction with symptomatic flexion of the spine; localization of the symptomatic segment; alleviation. **a**, Test start. **b**, Test end.

The change in symptoms can be demonstrated exactly:

- provocation of pain (Fig. 7.12a and b, film 34)
- alleviation of pain (Fig. 7.13a and b, film 35).

Assessment			
Goal	**Provocation of pain**	**Alleviation of pain**	**Remarks**
Starting position	Flexion of the spine to a position immediately before symptoms appear	Flexion of the spine to a position immediately after symptoms have appeared	Trunk remains in starting position
Test movement	Push via laminae or spinous processes of	For segments L2–L5, push via laminae or	

Goal	Provocation of pain	Alleviation of pain	Remarks
	L5–L2 in ventrocranial direction, starting caudally	spinous processes of L3–L5 in ventrocranial direction, starting cranially. For segment L5, via sacral base in ventral direction	
Neural involvement	Proximal and/or distal component without change of position in the relevant area	Proximal and/or distal component without change of position in the relevant area	
Explanation	The symptoms are provoked when the cranial vertebra in the segment is moved (flexion in the affected segment)	The symptoms are alleviated when the caudal vertebra in the segment is moved (extension in the affected segment)	
Additional data to support the hypothesis	General and specific mobility of the lumbar spine History (e.g., symptom behaviour, type of complaints, 24-hour behaviour) Specific palpation Neurodynamic tests (if specific provocation and alleviation indicate neural involvement) Reproducibility of test results Test treatment Imaging procedures (CT, MRI)		

Localization, lumbosacral junction – extension

Pain-provoking movement (Fig. 7.14)

- Extension of the spine provokes pain at the lumbosacral junction.
- Area localization hints at the lumbosacral junction.

Although functional demonstration was performed in standing, it is assumed in this example that the same symptoms can be reproduced in the prone position. If, however, symptoms cannot be reproduced exactly in that position or if other symptoms are reproduced, it is questionable whether results found in this way are related to the patient's functional problem.

The change in symptoms can be demonstrated exactly:

- provocation of pain (Fig. 7.15a and b, film 36)
- alleviation of pain (Fig. 7.16a and b, film 37).

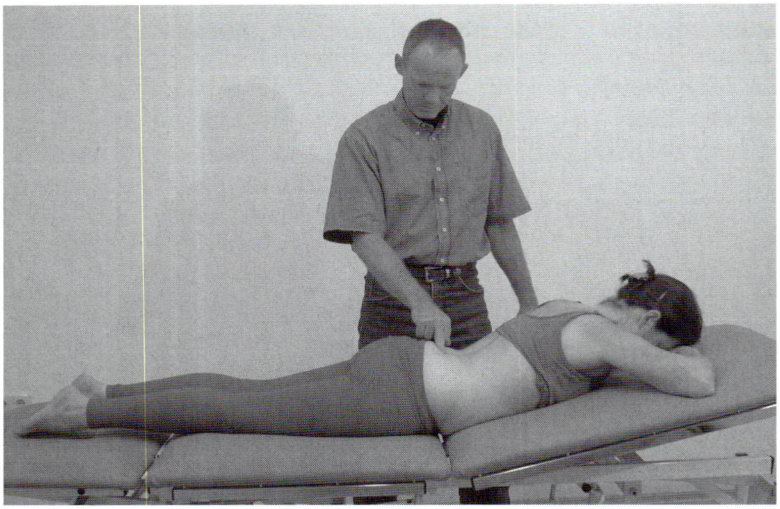

Figure 7.14 Symptom-provoking movement: extension of the spine provokes pain at the lumbosacral junction.

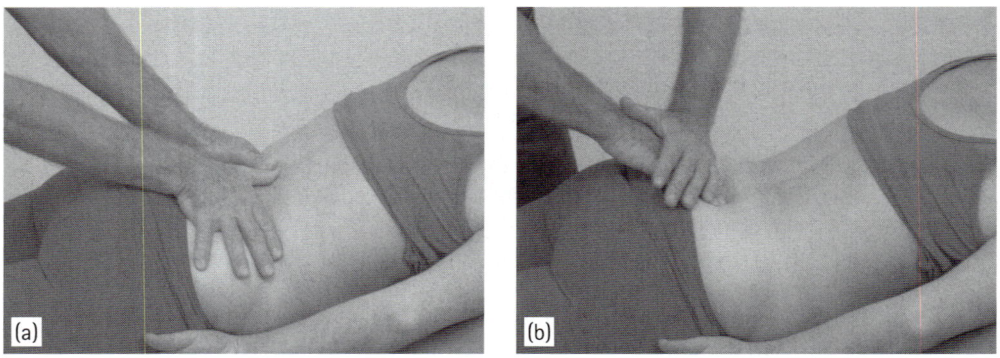

Figure 7.15a and b Specific provocation and alleviation in the area of the lumbosacral junction with symptomatic extension of the spine; localization of the symptomatic segment; provocation. **a**, Test start. **b**, Test end.

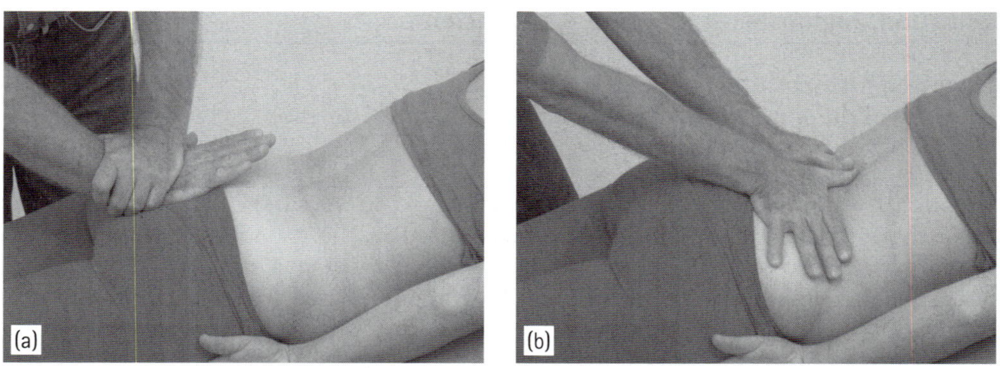

Figure 7.16a and b Specific provocation and alleviation in the area of the lumbosacral junction with symptomatic extension of the spine; localization of the symptomatic segment; alleviation. **a**, Test start. **b**, Test end.

Assessment			
Goal	**Provocation of pain**	**Alleviation of pain**	**Remarks**
Starting position	Extension of the spine to a position immediately before symptoms appear	Extension of the spine to a position immediately after symptoms have appeared	
Test movement	Push via laminae or spinous processes of L3–L5 in ventrocranial direction, starting cranially, then pushing sacrum via its base in ventrocaudal direction (extension L5)	Push via apex of sacrum in ventral direction (flexion L5), and then via laminae or spinous processes of L4–L2 in ventrocranial direction, starting caudally. If spinous process of L5 is easily accessible, flexion in segment L5 may also be achieved by push via spinous process of L5	It is the authors' experience that the spinous process of L5 is usually difficult to access. Therefore, in most cases the sacrum is used to move segment L5
Neural involvement	Proximal and/or distal component without change of position in the relevant area	Proximal and/or distal component without change of position in the relevant area	
Explanation	The symptoms are provoked when the caudal vertebra in the segment is moved (extension in the affected segment)	The symptoms are alleviated when the cranial vertebra in the segment is moved (flexion in the affected segment)	
Additional data to support the hypothesis	General and specific mobility of the lumbar spine History (e.g., symptom behaviour, type of complaints, 24-hour behaviour) Specific palpation Neurodynamic tests (if specific provocation and alleviation indicate neural involvement) Reproducibility of test results Test treatment Imaging procedures (CT, MRI)		

GENERAL MOVEMENT TESTS

General movement tests identify, quantify, and qualify individual anatomical movements and, in part, movement combinations in the area presumed. The individual manual therapy concepts have respective protocols at their disposal, which more or less have the same goals.

Information gained in this way is used for checking or modifying the relevant hypotheses developed on the basis of the anamnesis and area localization and will help in determining how to proceed.

General question: Is there enough information available to skip general movement tests?	
No	Yes
⇓	⇓
Performance of the general movement tests	• Additional tests • Test treatment

In view of the described clinical presentation and the results of area localization, general movement tests of the following regions seem to be useful.

Lumbar spine		
	Active	Passive
Lumbar spine in general	Flexion Extension Rotation (to the right and left) Lateral flexion (to the right and left)	Flexion Extension Rotation (to the right and left) Lateral flexion (to the right and left)
Movement combinations lumbar spine in general	Symptomatic movements of the lumbar spine	Symptomatic movements of the lumbar spine

TREATMENT EXAMPLE, LUMBAR SPINE – HYPERMOBILITY OF L5

SYMPTOMATIC MOVEMENT

Movement of the lumbar spine into extension provokes pain in the area of the lumbosacral junction.

ASSESSMENTS

Area localization

Area localization hints at the lumbar spine, without neural involvement. There is no contraindication for movement.

Specific provocation and alleviation

Specific provocation and alleviation hints at a provocation of symptoms by movement of L5 into extension.

Specific mobility

Specific mobility tests show angular hypermobility of L5 in extension with simultaneously increased translatory mobility in anterior-posterior direction at rest and, in addition, angular hypomobility of L1 and L2 in extension.

Palpation

Palpation indicates increased tenderness of tissues around segment L5. Paravertebral muscles in the area of the thoracolumbar junction show definitely increased tension and slightly increased tenderness as compared with neighbouring sections.

HYPOTHESIS

A painful hypermobility of L5 in extension with simultaneously restricted extension in L1 and L2 is suspected (Fig. 7.17).

GENERAL WAY OF PROCEEDING IN THE TREATMENT OF LUMBAR HYPERMOBILITY/INSTABILITY

Based on our understanding of painful hypermobility, local therapy procedures in the symptom-provoking area aim at decreasing tenderness (alleviation of pain). In everyday clinical practice, all kinds of movement which do not go to the end range of the symptomatic movement have proved useful for this purpose.

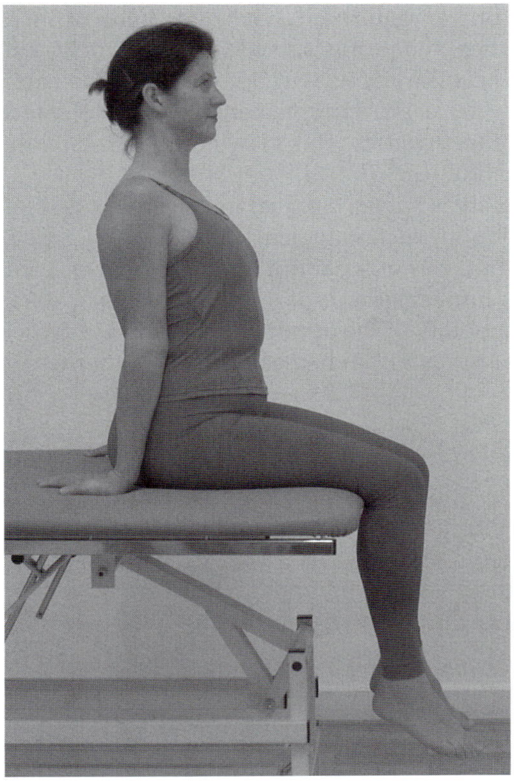

Figure 7.17 Symptom-provoking movement: extension of the spine provokes pain at the lumbosacral junction.

The selection of techniques (active and/or passive procedures including physical treatment modalities) depends, among other things, on the therapist as well as the patient, on the therapist's clinical experience, but primarily on reassessment. This means that even if all preconditions on the part of therapist and patient have been met, it is of no use to continue the technique if reassessment is negative.

Treatment of hypermobility consists mainly in stabilizing the hypermobile segment and in reducing the load on the symptomatic joint by treating contributing factors. These may consist of shortened muscles, hypomobile, functionally interconnected areas, habitual postures and movements, as well as insufficient local or general endurance.

Stabilization of the hypermobile segment is done primarily by improving proprioception (processing of afferent input regarding position and movement) as well as coordination (muscular control) with different forms of motor load on the segment. To this end, treatment starts at a joint position which the patient is still well able to control. End positions of the joint are avoided so as to not further stress the irritated structures. The treatment of contributing factors is an indispensable and complex process, which is often underestimated. Apart from local, often mobilizing measures, it frequently includes a change of movement patterns.

With markedly painful presentations, it may be necessary to start or accompany treatment with some external mechanical stabilization (e.g., lumbar spine bandage, tape) so as to prevent constant (even if not consciously perceived) irritation of the affected segment.

The structure of a stabilization programme that has proved efficient in clinical practice, in the authors' experience, is represented in Figure 7.18. Different schools put different emphasis on the measures listed there. First of all, it is of crucial importance to know the patient's requirements regarding his or her movement apparatus and then to identify the deficits which prevent successful performance of the required movements. Some of these deficits do not automatically disappear even when symptoms subside. These deficits will have to be remedied to such a degree that the necessary load will become tolerable again without compensatory mechanisms. This as well as an improvement in load tolerance beyond the necessary extent will possibly reduce recurrences. This view is supported by the authors' clinical experience and by the study of Hides (1996).

The overall management of painful hypermobility is not part of this book. Here, discussion will be restricted to the treatment of those contributing factors which, in the authors' experience, are very often clinically relevant to the hypothesis of a painful hypermobility of L5 in extension. Most often, hypomobility of the upper lumbar spine is of relevance. Below, we will first describe exemplary techniques to improve mobility of the upper lumbar spine, and then local treatment of the symptomatic hypermobile segment L5 aimed at reducing tenderness in this symptomatic segment.

RELAXATION TECHNIQUES

Soft tissue techniques

PARAVERTEBRAL MUSCLES, RIGHT SIDE (LATERAL FLEXION)

Therapy technique (film 38)

Patient's starting position:

- lying on the left side, lumbar spine adjusted in neutral position (Fig. 7.19a).

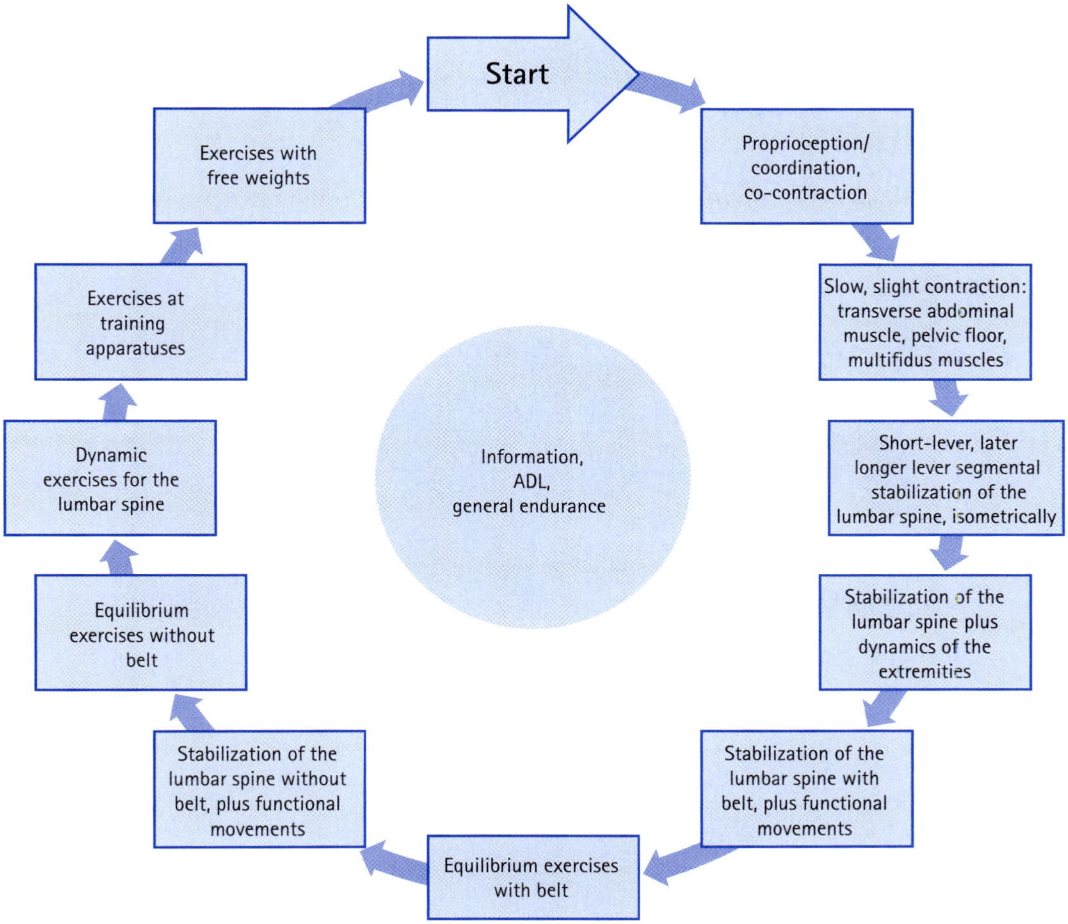

Figure 7.18 Structure of lumbar stabilization training.

Therapist's starting position:

- standing, in front of the patient, at the level of the patient's lumbar spine
- hands touch with finger tips the paravertebral muscles of the patient's upper side, immediately lateral of the spinous processes, forearms rest on the patient's thorax or on the right side of the patient's pelvis
- trunk is in contact with patient's pelvis and the anterior part of the patient's thighs.

Movement:

- passive lateral flexion of the lumbar spine by simultaneous push of both the therapist's forearms in cranial and caudal direction and simultaneous movement of trunk in a caudal direction (Fig. 7.19b)
- during this movement, finger tips exert pressure in a ventrolateral direction on the muscles that are to be treated
- then releasing pressure, and back to starting position.

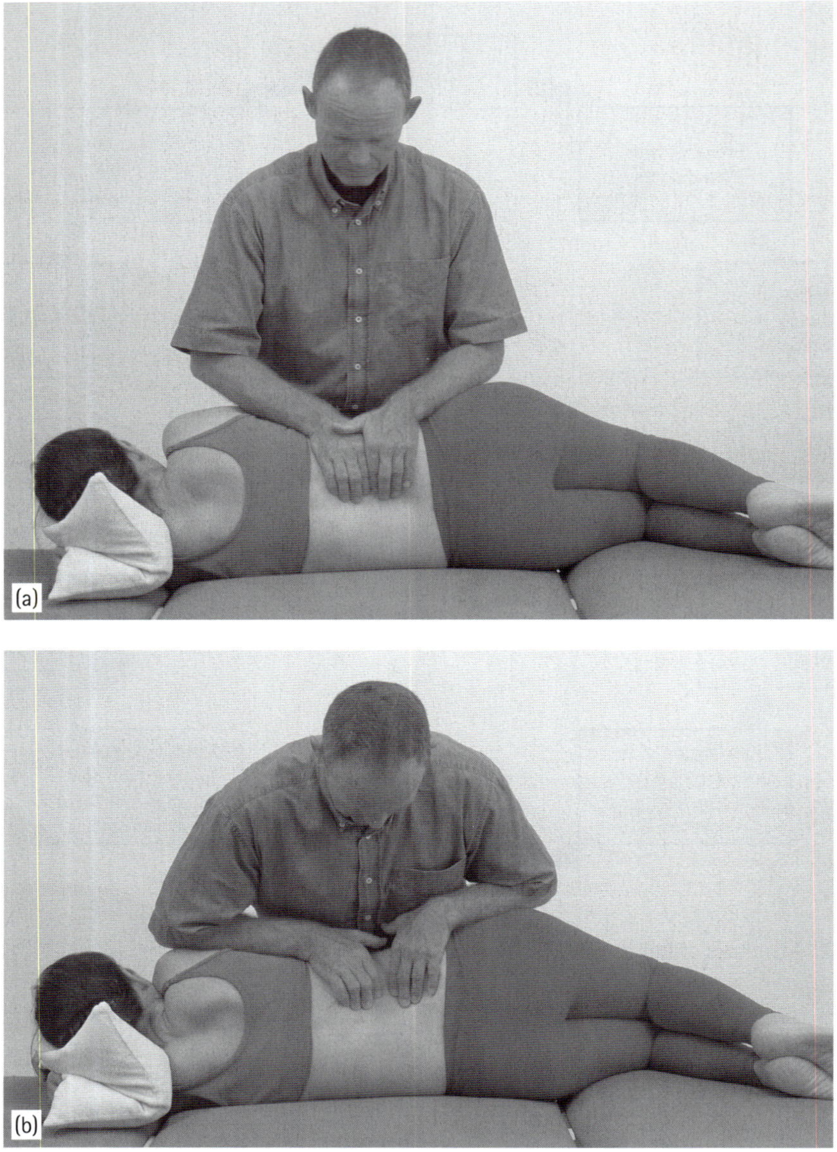

Figure 7.19a and b Soft tissue technique; right paravertebral muscles; lateral flexion; therapy technique. a, Starting position. b, End position.

Self-exercise (film 39)

Patient's starting position:

- sitting, knuckles of left hand, coming from left side, contact the medial edge of the paravertebral muscles in the area of the right side of the thoracolumbar junction (Fig. 7.20a)
- right hand, coming from right side, grasps left hand for reinforcement.

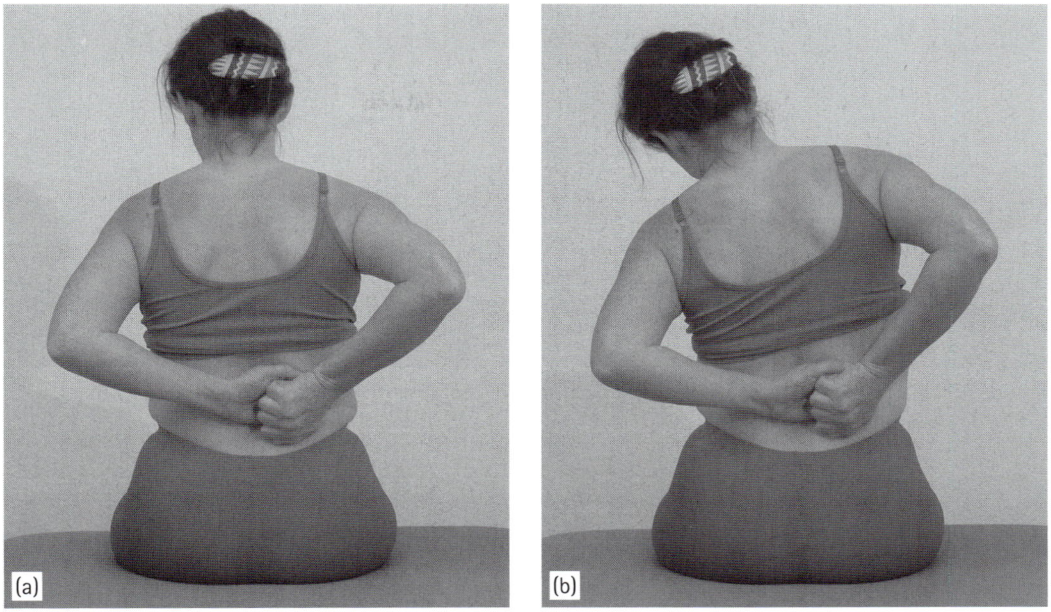

Figure 7.20a and b Soft tissue technique; right paravertebral muscles; lateral flexion; self-exercise. a, Starting position. b, End position.

Movement:

- movement of both hands in anterior direction and to the right creates pressure against the right paravertebral muscles from left side (Fig. 7.20b)
- pressure is maintained, and the section of the spine to be treated is moved into lateral flexion to the left
- then releasing pressure, and back to starting position.

PARAVERTEBRAL MUSCLES, RIGHT SIDE (ROTATION)

Therapy technique (film 40)

Patient's starting position:

- lying on the left side, arms folded in front of the chest, spine adjusted in neutral position in the sagittal plane (Fig. 7.21a)
- legs resting one over the other, slightly flexed in hips and knees.

Therapist's starting position:

- standing, in front of the patient
- fixing patient's pelvis between therapist's thorax and left forearm while contacting patient's paravertebral muscles with thenar of left hand
- right hand resting on patient's folded arms, at the right side.

Movement:

- passive rotation of patient's thorax to the right, while simultaneously exerting manual pressure on patient's paravertebral muscles, right side (Fig. 7.21b)
- releasing pressure, and back to starting position.

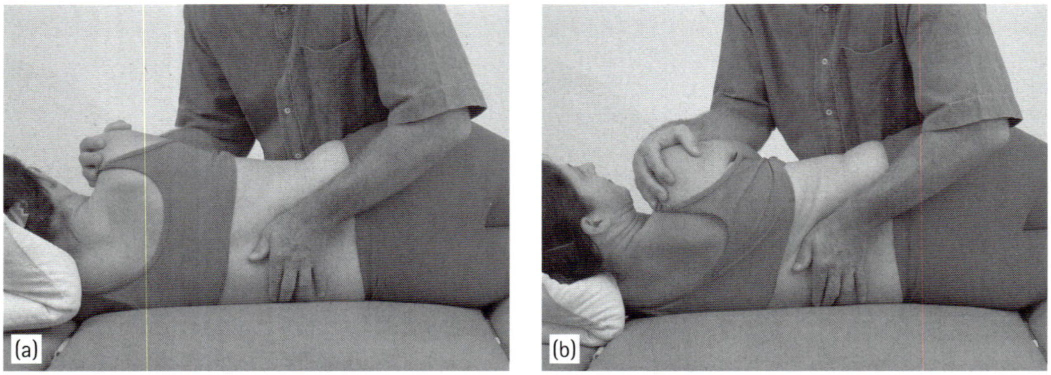

Figure 7.21a and b Soft tissue technique; right paravertebral muscles; rotation; therapy technique. a, Starting position. b, End position.

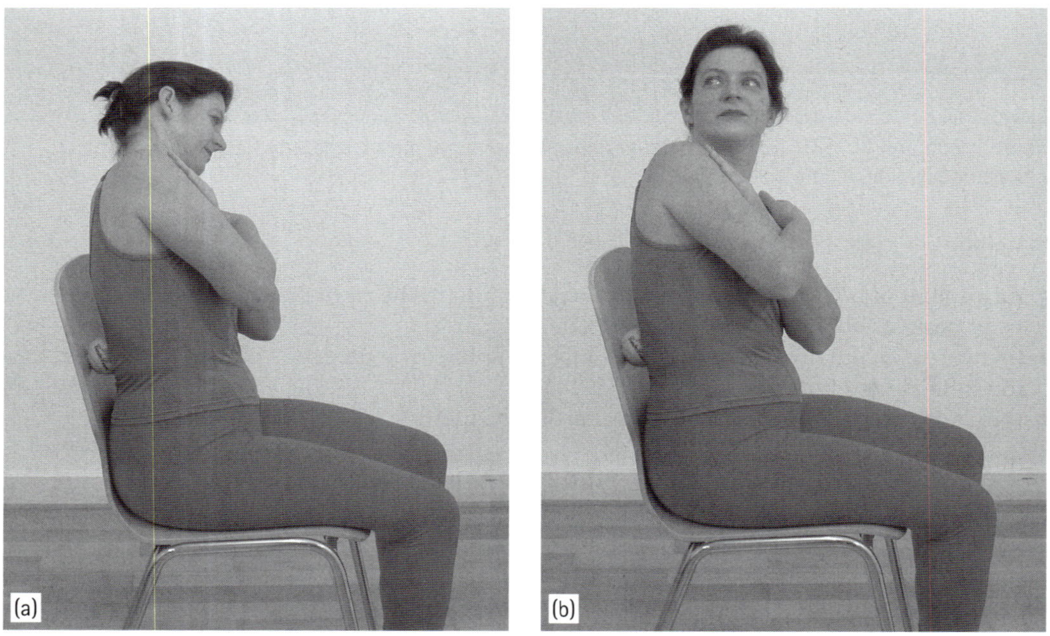

Figure 7.22a and b Soft tissue technique; right paravertebral muscles; rotation; self-exercise. a, Starting position. b, End position.

Note: If the patient is not able to relax or if performance of the movement seems too difficult, this soft tissue technique can also be performed assistively.

Self-exercise (film 41)

Patient's starting position:

- sitting on a chair (Fig. 7.22a)
- a tennis ball placed between right paravertebral muscles and back of the chair

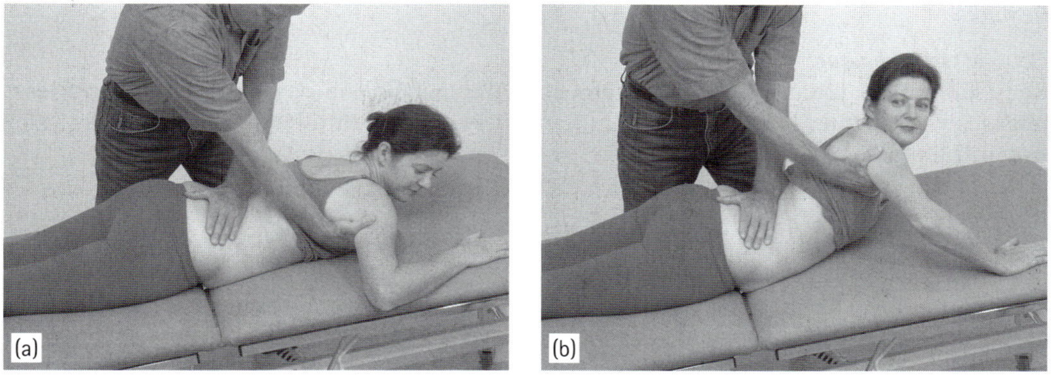

Figure 7.23a and b Soft tissue technique; right paravertebral muscles; rotation; therapy technique. a, Starting position. b, End position.

- arms folded in front of the chest
- lumbar spine pre-positioned in extension and lateral flexion.

Movement:

- increasing pressure by pushing feet against the floor and pushing thorax backwards against the ball (Fig. 7.22b)
- maintaining pressure, extension, and lateral flexion to the left while moving the spine into rotation to the right
- releasing pressure, and back to starting position.

PARAVERTEBRAL MUSCLES, RIGHT SIDE (ROTATION)

Therapy technique (film 42)

Patient's starting position:

- prone, head rotated to the right (Fig. 7.23a)
- left arm resting beside the body, right arm positioned in such a way that the right hand is placed beside or above the right shoulder.

Therapist's starting position:

- standing, at the patient's left side
- contacting patient's lumbar paravertebral muscles with hypothenar of left hand
- placing right hand from anterior under patient's right shoulder.

Movement:

- via right arm, the patient lifts the thorax from the plinth, while the therapist supports this movement and achieves rotation to the right and lateral flexion to the left in extension by pulling in a dorsomedial direction (Fig. 7.23b)
- during this assistive movement, therapist's left hand exerts pressure on patient's right paravertebral muscles
- then releasing pressure, and back to starting position.

Remarks

Goals of the technique
Reduction of the tonicity and improvement of the metabolism of the lumbar paravertebral muscles with painful hypermobility of L5 in extension and simultaneously restricted extension in L1 and L2.

Performance
Treatment is done within the pain-free range of movement. As the treatment techniques are performed without *specific fixation*, transferred movement has to be considered when the indication for the technique is determined, and loading L5 in end-range positions should be avoided.

Dosage
Both with acute and with chronic presentations, these techniques should always be pain-free.

Choice of technique
The selection of the technique depends, among other things, on the therapist as well as the patient, on the therapist's clinical experience, but primarily on reassessment. This means that even if all preconditions on the part of therapist and patient have been met, it is of no use to continue the technique if reassessment is negative.

Contributing factors
For a satisfactory solution of the patient's current problems it is important to consider the contributing factors and include them in the treatment.

The authors will, however, not go into a description of the various possibilities and their complex contexts as this would exceed the scope of the present book.

MOBILIZATION TECHNIQUES (SUPPORTING AREAS)

Active procedures

ACTIVE MOBILIZATION

Extension

Therapy technique (film 43)
Patient's starting position:

- prone, hands propped up at shoulder level or higher, L2 fixed by a wedge (Fig. 7.24a).

Therapist's starting position:

- standing, at the patient's side
- exerting pressure with the wedge against the lamina of L2.

Movement:

- against the fixation by the wedge, the patient tries to actively extend (Fig. 7.24b)
- extension is supported by the patient extending both the arms.

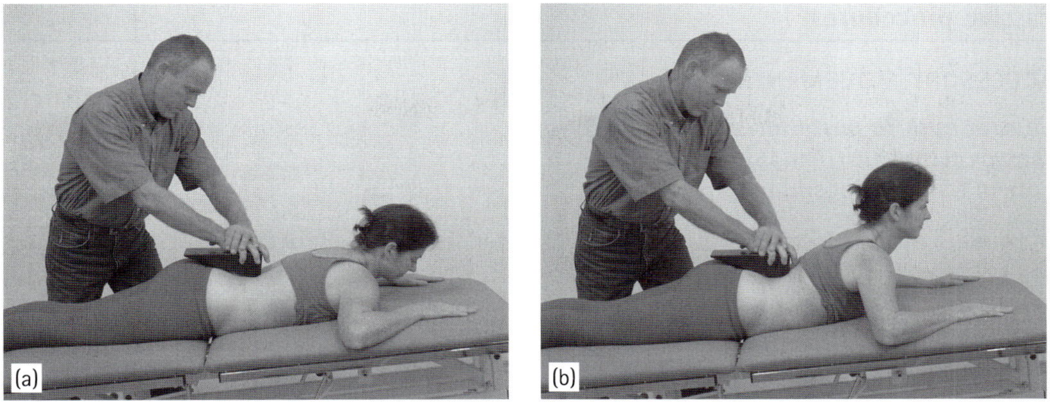

Figure 7.24a and b Active mobilization; extension (L1); therapy technique. **a**, Starting position. **b**, End position.

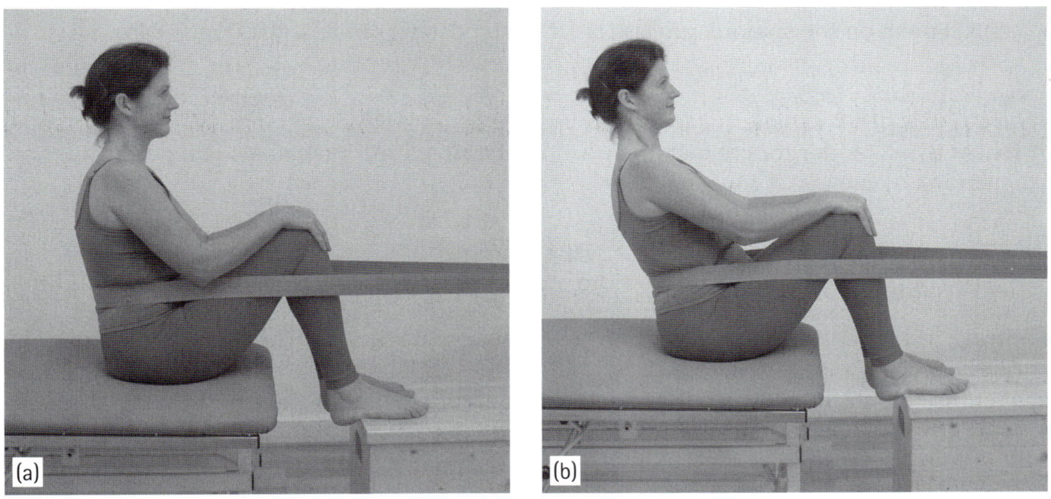

Figure 7.25a and b Active mobilization; extension (L1); self-exercise. **a**, Starting position. **b**, End position.

Self-exercise (film 44)

Patient's starting position:

- sitting on a chair, hips and knees flexed until lower lumbar spine is in flexion (Fig. 7.25a)
- feet placed on a stool
- a belt goes around the patient from anterior and fixes L2 in a ventral direction
- hands resting on the thighs.

Movement:

- extension of the spine above the fixation (Fig. 7.25b)
- the extension movement is supported by pushing the hands against the thighs
- then pressure is released, and back to starting position.

Passive procedures

ACCESSORY MOVEMENTS

Central push in posterior–anterior direction

Therapy technique (film 45)

Patient's starting position:

- prone, a firm cushion supporting patient's lower abdomen (slight flexion of the lower lumbar spine) (Fig. 7.26a).

Therapist's starting position:

- standing, at the patient's side
- the hypothenar of the right hand placed on the spinous process of L2; this contact is supported by the left hand.

Movement:

- central push on the spinous process of L2 from posterior to anterior (Fig. 7.26b).

> ***Note:*** Push of L2 in anterior direction leads to extension in segment L1. If the spinous process is too tender for contact, the push in anterior direction can also be performed via the lamina by means of a wedge.

Self-exercise (film 46)

Patient's starting position:

- sitting on a chair, feet placed on a stool for flexion of the lower lumbar spine (Fig. 7.27a)
- a tennis ball placed between the spinous process of L2 and the back of the chair
- arms crossed over the chest or resting on the thighs.

Movement:

- increasing pressure on the ball by pushing the feet towards the floor and pushing the trunk backwards against the ball (Fig. 7.27b); this exerts central pressure on L2 in a posterior–anterior direction
- releasing pressure, and back to starting position.

> ***Note:*** If the spinous process is too tender for contact, instead of the tennis ball a wedge can be laid over the lamina of L2.

Transversal push

Therapy technique (film 47)

Patient's starting position:

- lying on the left side (Fig. 7.28a)
- lumbar spine pre-positioned in extension without irritating the symptomatic segment.

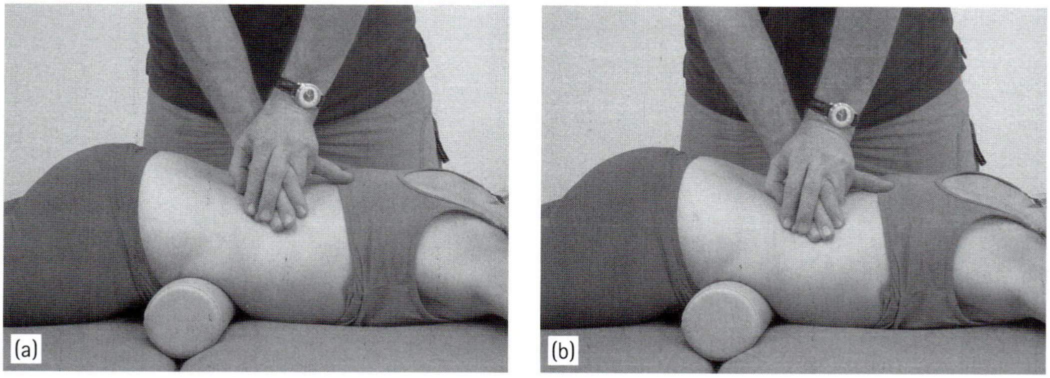

Figure 7.26a and b Accessory movement; central push in posterior–anterior direction (L2); therapy technique. **a**, Starting position. **b**, End position.

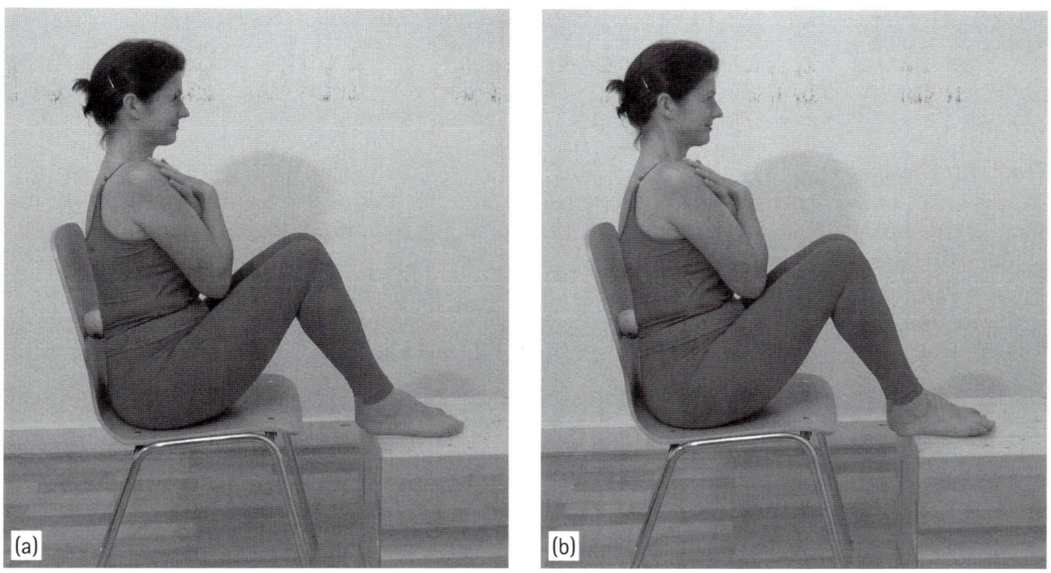

Figure 7.27a and b Accessory movement; central push in posterior–anterior direction (L2); self-exercise. **a**, Starting position. **b**, End position.

Therapist's starting position:

- standing, in front of the patient
- hypothenar of the right hand placed on patient's costal process of L2, supporting this contact with the left hand.

Movement:

- transversal push on the costal process of L2 from right to left (Fig. 7.28b).

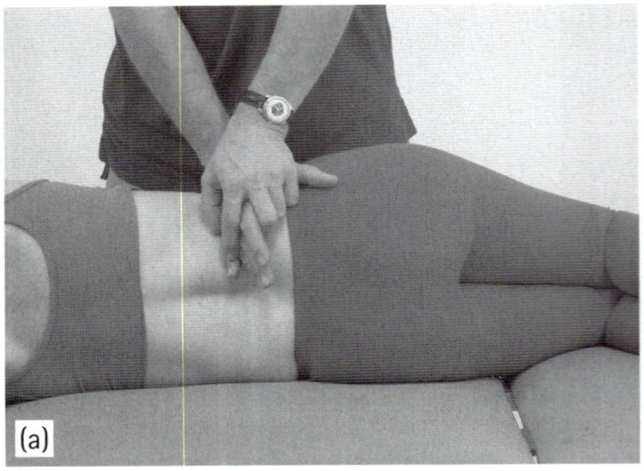

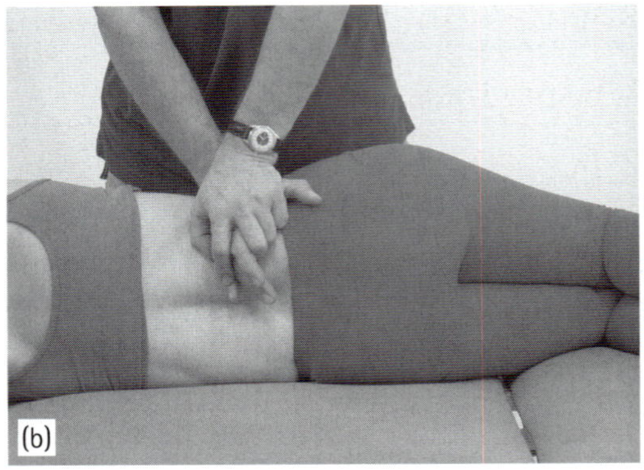

Figure 7.28a and b Accessory movement; transversal push (L2); therapy technique. **a**, Starting position. **b**, End position.

> ***Note:*** As, with this presentation, a globally restricted extension of the affected segments is assumed, the technique has to be applied in side-lying position, left and right.

Remarks

Goals of the technique

With painful hypermobility of L5 in extension, these techniques serve to improve hypomobility of the thoracolumbar junction (contributing factor) by mobilization of non-symptomatic tissue.

Performance

The more tissue resistance to be overcome by mobilization, the more important the fixation.

Dosage

As in this example the approach is treatment of a contributing factor adjacent to the symptomatic tissue, the symptomatic area may be put under stress due to continuing movement or inexact performance of the technique. Therefore, great care has to be taken not to reproduce the patient's symptoms. Dosage is determined by the expected training state of the tissue and, above all, by reassessment.

Choice of technique

The selection of the technique depends, among other things, on the therapist as well as the patient, on the therapist's clinical experience, but primarily on reassessment. So even if all preconditions on the part of therapist and patient have been met, it is of no use to continue the technique if reassessment is negative.

Contributing factors

For a satisfactory solution of the patient's current problems it is important to consider the contributing factors and include them in the treatment.

The authors will, however, not go into a description of the various possibilities and their complex contexts as this would exceed the scope of the present book.

MOBILIZATION TECHNIQUES (SYMPTOMATIC AREA)

Active procedures

ACTIVE MOBILIZATION WITH ACCESSORY MOVEMENT
Extension with ventrocranial push on L5, in prone position

Therapy technique (film 300)
Patient's starting position:

- prone (Fig. 7.29a)
- a cushion under the lumbar spine ensures flexion of the symptomatic area.

Therapist's starting position:

- standing, at the patient's side
- contact with both thumbs on patient's spinous process of L5.

Movement:

- pushing L5 in a ventrocranial direction and then moving the lumbar spine into extension (Fig. 7.29b)
- extension is initiated from caudal via tilting of the pelvis
- then the spine is guided back into starting position and pressure is released.

Self-exercise (film 301)
Patient's starting position:

- sitting, lumbar spine flexed (Fig. 7.30a)
- contact on the spinous process of L5 with the proximal phalanx of the second finger, from caudal.

Movement:

- pressure on the spinous process of L5 in a ventrocranial direction (Fig. 7.30b)
- while pressure is maintained, the lumbar spine is moved into extension by tilting the pelvis
- back to starting position and releasing pressure.

Remarks

Goals of the technique
With painful hypermobility of L5, these techniques serve to:

- reduce tonicity and improve the metabolism of the affected tissues
- restore pain-free function (change the input to the respective centres in the central nervous system).

Performance
The patient's typical symptoms provoked by extension should not be reproduced by these techniques.

Dosage
Pressure on the spinous process of L5 may meet with a sensitive reaction, due to sensitized tissue. But movement into extension must not be painful.

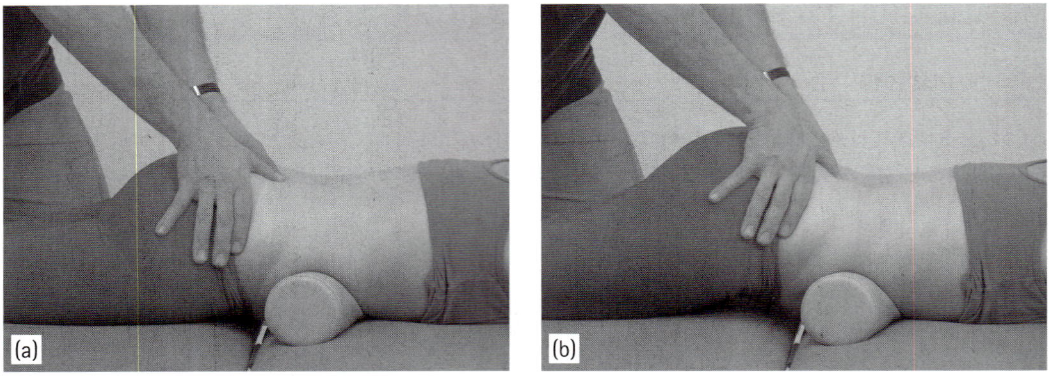

Figure 7.29a and b Active mobilization with accessory movement; ventrocranial push on L5 with subsequent movement of the lumbar spine into extension (prone position); therapy technique. **a**, Starting position. **b**, End position.

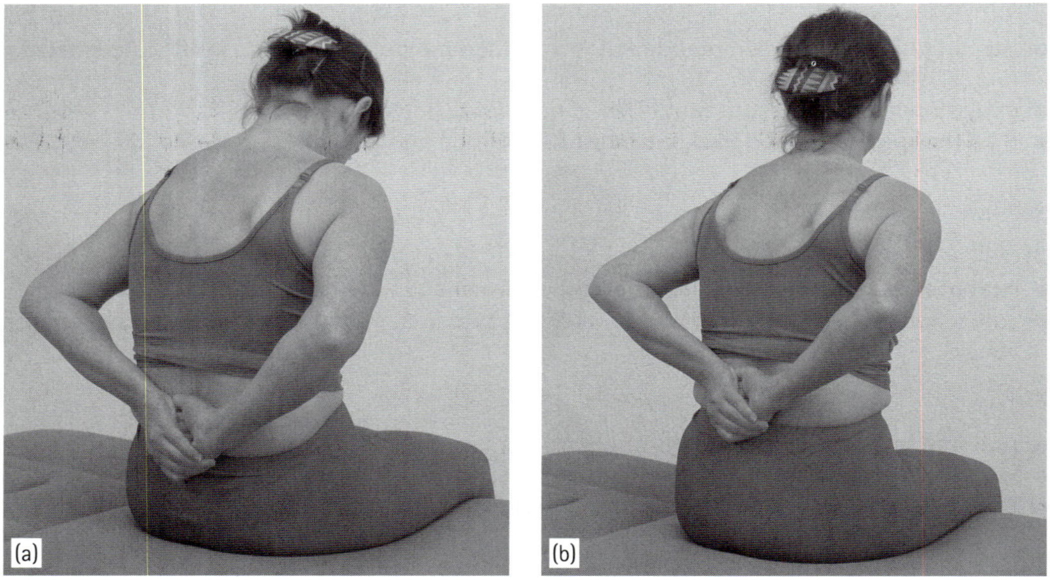

Figure 7.30a and b Active mobilization with accessory movement; ventrocranial push on L5 with subsequent movement of the lumbar spine into extension (sitting); self-exercise. **a**, Starting position. **b**, End position.

Choice of technique

The selection of the technique depends, among other things, on the therapist as well as the patient, on the therapist's clinical experience, but primarily on reassessment. This means that even if all preconditions on the part of therapist and patient have been met, it is of no use to continue the technique if reassessment is negative.

Contributing factors

For a satisfactory solution of the patient's current problems it is important to consider the contributing factors and include them in the treatment.

The authors will, however, not go into a description of the various possibilities and their complex contexts as this would exceed the scope of the present book.

Chapter 8

Buttocks and dorsolateral thigh

CHAPTER CONTENTS

AREA LOCALIZATION

IDENTIFICATION OF THE POTENTIALLY AFFECTED AREA BY DEMONSTRATION OF A SYMPTOMATIC FUNCTIONAL MOVEMENT/POSITION

Based on the information gained from the anamnesis so far, the therapist ascertains more details about potentially affected sections. This is done by means of area localization, which represents the beginning of the physical examination. Information gained in this way is used to check or modify the relevant hypotheses developed on the basis of the anamnesis and will determine how to proceed.

The way area localization is performed is explained by means of two examples. In both, the patient feels pain in the area of buttocks and dorsolateral thigh. Clinical experience and known clinical patterns suggest primarily the following areas as potential origins of the current complaints:

- lumbar spine
- neural structures.

General question: Is there enough information available to bypass area localization?	
No	Yes
⇓	⇓
Performance of area localization	• General movement tests • Additional tests • Test treatment

Example 1: Flexion

Symptom area: buttocks/dorsolateral thigh, right side
Symptom provocation: flexion of the spine (Fig. 8.1)

With this presentation, clinical experience suggests primarily the lumbar spine and the neural structures as symptom-provoking areas.

Below, examples illustrate how to differentiate between these areas. To this end, area localization is first attempted by means of active movements alone. If this is not possible, tests will be performed by means of assistive movements.

Hypothesis 1: The symptom-provoking area is the neural structures

Differentiation: neural involvement vs. lumbar spine/sacroiliac joint (SIJ).

The change in symptoms can be demonstrated exactly:

- provocation of pain (Fig. 8.2a and b, film 48)
- alleviation of pain (Fig. 8.3a and b, film 49).

The result of area localization should be verified by further specific tests; otherwise the result remains in doubt.

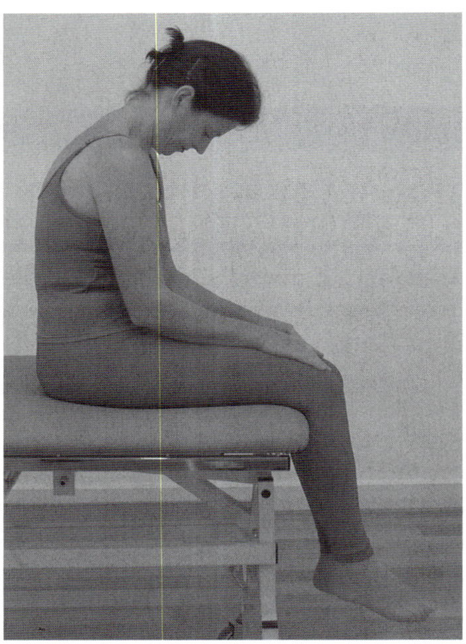

Figure 8.1 Symptom-provoking movement: flexion of the spine provokes pain in the buttocks and dorsolateral thigh, right side.

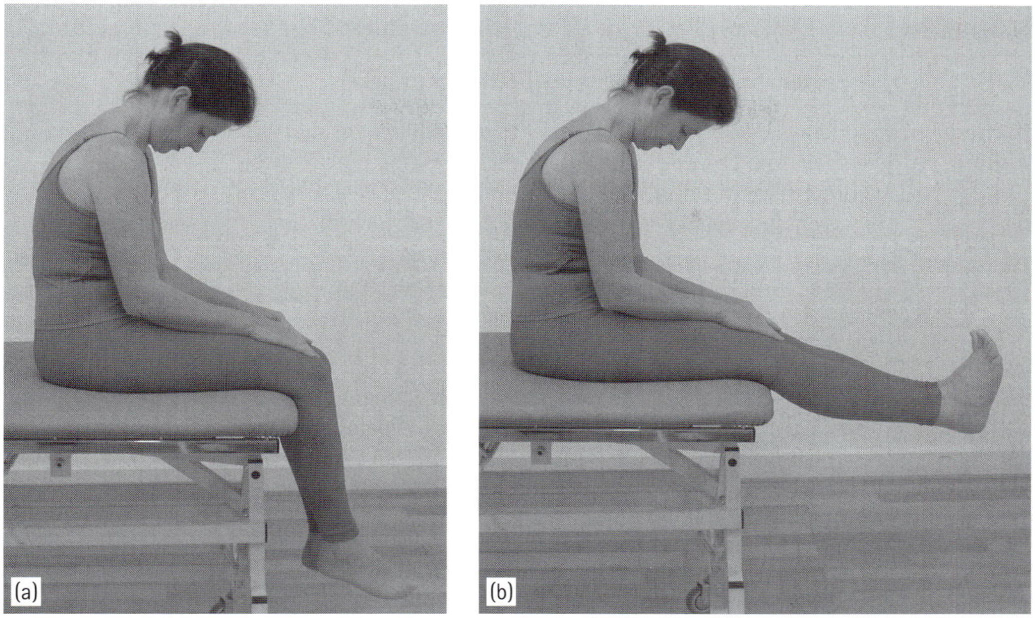

Figure 8.2a and b Area localization with symptomatic movement of the spine into flexion; differentiation between neural structures and lumbar spine/SIJ; provocation. **a**, Starting position. **b**, End position.

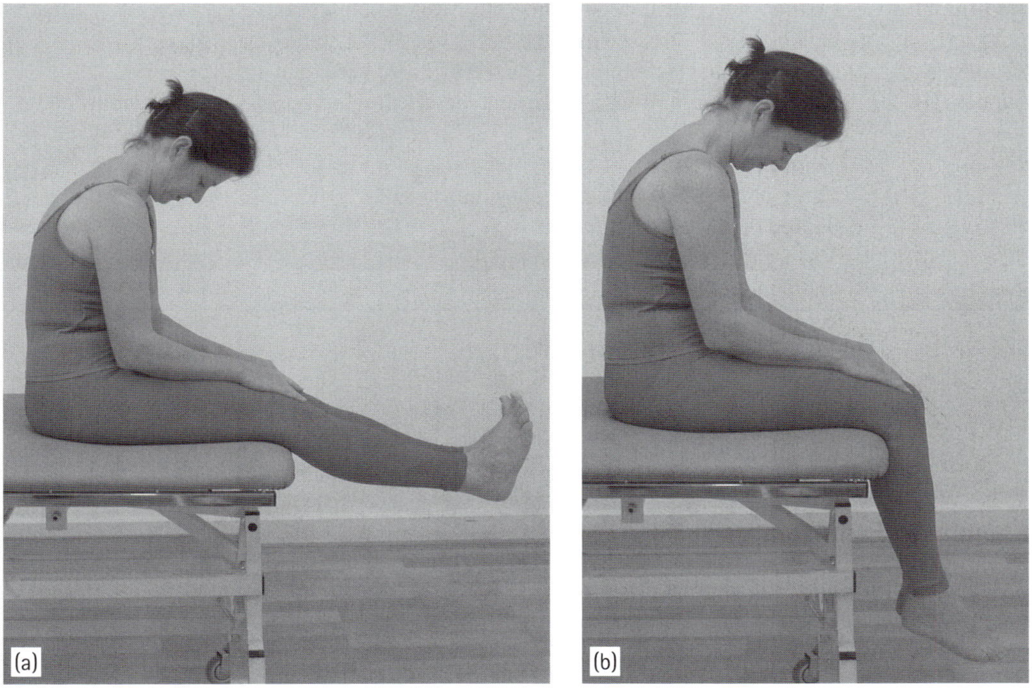

Figure 8.3a and b Area localization with symptomatic movement of the spine into flexion; differentiation between neural structures and lumbar spine/SIJ; alleviation. **a**, Starting position. **b**, End position.

Assessment

Goal	Provocation of pain	Alleviation of pain	Remarks
Starting position	Flexion of the spine to a position immediately before symptoms appear	With bilateral extension of the knees and dorsal flexion of the ankles, flexion of the spine to a position immediately after symptoms have appeared	
Test movement	Bilateral extension of the knees, dorsal flexion of the ankles, in sitting	Bilateral flexion of the knees reduces the tension on the neural structures produced by the starting position	
Explanation	The test movement increases tension in the neural structures	The test movement reduces tension in the neural structures	If the patient's typical pain is changed by these manoeuvres, this suggests at least an involvement of the neural structures
Additional data to support the hypothesis	Further movements of proximal or distal components to increase neural tension which are not directly involved in flexion of the spine General and specific mobility of the affected area History (e.g., symptom behaviour, type of complaints, 24-hour behaviour) Palpation Neurodynamic tests Nerve provocation tests (e.g., bow string sign) Reproducibility of test results Test treatment Imaging procedures (CT, MRI)		

Example 2: Extension

Symptom area: buttocks/dorsolateral thigh
Symptom provocation: extension, lateral flexion, and rotation of the spine to the right (Fig. 8.4)

With this presentation, clinical experience suggests primarily the lumbar spine and the neural structures as symptom-provoking areas.

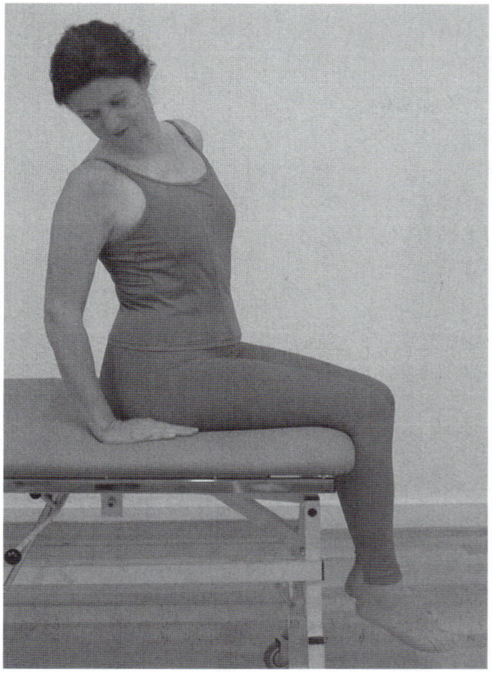

Figure 8.4 Symptom-provoking movement: extension, lateral flexion, and rotation of the spine to the right provokes pain in the buttocks and dorsolateral thigh, right side.

Below, examples illustrate how to differentiate between these areas. To this end, area localization is first attempted by means of active movements alone. If this is not possible, tests will be performed by means of assistive movements.

Hypothesis 1: The symptom-provoking area is the neural structures

Differentiation: neural involvement vs. lumbar spine.

The change in symptoms can be demonstrated exactly:

- provocation of pain (Fig. 8.5a and b, film 50)
- alleviation of pain (Fig. 8.6a and b, film 51).

The result of area localization should be verified by further specific tests; otherwise the result remains in doubt.

QUICK CHECK – SYMPTOMS, BUTTOCKS/DORSOLATERAL THIGH

See Figures 8.7–8.9: if neither the area nor a symptom-provoking or symptom-reducing action is known, the quick check is used to try to load individual potential areas with specific biomechanically provocative movement combinations. The chosen movement combinations correspond with the straining and often symptom-provoking movements of the individual sections.

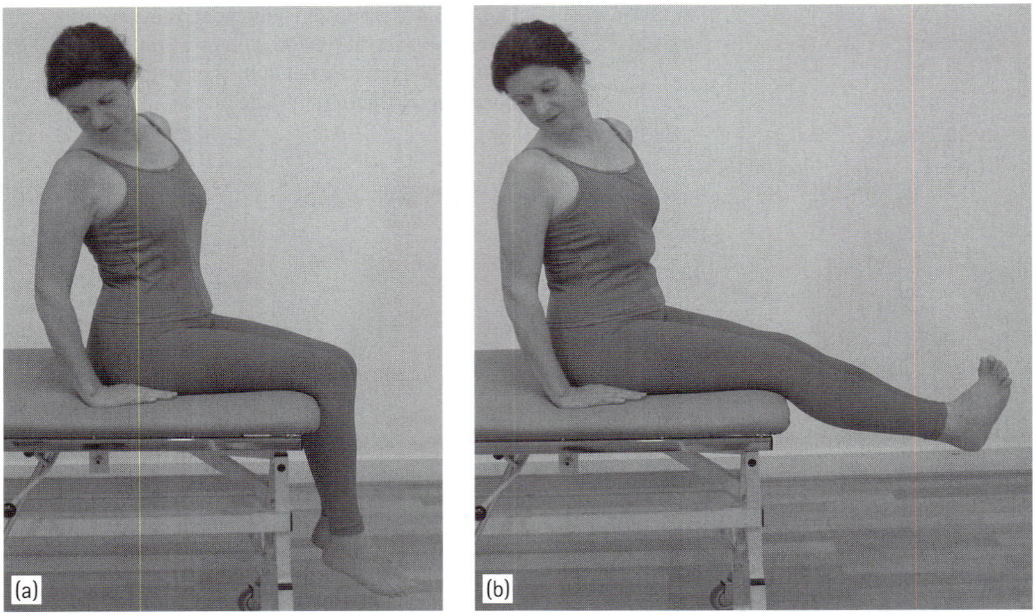

Figure 8.5a and b Area localization with symptomatic movement of the spine into extension, lateral flexion and rotation to the right; differentiation between neural structures and lumbar spine; provocation. a, Starting position. b, End position.

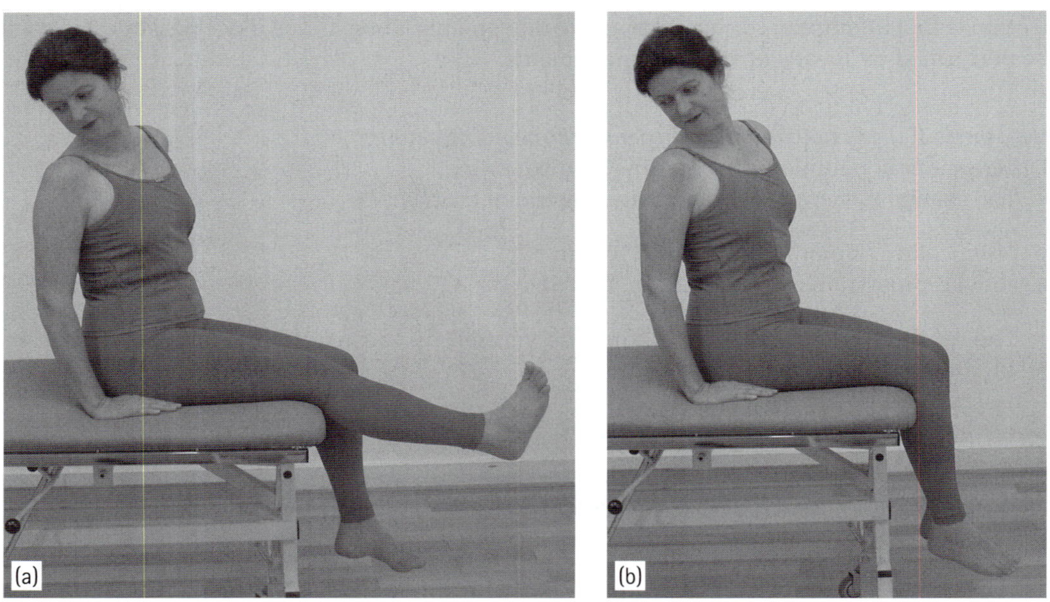

Figure 8.6a and b Area localization with symptomatic movement of the spine into extension, lateral flexion and rotation to the right; differentiation between neural structures and lumbar spine; alleviation. a, Starting position. b, End position.

Assessment			
Goal	**Provocation of pain**	**Alleviation of pain**	**Remarks**
Starting position	Extension, lateral flexion, and rotation of the spine to the right, to a position immediately before symptoms appear	With the right knee pre-positioned in extension and the right ankle in dorsal flexion, extension, lateral flexion, and rotation of the spine to the right, to a position immediately after symptoms have appeared	Provocation of the symptoms will reduce symptoms in the right leg. Repeated pain provocation via right leg alone will also reproduce symptoms in the right leg. Therefore, alleviation manoeuvres are done via the right leg, too
Test movement	Bilateral and unilateral extension of the knees and dorsal flexion of the ankles, in sitting	Flexion of the right knee, which reduces the tension in the neural structures produced by the starting position	
Explanation	The test movement increases tension in the neural structures	The test movement reduces tension in the neural structures	If the typical pain is provoked or alleviated by these manoeuvres, this suggests at least an involvement of the neural structures
Additional data to support the hypothesis	Further movements of proximal and distal components to increase neural tension which are not directly involved in flexion of the spine General and specific mobility of the affected area History (e.g., symptom behaviour, type of complaints, 24-hour behaviour) Palpation Neurodynamic tests Nerve provocation tests (e.g., bow string sign) Reproducibility of test results Test treatment Imaging procedures (CT, MRI)		

LUMBAR SPINE

Movement (*film 226*)

- Extension/lateral flexion to the right, and rotation to the same as well as to the opposite side, with overpressure (Fig. 8.7a and b)
- Extension/lateral flexion to the left, and rotation to the same as well as to the opposite side, with overpressure (Fig. 8.8a and b).

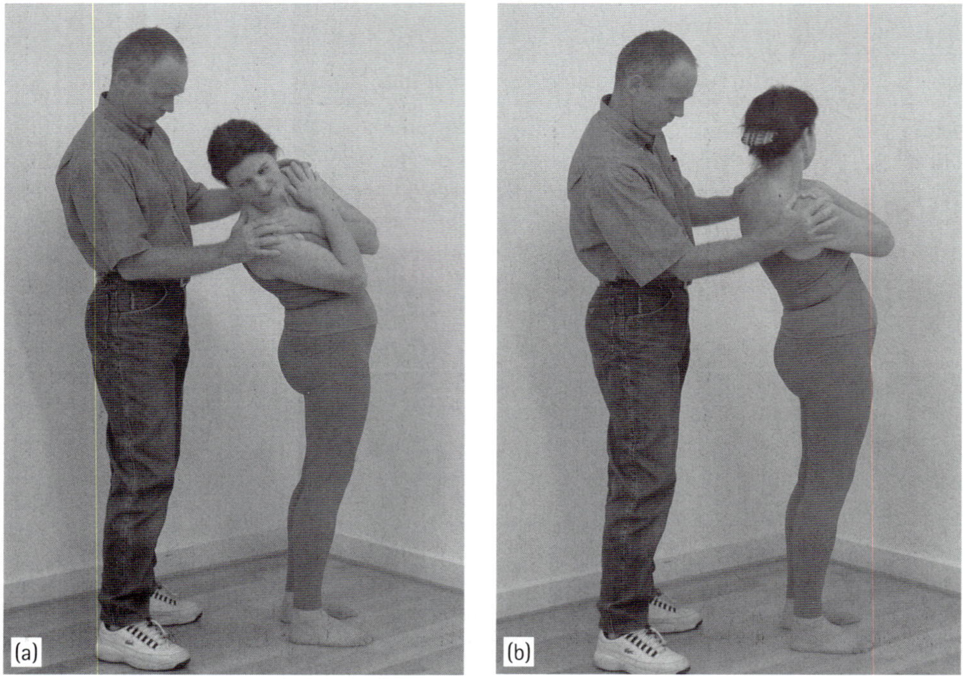

Figure 8.7a and b Quick check lumbar spine; extension, lateral flexion to the right. **a**, Rotation to the same side. **b**, Rotation to the opposite side.

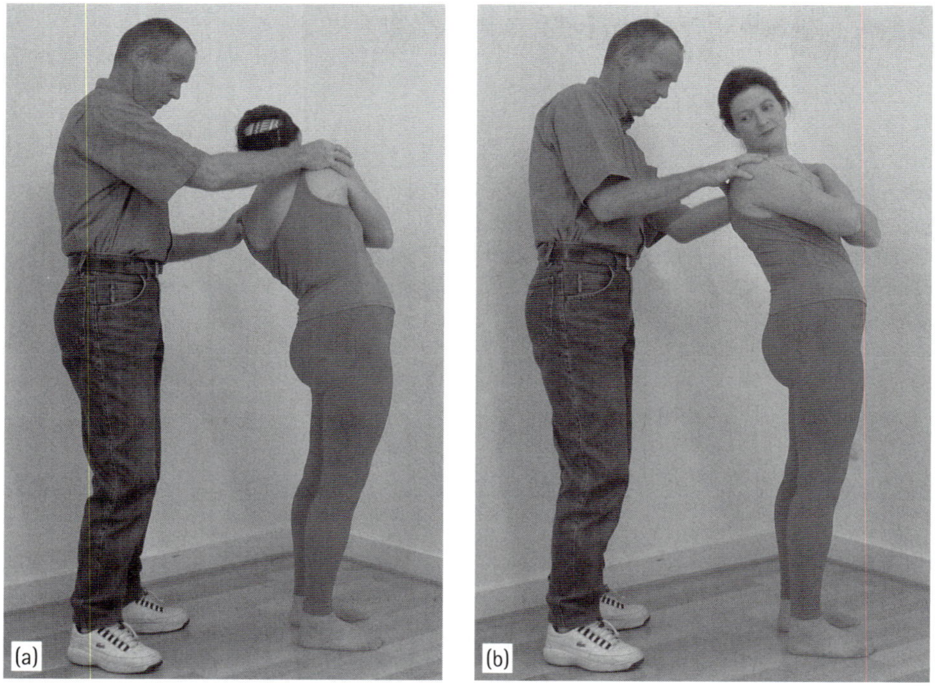

Figure 8.8a and b Quick check lumbar spine; extension, lateral flexion to the left. **a**, Rotation to the same side. **b**, Rotation to the opposite side.

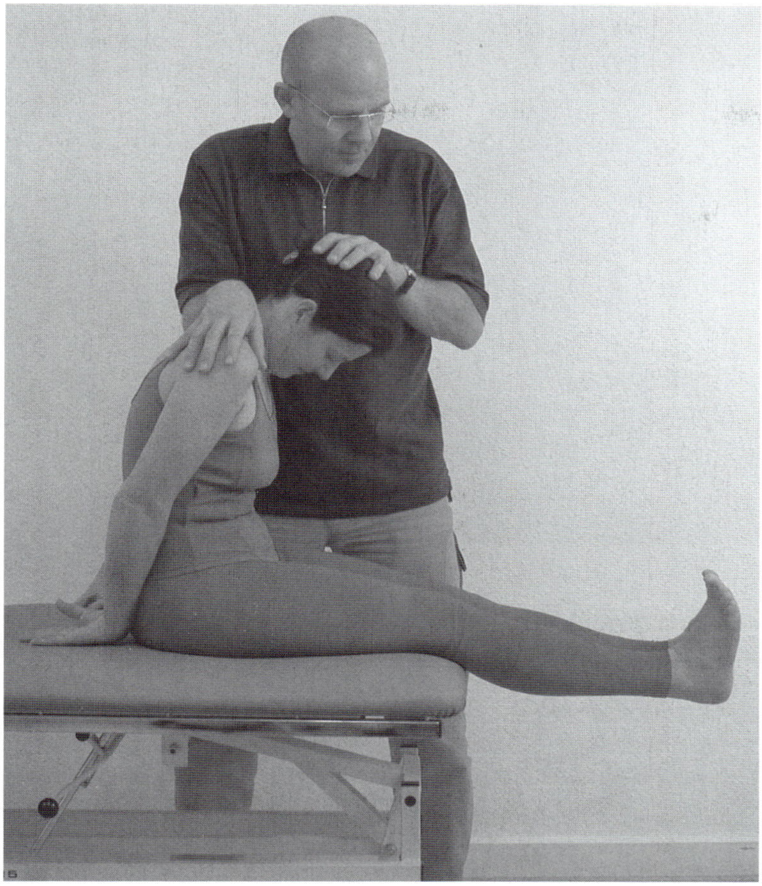

Figure 8.9 Quick check neurodynamics; slump test.

NEURAL STRUCTURES

Tension tests

- Slump test (Fig. 8.9, film 616)
- Straight leg raise (SLR; Fig. 8.10, film 618).

Note: Even an area that proves negative in the quick check may possibly be symptom-provoking (another movement combination, or passive overpressure may be required).

SPECIFIC PROVOCATION AND ALLEVIATION

Specific provocation and alleviation allows one to differentiate within an articular complex and to identify the symptom-provoking movement direction(s).

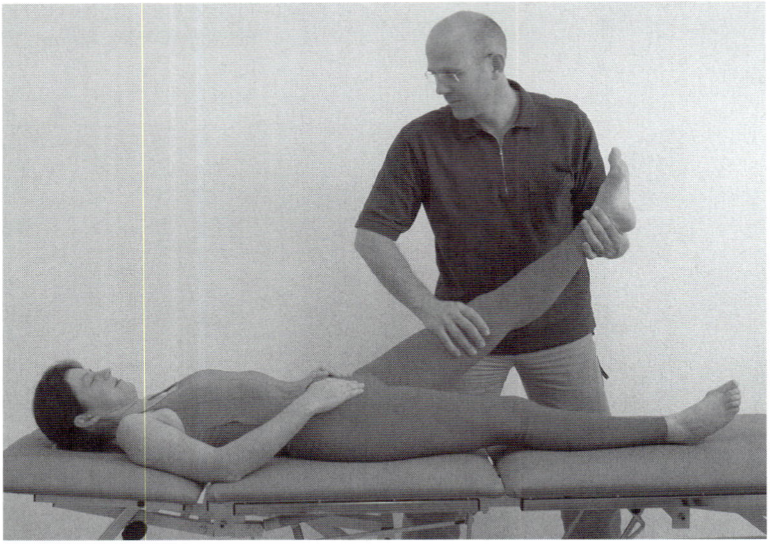

Figure 8.10 Quick check neurodynamics; straight leg raise (SLR) test.

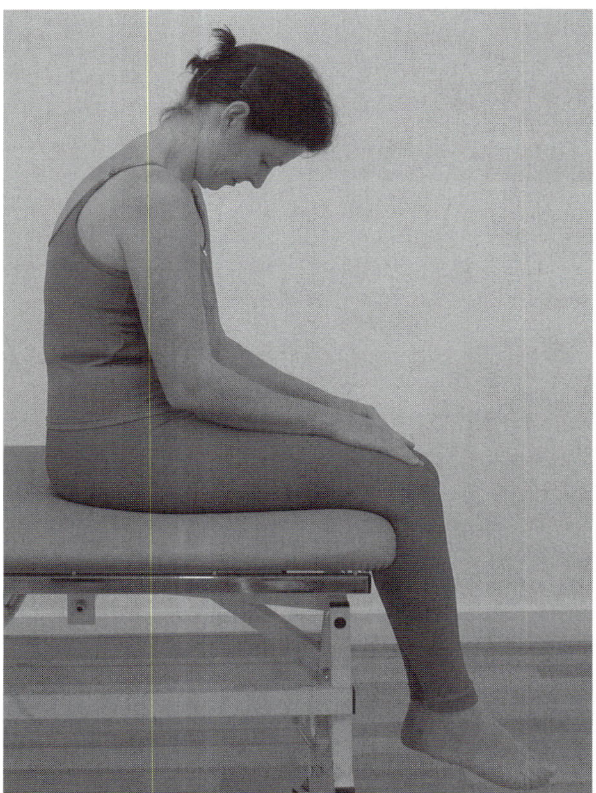

Figure 8.11 Symptom-provoking movement: flexion of the spine provokes pain in the buttocks and dorsolateral thigh, right side.

SPECIFIC PROVOCATION AND ALLEVIATION, LUMBAR SPINE

Localization, lumbar spine – flexion

Pain-provoking movement (Fig. 8.11)

- Flexion of the lumbar spine provokes pain in the buttocks and dorsolateral thigh.
- Area localization hints at the lumbar spine with neural involvement.

History and current clinical presentation hint at an acute discogenic dysfunction with neural involvement, which requires caution with the further examination. For this reason, a starting position is chosen for further differentiation tests where the stress for the patient seems as low as possible.

The change in symptoms can be demonstrated exactly:

- provocation of pain (Fig. 8.12a and b, film 52)
- alleviation of pain (Fig. 8.13a and b, film 53).

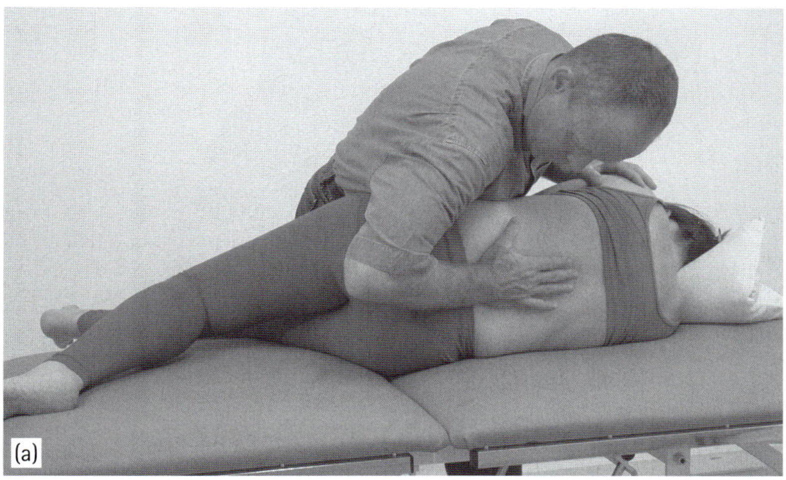

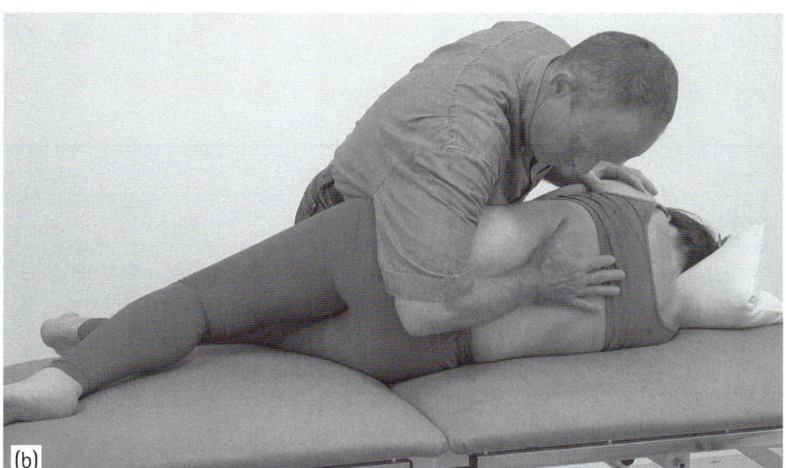

Figure 8.12a and b Specific provocation and alleviation in the area of buttocks and dorsolateral thigh, right side, with symptomatic flexion of the spine; localization of the symptomatic segment; provocation. **a**, Test start. **b**, Test end.

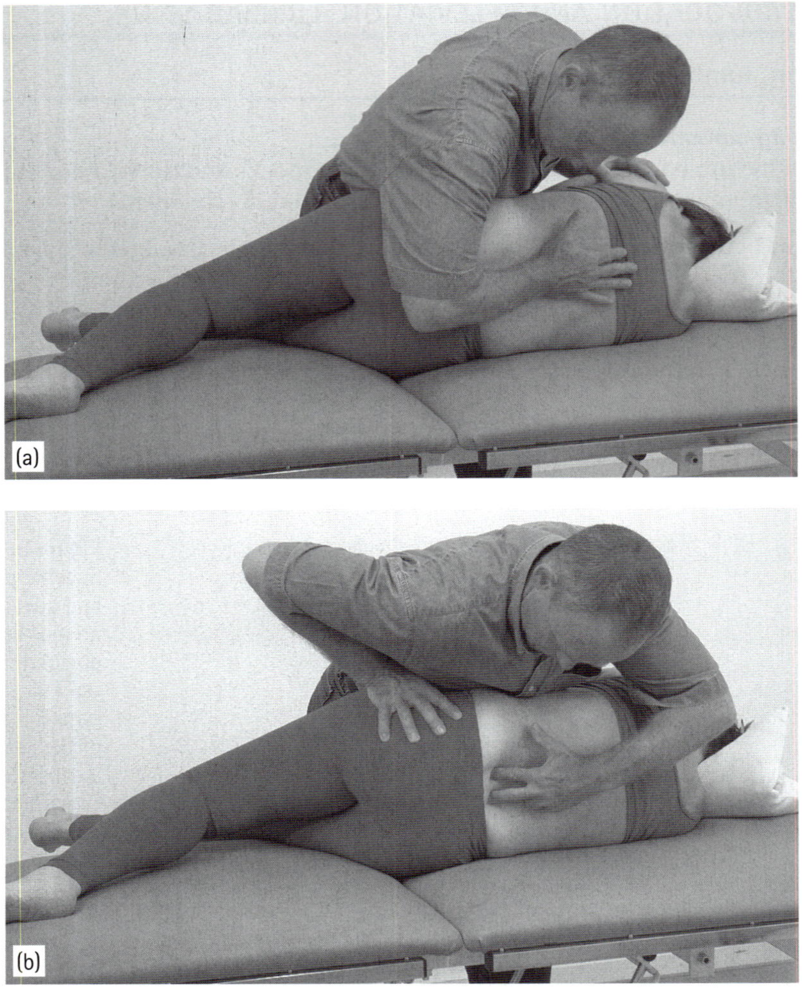

Figure 8.13a and b Specific provocation and alleviation in the area of the buttocks and dorsolateral thigh, right side, with symptomatic flexion of the spine; localization of the symptomatic segment; alleviation. **a**, Test start. **b**, Test end.

Assessment

Goal	Provocation of pain	Alleviation of pain	Remarks
Starting position	Side-lying, the lumbar spine pre-positioned in flexion in a position immediately before symptoms appear, extension of the right knee joint (increase in neural tension) to a	Side-lying, the lumbar spine pre-positioned in flexion in a position immediately before symptoms appear. Then extension of the right knee joint (increase in neural tension) to a	The patient's pelvis is stabilized by the therapist's upper trunk

Goal	Provocation of pain	Alleviation of pain	Remarks
	position immediately before symptoms appear	position immediately after symptoms have appeared	
Test movement	Pushing the vertebra via lamina or spinous process in ventrocranial direction, starting caudally (L5–L2)	Pushing the vertebra via lamina or spinous process in ventrocranial direction, starting cranially (L3–L5). To achieve less flexion in segment L5, the sacral base has to be shifted in ventral direction	Care has to be taken that the pelvis remains immobile during the push in ventrocranial direction. If the pelvis moves, it has to be fixed manually or by a belt
Neural involvement	Proximal and/or distal component without change of position in the relevant area	Proximal and/or distal component without change of position in the relevant area	
Explanation	The symptoms are provoked when the cranial vertebra in the segment is moved (flexion in the affected segment)	The symptoms are alleviated when the caudal vertebra in the segment is moved (extension in the affected segment)	
Additional data to support the hypothesis	General and specific mobility of the lumbar spine History (e.g., symptom behaviour, type of complaints, 24-hour behaviour) Specific palpation Nerve mobility tests (if specific provocation and alleviation indicate neural involvement) Reproducibility of test results Test treatment Imaging procedures (CT, MRI)		

Localization, lumbar spine – extension/lateral flexion to the right/rotation to the right

Pain-provoking movement (Fig. 8.14)

- Extension/lateral flexion to the right/rotation to the right of the lumbar spine provokes pain in the buttocks and dorsolateral thigh.
- Area localization hints at the lumbar spine.

The change in symptoms can be demonstrated exactly:

- provocation of pain (Fig. 8.15a and b, film 54)
- alleviation of pain (Fig. 8.16a and b, film 55).

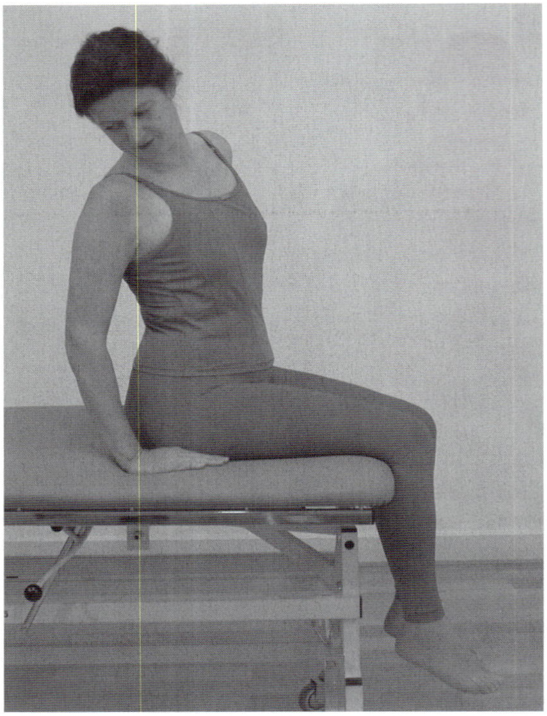

Figure 8.14 Symptom-provoking movement: extension, lateral flexion to the right, rotation to the right of the spine provokes pain in buttocks and dorsolateral thigh, right side.

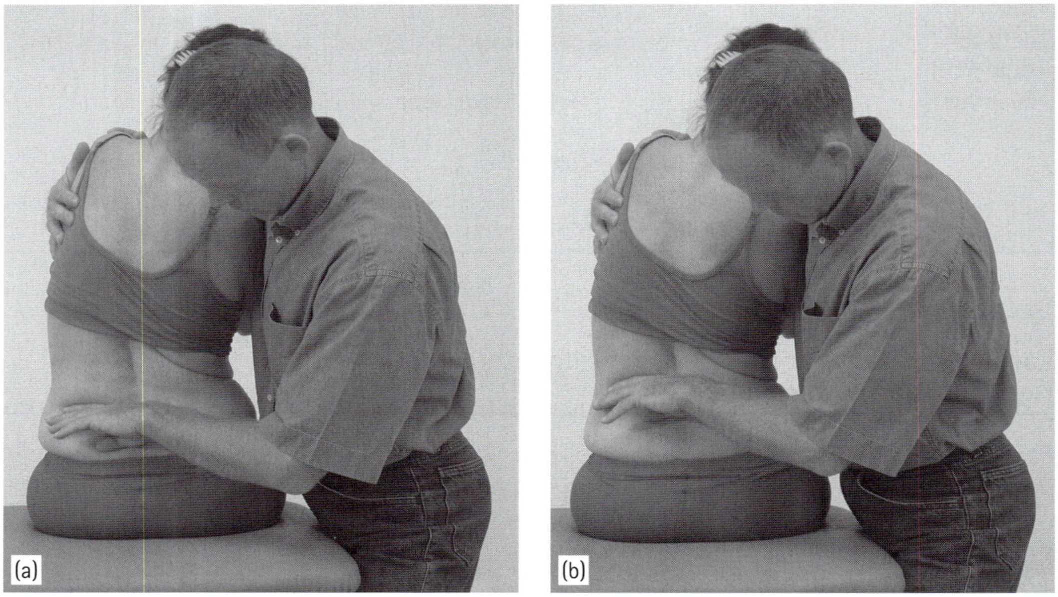

Figure 8.15a and b Specific provocation and alleviation in the area of the spine with symptomatic extension, lateral flexion to the right, rotation to the right of the spine; localization of the symptomatic segment; provocation. **a**, Test start. **b**, Test end.

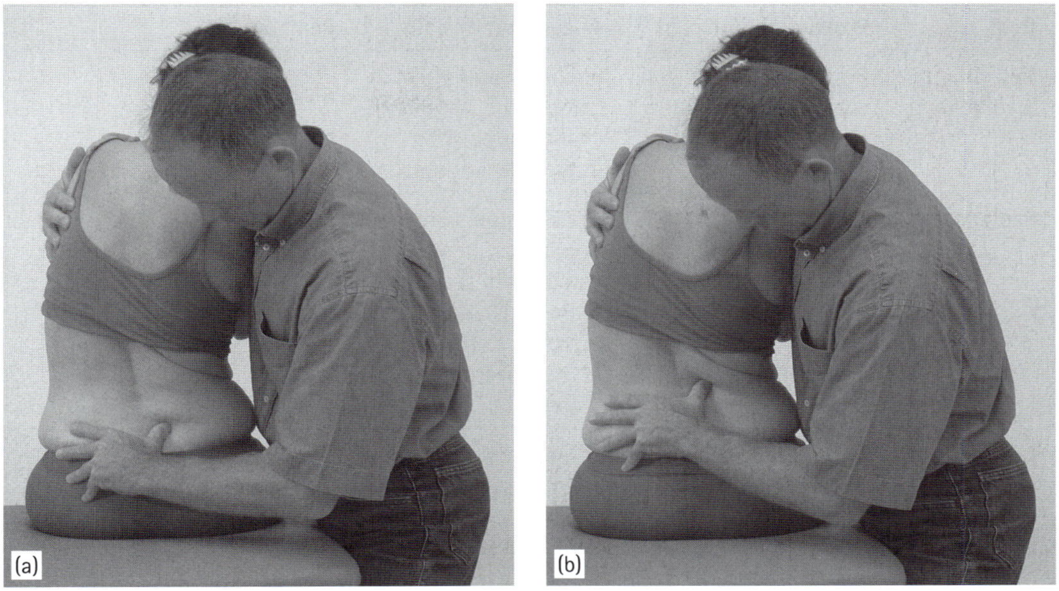

Figure 8.16a and b Specific provocation and alleviation in the area of the spine with symptomatic extension, lateral flexion to the right, rotation to the right of the spine; localization of the symptomatic segment; alleviation. **a**, Test start. **b**, Test end.

Assessment			
Goal	**Provocation of pain**	**Alleviation of pain**	**Remarks**
Starting position	Sitting, lumbar spine in extension/lateral flexion to the right/ rotation to the right to a position immediately before symptoms appear	Sitting, lumbar spine in extension/lateral flexion to the right/ rotation to the right to a position immediately after symptoms have appeared	Trunk remains in starting position
Test movement	Pushing the vertebra via the left transverse process into rotation to the right, starting caudally (L5–L2)	Pushing the vertebra via the right transverse process into rotation to the left, starting caudally (L5–L2)	If differentiation is performed by pushing the vertebra into rotation to the right, provocation has to start caudally. With alleviation, differentiation is performed by push of the cranial vertebra in the segment into rotation to the left. Otherwise, L5 would have to be pushed via the sacrum to move the segment

Goal	Provocation of pain	Alleviation of pain	Remarks
Neural involvement	Proximal and/or distal component without change of position in the relevant area	Proximal and/or distal component without change of position in the relevant area	
Explanation	The symptoms are provoked when the cranial vertebra in the segment is moved (rotation to the right in the affected segment)	The symptoms are alleviated when the cranial vertebra in the segment is moved (rotation to the left in the affected segment)	
Additional data to support the hypothesis	General and specific mobility of the lumbar spine History (e.g., symptom behaviour, type of complaints, 24-hour behaviour) Specific palpation Neurodynamic tests (if specific provocation and alleviation indicate neural involvement) Reproducibility of test results Test treatment Imaging procedures (CT, MRI)		

GENERAL MOVEMENT TESTS

General movement tests identify, quantify, and qualify anatomical individual movements and, in part, movement combinations in the area concerned. The individual manual therapy concepts have respective protocols at their disposal, which more or less have the same goals.

Information gained in this way is used for checking or modifying the relevant hypotheses developed on the basis of anamnesis and area localization and will help in determining how to proceed.

General question: Is there enough information available to bypass general movement tests?	
No	Yes
⇓	⇓
Performance of the general movement tests	• Additional tests • Test treatment

In view of the described clinical presentation and the results of area localization, general movement tests of the following regions seem to be useful.

Lumbar spine		
	Active	Passive
Lumbar spine in general	Flexion Extension Rotation (to the right and left) Lateral flexion (to the right and left)	Flexion Extension Rotation (to the right and left) Lateral flexion (to the right and left)
Movement combinations lumbar spine in general	Symptomatic movements of the lumbar spine	Symptomatic movements of the lumbar spine

TREATMENT EXAMPLE, LUMBAR SPINE: ACUTE RADICULAR SYNDROME

SYMPTOMATIC MOVEMENT

Movement of the lumbar spine into flexion provokes pain in the buttocks and the dorsolateral thigh.

ASSESSMENTS

Area localization

Area localization hints at the lumbar spine with neural involvement. There is no contraindication for movement. But because of the irritability of the current presentation, caution is required.

Neurology

Neurological examination yields the following data:

Function:

- key muscles: weakening of the extensor hallucis longus muscle
- sensitivity: hypoaesthesia in dermatome L5
- reflexes: slight hyporeflexia of the Achilles tendon reflex.

Neurodynamics:

- SLR: lifting the extended right leg (SLR) shows changed quality and quantity of movement (resistance behaviour during movement) as well as changed sensory response (area and type of sensation) as compared with the left side
- slump test: examination with the slump test shows that the patient's typical symptoms can be reproduced by movement of the right knee into extension.

General movement tests

Due to the irritability of the current presentation, only a few movement directions of the whole protocol are selected for further examination (flexion/extension/lateral flexion to the left and right).

It is seen that flexion is the movement which is most clearly restricted and which significantly increases the patient's typical symptoms (buttocks and dorsolateral thigh), whereas movement into extension reduces radiation of pain into the dorsolateral thigh, and although the symptoms in the buttocks increase a little, the symptom area is shifted in a central direction. With symptom provocation by flexion, the distance between finger tips and upper patellar edge amounts to 5 cm (about 2 inches).

Specific provocation and alleviation

In the described situation, specific provocation and alleviation in flexion to localize the symptomatic segment is not performed since it would not yield any relevant information for the patient's current management. Neural involvement as well as the patient's medical history hint at a discogenic cause of the presentation.

To check this hypothesis, movement directions will be used for further differentiation which are characteristic of an acute discogenic presentation (traction/compression). The patient shows that the symptoms can be alleviated by traction and increased by compression.

Specific mobility

Specific mobility is not tested since the presentation is an acute one.

Palpation

Palpation indicates increased tension and increased tenderness of the lumbar paravertebral muscles as compared with the opposite side. The patient shows a positive *bow string sign* on the right side.

HYPOTHESIS

An acute lumboradicular syndrome of discogenic origin is suspected (Fig. 8.17).

MOBILIZATION TECHNIQUES

Active procedures

ACTIVE MOBILIZATION

Repeated extension, in lying

Self-exercise (film 56)

Patient's starting position:

- prone (Fig. 8.18a) (if necessary a roll may be placed under the distal lower legs)
- both hands placed beside the shoulders
- back muscles as relaxed as possible.

Movement:

- via extension of the elbows, the trunk is slowly lifted, from the cranial to caudal end (Fig. 8.18b)
- then back to starting position.

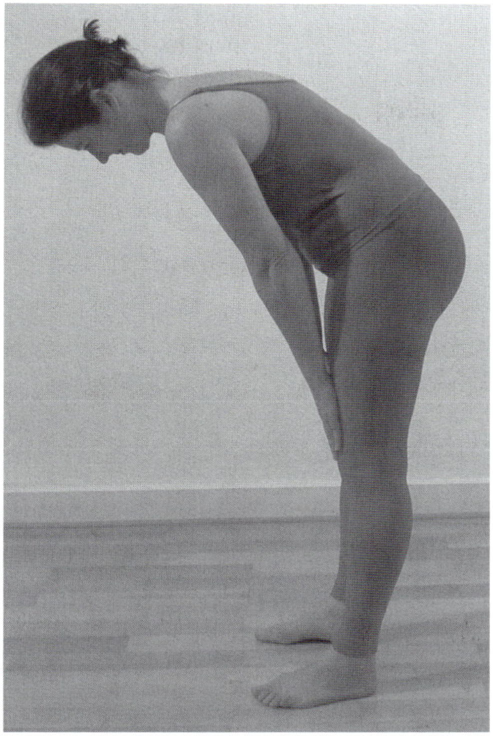

Figure 8.17 Symptom-provoking movement: flexion of the spine provokes pain in the buttocks and dorsolateral thigh, right side.

Remarks

Goals of the technique

With an acute lumboradicular syndrome of discogenic origin, this technique serves to reduce derangement (McKenzie 1998).

Performance

The following points have been observed:

- the back muscles do not support the lifting of the trunk
- the pelvis has to remain on the supporting surface
- the symptoms must not peripheralize (shift of the radiating symptoms in a distal direction).

Dosage

With repeated extension, the central symptoms in the back may increase. This is no reason to stop the exercise.

In the authors' opinion, in a presentation with no symptoms appearing in prone position, movement into extension should be performed up to the position where back pain just starts (P1). If, however, symptoms appear in prone position, movement is performed up to the first increase in symptoms. If no increase in symptoms occurs during full-range extension, movement can continue up to the position where the pelvis is just at the point of leaving the supporting surface.

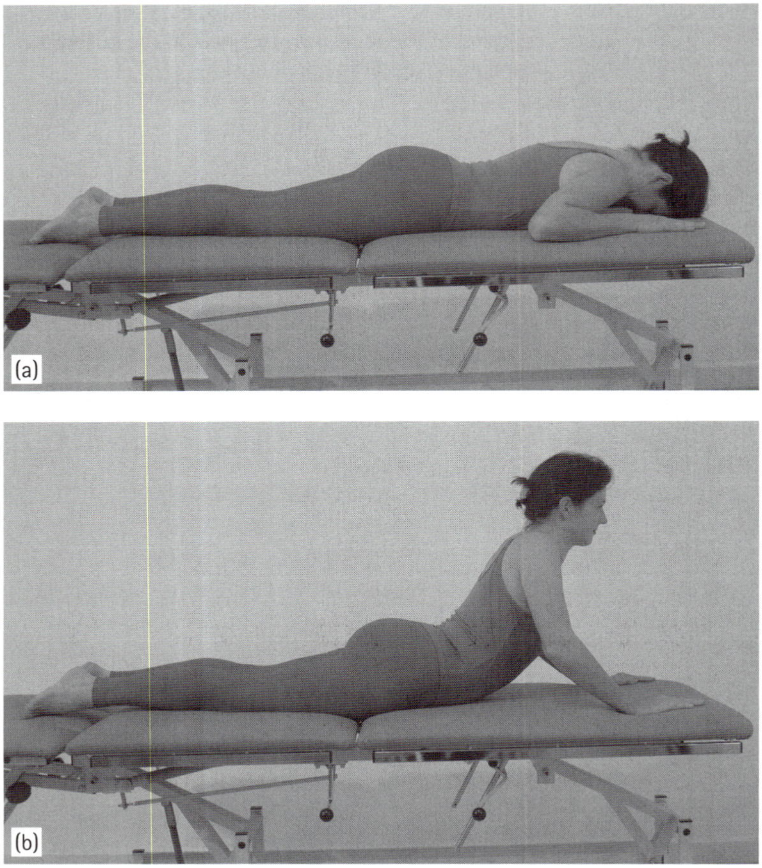

Figure 8.18a and b Active mobilization; repeated extension in lying; self-exercise. a, Starting position. b, End position.

For further information about dosage, modification of the technique, and further progression, the reader is referred to the work of Robin McKenzie (McKenzie 1998).

Choice of technique

The selection of the technique depends, among other things, on the therapist as well as the patient, on the therapist's clinical experience, but primarily on reassessment. This means that even if all preconditions on the part of therapist and patient seem to be met, it is of no use to continue the technique if reassessment is negative.

To preserve achieved treatment results in this acute phase and to avoid worsening of the condition due to negative movement input, it is often useful to support the lumbar spine externally with a firm belt so as to restrict its movements.

Contributing factors

For a satisfactory solution of the patient's current problems it is important to consider the contributing factors and include them in the treatment.

The authors will, however, not go deeper into a description of the various possibilities and their complex contexts as this would exceed the scope of the present book.

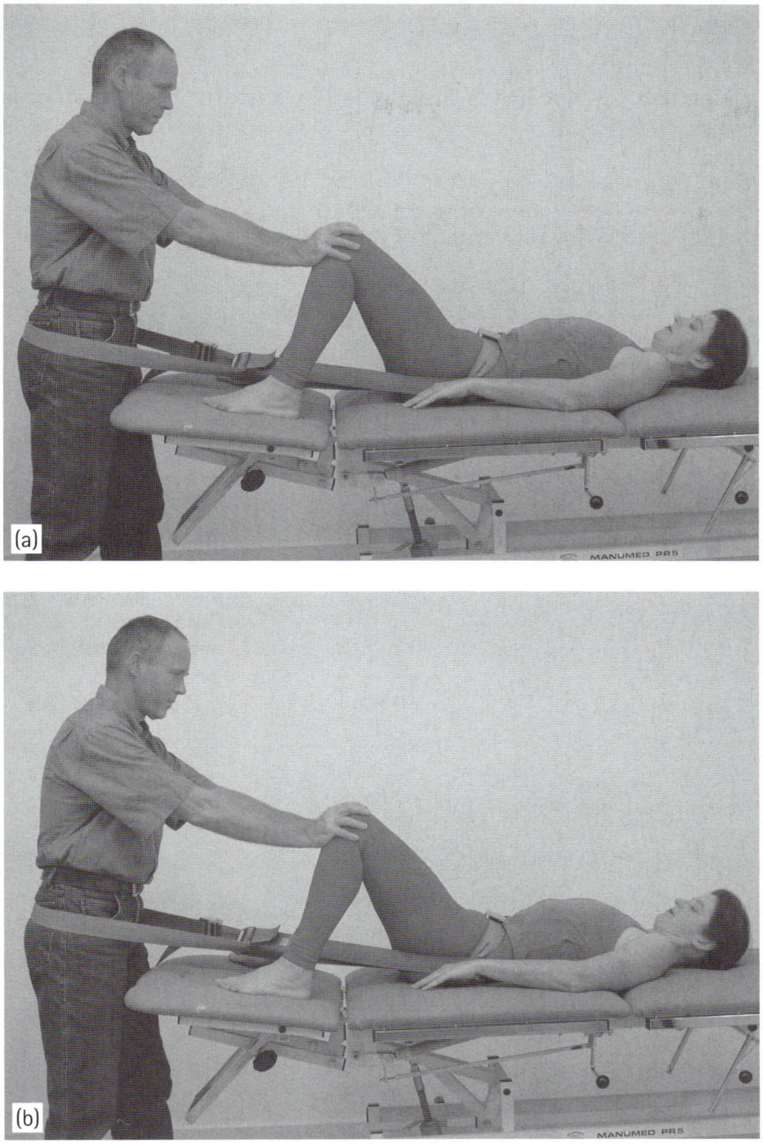

Figure 8.19a and b
Translatory movement; traction; therapy technique. a, Starting position. b, End position.

Passive procedures

TRANSLATORY MOVEMENTS

Traction

Therapy technique (film 57)

Patient's starting position:

- supine, adjusted in a position as symptom-free as possible (Fig. 8.19a)
- the pelvis is surrounded by a fixation belt (pelvic belt).

Therapist's starting position:

- standing, at the foot end of the plinth
- a fixation belt linked to the patient's pelvic belt is surrounded by a further belt which goes around the therapist's pelvis.

Movement:

- traction of the lumbar spine by backward movement of the therapist's pelvis (Fig. 8.19b).

Self-exercise (film 58)

Patient's starting position:

- supine, adjusted in a position as symptom-free as possible (Fig. 8.20a).

Movement:

- traction of the lumbar spine by pushing the arms against the thighs (as close to the pelvis as possible; Fig. 8.20b).

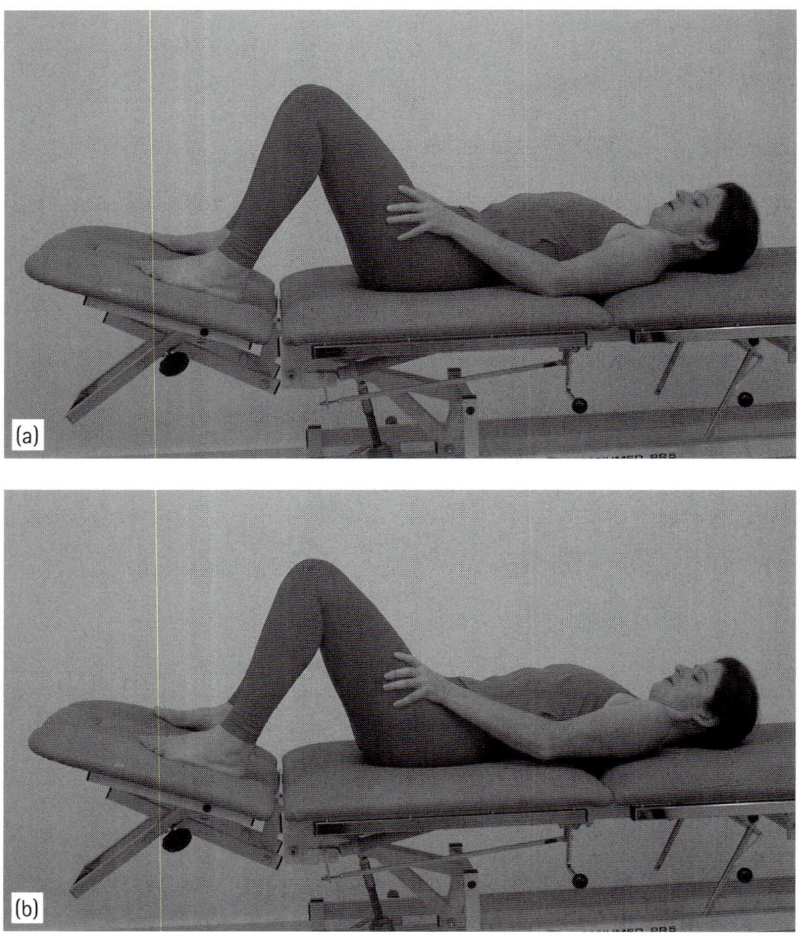

Figure 8.20a and b Translatory movement; traction; self-exercise. a, Starting position. b, End position.

ANGULAR MOVEMENTS

Internal rotation of the hip joint (neural mobilization)

Therapy technique (film 59)

Patient's starting position:

- supine, in a position as symptom-free as possible (Fig. 8.21a)
- hip joint pre-positioned in external rotation.

Therapist's starting position:

- standing, at the patient's side.

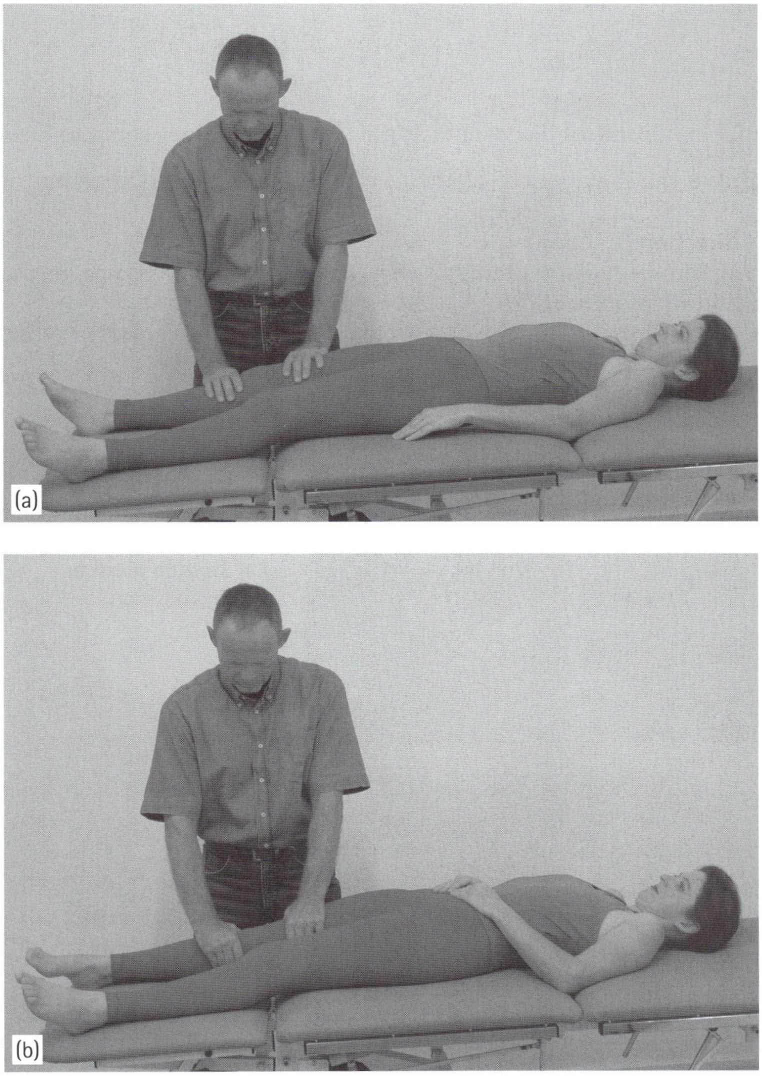

Figure 8.21a and b
Passive angular movement; internal rotation of the hip joint; therapy technique.
a, Starting position.
b, End position.

Movement:

- passive movement of patient's hip joint into internal rotation by rolling patient's leg over the plinth (Fig. 8.21b)
- then moving the leg back to starting position.

Self-exercise (film 60)

Patient's starting position:

- supine, in a position as symptom-free as possible (Fig. 8.22a)
- the hip joint pre-positioned in external rotation.

Movement:

- active movement of the hip joint into internal rotation by rolling the leg over the plinth (Fig. 8.22b)
- then moving the leg back to starting position.

Remarks

Goals of the technique

With an acute lumboradicular syndrome of discogenic origin, these techniques serve to:

- reduce tonicity and improve the metabolism of the affected tissues by mobilization of symptomatic tissue:
  - in symptom-reducing direction (traction)
  - by application of a symptom-provoking stimulus with dose adjusted according to the current load tolerance (neural mobilization)
- restore pain-free function (change the input to the respective centres of the central nervous system (CNS)).

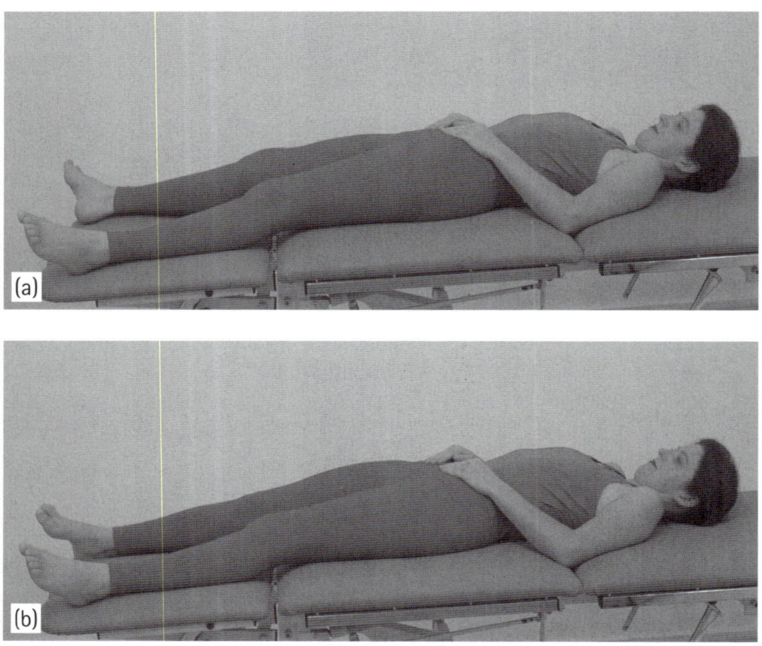

Figure 8.22a and b
Passive angular movement; internal rotation of the hip joint; self-exercise.
a, Starting position.
b, End position.

Performance

The patient's typical symptoms must *not* be reproduced by the demonstrated techniques during the acute phase.

Dosage

The described acute presentation (predominantly peripheral-nociceptive) corresponds with the inflammation phase and therefore requires the following dosage for the described techniques targeting the symptomatic tissue.

Acute presentation (predominantly peripheral pain mechanisms)			
Phase	Limitation of movement due to pain and resistance	Concept	Movement grade
Inflammation phase	No pain	Kaltenborn–Evjenth	Up to the beginning of II
	No resistance	Maitland	Up to II

Choice of technique

The selection of the technique depends, among other things, on the therapist as well as the patient, on the therapist's clinical experience, but primarily on reassessment. This means that even if all preconditions on the part of therapist and patient seem to be met, it is of no use to continue the technique if reassessment is negative.

To preserve achieved treatment results in this acute phase and to avoid worsening of the state due to negative movement input, it is often useful to support the lumbar spine externally with a firm belt (lumbar corset) so as to restrict its movements.

Contributing factors

For a satisfactory solution of the patient's current problems it is important to consider the contributing factors and include them in the treatment.

The authors will, however, not go deeper into a description of the various possibilities and their complex contexts as this would exceed the scope of the present book.

TREATMENT EXAMPLE, LUMBAR SPINE: SUBACUTE RADICULAR SYNDROME

SYMPTOMATIC MOVEMENT

Movement of the lumbar spine into flexion provokes pain in the buttocks and dorsolateral thigh.

ASSESSMENTS

Area localization

Area localization hints at the lumbar spine with neural involvement. There is no contraindication for movement.

Neurology

Neurological examination yields the following data:

Function:

- key muscles: weakening of the extensor hallucis longus muscle
- sensitivity: hypoaesthesia in dermatome L5
- reflexes: slight hyporeflexia of the Achilles tendon reflex.

Neurodynamics:

- SLR: lifting the extended right leg (SLR) shows changed quality of movement (resistance behaviour during movement) as well as changed sensory response (area and type of sensation) as compared with the left side
- slump test: examination with the slump test shows that the patient's typical symptoms can be reproduced by movement of the right knee into extension.

Specific provocation and alleviation

Specific provocation and alleviation hints at symptom provocation by L4 in flexion, with neural involvement.

Specific mobility

Specific mobility tests indicate hypomobility of L4 in flexion and rotation to the right.

Palpation

Palpation shows increased tension and increased tenderness of the right lumbar paravertebral muscles as compared with the opposite side. The patient shows a positive *bow string sign* on the right side (provocation of the patient's typical symptoms by pressure on the tibial nerve put under tension in the popliteal region of the affected side).

HYPOTHESIS

A subacute lumboradicular syndrome of discogenic origin, with restricted specific mobility of L4 into flexion and rotation to the right is suspected (Fig. 8.23).

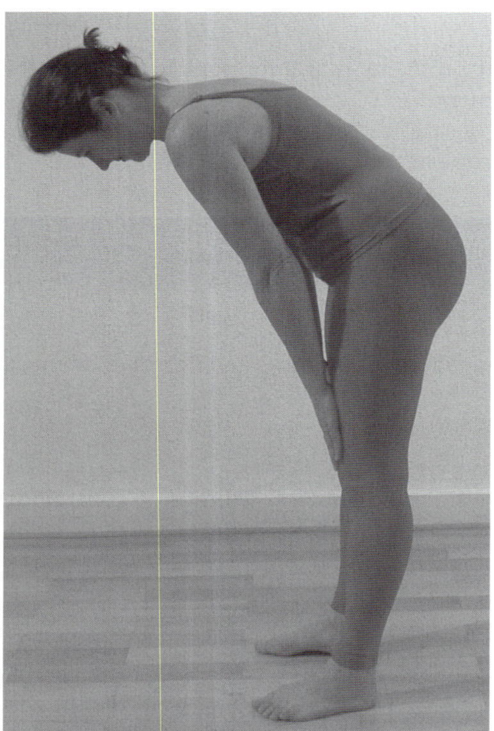

Figure 8.23 Symptom-provoking movement: flexion of the spine provokes pain in the buttocks and dorsolateral thigh, right side.

RELAXATION TECHNIQUES

Hold–relax techniques

MOVEMENT-DIRECTED CONTRACTION IN THE DIRECTION OPPOSING THE PAINFUL AND/OR RESTRICTED DIRECTION

Therapy technique (film 61)

Patient's starting position:

- sitting on the plinth, arms folded in front of the chest (Fig. 8.24a).

Therapist's starting position:

- standing, at the patient's right side
- fixing the patient's thorax by grasping the patient's shoulder girdle from the front.

Movement:

- adjusting the spine in flexion and rotation to the right (Fig. 8.24b)
- in this position, the therapist tries to move the spine further into flexion and rotation to the right, while the patient prevents this movement by muscle contraction.

Self-exercise (film 62)

Patient's starting position:

- sitting on a chair, spine pre-positioned in flexion and rotation to the right (Fig. 8.25a)
- a belt tied around the right front leg of the chair is grasped with the hands.

Movement:

- extension and rotation of the spine to the left against fixation (Fig. 8.25b).

MOVEMENT-DIRECTED CONTRACTION IN THE PAINFUL AND/OR RESTRICTED DIRECTION

Therapy technique (film 63)

Patient's starting position:

- sitting on the plinth, arms folded in front of the chest (Fig. 8.26a).

Therapist's starting position:

- standing, at the patient's right side
- fixing the patient's thorax by grasping the patient's shoulder girdle and thorax from the front.

Movement:

- adjusting the spine in flexion and rotation to the right (Fig. 8.26b)
- in this position, the therapist tries to move back into extension and rotation to the left, while the patient prevents this movement by muscle contraction.

Self-exercise (film 64)

Patient's starting position:

- sitting on a chair, pre-positioned in flexion and rotation to the right (Fig. 8.27a)
- the left hand is placed on the thigh while the right hand takes hold of the left wrist.

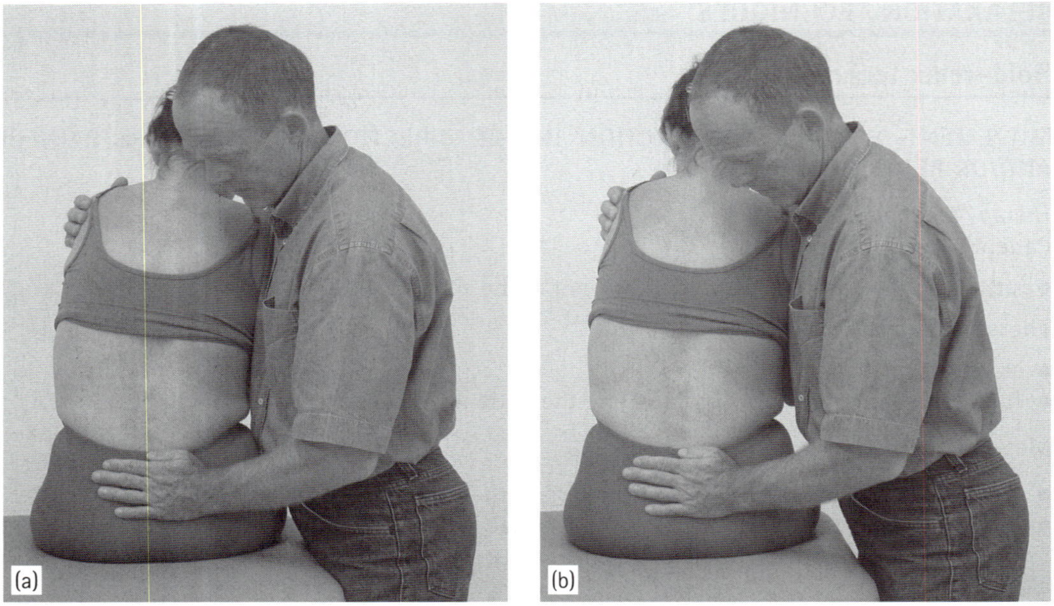

Figure 8.24a and b Hold–relax technique; movement-directed contraction in the direction opposing the painful and/or restricted direction; therapy technique. a, Starting position. b, End position.

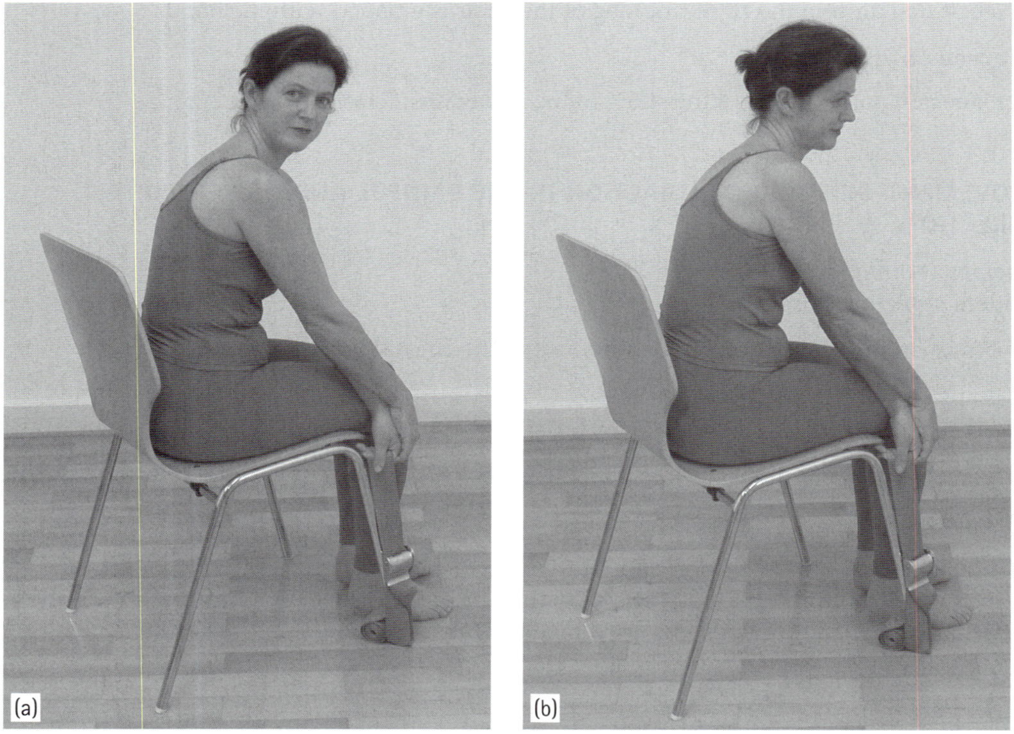

Figure 8.25a and b Hold–relax technique; movement-directed contraction in the direction opposing the painful and/or restricted direction; self-exercise. a, Starting position. b, End position.

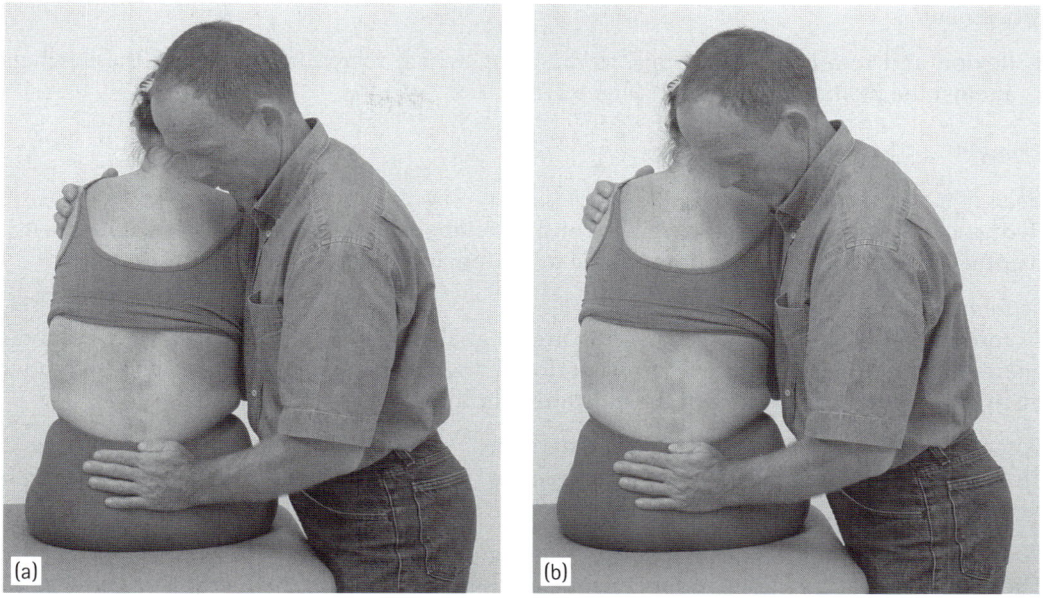

Figure 8.26a and b Hold–relax technique; movement-directed contraction in the painful and/or restricted direction; therapy technique. **a**, Starting position. **b**, End position.

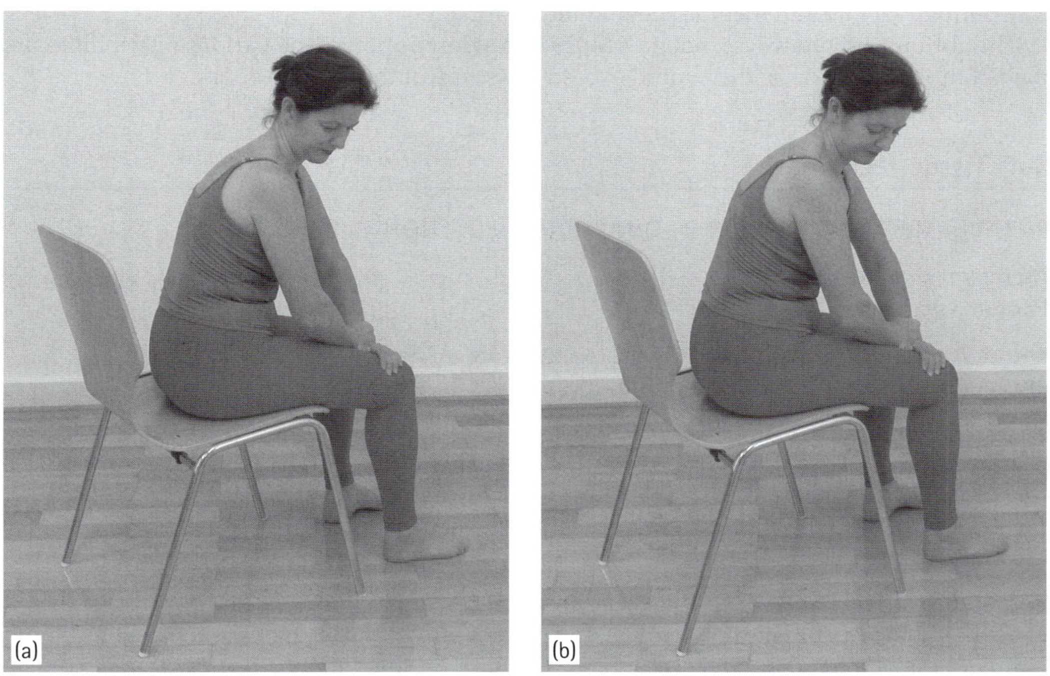

Figure 8.27a and b Hold–relax technique; movement-directed contraction in the painful and/or restricted direction; self-exercise. **a**, Starting position. **b**, End position.

Movement:

- flexion and rotation of the trunk to the right, which increasingly presses the left hand against the fixation on the thigh (Fig. 8.27b).

Remarks

Goals of the technique
Reduction of tonicity and improvement of the metabolism of the periarticular tissues with a painful movement restriction of the spine in flexion and rotation to the right.

Performance
According to irritability or the desired treatment goal, the joint to be treated is pre-positioned before treatment. As the self-exercise is performed without *specific fixation*, transferred movement has to be considered when the indication for the exercise is determined.

Dosage (regarding the affected symptomatic structure)
Neither with adjustment nor with contraction must the patient's typical symptoms be reproduced.

Choice of technique
The selection of the technique depends, among other things, on the therapist as well as the patient, on the therapist's clinical experience, but primarily on reassessment. This means that even if all preconditions on the part of therapist and patient seem to be met, it is of no use to continue the technique if reassessment is negative.

Contributing factors
For a satisfactory solution of the patient's current problems it is important to consider the contributing factors and include them in the treatment.

The authors will, however, not go deeper into a description of the various possibilities and their complex contexts as this would exceed the scope of the present book.

Soft tissue techniques

PARAVERTEBRAL MUSCLES, IN QUADRUPED POSITION

Therapy technique (film 65)
Patient's starting position:

- quadruped position, at the end of the plinth (Fig. 8.28a)
- the feet protrude beyond the plinth.

Therapist's starting position:

- standing, behind the patient
- both hands placed over the patient's lumbar paravertebral muscles.

Movement:

- pressure on the paravertebral muscles in a ventrocranial direction (Fig. 8.28b)
- against this pressure of the therapist, the patient moves the buttocks to the heels. Thereby, the therapist's hands glide in a cranial direction on the patient's back without reducing pressure on the soft tissues
- then releasing pressure, and back to starting position.

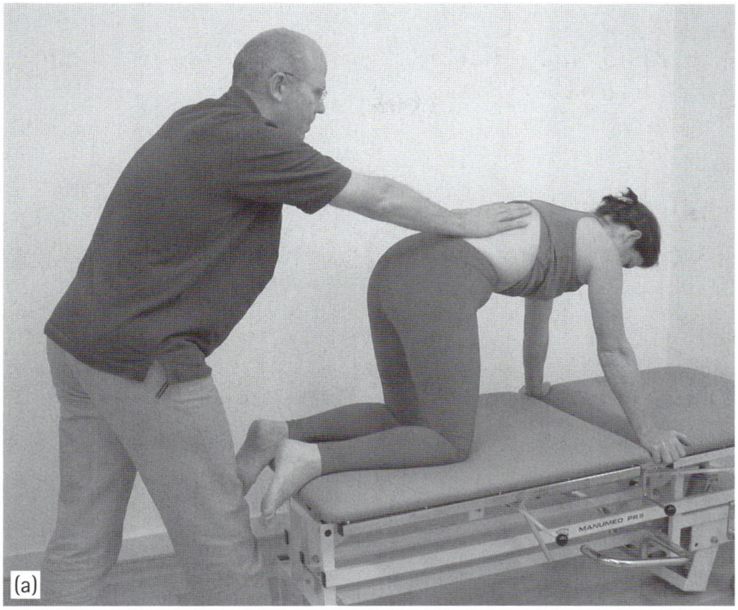

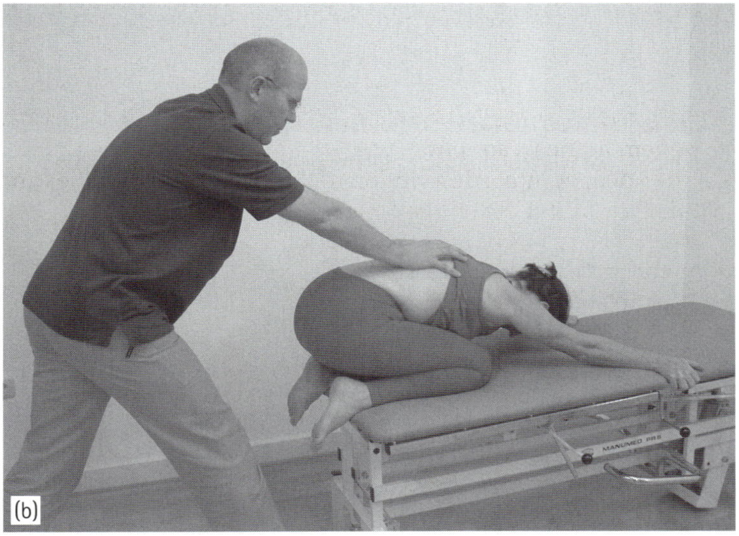

Figure 8.28a and b
Soft tissue technique; paravertebral muscles bilaterally; therapy technique. **a**, Starting position. **b**, End position.

Self-exercise (film 66)

Patient's starting position:

- sitting on a chair (Fig. 8.29a)
- two tennis balls in a sock placed between the paravertebral muscles and the back of the chair
- arms folded in front of the chest.

Movement:

- increasing the pressure on the balls by pushing the feet against the floor and pushing the thorax backwards against the balls (Fig. 8.29b)

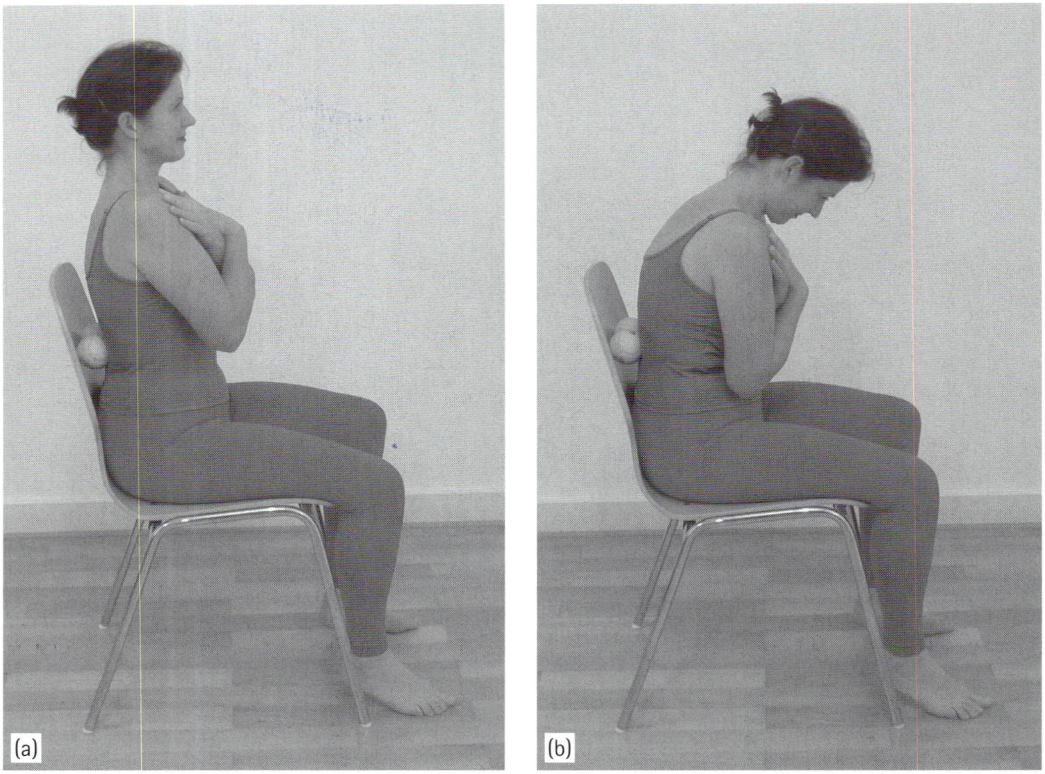

Figure 8.29a and b Soft tissue technique; paravertebral muscles bilaterally; self-exercise. a, Starting position. b, End position.

- moving the spine into flexion while maintaining pressure
- then releasing pressure, and back to starting position.

PARAVERTEBRAL MUSCLES, RIGHT SIDE, IN PRONE POSITION

Therapy technique (film 67)

Patient's starting position:

- prone, on the plinth (Fig. 8.30a)
- spine pre-positioned in flexion (cushion under the abdomen), slight lateral flexion to the left.

Therapist's starting position:

- standing, at the patient's left side, at the level of the pelvis
- grasping the patient's pelvis ventrally with right hand, at the level of the anterior superior iliac spine, while contacting the patient's right lumbar paravertebral muscles with the thenar of the left hand.

Movement:

- passive rotation of the pelvis to the right with simultaneous manual pressure on the paravertebral muscles, right side (Fig. 8.30b)
- releasing pressure, and back to starting position.

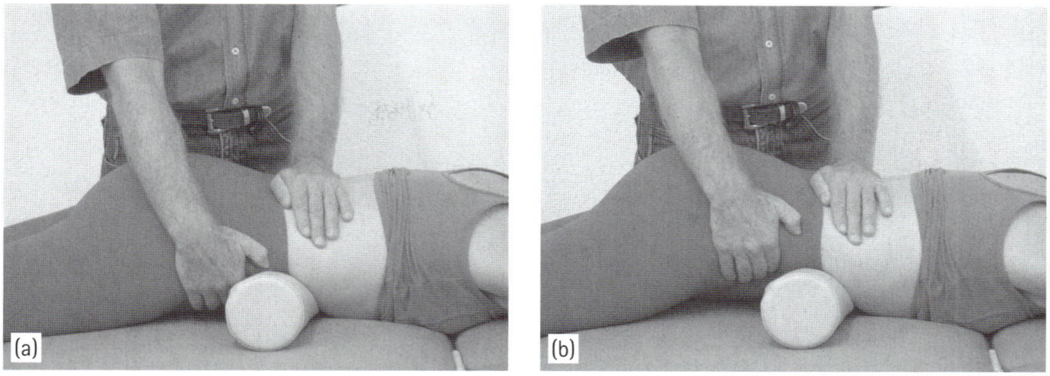

Figure 8.30a and b Soft tissue technique; right paravertebral muscles; therapy technique. a, Starting position. b, End position.

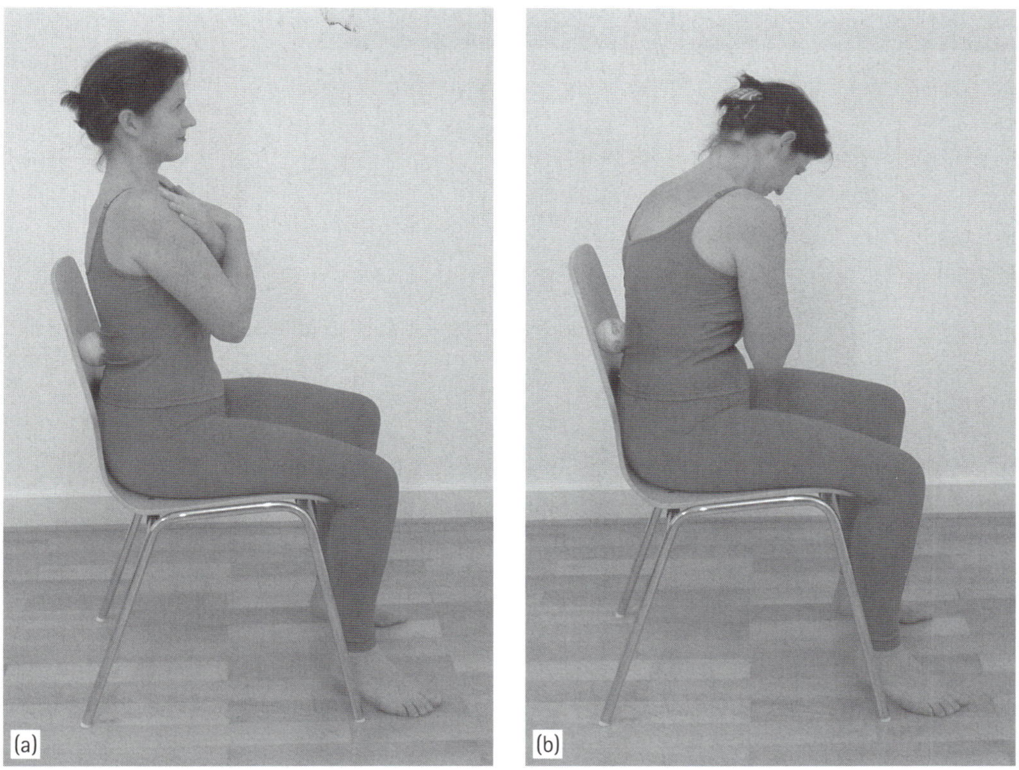

Figure 8.31a and b Soft tissue technique; right paravertebral muscles; self-exercise. a, Starting position. b, End position.

Self-exercise (film 68)

Patient's starting position:

- sitting on a chair (Fig. 8.31a)
- a tennis ball placed between right paravertebral muscles and back of the chair
- arms folded in front of the chest.

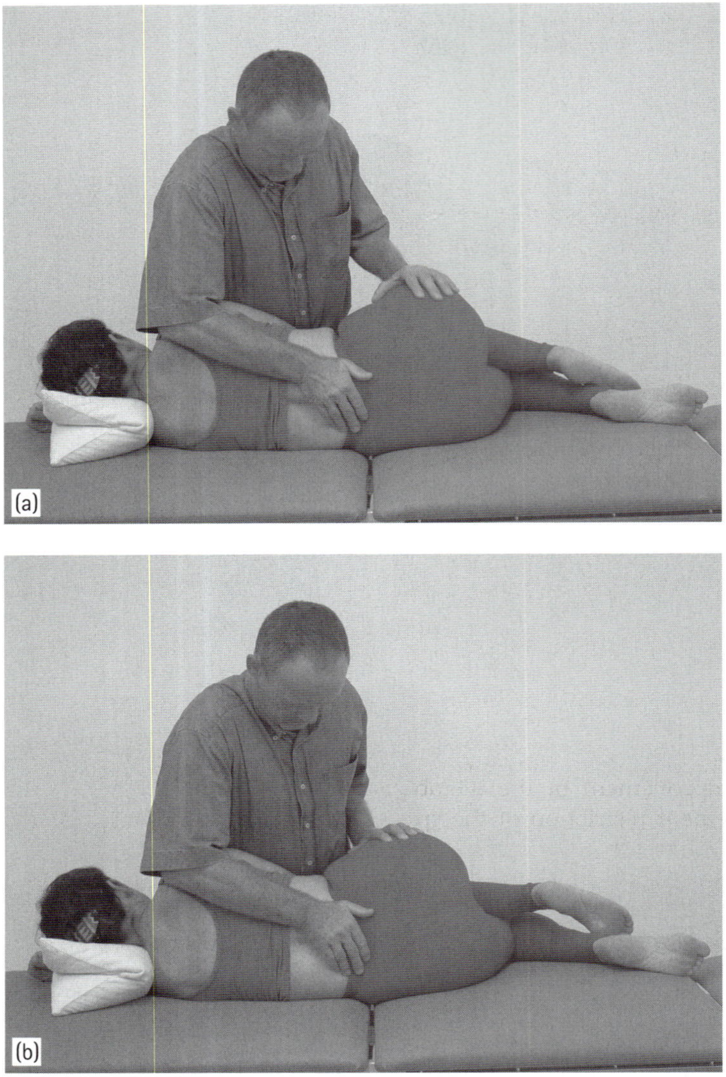

Figure 8.32a and b Soft tissue technique; right paravertebral muscles; therapy technique.
a, Starting position.
b, End position.

Movement:

- increasing the pressure on the ball by pushing the feet against the floor and pushing the thorax backwards against the ball (Fig. 8.31b)
- moving spine into flexion and rotation to the left while maintaining pressure
- then releasing pressure, and back to starting position.

PARAVERTEBRAL MUSCLES, RIGHT SIDE, IN SIDE-LYING POSITION

Therapy technique (film 69)

Patient's starting position:

- lying on the left side (Fig. 8.32a)
- arms folded in front of the chest

- the spine pre-positioned in flexion and lateral flexion to the right
- knee of the upper, right leg placed somewhat in front of the lower, left leg.

Therapist's starting position:

- standing, in front of the patient
- therapist's thorax leaning, for fixation, against patient's arms, while the thenar of therapist's right hand contacts patient's paravertebral muscles
- therapist's left hand resting on right side of patient's pelvis.

Movement:

- passive movement of the pelvis in ventrocranial direction (rotation of pelvis to the left – rotation of lumbar spine to the right) with simultaneous manual pressure on the paravertebral muscles, right side (Fig. 8.32b)
- releasing pressure, and back to starting position.

> ***Note:*** If the patient is not able to relax or if performance of the movement seems too difficult, this soft tissue technique can also be performed assistively.

Remarks

Goals of the technique

Reduction of tonicity and improvement of the metabolism of the lumbar paravertebral muscles with a painful movement restriction of the spine into flexion and rotation to the right.

Performance

Treatment is done in the pain-free range of movement. As the treatment techniques are performed without *specific fixation*, transferred movement has to be considered when the indication for the technique is determined.

Dosage (regarding the affected symptomatic structure)

Both with an acute and with a chronic presentation, application of these techniques should always be pain-free.

Choice of technique

The selection of the technique depends, among other things, on the therapist as well as the patient, on the therapist's clinical experience, but primarily on reassessment. This means that even if all preconditions on the part of therapist and patient seem to be met, it is of no use to continue the technique if reassessment is negative.

Contributing factors

For a satisfactory solution of the patient's current problems it is important to consider the contributing factors and include them in the treatment.

The authors will, however, not go deeper into a description of the various possibilities and their complex contexts as this would exceed the scope of the present book.

MOBILIZATION TECHNIQUES

Active procedures

ACTIVE MOBILIZATION

Rotation of L4 to the right, in side-lying position

Therapy technique (film 70)

Patient's starting position:

- side-lying position (Fig. 8.33a)
- lumbar spine in flexion and slight lateral flexion to the right
- the left hand placed on the right thigh, the right holding in the back of the neck.

Therapist's starting position:

- standing, behind the patient
- contact with the ulnar edge of the left hand on the costal process of L5.

Movement:

- rotation of the lumbar spine to the right (Fig. 8.33b).

Rotation of L4 to the right, in sitting

Therapy technique (film 71)

Patient's starting position:

- sitting (Fig. 8.34a)
- lumbar spine in flexion and slight lateral flexion to the right
- arms folded in front of the chest.

Therapist's starting position:

- standing, behind the patient
- a belt running, for fixation, around patient's pelvis from anterior and around therapist's pelvis from posterior
- contact with both thumbs on the right costal process of L5
- shifting therapist's pelvis in posterior direction to fix patient's pelvis.

Movement:

- pressure of both thumbs in anterior direction against right costal process of L5 to fix L5, and subsequent active rotation of the lumbar spine to the right (Fig. 8.34b).

Self-exercise (film 72)

Patient's starting position:

- sitting on a chair (Fig. 8.35a)
- a tennis ball placed at the level of L5 (possibly marked by tape to be more easily identified by the patient) between right paravertebral muscles and back of the chair
- arms folded in front of chest.

Movement:

- increasing the pressure on the ball by pushing the feet against the floor and pushing the thorax backwards against the ball (Fig. 8.35b)

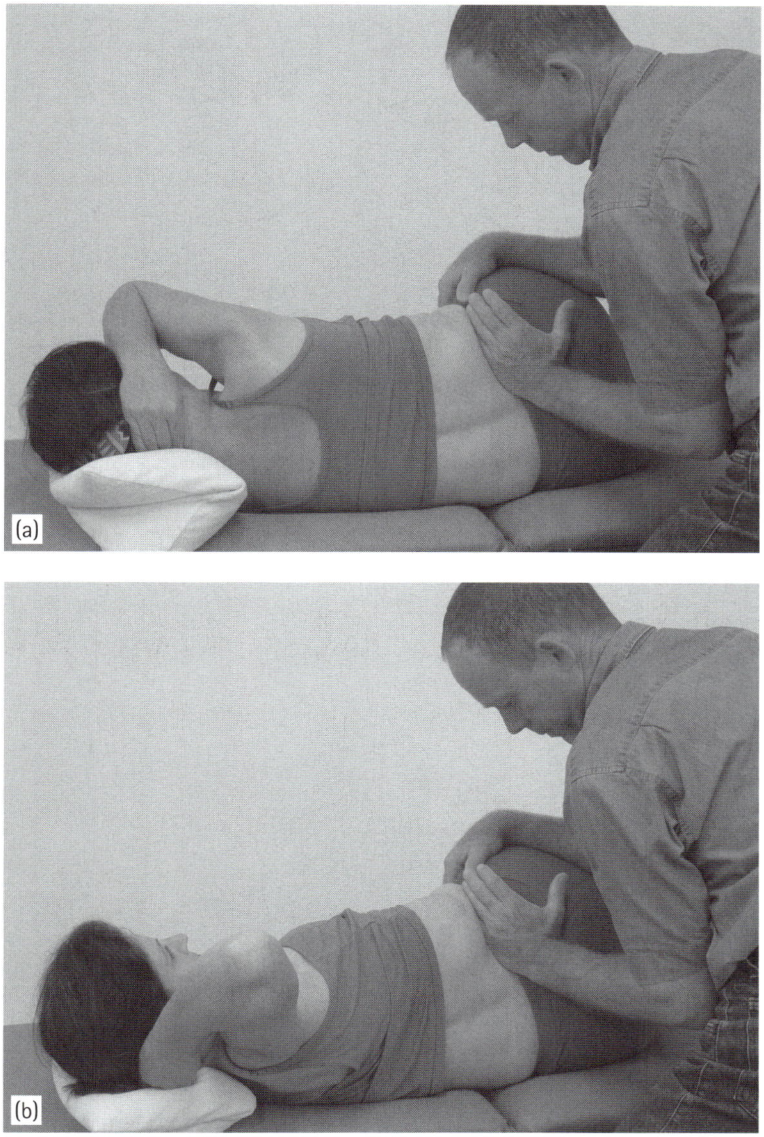

Figure 8.33a and b Active mobilization; rotation to the right (side-lying); therapy technique. **a**, Starting position. **b**, End position.

- moving spine into lateral flexion to the right, rotation to the right, and slight flexion, while maintaining pressure
- then releasing pressure, and back to starting position.

Note: As flexion is the predominant symptom-provoking component, flexion is not emphasized too much in this phase of the current presentation. This 'precautionary measure' is recommended because of the lack of control in self-exercise.

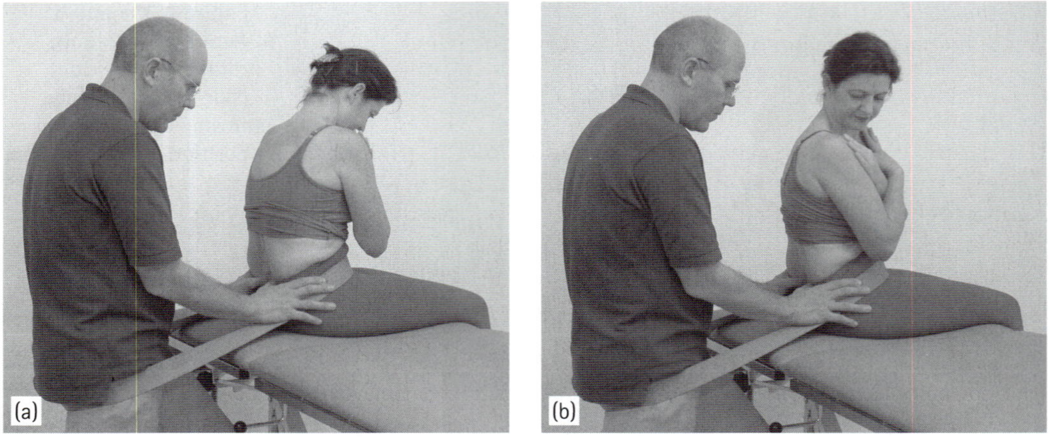

Figure 8.34a and b Active mobilization; rotation to the right (sitting); therapy technique. a, Starting position. b, End position.

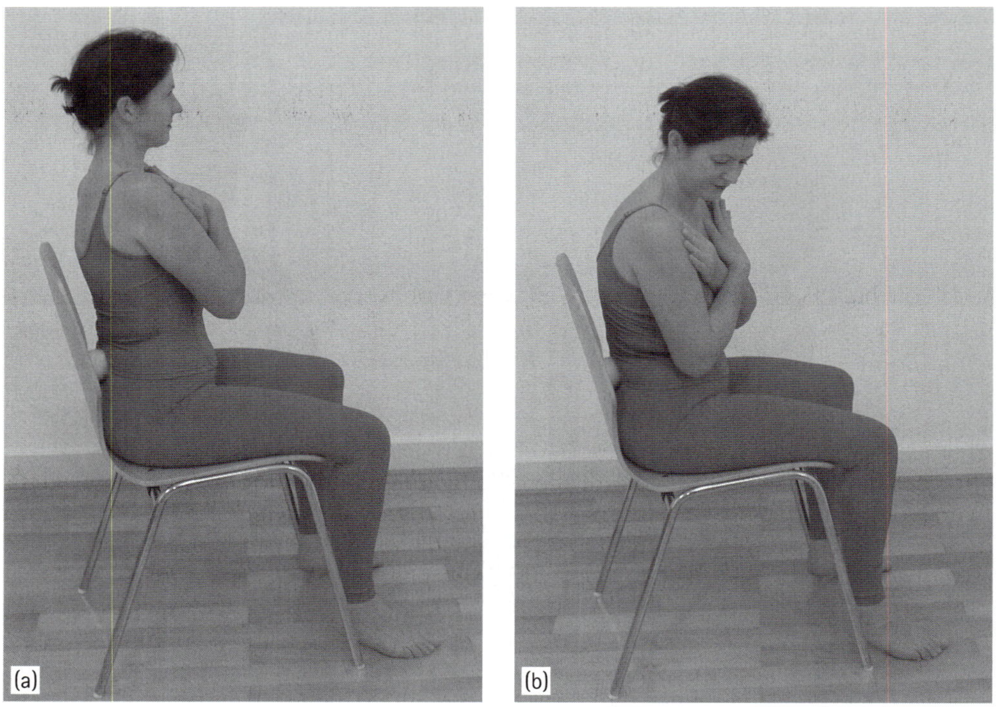

Figure 8.35a and b Active mobilization; rotation to the right (sitting); self-exercise. a, Starting position. b, End position.

Remarks

Goals of the technique

With a subacute lumboradicular syndrome of discogenic origin, these techniques serve to reduce tonicity and improve the metabolism of the affected tissues, by mobilizing symptomatic tissue to apply a symptom-provoking stimulus dosed according to the current load tolerance.

Performance
The demonstrated techniques should not reproduce the symptoms in the leg in this subacute phase.

Dosage
The described subacute presentation (predominantly peripheral-nociceptive) corresponds with the proliferation phase as well as with the first section of the remodelling phase and therefore requires the following dosage for the techniques described. As flexion is the symptom-provoking component, this movement component is employed very carefully at the assumed healing stage. In later phases, the individual movement directions will often be chosen in a different sequence, to improve the loading capacity of the symptomatic tissue.

Phase	Limitation of movement due to pain and resistance	Concept	Movement grade
Proliferation phase	Up to P1	Kaltenborn-Evjenth	Up to the 1st third of II
	Slowly progressing up to low resistance	Maitland	Up to III$^-$
Remodelling/organization phase	Slowly progressing up to maximum resistance	Kaltenborn-Evjenth	Up to III
	(Note: duration of turnover!)	Maitland	Up to IV^{++} or III^{++}

Note: The chances of a disturbed (delayed) course of healing and the consequences for the loading capacity of the tissue (e.g., diabetes, old age, partial or general immobilization) have to be considered.

Choice of technique
The selection of the technique depends, among other things, on the therapist as well as the patient, on the therapist's clinical experience, but primarily on reassessment. This means that even if all preconditions on the part of therapist and patient seem to be met, it is of no use to continue the technique if reassessment is negative.

Contributing factors
For a satisfactory solution of the patient's current problems it is important to consider the contributing factors and include them in the treatment.

The authors will, however, not go deeper into a description of the various possibilities and their complex contexts as this would exceed the scope of the present book.

ACTIVE MOBILIZATION PLUS ACCESSORY MOVEMENT

Neural mobilization with ventrocranial push on L4, in side-lying position

Therapy technique (film 73)
Patient's starting position:

- lying on the left side (Fig. 8.36a)
- hips and knees flexed
- the spine may be pre-positioned in flexion to achieve greater neural pretension.

Therapist's starting position:

- standing, in front of the patient
- contact with the wedge on the laminae of L4.

Movement:

- pushing L4 in a ventrocranial direction, then having the patient move the foot into dorsal flexion and the knee into extension (Fig. 8.36b)
- then having the patient move leg back, and releasing pressure.

Neural mobilization with ventrocranial push on L4, in sitting

Therapy technique (film 74)

Patient's starting position:

- sitting (Fig. 8.37a)
- a belt loop running around patient's pelvis from anterior and around the therapist's pelvis from posterior.

Therapist's starting position:

- standing, behind the patient
- contact with the thumbs on the patient's spinous process of L4

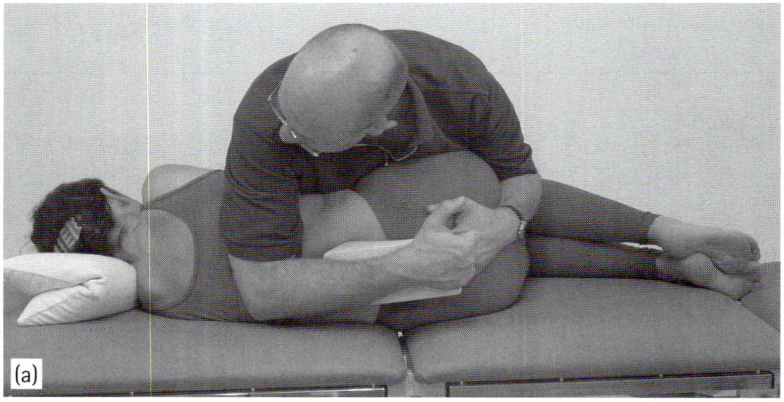

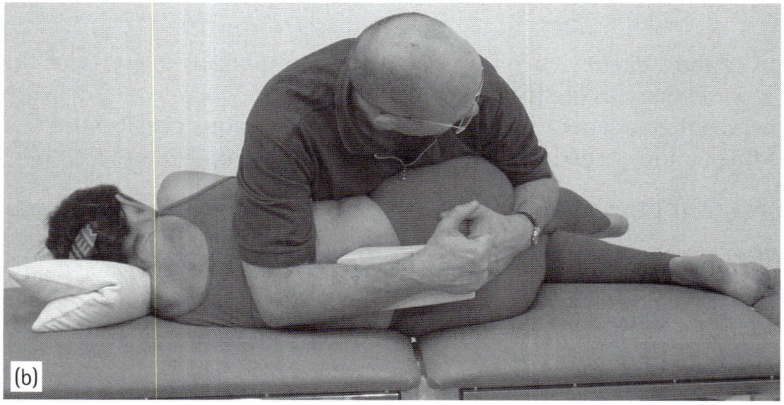

Figure 8.36a and b Active mobilization with accessory movement; neural mobilization with ventrocranial push on L4 (side-lying); therapy technique. **a**, Starting position. **b**, End position.

- the belt is tensed by the therapist leaning back, which provides an abutment for the thumb pressure.

Movement:

- pushing L4 in a ventrocranial direction, then having the patient move the foot into dorsal flexion and the knee into extension (Fig. 8.37b)
- then having the patient move the leg back, and releasing pressure.

Self-exercise (film 75)

Patient's starting position:

- sitting (Fig. 8.38a)
- contacting the spinous process of L4 caudally with the proximal phalanx of the second finger (position may be marked by tape).

Movement:

- pressure on spinous process of L4 in a ventrocranial direction (Fig. 8.38b)
- moving lumbar spine into flexion by tilting pelvis in a posterior direction, while maintaining pressure
- in this position, moving right foot into dorsal flexion and right knee into extension
- moving back and leg back into starting position, and releasing pressure.

Flexion with transversal push on L4, in side-lying

Therapy technique (film 76)

Patient's starting position:

- lying on the right side (Fig. 8.39a)
- hips and knees slightly flexed
- spine may be pre-positioned in flexion, from cranial, so as to achieve greater neural pretension.

Therapist's starting position:

- standing, in front of the patient
- contact with ulnar edge of left hand on patient's costal process of L4.

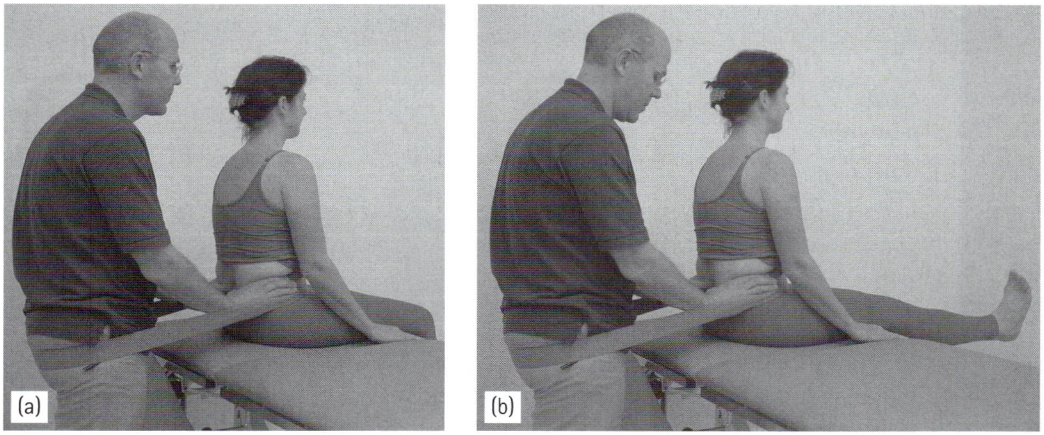

Figure 8.37a and b Active mobilization with accessory movement; neural mobilization with ventrocranial push on L4 (sitting); therapy technique. **a**, Starting position. **b**, End position.

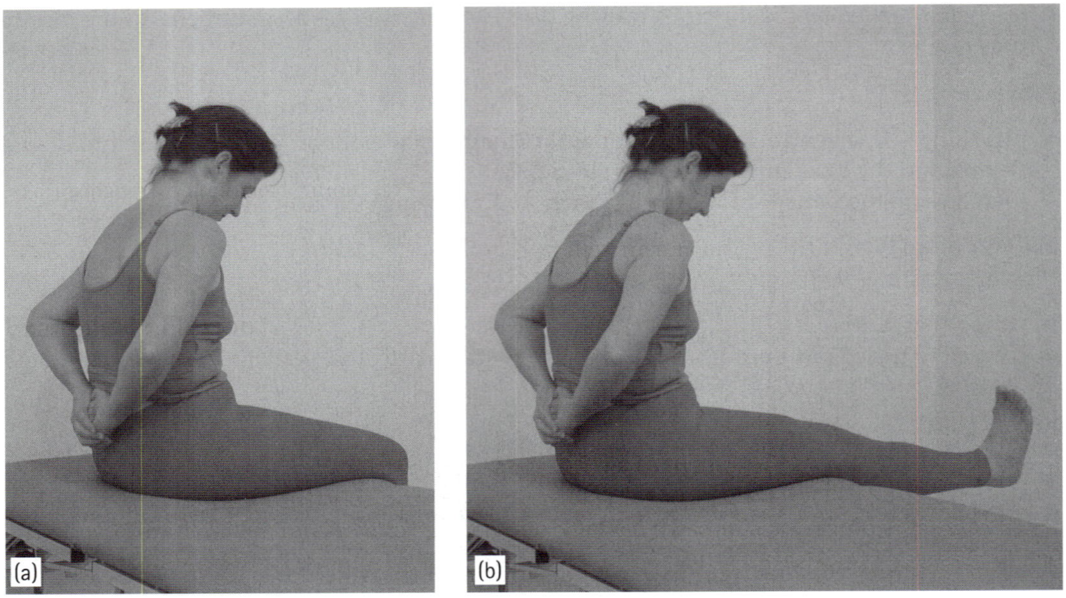

Figure 8.38a and b Active mobilization with accessory movement; neural mobilization with ventrocranial push on L4 (sitting); self-exercise. a, Starting position. b, End position.

Movement:

- transversal push of L4 to the right, then moving left hip into flexion so far that the movement continues into the lumbar spine (Fig. 8.39b)
- moving leg back, and releasing pressure.

> *Note:* If the actual force and size relations of patient/therapist do not allow this one-armed mobilization technique, the transversal push should be done with both arms. In that case, the patient has to move the left leg himself/herself. It is best if the therapist stands behind the patient so as not to impede movement of the leg.

Self-exercise (film 77)

Patient's starting position:

- standing beside the plinth (Fig. 8.40a)
- a belt runs around patient's trunk at the level of L4 and is fixed to some firm object
- right hand supporting against the plinth
- the belt length is such that the elbow is slightly flexed.

Movement:

- shifting weight onto left leg with simultaneous push via right hand leads to a transversal pushing of L4 to the right by the belt (Fig. 8.40b)
- moving right hip into flexion so far that movement continues into lumbar spine, while maintaining transversal push
- moving leg back into starting position, and releasing pressure.

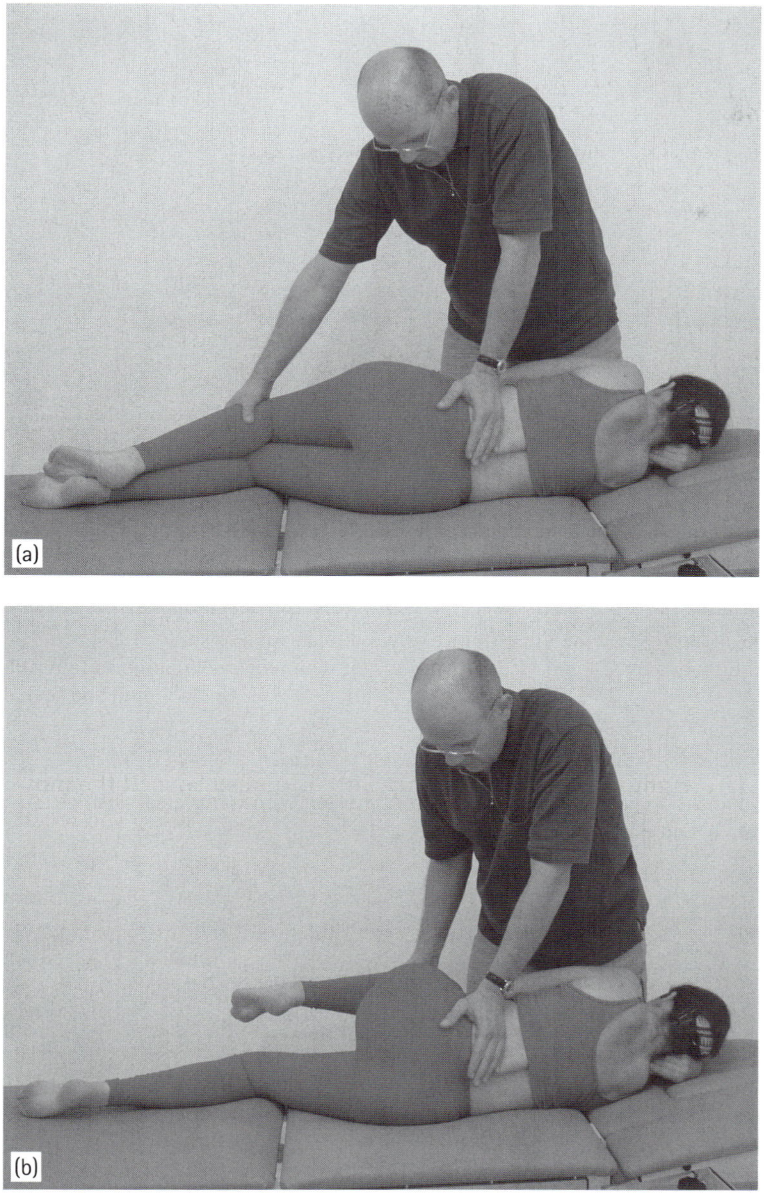

Figure 8.39a and b
Active mobilization with accessory movement; flexion with transversal push on L4 (side-lying); therapy technique.
a, Starting position.
b, End position.

Flexion with ventrocranial push on L4, quadruped position

Therapy technique (film 78)

Patient's starting position:

- quadruped position, at the end of the plinth (Fig. 8.41a)
- feet protruding beyond the plinth.

Therapist's starting position:

- standing, behind the patient
- both thumbs placed on patient's spinous process of L4.

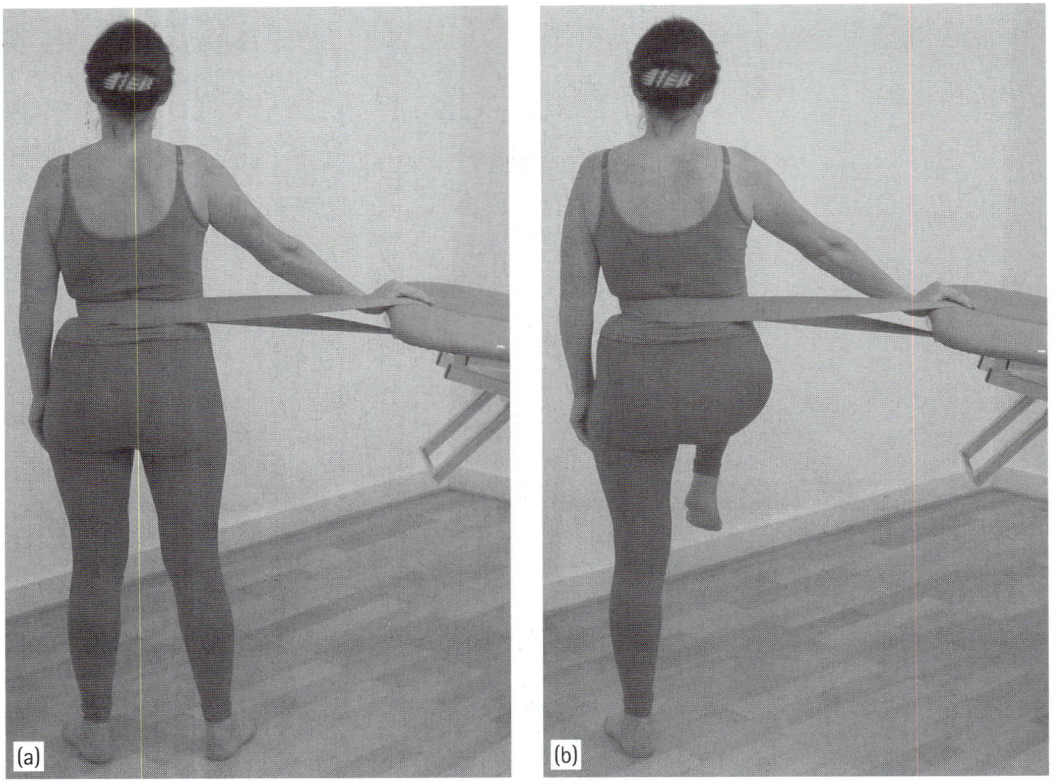

Figure 8.40a and b Active mobilization with accessory movement; flexion with transversal push on L4; self-exercise. a, Starting position. b, End position.

Movement:

- pressure on the spinous process of L4 in a ventrocranial direction (Fig. 8.41b)
- patient moves buttocks towards the heels without changing position of the hands, while pressure is maintained
- then back to starting position, and releasing pressure.

Flexion with ventrocranial push on L4, in sitting

Therapy technique (film 79)

Patient's starting position:

- sitting (Fig. 8.42a)
- a belt loop running around patient's pelvis from the front and around therapist's pelvis from behind.

Therapist's starting position:

- standing, behind the patient
- contact with hypothenar on patient's spinous process of L4
- by leaning back, the therapist tenses the belt, which provides an abutment for hypothenar pressure.

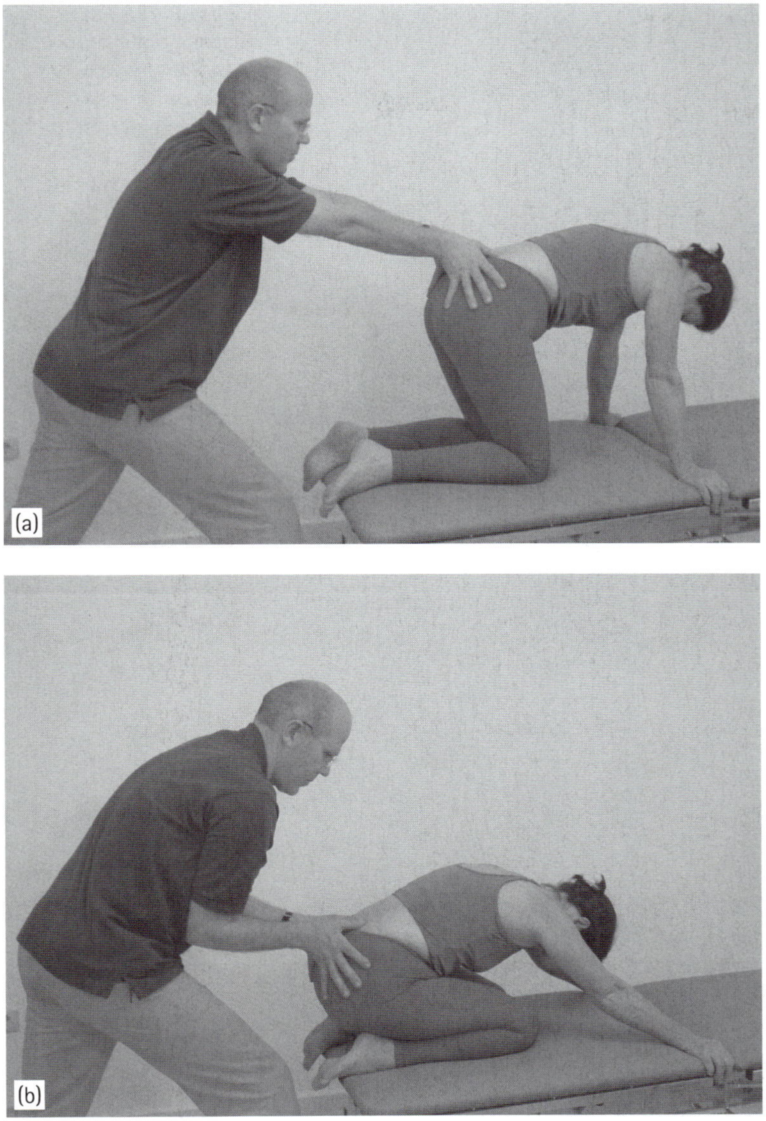

Figure 8.41a and b
Active mobilization with accessory movement; flexion with ventrocranial push on L4 (quadruped position); therapy technique.
a, Starting position.
b, End position.

Movement:

- pushing L4 in ventrocranial direction, then having patient move spine into flexion (Fig. 8.42b)
- having patient move spine back, and releasing the push.

Self-exercise (film 80)

Patient's starting position:

- sitting (Fig. 8.43a)
- contacting the spinous process of L4 caudally with the proximal phalanx of the second finger (position may be marked by tape).

Movement:

- pressure on spinous process of L4 in a ventrocranial direction (Fig. 8.43b)

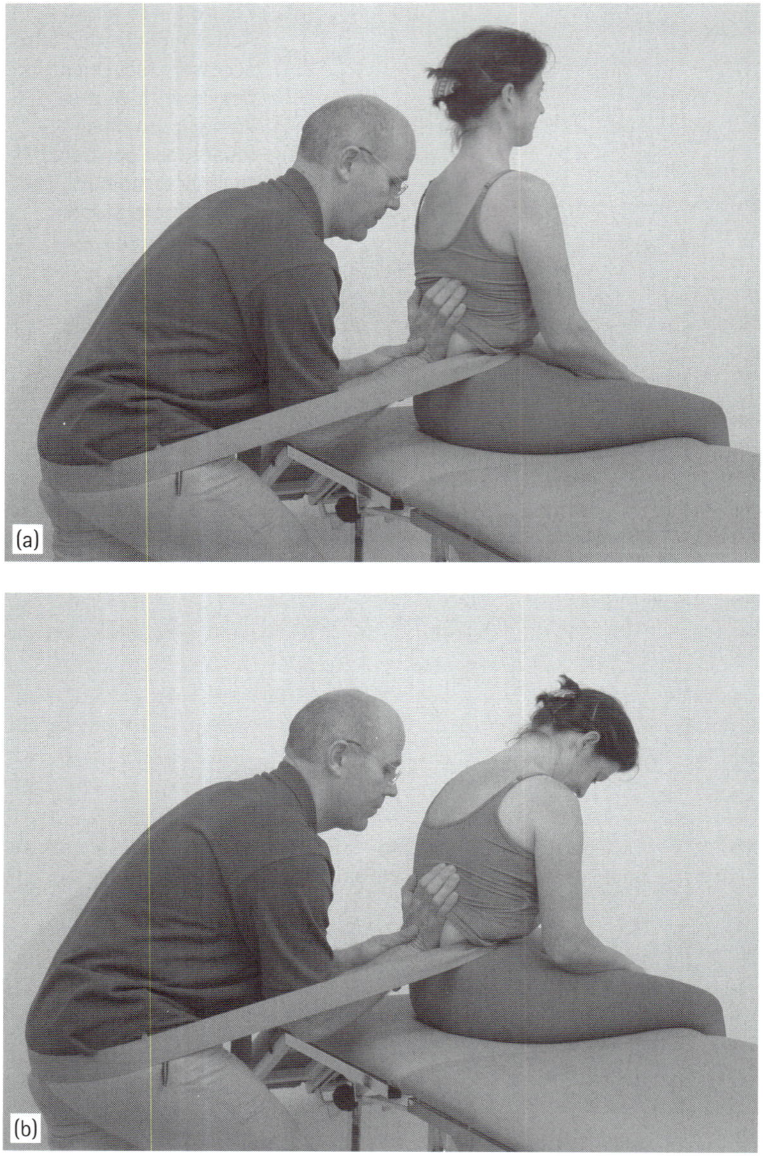

Figure 8.42a and b
Active mobilization with accessory movement; flexion with ventrocranial push on L4 (sitting); therapy technique. **a**, Starting position. **b**, End position.

- moving lumbar spine into flexion by tilting pelvis in a posterior direction, while maintaining pressure
- back to starting position, and releasing pressure.

Remarks

Goals of the technique

With a subacute lumboradicular syndrome of discogenic origin, these techniques serve to:

- reduce tonicity and improve the metabolism of the affected tissues
- restore pain-free function (perhaps through changing the input to the respective centres of the CNS).

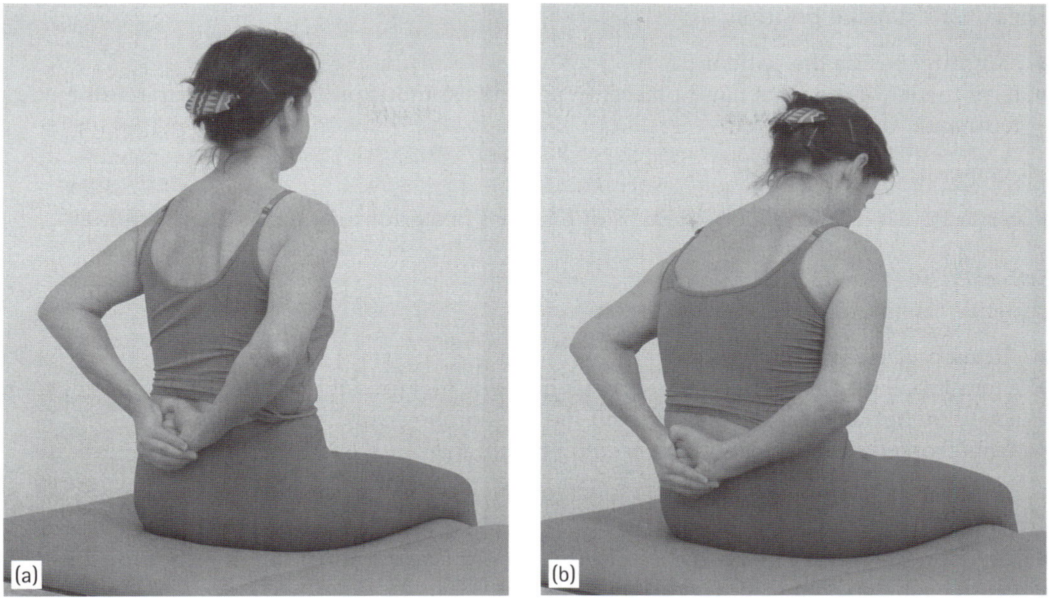

Figure 8.43a and b Active mobilization with accessory movement; flexion with ventrocranial push on L4 (sitting); self-exercise. **a**, Starting position. **b**, End position.

Performance
The demonstrated techniques should not reproduce the patient's typical symptoms.

Dosage
With the described clinical presentation, too early a vertical load on the spine may worsen the situation. By changing the vertical load – as shown in these techniques – the dosage can be adjusted accordingly after reassessment.

Choice of technique
The selection of the technique depends, among other things, on the therapist as well as the patient, on the therapist's clinical experience, but primarily on reassessment. This means that even if all preconditions on the part of therapist and patient seem to be met, it is of no use to continue the technique if reassessment is negative.

Contributing factors
For a satisfactory solution of the patient's current problems it is important to consider the contributing factors and include them in the treatment.

The authors will, however, not go deeper into a description of the various possibilities and their complex contexts as this would exceed the scope of the present book.

Passive procedures

ACCESSORY MOVEMENTS

Central push in posterior–anterior direction

Therapy technique (film 81)
Patient's starting position:

- prone (Fig. 8.44a).

Therapist's starting position:

- standing, beside the patient
- hypothenar of the right hand placed on patient's spinous process of L4, grip reinforced by left hand.

Movement:

- central push on the spinous process of L4, from posterior to anterior (Fig. 8.44b).

Self-exercise (film 82)

Patient's starting position:

- sitting on a chair (Fig. 8.45a)
- a tennis ball placed between the spinous process of L4 (possibly marked by tape to be more easily identifiable for the patient) and the back of the chair
- arms crossed over the chest or placed on the thighs.

Movement:

- increasing the pressure on the ball by pushing the feet against the floor and pushing the trunk backwards against the ball (Fig. 8.45b)
- this results in central pressure on L4 in a posterior-anterior direction
- releasing pressure, and back to starting position.

Unilateral push in posterior-anterior direction

Therapy technique (film 83)

Patient's starting position:

- prone (Fig. 8.46a).

Therapist's starting position:

- standing, at the patient's left side
- hypothenar of the right hand placed on patient's right costal process of L4, grip reinforced by left hand.

Movement:

- unilateral push on the costal process of L4, right side, from posterior to anterior (Fig. 8.46b).

Self-exercise (film 84)

Patient's starting position:

- sitting on a chair (Fig. 8.47a)
- a tennis ball placed between the costal process of L4, right side (possibly marked by tape to be more easily identifiable for the patient), and the back of the chair
- arms crossed over the chest or placed on the thighs.

Movement:

- increasing the pressure on the ball by pushing the feet against the floor and pushing the trunk backwards against the ball (Fig. 8.47b)
- this results in unilateral pressure on L4, right side, in a posterior-anterior direction
- releasing pressure, and back to starting position.

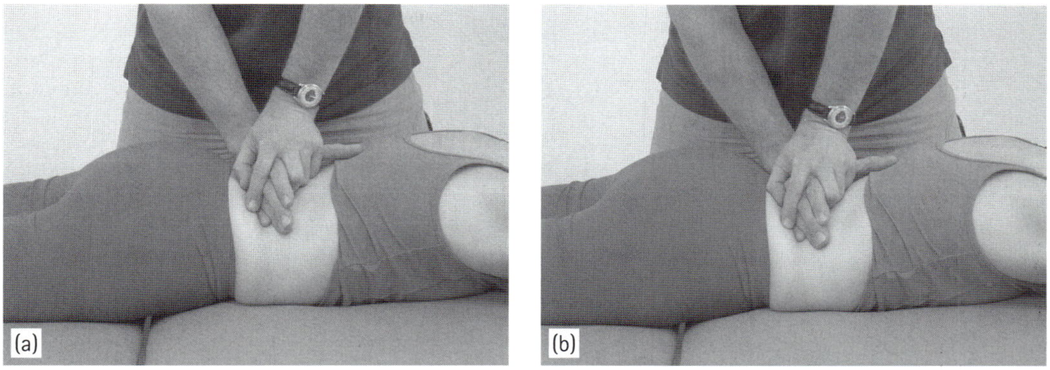

Figure 8.44a and b Accessory movement; central push in posterior–anterior direction (L4); therapy technique. a, Starting position. b, End position.

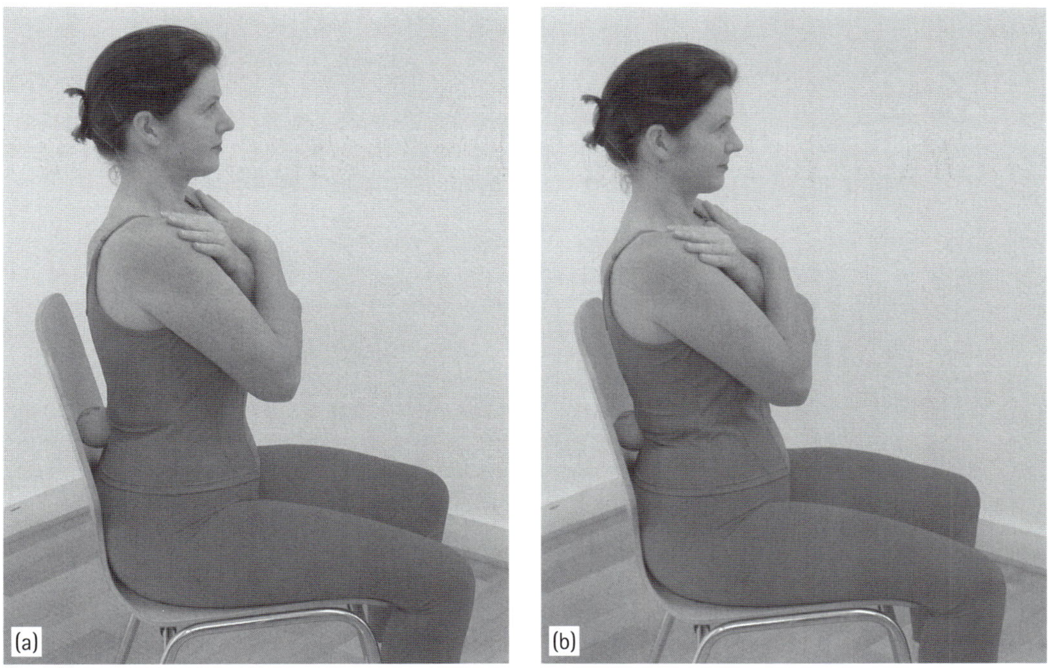

Figure 8.45a and b Accessory movement; central push in posterior–anterior direction (L4); self-exercise. a, Starting position. b, End position.

UNILATERAL PUSH IN POSTERIOR–ANTERIOR DIRECTION WITH NEURAL PRETENSIONING

Therapy technique (film 85)

Patient's starting position:

- prone, at the right side of the plinth (Fig. 8.48a)
- the right leg, extended at the knee, stands on the floor so as to bring the structures of the sacral plexus under tension
- the symptoms must not be reproduced by the chosen starting position.

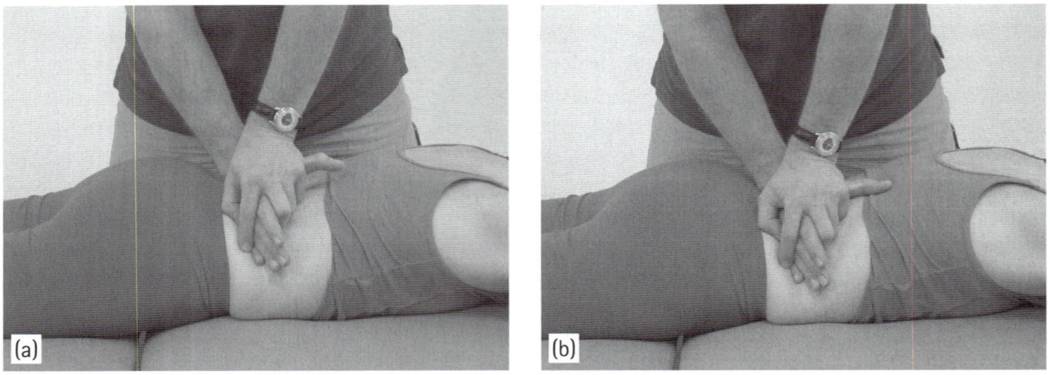

Figure 8.46a and b Accessory movement; unilateral push in posterior–anterior direction (L4); therapy technique. a, Starting position. b, End position.

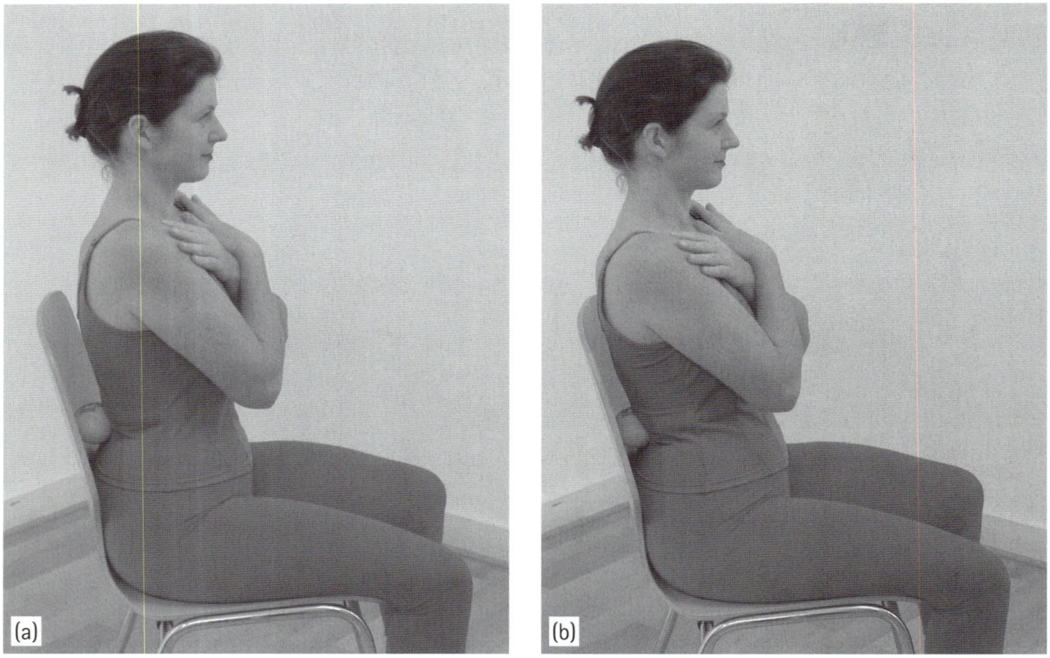

Figure 8.47a and b Accessory movement; unilateral push in posterior–anterior direction (L4); self-exercise. a, Starting position. b, End position.

Therapist's starting position:

- standing, at the patient's right side and behind the patient
- both thumbs placed on the patient's costal processes of L4.

Movement:

- unilateral push on the costal process of L4, right side, from posterior to anterior (Fig. 8.48b).

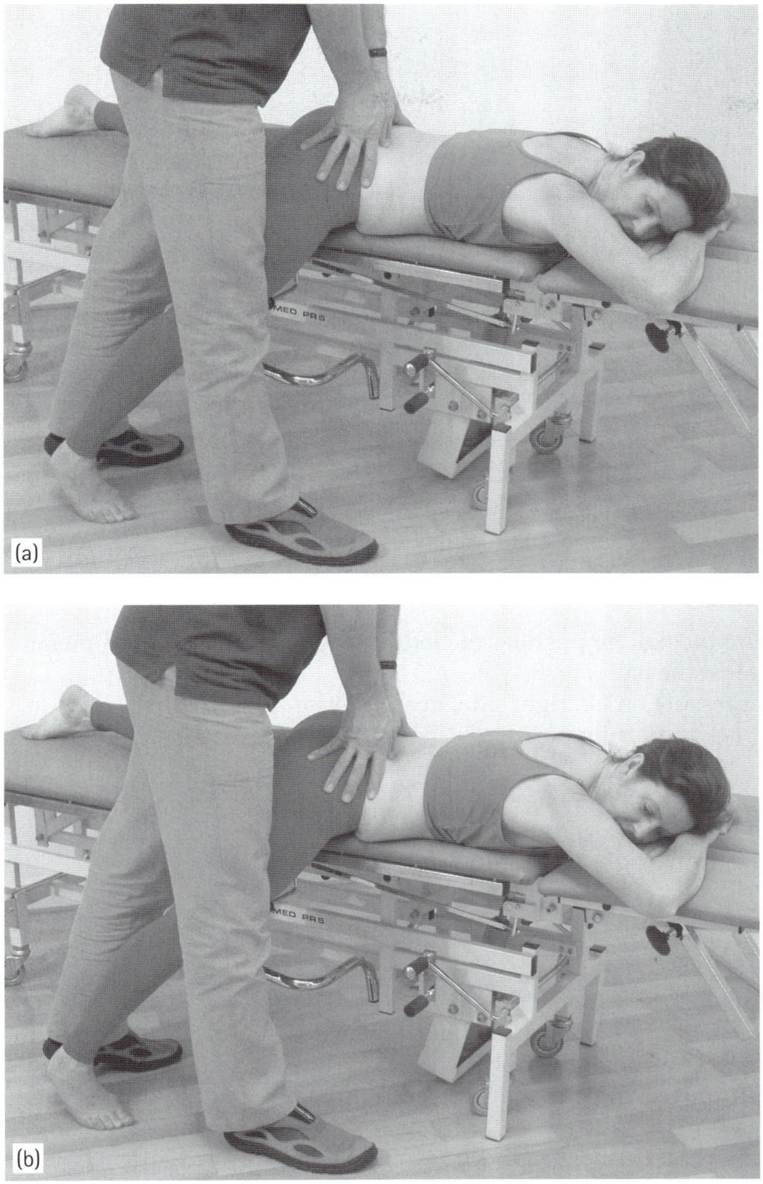

Figure 8.48a and b
Accessory movement; unilateral push in posterior–anterior direction with neural pretensioning; therapy technique. **a**, Starting position. **b**, End position.

Self-exercise (film 86)

Patient's starting position:

- sitting on a chair (Fig. 8.49a)
- the right leg extended at the knee and supported on a stool so as to bring the structures of the sacral plexus under tension
- the symptoms must not be reproduced by the chosen starting position
- a tennis ball placed between the right costal process of L4 (possibly marked by tape to be more easily identifiable for the patient) and the back of the chair
- arms crossed over the chest or placed on the thighs.

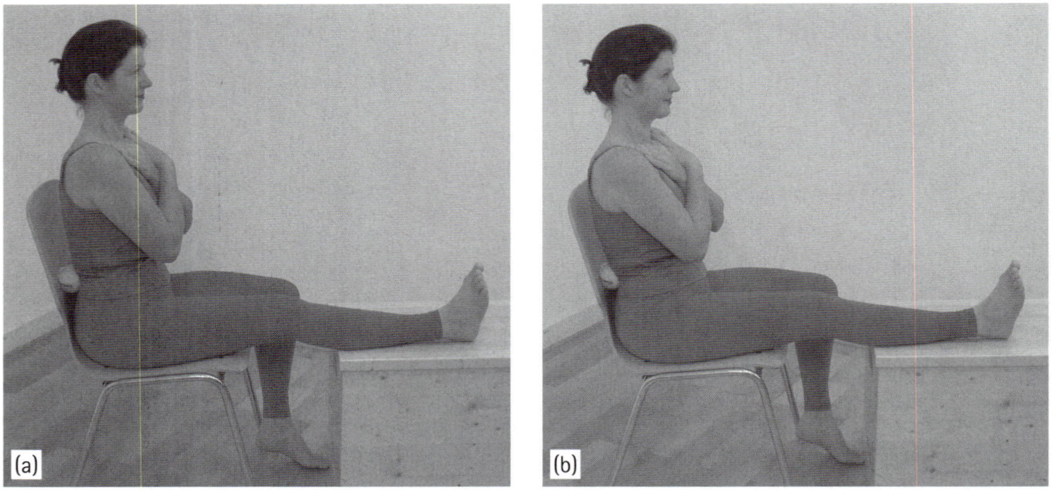

Figure 8.49a and b Accessory movement; unilateral push in posterior–anterior direction with neural pretensioning; self-exercise. **a**, Starting position. **b**, End position.

Movement:

- increasing the pressure on the ball by pushing the left foot against the floor and pushing the trunk backwards against the ball (Fig. 8.49b)
- this results in unilateral pressure on L4, right side, in a posterior-anterior direction
- releasing pressure, and back to starting position.

ANGULAR MOVEMENTS

Rotation of L4 to the right, in flexion, from side-lying position

Therapy technique (film 87)

Patient's starting position:

- lying on the left side (Fig. 8.50a)
- legs flexed in hips and knees, lumbar spine pre-positioned in flexion
- pelvis resting on the adjustable foot part of the plinth, which is slightly lifted to put the lumbar spine in slight lateral flexion to the right
- the lumbar spine is then moved into rotation to the right, from cranial, until rotation arrives at L4 (palpation)
- the right hip is flexed somewhat further, i.e. the leg is slightly put forward.

Therapist's starting position:

- standing, in front of the patient, patient's thorax fixed by therapist's body from the front side
- contacting patient's spinous process of L4 from right side with right hand and fixing it towards the left
- contacting patient's spinous process of L5 from left side with left hand
- left forearm rests on right side of patient's pelvis.

Movement:

- pulling right side of pelvis in anterior and cranial direction while pulling spinous process of L5 to the right with left hand (Fig. 8.50b)

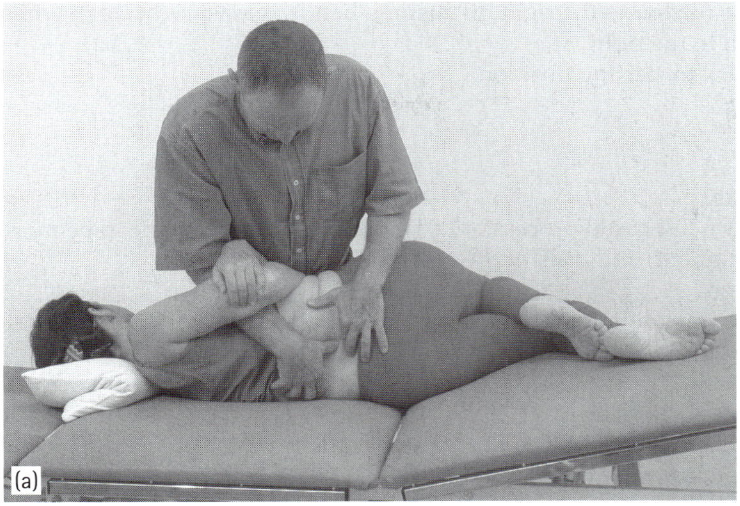

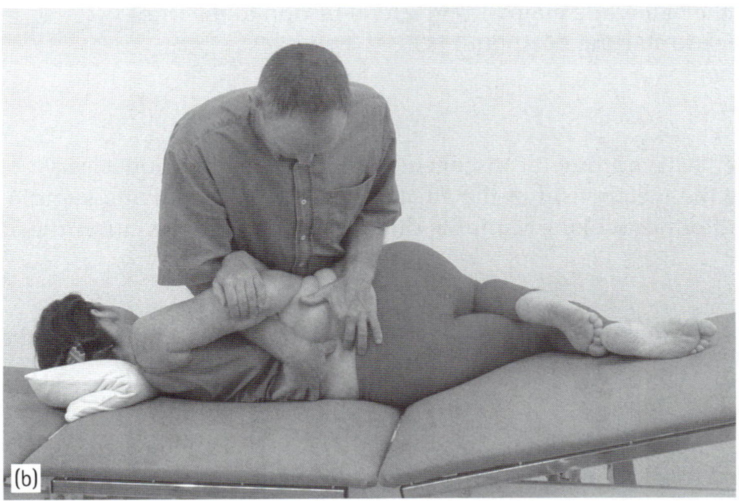

Figure 8.50a and b
Passive angular movement; rotation of L4 to the right (side-lying); therapy technique. **a**, Starting position. **b**, End position.

- this rotates and lateroflexes L4 to the right
- back to starting position.

Self-exercise 1 (film 88)

Patient's starting position:

- sitting on a chair (Fig. 8.51a)
- a tennis ball placed between right costal process of L5 (possibly marked by tape to be more easily identifiable for the patient) and back of the chair
- hands resting at the right side of right thigh
- adjusting lumbar spine in flexion, lateral flexion and rotation to the right, from cranial, until clear pressure of the tennis ball is felt.

Movement:

- increasing the pressure on the ball by pushing right leg against the floor and pushing right side of pelvis backwards against the ball (Fig. 8.51b)

- then rotating lumbar spine further to the right by pushing hands against right thigh while maintaining lateral flexion to the right
- releasing pressure, and back to starting position.

Self-exercise 2 (film 89)

Patient's starting position:

- sitting on a chair (Fig. 8.52a)
- a tennis ball placed between left costal process of L4 (possibly marked by tape to be more easily identifiable for the patient) and back of the chair
- hands resting on right thigh
- adjusting lumbar spine in flexion, lateral flexion and rotation to the right, from cranial, until clear pressure of the tennis ball is felt.

Movement:

- fixing lumbar spine in the adjusted position of rotation to the right by pushing with the arms against the right thigh, towards the knee (Fig. 8.52b)
- increasing pressure on the ball by pushing left leg against the floor and pushing left side of pelvis backwards against the ball while maintaining lateral flexion to the right
- releasing pressure, and back to starting position.

Remarks

Goals of the technique

With a subacute lumboradicular syndrome of discogenic origin, these techniques serve to reduce tonicity and improve the metabolism of the affected tissues, by mobilizing symptomatic tissue to apply a symptom-provoking stimulus dosed according to the current load tolerance.

Performance

The demonstrated techniques should not reproduce the symptoms in the leg in this subacute phase.

Dosage

The described subacute presentation (predominantly peripheral-nociceptive) corresponds with the proliferation phase as well as with the first section of the remodelling phase and therefore requires the following dosage for the techniques described.

Phase	Limitation of movement due to pain and resistance	Concept	Movement grade
Proliferation phase	Up to P1	Kaltenborn–Evjenth	Up to the 1st third of II
	Slowly progressing up to low resistance	Maitland	Up to III^{-}
Remodelling/organization phase	Slowly progressing up to maximum resistance	Kaltenborn–Evjenth	Up to III
	(Note: duration of turnover !)	Maitland	Up to IV^{++} or III^{++}

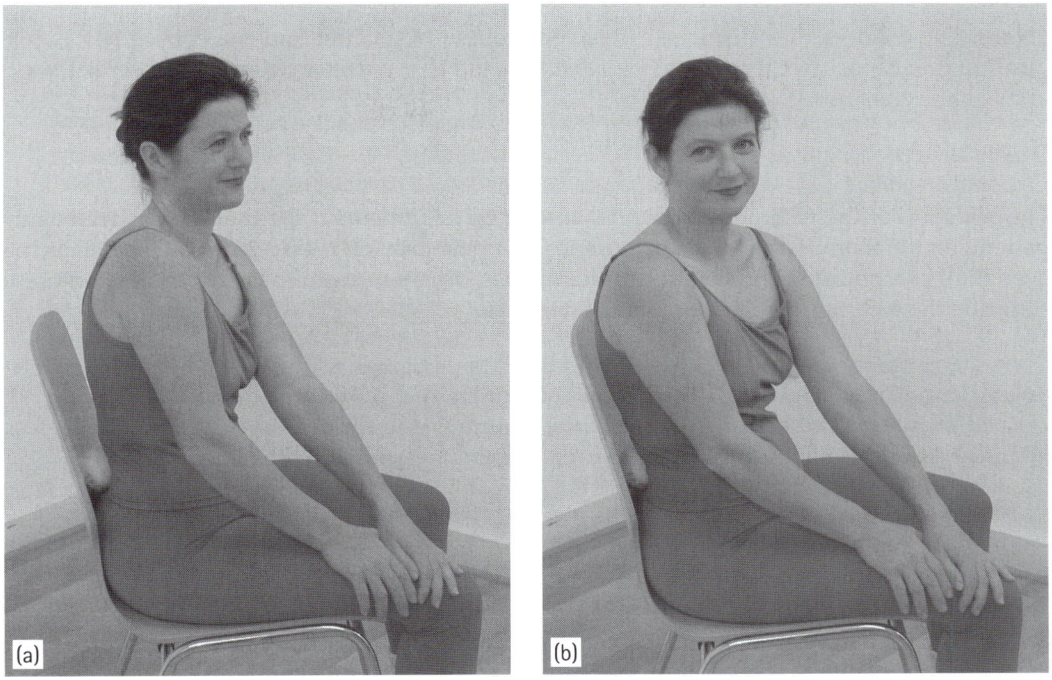

Figure 8.51a and b Passive angular movement; rotation of L4 to the right; self-exercise 1. **a**, Starting position. **b**, End position.

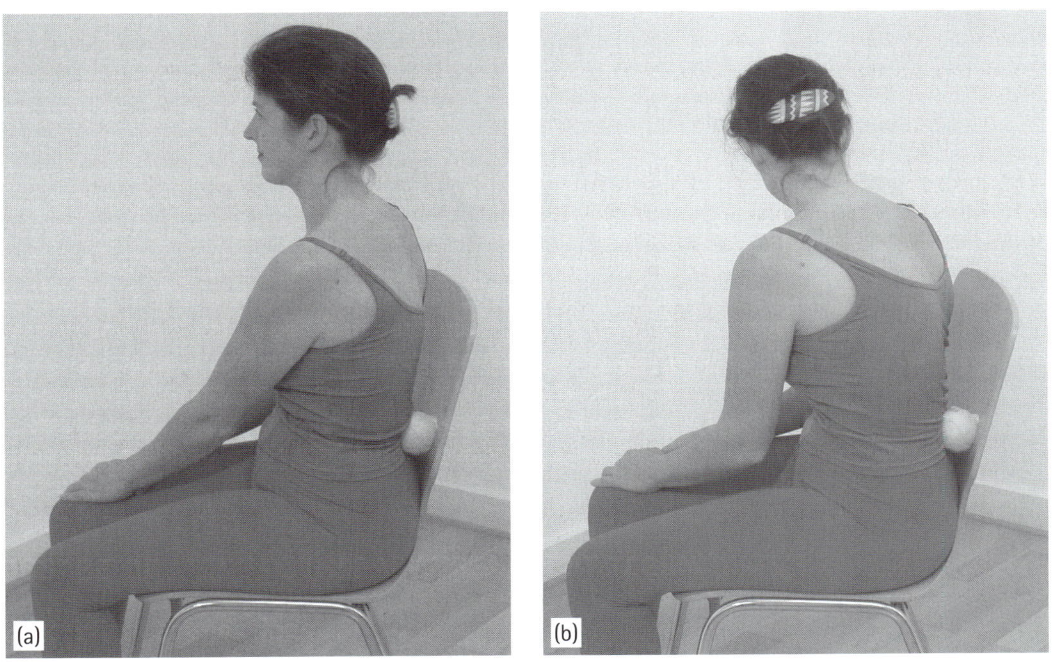

Figure 8.52a and b Passive angular movement; rotation of L4 to the right; self-exercise 2. **a**, Starting position. **b**, End position.

Note: The chances of a disturbed (delayed) course of healing and the consequences for the loading capacity of the tissue (e.g., diabetes, old age, partial or general immobilization) have to be considered.

Choice of technique

The selection of the technique depends, among other things, on the therapist as well as the patient, on the therapist's clinical experience, but primarily on reassessment. This means that even if all preconditions on the part of therapist and patient seem to be met, it is of no use to continue the technique if reassessment is negative.

Note: Regarding technique 'Rotation of L4 to the right in flexion – self-exercises 1 and 2': If in self-exercise 1 the pressure of the tennis ball over the right costal process of L5 is too painful, application of self-exercise 2 is recommended, and vice versa.

Contributing factors

For a satisfactory solution of the patient's current problems it is important to consider the contributing factors and include them in the treatment.

The authors will, however, not go deeper into a description of the various possibilities and their complex contexts as this would exceed the scope of the present book.

Chapter 9

Groin

CHAPTER CONTENTS

AREA LOCALIZATION

IDENTIFICATION OF THE POTENTIALLY AFFECTED AREA BY DEMONSTRATION OF A SYMPTOMATIC FUNCTIONAL MOVEMENT/POSITION

Based on the information gained from the anamnesis so far, the therapist ascertains more details about potentially affected sections. This is done by means of area localization, which represents the beginning of the physical examination. Information gained in this way is used to check or modify the relevant hypotheses developed on the basis of the anamnesis and will determine further proceedings.

Area localization is explained by means of four examples. In all four examples, the patient feels pain in the area of the groin. Clinical experience and known clinical patterns suggest primarily the following sections as potential sources of the current complaints:

- lumbar spine/sacroiliac joint (SIJ)
- hip complex
- neural structures.

General question: Is there enough information available to bypass area localization?	
No	Yes
⇓	⇓
Performance of area localization	• General movement tests • Additional tests • Test treatment

Example 1: Turning the trunk to the right

Symptom area: groin, right side
Symptom provocation: turning the trunk to the right with fixed right stance leg (Fig. 9.1)

With this presentation, clinical experience suggests primarily the hip complex, lumbar spine/SIJ, and neural structures as symptom-provoking areas.

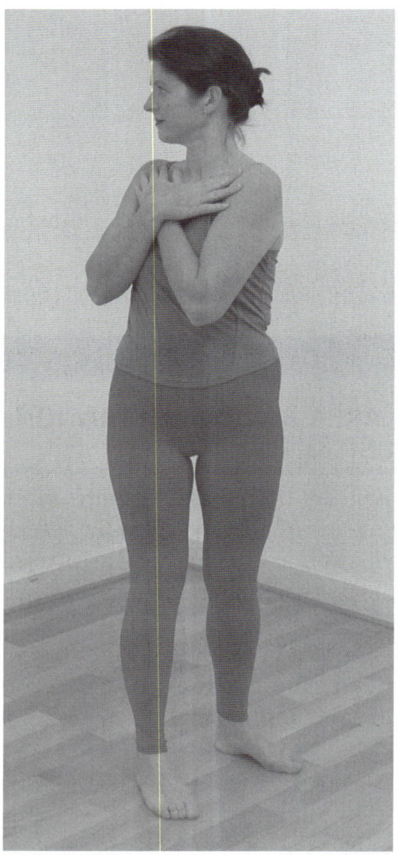

Figure 9.1 Symptom-provoking movement: turning the trunk to the right provokes pain in the right groin.

Below, examples illustrate how to differentiate between these areas. To this end, the therapist performs area localization by means of active movements alone. If this is not possible, tests will be performed by means of passive movements.

Hypothesis 1: The symptom-provoking area is the hip complex
Differentiation: hip complex vs. lumbar spine/SIJ.

The change in symptoms can be demonstrated exactly:

- provocation of pain (Fig. 9.2a and b, film 90)
- alleviation of pain (Fig. 9.3a and b, film 91).

The result of area localization has to be verified by further specific tests; otherwise the result remains in doubt.

Assessment

Goal	Provocation of pain	Alleviation of pain	Remarks
Starting position	Standing on the right leg, and rotation of the trunk to the right, to a position immediately before symptoms appear	Standing on the right leg, and rotation of the trunk to the right, to a position immediately after symptoms have appeared	
Test movement	Turning the pelvis to the right	Turning the pelvis to the left	The shoulder girdle is fixed by the therapist
Explanation	Turning the pelvis to the right increases internal rotation of the right hip joint	Turning the pelvis to the left reduces internal rotation of the right hip joint	
Additional data to support the hypothesis	General and specific mobility of hip joint, lumbar spine, and SIJ History (e.g., symptom behaviour, type of complaints, 24-hour behaviour) Palpation Reproducibility of test results Test treatment Imaging procedures (CT, MRI)		

Hypothesis 2: The symptom-provoking area is the neural structures
Differentiation: neural involvement vs. hip complex.

The change in symptoms can be demonstrated exactly:

- provocation of pain (Fig. 9.4a and b, film 92)
- alleviation of pain (Fig. 9.5a and b, film 93).

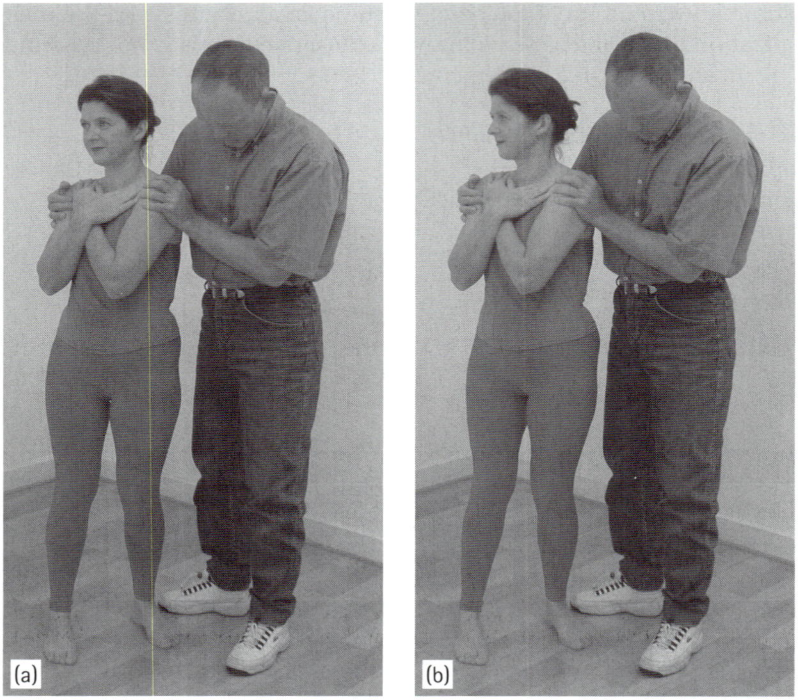

Figure 9.2a and b
Area localization with symptomatic turning of the trunk to the right; differentiation between hip complex, SIJ, and lumbar spine; provocation.
a, Starting position.
b, End position.

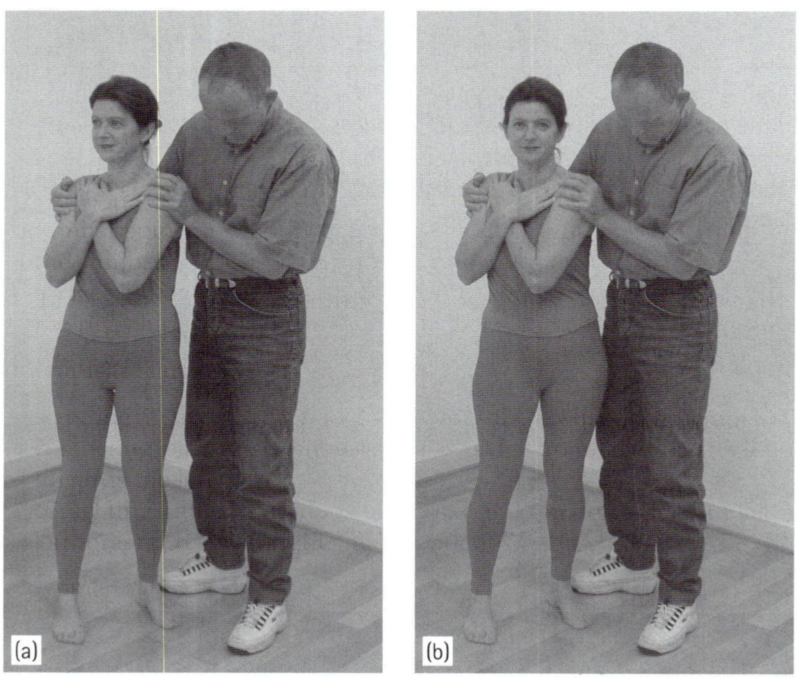

Figure 9.3a and b
Area localization with symptomatic turning of the trunk to the right; differentiation between hip complex, SIJ, and lumbar spine; alleviation.
a, Starting position.
b, End position.

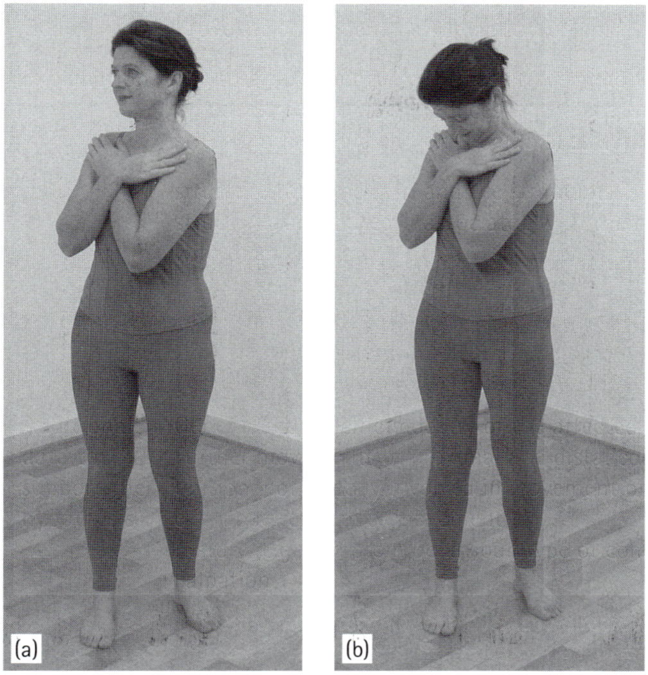

Figure 9.4a and b Area localization with symptomatic turning of the trunk to the right; differentiation between neural structures and hip complex; provocation. **a**, Starting position. **b**, End position.

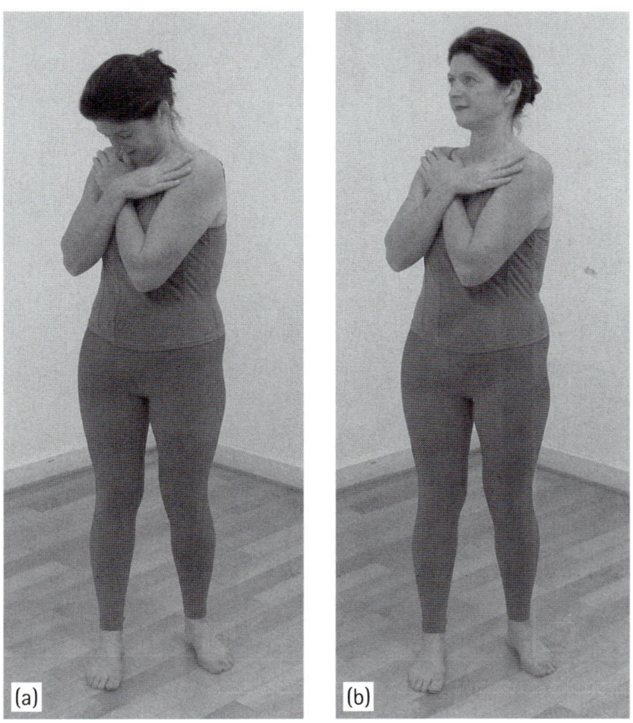

Figure 9.5a and b Area localization with symptomatic turning of the trunk to the right; differentiation between neural structures and hip complex; alleviation. **a**, Starting position. **b**, End position.

The result of area localization has to be verified by further specific tests; otherwise the result remains in doubt.

Assessment			
Goal	**Provocation of pain**	**Alleviation of pain**	**Remarks**
Starting position	Standing on the right leg, and rotation of the trunk to the right, to a position immediately before symptoms appear	With the cervical spine pre-positioned in flexion standing on the right leg, and rotation of the trunk to the right, to a position immediately after symptoms have appeared	
Test movement	Flexion of the cervical spine	Moving the cervical spine back	
Explanation	The test movement produces mechanical stress on the neural structures and the structures associated with them	The test movement reduces mechanical stress on the neural structures and the structures associated with them	If the typical pain is provoked or alleviated by these manoeuvres without changing the starting position, this suggests at least an involvement of the neural structures. The same manoeuvre can be applied when lumbar spine or SIJ is responsible for the symptoms
Additional data to support the hypothesis	General and specific mobility of the affected area Further movement of proximal and distal components to increase neural tension, not directly involved in movement of the backwards, e.g., upper extremity movement History (e.g., symptom behaviour, type of complaints, 24-hour behaviour) Palpation Neurodynamic tests Reproducibility of test results Test treatment Imaging procedures (CT, MRI)		

Hypothesis 3: The symptom-provoking area is the hip complex
Differentiation: hip complex vs. SIJ vs. lumbar spine.

The change in symptoms can be demonstrated exactly. Although functional demonstration was performed in standing, in this example it is assumed that the same symptoms can be reproduced by internal rotation of the right leg from a prone position. If no exact reproduction of symptoms in this position is possible or if other symptoms are reproduced, it is questionable whether results gained in this way are associated with the patient's functional problem:

- provocation of pain (Figs 9.6a and b, 9.7a and b, 9.8a and b, film 94)
- alleviation of pain (Figs 9.9a and b, 9.10a and b, 9.11a and b, film 95).

The result of area localization has to be verified by further specific tests; otherwise the result remains in doubt.

Assessment			
Goal	**Provocation of pain**	**Alleviation of pain**	**Remarks**
Starting position	Prone, internal rotation of right hip joint without fixation of the pelvis, to a position immediately before symptoms appear	Prone, internal rotation of right hip joint without fixation of the pelvis, to a position immediately after symptoms have appeared	
Test movement	Push to the left: ● contact with the ilium ● contact with the sacrum ● contact with the spinous processes L5–L1	Push to the right: ● contact with the sciatic tuberosity ● contact with the sacrum ● contact with the spinous processes L5–L1	
Explanation	The test movements provoke: ● the hip complex ● in addition to the hip complex the SIJ ● in addition to the hip complex and SIJ the lumbar spine	The test movements alleviate: ● the hip complex ● in addition to the hip complex the SIJ ● in addition to the hip complex and SIJ the lumbar spine	
Additional data to support the hypothesis	General and specific mobility of hip joint, lumbar spine, and SIJ History (e.g., symptom behaviour, type of complaints, 24-hour behaviour) Palpation Reproducibility of test results Test treatment Imaging procedures (CT, MRI)		

Note: If, based on the information from the anamnesis, the lumbar spine is considered to be the symptom-provoking area, its upper segments are the most probable sources of symptoms (referred pain from the lumbar spine at the groin rather suggests the upper lumbar segments).

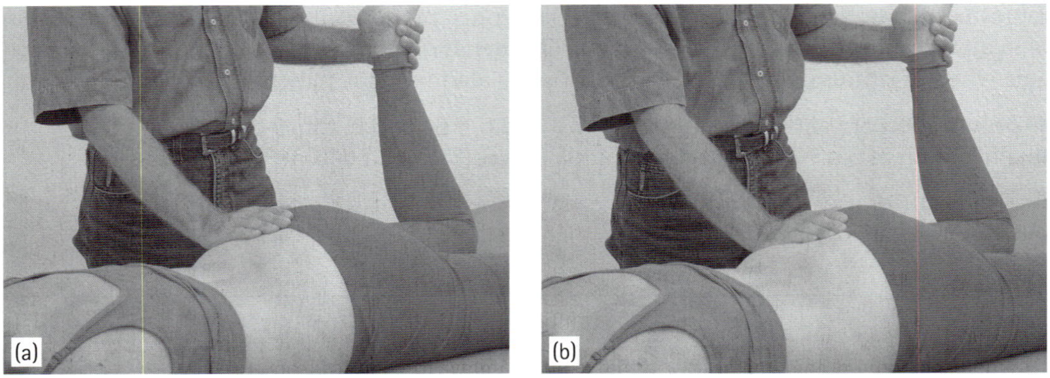

Figure 9.6a and b Area localization with symptomatic internal rotation of the hip joint in prone position; differentiation between hip complex, SIJ, and lumbar spine; first step: ilium; provocation. **a**, Starting position. **b**, End position.

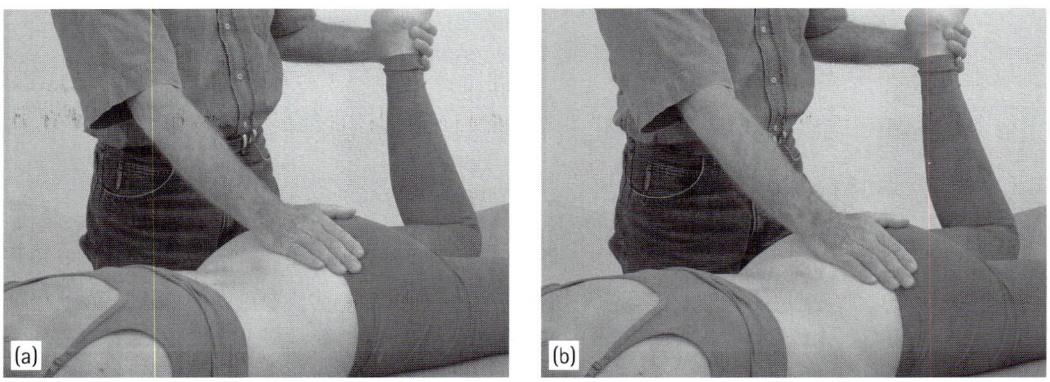

Figure 9.7a and b Area localization with symptomatic internal rotation of the hip joint in prone position; differentiation between hip complex, SIJ, and lumbar spine; second step: sacrum; provocation. **a**, Starting position. **b**, End position.

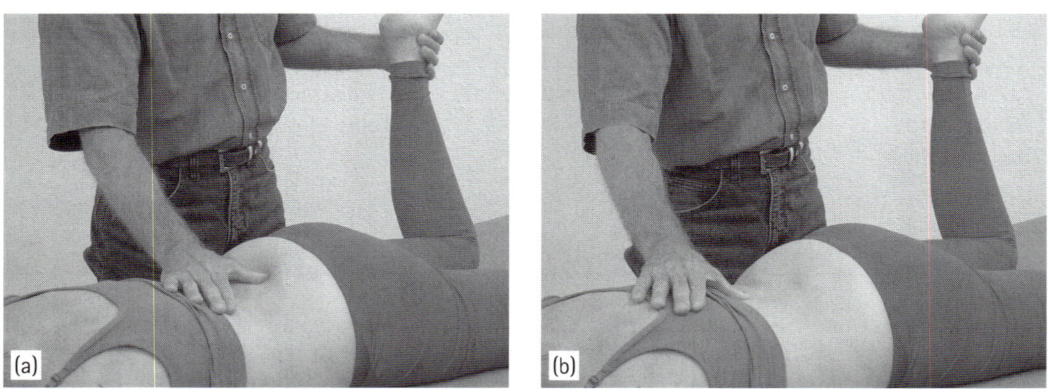

Figure 9.8a and b Area localization with symptomatic internal rotation of the hip joint in prone position; differentiation between hip complex, SIJ, and lumbar spine; third step: lumbar spine; provocation. **a**, Starting position. **b**, End position.

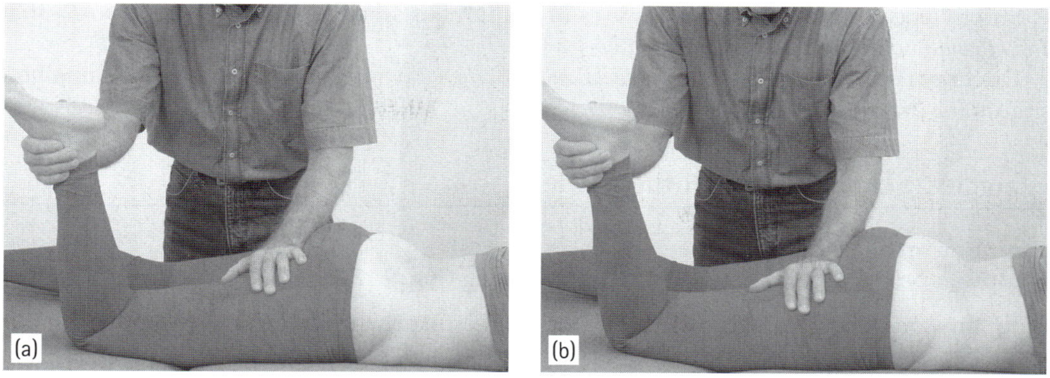

Figure 9.9a and b Area localization with symptomatic internal rotation of the hip joint in prone position; differentiation between hip complex, SIJ, and lumbar spine; first step: ilium; alleviation. **a**, Starting position. **b**, End position.

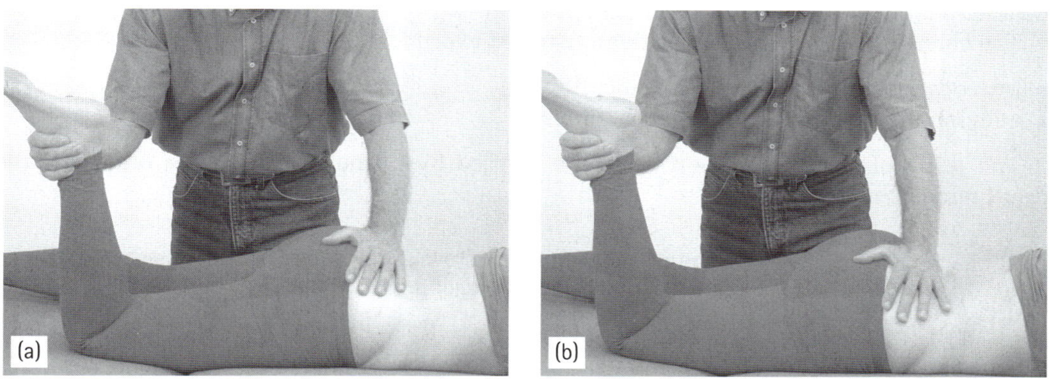

Figure 9.10a and b Area localization with symptomatic internal rotation of the hip joint in prone position; differentiation between hip complex, SIJ, and lumbar spine; second step: sacrum; alleviation. **a**, Starting position. **b**, End position.

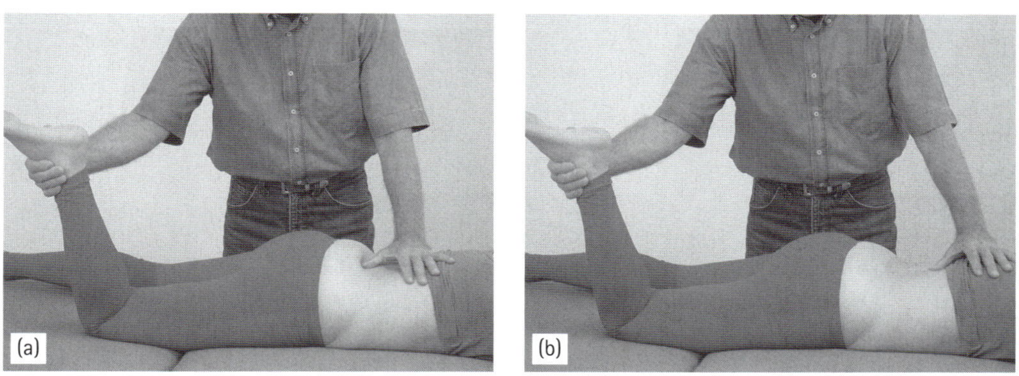

Figure 9.11a and b Area localization with symptomatic internal rotation of the hip joint in prone position; differentiation between hip complex, SIJ, and lumbar spine; third step: lumbar spine; alleviation. **a**, Starting position. **b**, End position.

Strictly speaking, the test manoeuvres of the lumbar spine are part of *specific provocation and alleviation* and not *area localization*.

Direct performance of *specific provocation and alleviation* at the lumbar spine is done here simply for practical reasons.

Example 2: Lunge step with the left leg

Symptom area: groin, right side
Symptom provocation: lunge step with the left leg (Fig. 9.12)

With this presentation, clinical experience suggests primarily the hip complex, lumbar spine/SIJ, and neural structures as symptom-provoking areas.

Below, examples illustrate how to differentiate between these areas. To this end, the therapist performs area localization by means of active movements alone. If this is not possible, tests will be performed by means of passive movements.

Hypothesis 1: The symptom-provoking area is the hip complex

Differentiation: hip complex vs. lumbar spine/SIJ.

The change in symptoms can be demonstrated exactly:

- provocation of pain (Fig. 9.13a and b, film 96)
- alleviation of pain (Fig. 9.14a and b, film 97).

The result of area localization has to be verified by further specific tests; otherwise the result remains in doubt.

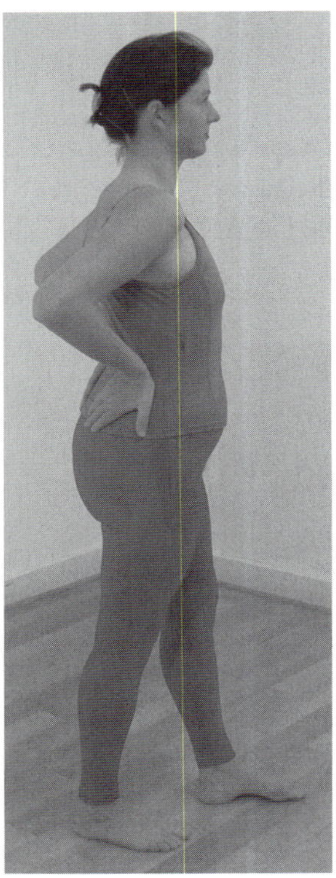

Figure 9.12 Symptom-provoking movement: a lunge step with the left leg provokes pain in the right groin.

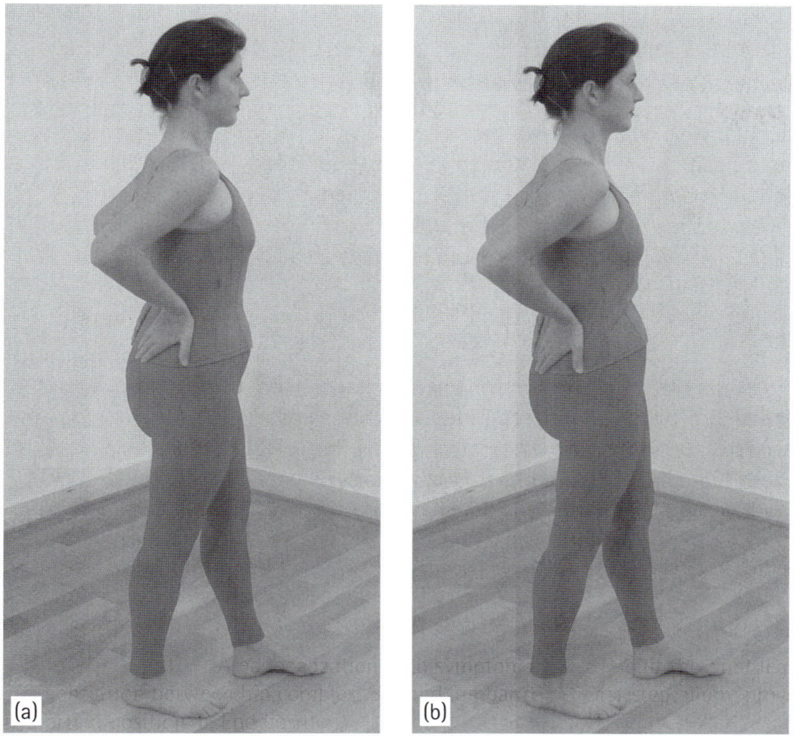

Figure 9.13a and b
Area localization with symptomatic lunge step with left leg; differentiation between hip complex, SIJ, and lumbar spine; provocation. **a**, Starting position. **b**, End position.

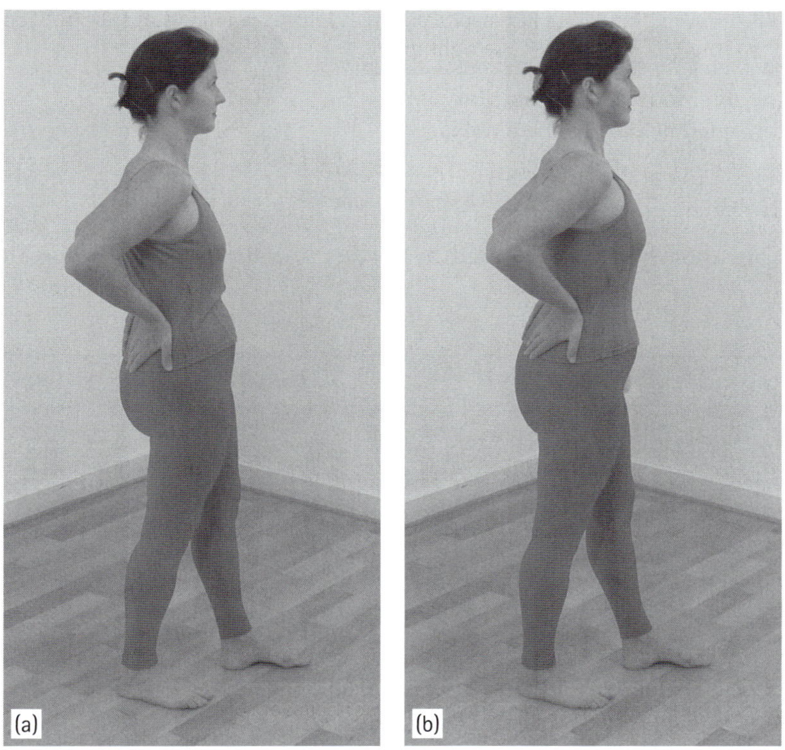

Figure 9.14a and b
Area localization with symptomatic lunge step with left leg; differentiation between hip complex, SIJ, and lumbar spine; alleviation. **a**, Starting position. **b**, End position.

Assessment			
Goal	**Provocation of pain**	**Alleviation of pain**	**Remarks**
Starting position	Lunge step with left leg, to a position immediately before symptoms appear	With the pelvis pre-positioned in a posterior tilt, lunge step with left leg, to a position immediately after symptoms have appeared	
Test movement	Tilting the pelvis in posterior direction	Tilting the pelvis in anterior direction	
Explanation	Tilting the pelvis in posterior direction increases extension in the right hip complex and reduces extension of lumbar spine/SIJ	Tilting the pelvis in anterior direction reduces extension in the right hip complex and increases extension of lumbar spine/SIJ	
Additional data to support the hypothesis	General and specific mobility of hip joint, lumbar spine, and SIJ History (e.g., symptom behaviour, type of complaints, 24-hour behaviour) Palpation Reproducibility of test results Test treatment Imaging procedures (CT, MRI)		

Hypothesis 2: The symptom-provoking area is the neural structures

Differentiation: neural involvement vs. hip complex.

The change in symptoms can be demonstrated exactly:

- provocation of pain (Fig. 9.15a and b, film 98)
- alleviation of pain (Fig. 9.16a and b, film 99).

The result of area localization has to be verified by further specific tests; otherwise the result remains in doubt.

Assessment			
Goal	**Provocation of pain**	**Alleviation of pain**	**Remarks**
Starting position	Lunge step with left leg, to a position immediately before symptoms appear	With the cervical spine pre-positioned in flexion, lunge step with left leg, to a position immediately after symptoms have appeared	
Test movement	Flexion of the cervical spine	Moving the cervical spine back	

Goal	Provocation of pain	Alleviation of pain	Remarks
Explanation	The test movement produces mechanical stress on the neural	The test movement reduces mechanical stress on the neural structures	If the typical pain is provoked or alleviated by these
	structures and the structures associated with them	and the structures associated with them	manoeuvres without changing the starting position, this suggests at least an involvement of the neural structures. The same manoeuvre can be applied when lumbar spine or SIJ is responsible for the symptoms
Additional data to support the hypothesis	General and specific mobility of the affected area Further movements of proximal and distal components to increase neural tension, not directly involved in movement of the head backwards, e.g., upper extremity movement History (e.g., symptom behaviour, type of complaints, 24-hour behaviour) Palpation Neurodynamic tests Reproducibility of test results Test treatment Imaging procedures (CT, MRI)		

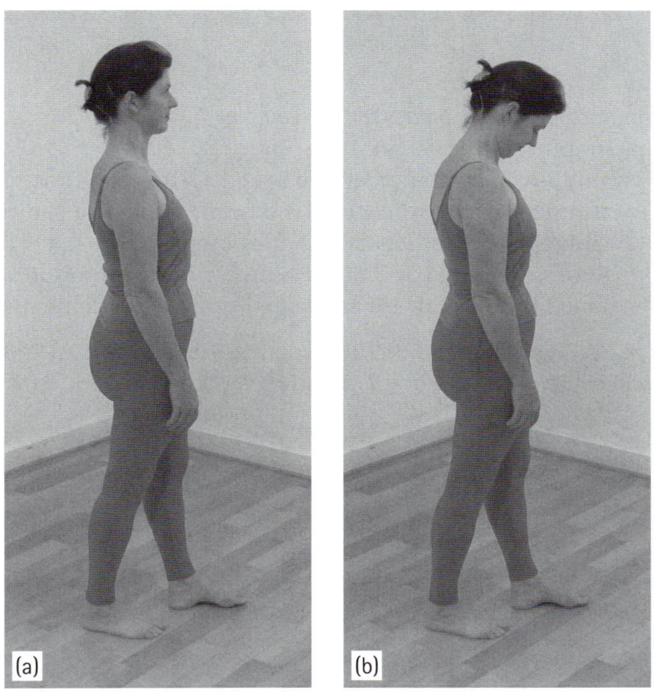

Figure 9.15a and b Area localization with symptomatic lunge step with left leg; differentiation between neural structures and hip complex; provocation. a, Starting position. b, End position.

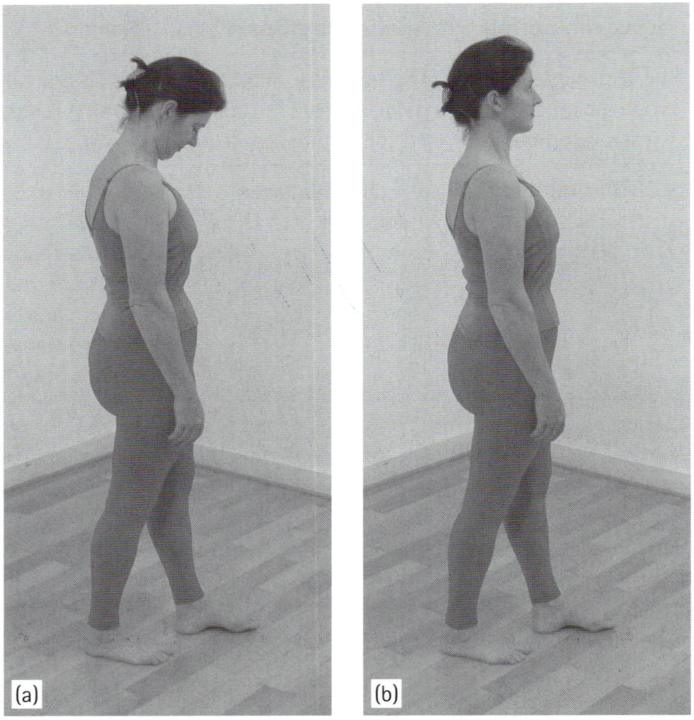

Figure 9.16a and b Area localization with symptomatic lunge step with left leg; differentiation between neural structures and hip complex; alleviation. a, Starting position. b, End position.

Hypothesis 3: The symptom-provoking area is the hip complex

Differentiation: hip complex vs. SIJ vs. lumbar spine.

The change in symptoms can be demonstrated exactly. Although functional demonstration was performed in standing, in this example it is assumed that the same symptoms can be reproduced by extension of the right leg from a prone position. If no exact reproduction of symptoms in this position is possible or if other symptoms are reproduced, it is questionable whether the results gained in this way are associated with the patient's functional problem:

- provocation of pain (Figs 9.17a and b, 9.18a and b, 9.19a and b, film 100)
- alleviation of pain (Figs 9.20a and b, 9.21a and b, 9.22a and b, film 101).

The result of area localization has to be verified by further specific tests; otherwise the result remains in doubt.

Assessment

Goal	Provocation of pain	Alleviation of pain	Remarks
Starting position	Prone, extension of right hip joint without fixation of the	Prone, extension of right hip joint without fixation of the	

Goal	Provocation of pain	Alleviation of pain	Remarks
	pelvis, to a position immediately before symptoms appear	pelvis, to a position immediately after symptoms have appeared	
Test movement	• Rotation of the ilium backwards • Pressure on the apex of the sacrum (counter-nutation) • Push in anterior-cranial direction on the spinous processes L2–L5, and then pressure on the sacral base (extension L5)	• Rotation of the ilium forwards • Pressure on the sacral base (nutation) • Push in anterior-cranial direction on the spinous processes L5–L1 • If the spinous process of L5 is not accessible for cranial push, flexion of L5 can finally be achieved by anterior push on the apex of the sacrum	
Explanation	The test movements provoke: • the hip complex • in addition to the hip complex the SIJ • in addition to the hip complex and SIJ the lumbar spine; the movement has to be started from cranial, since otherwise differentiation is not selective	The test movements alleviate: • the hip complex • in addition to the hip complex the SIJ • in addition to the hip complex and SIJ the lumbar spine	
Additional data to support the hypothesis	General and specific mobility of hip joint, lumbar spine, and SIJ History (e.g., symptom behaviour, type of complaints, 24-hour behaviour) Palpation Reproducibility of test results Test treatment Imaging procedures (CT, MRI)		

Note: If, based on the information from the anamnesis, the lumbar spine is considered to be the symptom-provoking area, its upper segments are the most probable sources of symptoms.

Strictly speaking, the test manoeuvres of the lumbar spine are part of *specific provocation and alleviation* and not *area localization*.

Direct performance of *specific provocation and alleviation* at the lumbar spine is done here simply for practical reasons.

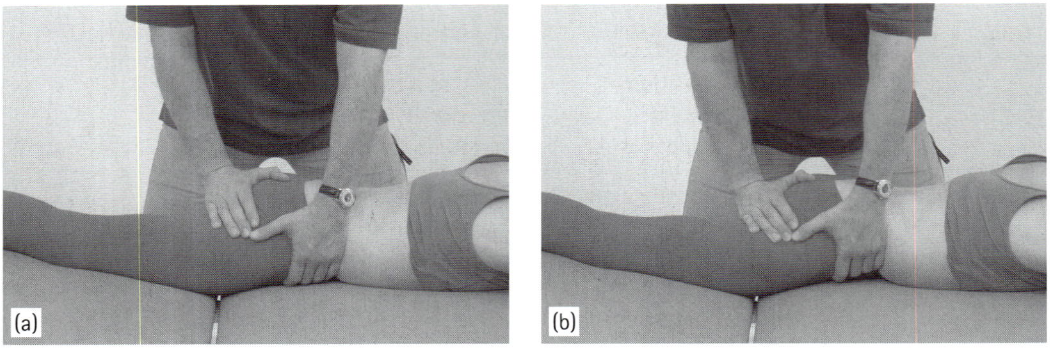

Figure 9.17a and b Area localization with symptomatic extension of the hip joint in prone position; differentiation between hip complex, SIJ, and lumbar spine; first step: hip complex provocation. **a**, Starting position. **b**, End position.

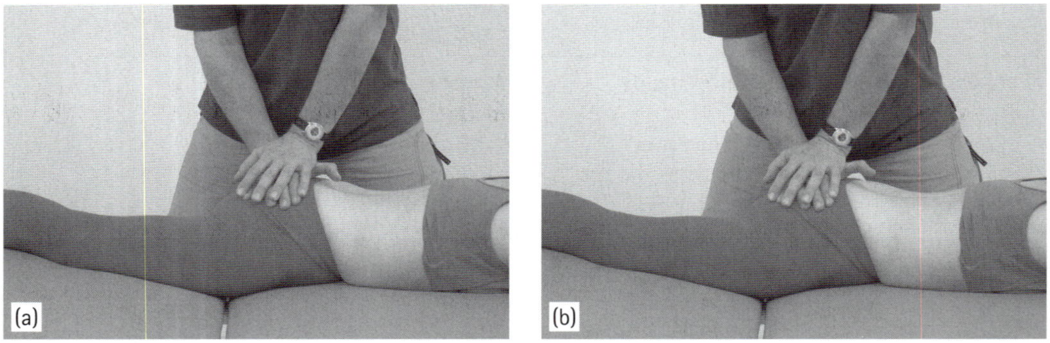

Figure 9.18a and b Area localization with symptomatic extension of the hip joint in prone position; differentiation between hip complex, SIJ, and lumbar spine; second step: SIJ provocation. **a**, Starting position. **b**, End position.

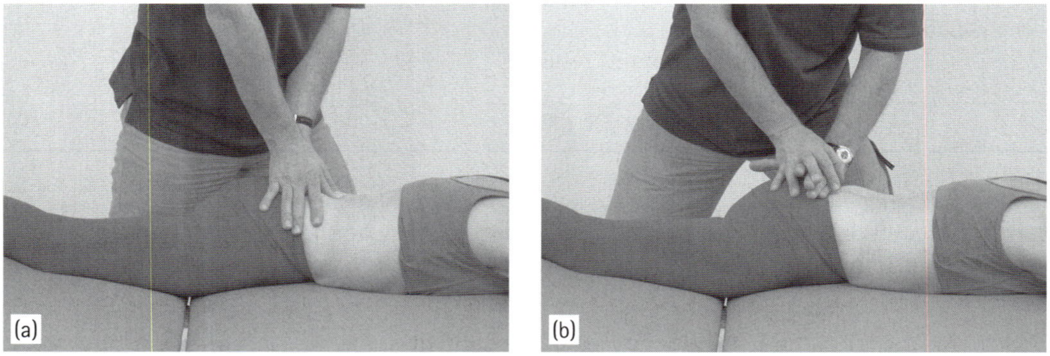

Figure 9.19a and b Area localization with symptomatic extension of the hip joint in prone position; differentiation between hip complex, SIJ, and lumbar spine; third step: lumbar spine provocation. **a**, Starting position. **b**, End position.

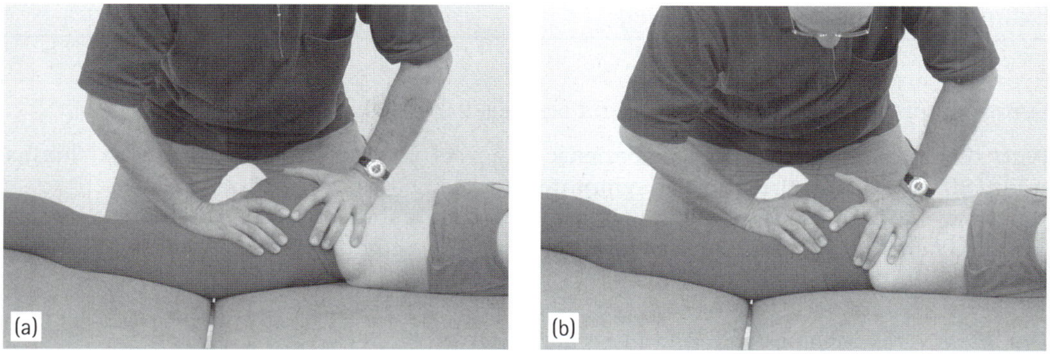

Figure 9.20a and b Area localization with symptomatic extension of the hip joint in prone position; differentiation between hip complex, SIJ, and lumbar spine; first step: hip complex; alleviation. **a**, Starting position. **b**, End position.

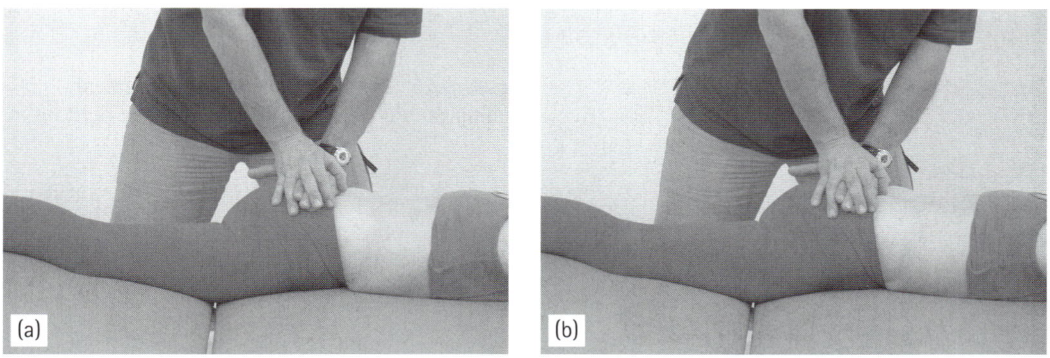

Figure 9.21a and b Area localization with symptomatic extension of the hip joint in prone position; differentiation between hip complex, SIJ, and lumbar spine; second step: SIJ; alleviation. **a**, Starting position. **b**, End position.

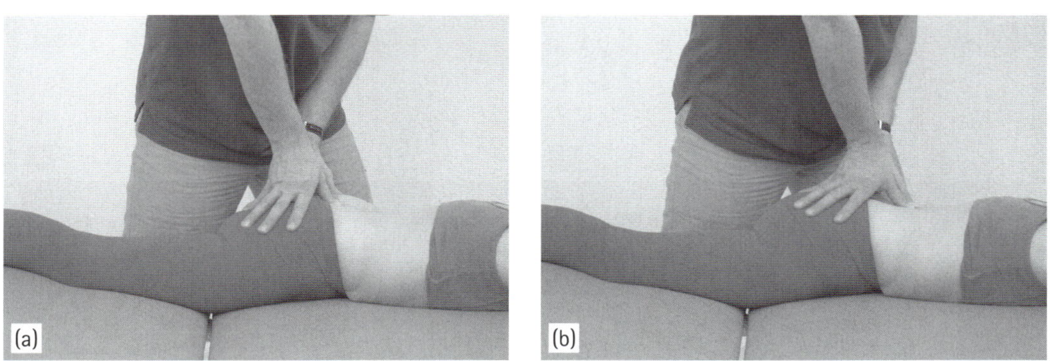

Figure 9.22a and b Area localization with symptomatic extension of the hip joint in prone position; differentiation between hip complex, SIJ, and lumbar spine; third step: lumbar spine; alleviation. **a**, Starting position. **b**, End position.

Example 3: Loading the right leg

Symptom area: groin, right side
Symptom provocation: loading the right leg (Fig. 9.23)

With this presentation, clinical experience suggests primarily the hip complex, lumbar spine/SIJ, and neural structures as symptom-provoking areas.

Below, one example is given showing how to differentiate between these areas. As it is assumed here that symptom provocation occurs due to a compression component, it is necessary to test with passive movements.

Hypothesis 1: The symptom-provoking area is the hip complex

Differentiation: hip complex vs. SIJ vs. lumbar spine.

The change in symptoms can be demonstrated exactly:

- provocation of pain (Figs 9.24a and b, 9.25a and b, 9.26a and b, film 102)
- alleviation of pain (Figs 9.27a and b, 9.28a and b, 9.29a and b, film 103).

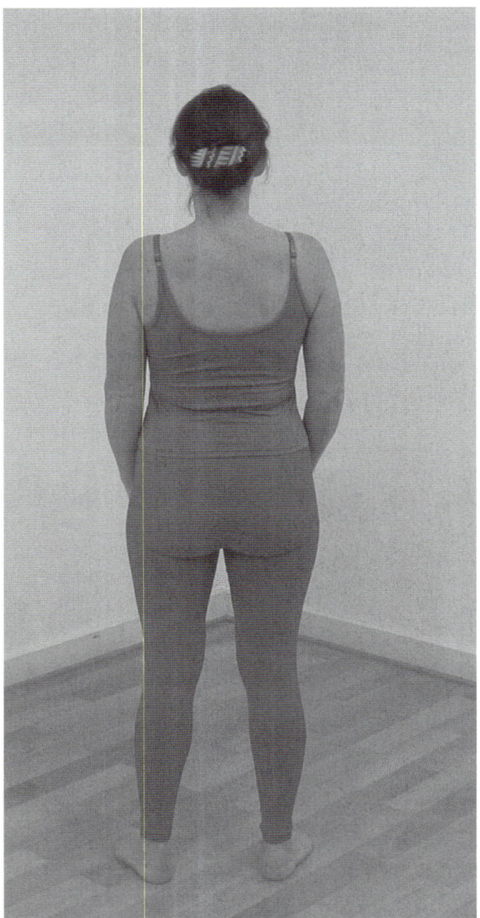

Figure 9.23 Symptom-provoking movement: loading the right leg provokes pain in the right groin.

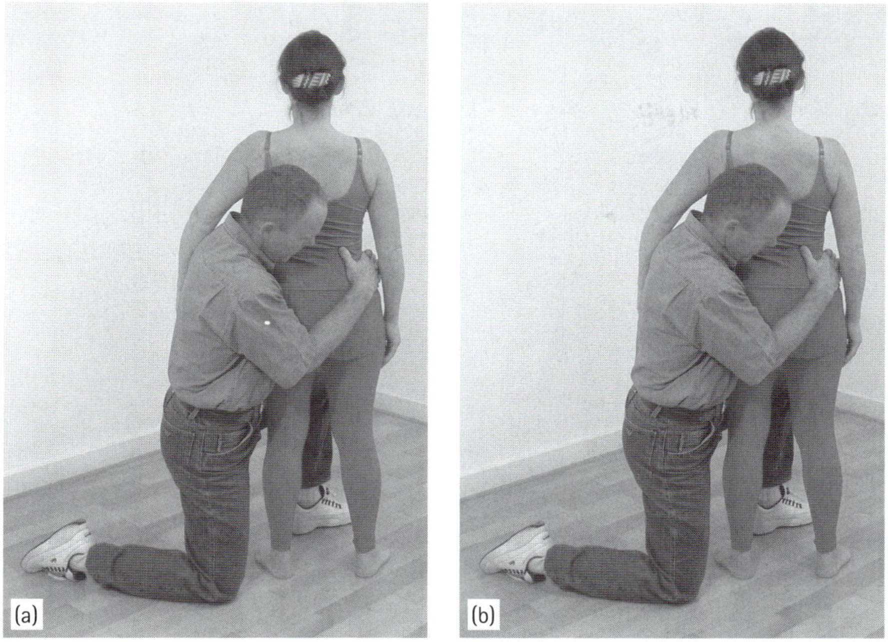

Figure 9.24a and b Area localization with symptomatic loading of the right leg in standing; differentiation between hip complex, SIJ, and lumbar spine; first step: ilium; provocation. a, Starting position. b, End position.

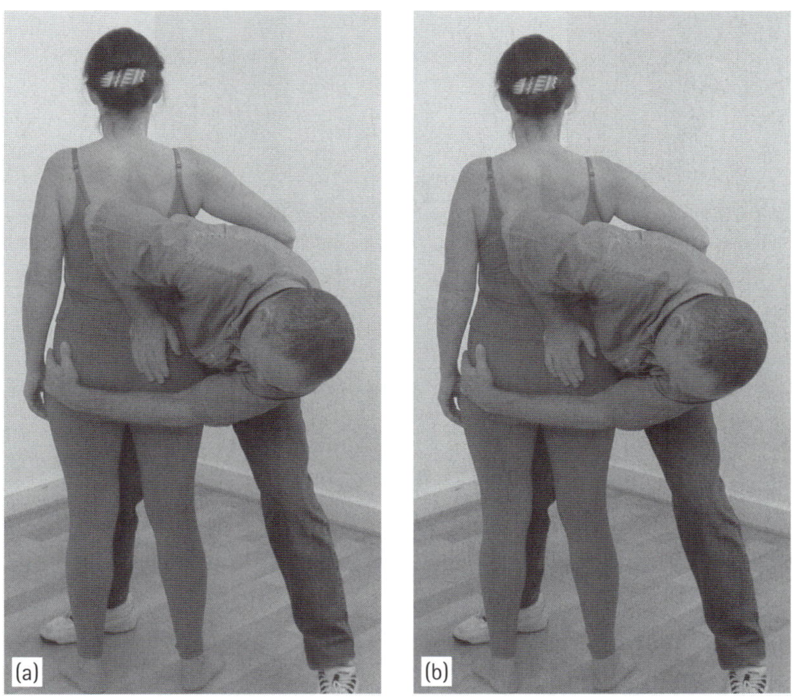

Figure 9.25a and b Area localization with symptomatic loading of the right leg in standing; differentiation between hip complex, SIJ, and lumbar spine; second step: sacrum; provocation. a, Starting position. b, End position.

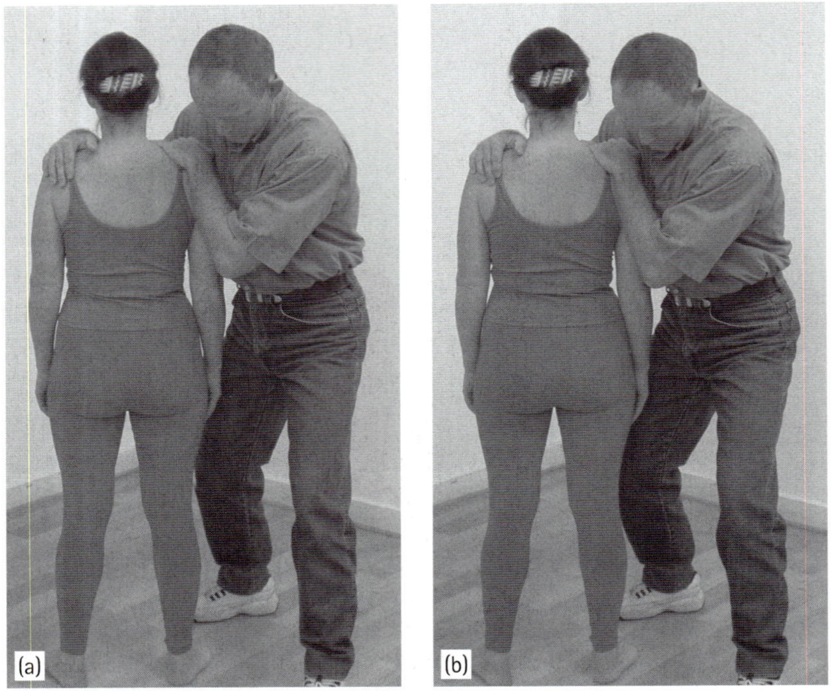

Figure 9.26a and b Area localization with symptomatic loading of the right leg in standing; differentiation between hip complex, SIJ, and lumbar spine; third step: lumbar spine; provocation. a, Starting position. b, End position.

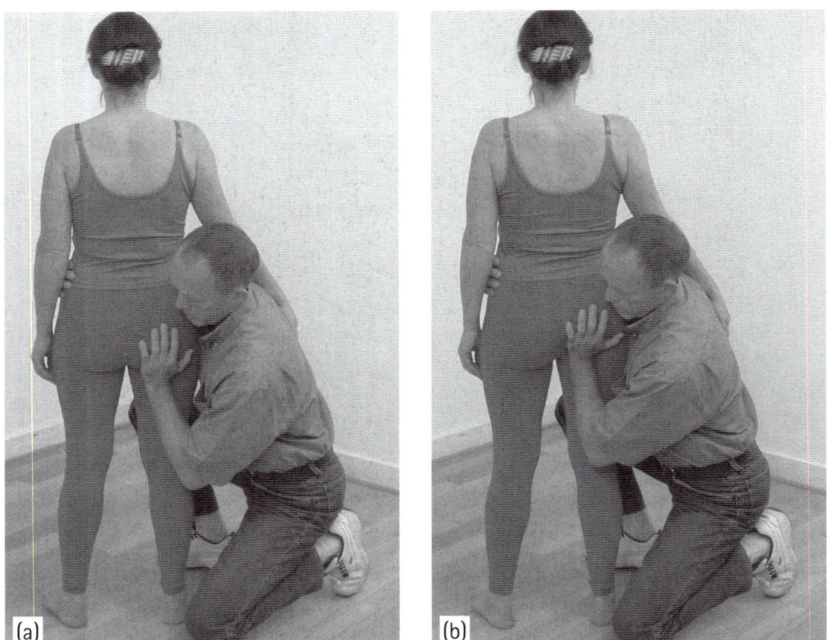

Figure 9.27a and b Area localization with symptomatic loading of the right leg in standing; differentiation between hip complex, SIJ, and lumbar spine; first step: ilium; alleviation. a, Starting position. b, End position.

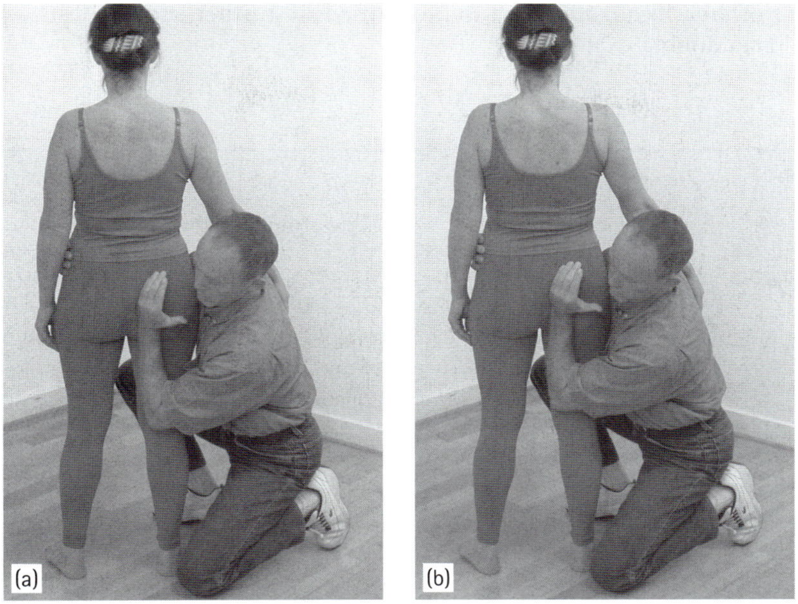

Figure 9.28a and b Area localization with symptomatic loading of the right leg in standing; differentiation between hip complex, SIJ, and lumbar spine; second step: sacrum; alleviation. **a**, Starting position. **b**, End position.

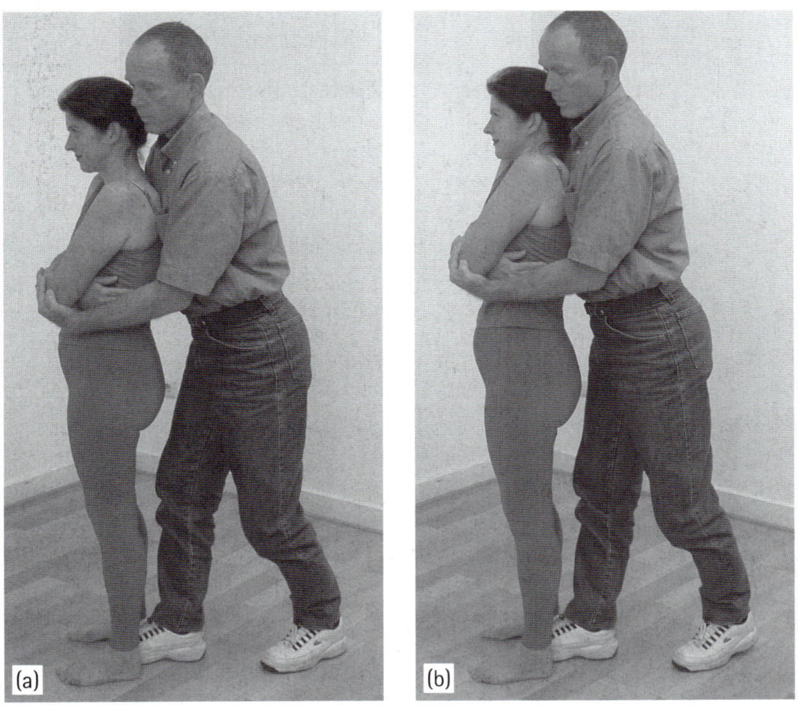

Figure 9.29a and b Area localization with symptomatic loading of the right leg in standing; differentiation between hip complex, SIJ, and lumbar spine; third step: lumbar spine; alleviation. **a**, Starting position. **b**, End position.

The result of area localization has to be verified by further specific tests; otherwise the result remains in doubt.

Assessment			
Goal	**Provocation of pain**	**Alleviation of pain**	**Remarks**
Starting position	Standing, loading the right leg to an extent immediately after symptoms have appeared	Standing, loading the right leg to an extent immediately after symptoms have appeared	Because with pre-positioning to a position before symptoms appear non-symptomatic parts of the affected joint may be compressed, a symptomatic position is also chosen for provocation
Test movement	• Push of the ilium in caudal direction • Push of the sacrum in caudal direction • Compression of the lumbar spine	• Push of the ilium in cranial direction • Push of the sacrum in cranial direction • Traction of the lumbar spine	
Explanation	The test movements provoke: • the hip complex • in addition to the hip complex the SIJ • in addition to the hip complex and SIJ the lumbar spine	The test movements alleviate: • the hip complex • in addition to the hip complex the SIJ • in addition to the hip complex and SIJ the lumbar spine	
Additional data to support the hypothesis	General and specific mobility of hip joint, lumbar spine, and SIJ History (e.g., symptom behaviour, type of complaints, 24-hour behaviour) Palpation Reproducibility of test results Test treatment Imaging procedures (CT, MRI)		

Note: If, based on the information from the anamnesis, the lumbar spine is considered to be the symptom-provoking area, its upper segments are the most probable sources of symptoms.

Example 4: Flexion

Symptom area: groin, right side
Symptom provocation: lifting the right foot to place it on a stool (Fig. 9.30)

With this presentation, clinical experience suggests primarily the hip complex, lumbar spine/SIJ, and neural structures as symptom-provoking areas.

Below, examples illustrate how to differentiate between these areas. To this end, the therapist performs area localization by means of active movements alone. If this is not possible, tests will be performed by means of passive movements.

Hypothesis 1: The symptom-provoking area is the hip complex

Differentiation: hip complex vs. lumbar spine/SIJ.

The change in symptoms can be demonstrated exactly:

- provocation of pain (Fig. 9.31a and b, film 104)
- alleviation of pain (Fig. 9.32a and b, film 105).

The result of area localization has to be verified by further specific tests; otherwise the result remains in doubt.

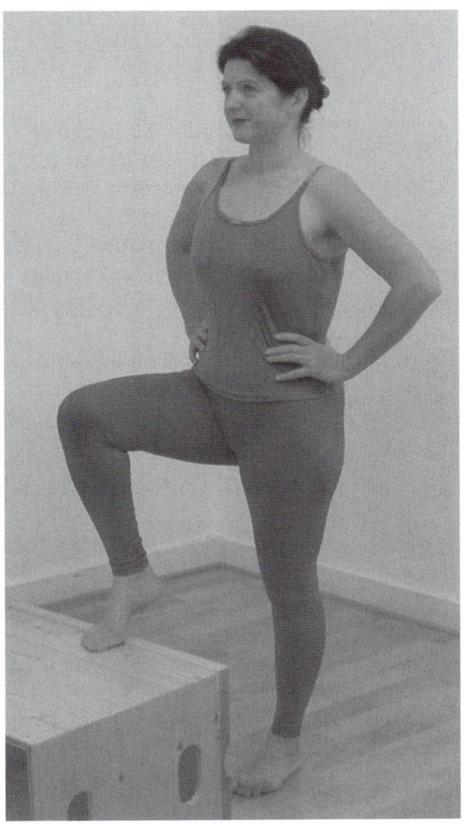

Figure 9.30 Symptom-provoking movement: flexion of the right hip joint provokes pain in the right groin.

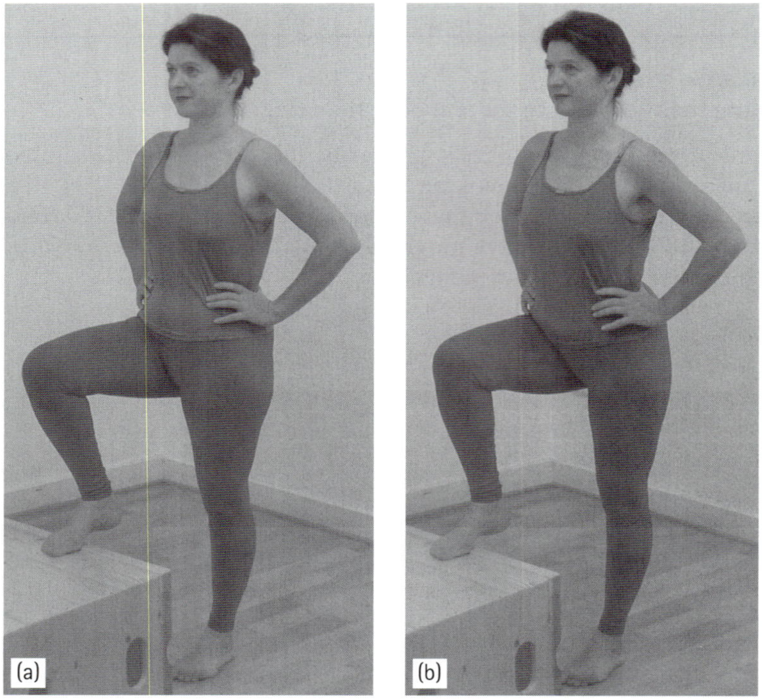

Figure 9.31a and b Area localization with symptomatic flexion of the right hip joint; differentiation between hip complex and lumbar spine/SIJ; provocation.
a, Starting position.
b, End position.

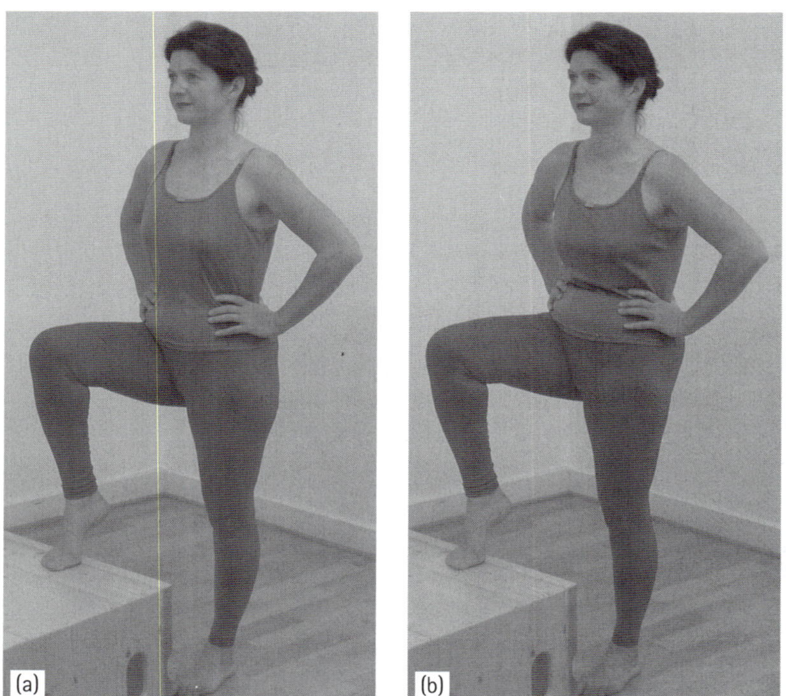

Figure 9.32a and b Area localization with symptomatic flexion of the right hip joint; differentiation between hip complex and lumbar spine/SIJ; alleviation.
a, Starting position.
b, End position.

Assessment			
Goal	**Provocation of pain**	**Alleviation of pain**	**Remarks**
Starting position	Standing, flexing right leg to a position immediately before symptoms appear	Standing, flexing right leg to a position immediately after symptoms have appeared	
Test movement	Tilting the pelvis in anterior direction	Tilting the pelvis in posterior direction	
Explanation	Tilting the pelvis in anterior direction increases flexion in the right hip complex and reduces the flexion of lumbar spine/SIJ	Tilting the pelvis in posterior direction reduces flexion in the right hip complex and increases the extension of lumbar spine/SIJ	
Additional data to support the hypothesis	General and specific mobility of hip joint, lumbar spine, and SIJ History (e.g., symptom behaviour, type of complaints, 24-hour behaviour) Palpation Reproducibility of test results Test treatment Imaging procedures (CT, MRI)		

Hypothesis 2: The symptom-provoking area is the neural structures

Differentiation: neural involvement vs. hip complex.

The change in symptoms can be demonstrated exactly:

- provocation of pain (Fig. 9.33a and b, film 106)
- alleviation of pain (Fig. 9.34a and b, film 107).

The result of area localization has to be verified by further specific tests; otherwise the result remains in doubt

Assessment			
Goal	**Provocation of pain**	**Alleviation of pain**	**Remarks**
Starting position	Standing, flexing right leg to a position immediately before symptoms appear	Flexion of the cervical spine, then standing, flexing right leg to a position immediately after symptoms have appeared	
Test movement	Flexion of the cervical spine	Moving the cervical spine back	
Explanation	The test movement produces mechanical stress on the neural	The test movement reduces mechanical stress on the neural	If the typical pain is provoked or alleviated by these

Goal	Provocation of pain	Alleviation of pain	Remarks
	structures and the structures associated with them	structures and the structures associated with them	manoeuvres without changing the starting position, this suggests at least an involvement of the neural structures. The same manoeuvre can be applied when lumbar spine or SIJ is responsible for the symptoms
Additional data to support the hypothesis	General and specific mobility of the affected area Further movements of proximal and distal components to increase neural tension, not directly involved in movement of the head backwards, e.g., upper extremity movement History (e.g., symptom behaviour, type of complaints, 24-hour behaviour) Palpation Neurodynamic tests Reproducibility of test results Test treatment Imaging procedures (CT, MRI)		

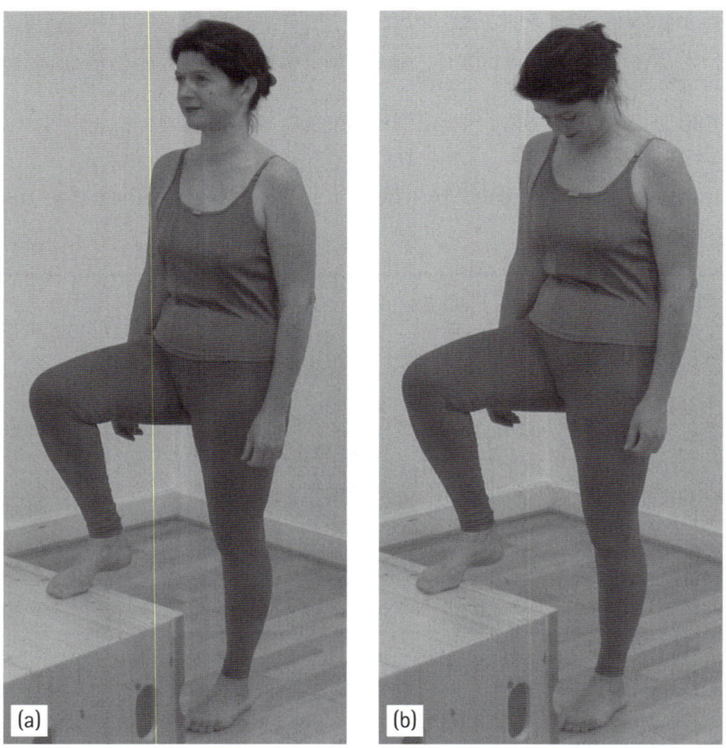

Figure 9.33a and b Area localization with symptomatic flexion of the right hip joint; differentiation between neural structures and hip complex; provocation.
a, Starting position.
b, End position.

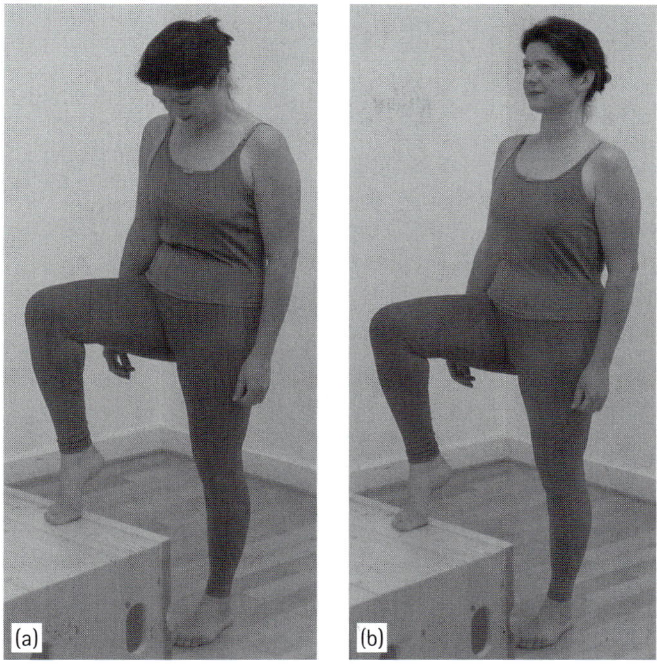

Figure 9.34a and b Area localization with symptomatic flexion of the right hip joint; differentiation between neural structures and hip complex; alleviation. **a**, Starting position. **b**, End position.

QUICK CHECK – SYMPTOMS, GROIN

If neither the area nor a symptom-provoking or symptom-reducing action is known, the quick check is used to try to load individual potential areas with specific biomechanically provocative movement combinations. The chosen movement combinations correspond with the straining and often symptom-provoking movements of the individual sections.

LUMBAR SPINE/SIJ

Movement (film 226)

- Extension/lateral flexion to the right, and rotation to the same as well as to the opposite side, with overpressure (Fig. 9.35a and b)
- Extension/lateral flexion to the left, and rotation to the same as well as to the opposite side, with overpressure (Fig. 9.36a and b).

Note: If the anamnesis suggests that flexion of the spine contributes to symptom provocation, the described movement combinations should, of course, be performed in flexion.

SIJ provocation tests in prone position (film 231)

- Sacrum, in anterior direction (Fig. 9.37)
- Ilium, in anterior direction (Fig. 9.38)
- Sacrum, in caudal direction (Fig. 9.39)
- Sacrum, in cranial direction (Fig. 9.40)
- Gapping, in posterior direction (Fig. 9.41)
- Gapping, in anterior direction (Fig. 9.42).

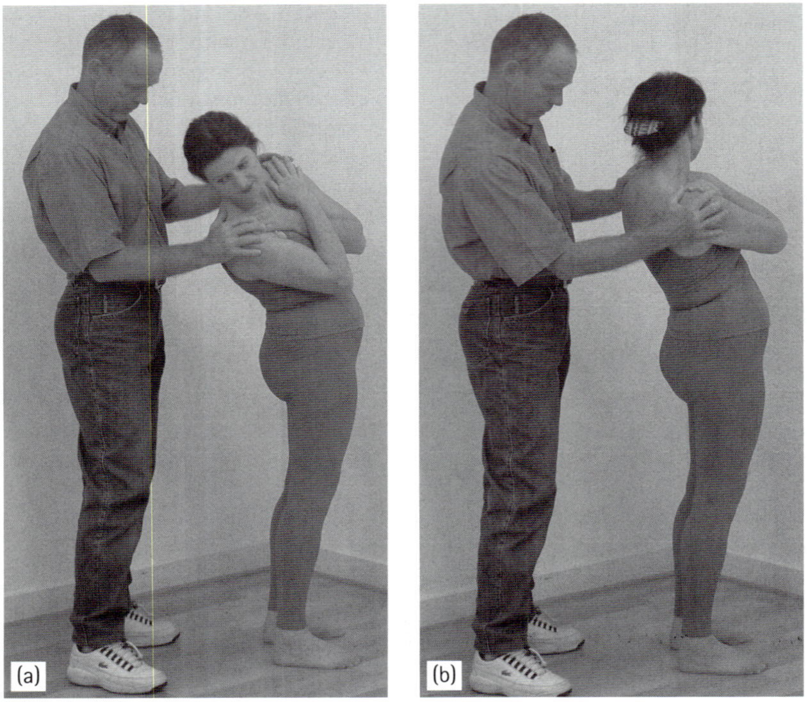

Figure 9.35a and b Quick check lumbar spine; extension, lateral flexion to the right. **a**, Rotation to the same side. **b**, Rotation to the opposite side.

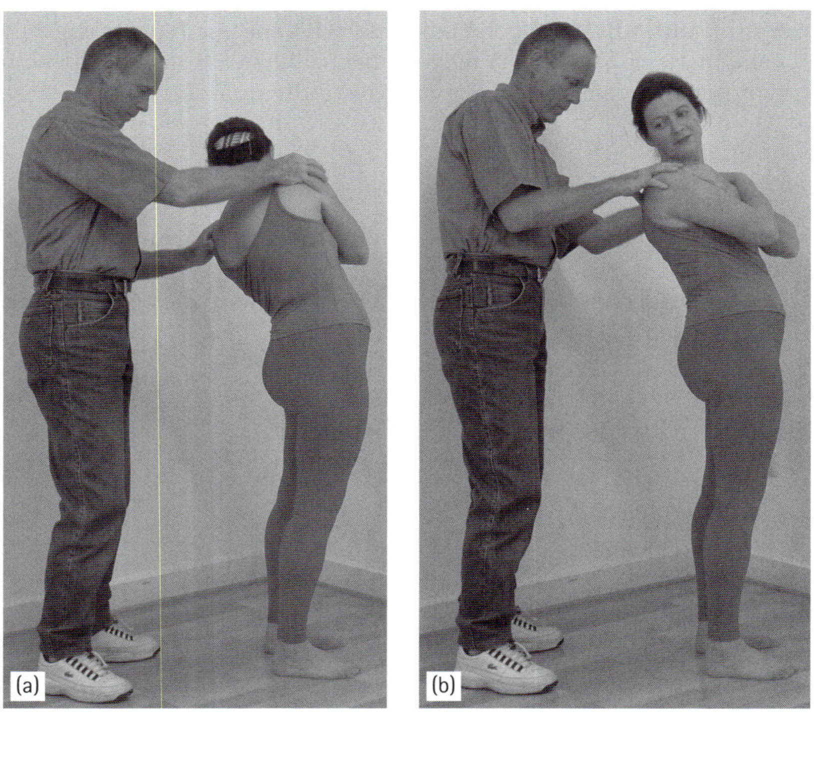

Figure 9.36a and b Quick check lumbar spine; extension, lateral flexion to the left. **a**, Rotation to the same side. **b**, Rotation to the opposite side.

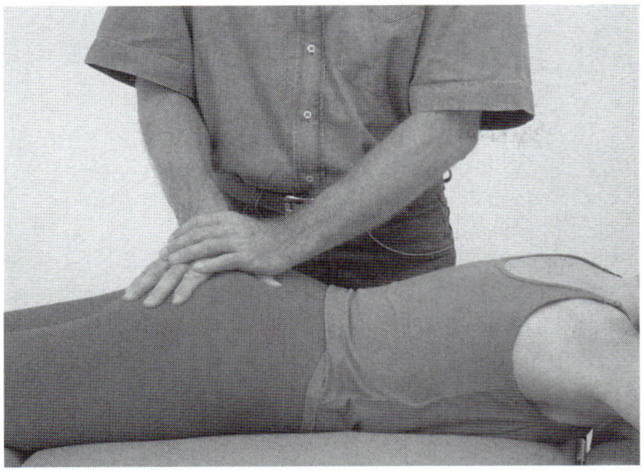

Figure 9.37 Quick check SIJ; sacrum, in anterior direction.

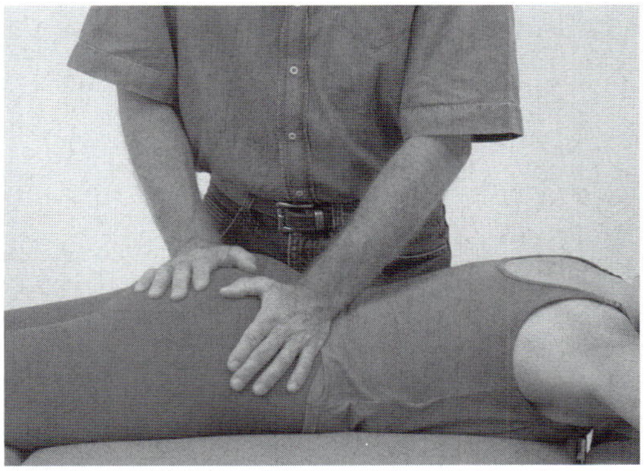

Figure 9.38 Quick check SIJ; ilium, in anterior direction.

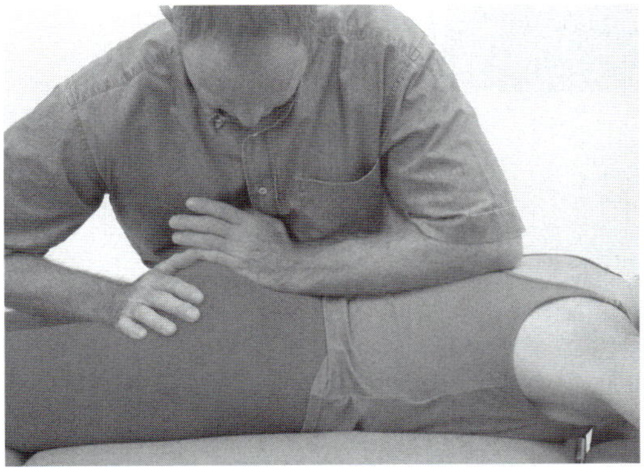

Figure 9.39 Quick check SIJ; sacrum, in caudal direction.

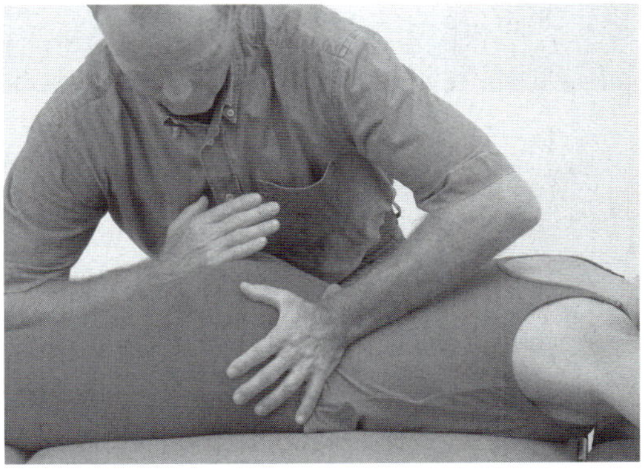

Figure 9.40 Quick check SIJ; sacrum, in cranial direction.

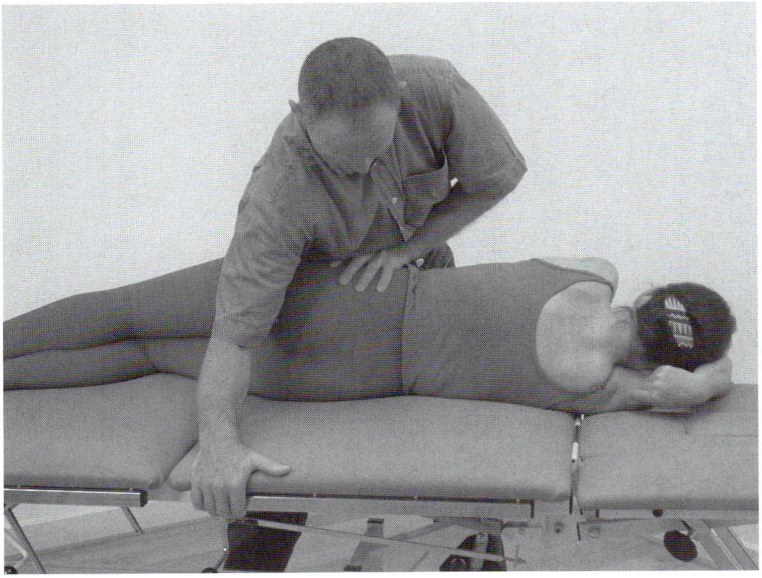

Figure 9.41 Quick check SIJ; gapping, in posterior direction.

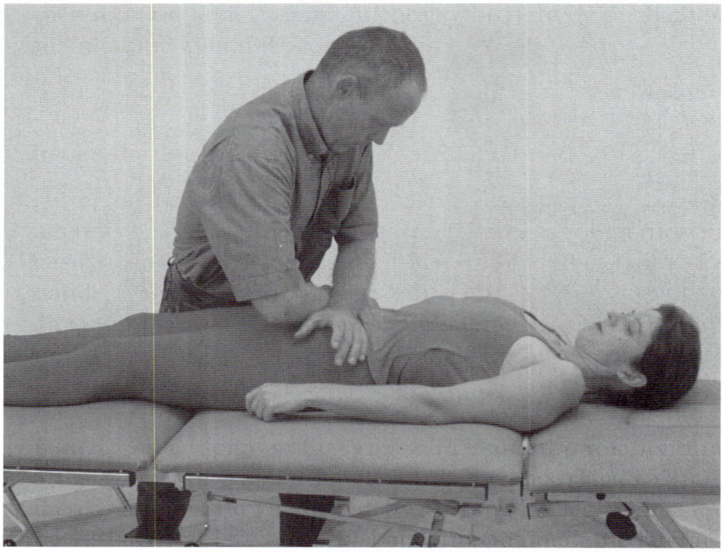

Figure 9.42 Quick check SIJ; gapping, in anterior direction.

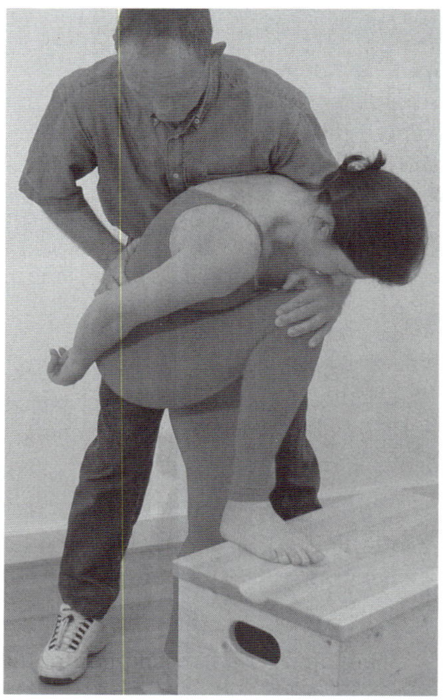

Figure 9.43 Quick check hip; flexion/adduction/ internal rotation.

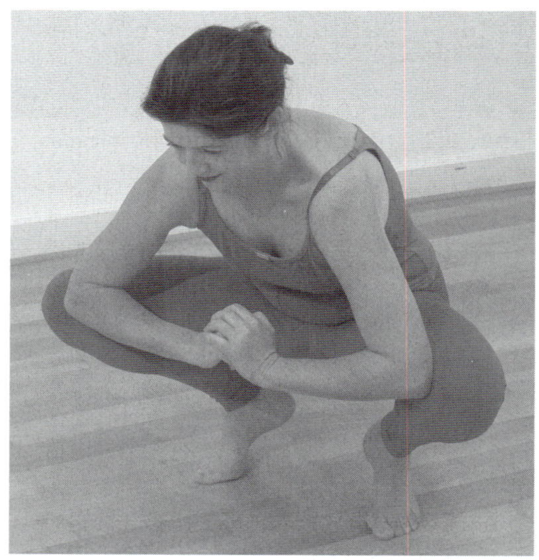

Figure 9.44 Quick check hip; flexion/abduction.

HIP

Movement (film 228)

- Flexion/adduction/internal rotation, with overpressure (Fig. 9.43)
- Flexion/abduction, with overpressure (Fig. 9.44).

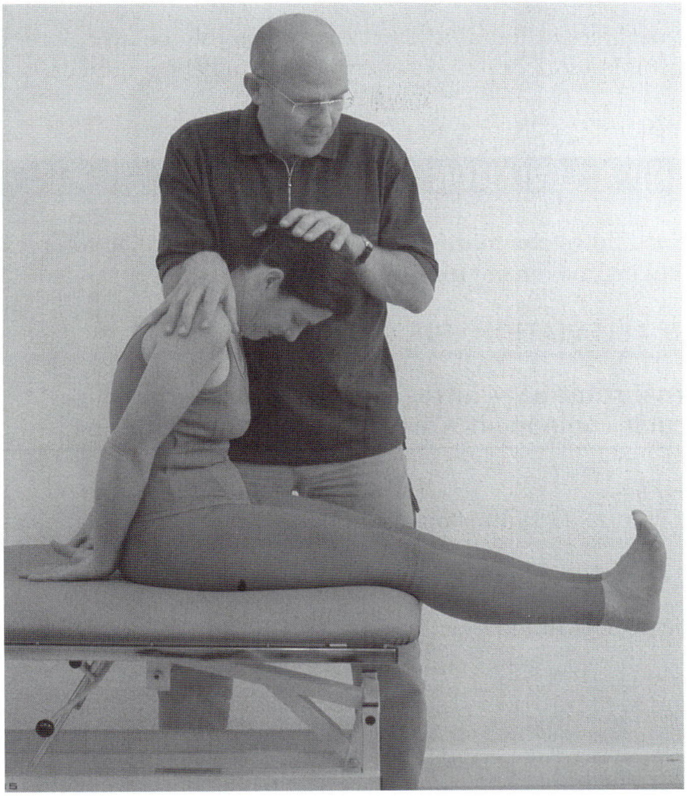

Figure 9.45 Quick check neurodynamics; slump (SLR) test.

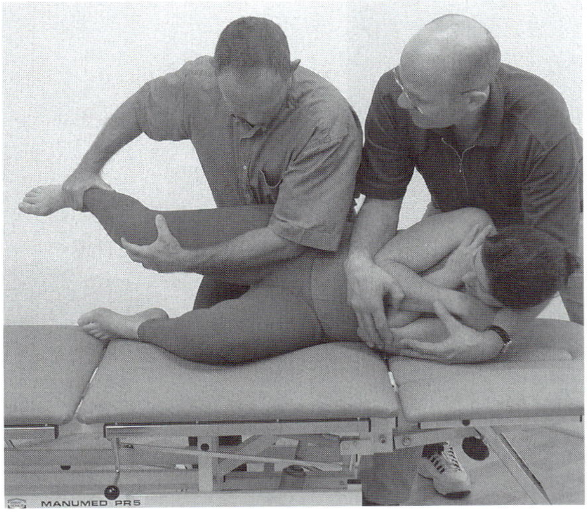

Figure 9.46 Quick check neurodynamics; prone knee bend (PKB) test.

NEURAL STRUCTURES

Tension tests

- Slump test (Fig. 9.45, film 616)
- PKB (prone knee bend; femoral nerve test; Fig. 9.46, film 241).

Note: Even an area that proves negative in the quick check may possibly be symptom-provoking (another movement combination, or passive overpressure may be required).

SPECIFIC PROVOCATION AND ALLEVIATION

Specific provocation and alleviation allows one to differentiate within an articular complex and to identify the symptom-provoking movement direction(s).

SPECIFIC PROVOCATION AND ALLEVIATION, HIP COMPLEX

Localization, hip joint – internal rotation – intra-articular (symptom provocation by an intra-articular component – weight-bearing aspect)

Pain-provoking movement (Fig. 9.47)

- Turning the trunk to the right with fixed right stance leg (loaded) provokes pain in the right groin.
- Area localization hints at the hip complex.

The change in symptoms can be demonstrated exactly:

- provocation of pain (Fig. 9.48a and b, film 108)
- alleviation of pain (Fig. 9.49a and b, film 109).

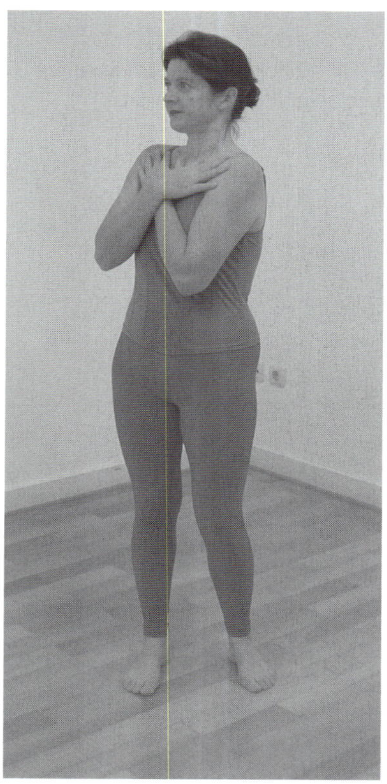

Figure 9.47 Symptom-provoking movement: turning the trunk to the right provokes pain in the right groin.

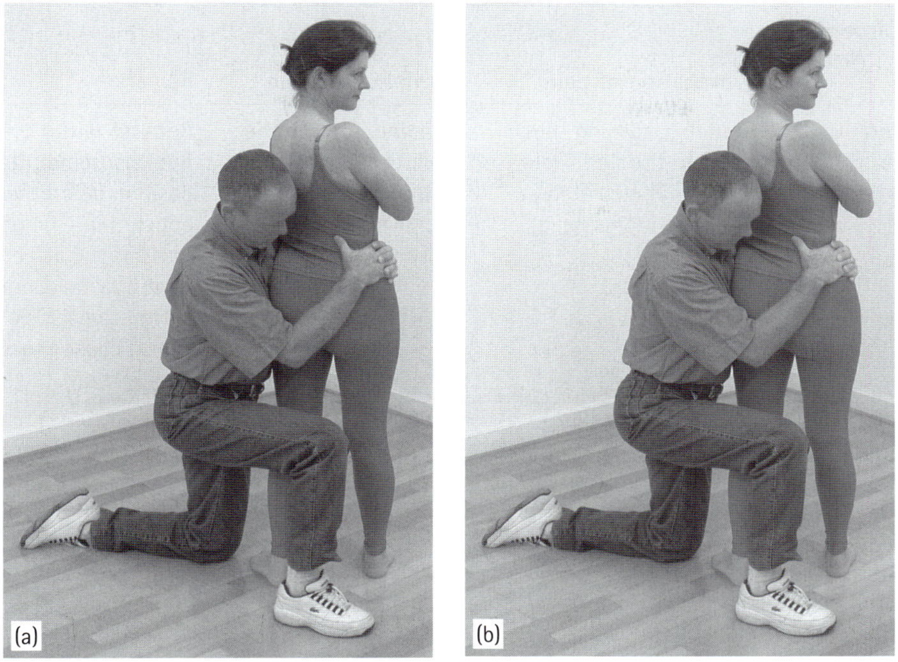

Figure 9.48a and b Specific provocation and alleviation in the area of the lumbosacral junction with symptomatic turning of the trunk to the right; localization, hip joint – internal rotation (intra-articular mechanism); provocation. a, Test start. b, Test end.

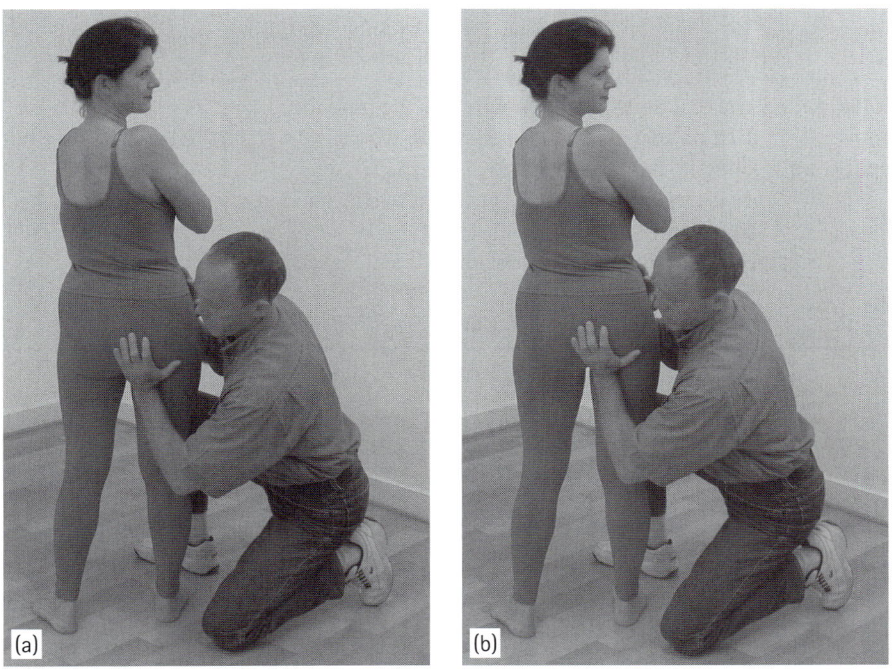

Figure 9.49a and b Specific provocation and alleviation in the area of the lumbosacral junction with symptomatic turning of the trunk to the right; localization, hip joint – internal rotation (intra-articular mechanism); alleviation. a, Test start. b, Test end.

Assessment			
Goal	**Provocation of pain**	**Alleviation of pain**	**Remarks**
Starting position	Standing, turning the trunk to the right, to a position immediately after symptoms have appeared	Standing, turning the trunk to the right, to a position immediately after symptoms have appeared	Because with pre-positioning to a position before symptoms appear non-symptomatic parts of the affected joint may be compressed, a symptomatic position is also chosen for provocation
Test movement	Compression in the weight-bearing part of the hip joint via ipsilateral ilium	Traction in the weight-bearing part of the hip joint via ipsilateral hip bone	
Neural involvement	Proximal and/or distal component without change of position in the relevant area	Proximal and/or distal component without change of position in the relevant area	
Explanation	This manoeuvre increases the intra-articular compression forces in the weight-bearing part of the hip joint	This manoeuvre reduces the intra-articular compression forces in the weight-bearing part of the hip joint	
Additional data to support the hypothesis	General and specific mobility of the hip joint History (e.g., symptom behaviour, type of complaints, 24-hour behaviour) Specific palpation Neurodynamic tests (if specific provocation and alleviation indicate neural involvement) Reproducibility of test results Test treatment Imaging procedures (CT, MRI)		

Localization, hip joint – internal rotation – movement as symptom-provoking component – rolling

Pain-provoking movement

- Turning the trunk to the right with fixed right stance leg provokes pain in the right groin.
- Area localization hints at the hip complex.

The change in symptoms can be demonstrated exactly. Although functional demonstration was performed in standing, it is assumed in this example that the same symptoms can be reproduced in prone position by internal rotation of the right leg. If, however, symptoms cannot be reproduced exactly in this position or if other symptoms are reproduced, it is questionable whether results found in this way are related to the patient's functional problem:

- provocation of pain (Fig. 9.50a and b, film 110)
- alleviation of pain (Fig. 9.51a and b, film 111).

Assessment

Goal	Provocation of pain	Alleviation of pain	Remarks
Starting position	Prone, right hip rotated internally to a position immediately before symptoms appear	Prone, right hip rotated internally to a position immediately after symptoms have appeared	
Test movement	Femur moves in anterior direction with fixed ilium	Ilium moves in anterior direction with fixed femur	Fixation is done by means of a wedge or sandbag
Neural involvement	Proximal and/or distal component without change of position in the relevant area	Proximal and/or distal component without change of position in the relevant area	
Explanation	It is assumed that symptomatic structures in the anterior area are provoked by the decentring of the femur due to rolling in anterior direction	Movement of the ilium in anterior direction leads to posterior glide of the femur, which takes load off symptomatic structures in the anterior area	
Additional data to support the hypothesis	General and specific mobility of the hip joint History (e.g., symptom behaviour, type of complaints, 24-hour behaviour) Specific palpation Neurodynamic tests (if specific provocation and alleviation indicate neural involvement) Reproducibility of test results Test treatment Imaging procedures (CT, MRI)		

Localization, hip joint – internal rotation – movement as symptom-provoking component – gliding

Pain-provoking movement

- Turning the trunk to the right with fixed right stance leg provokes pain in the right groin.
- Area localization hints at the hip complex.

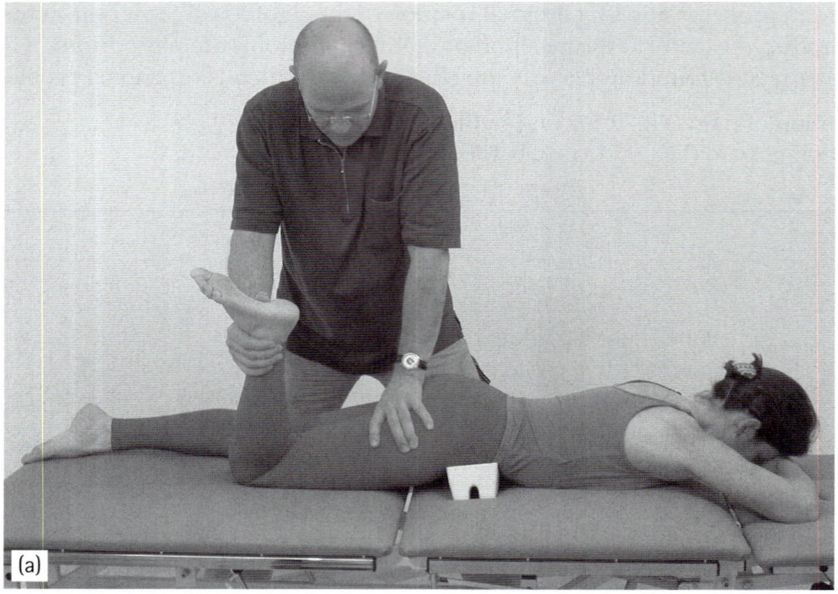

(a)

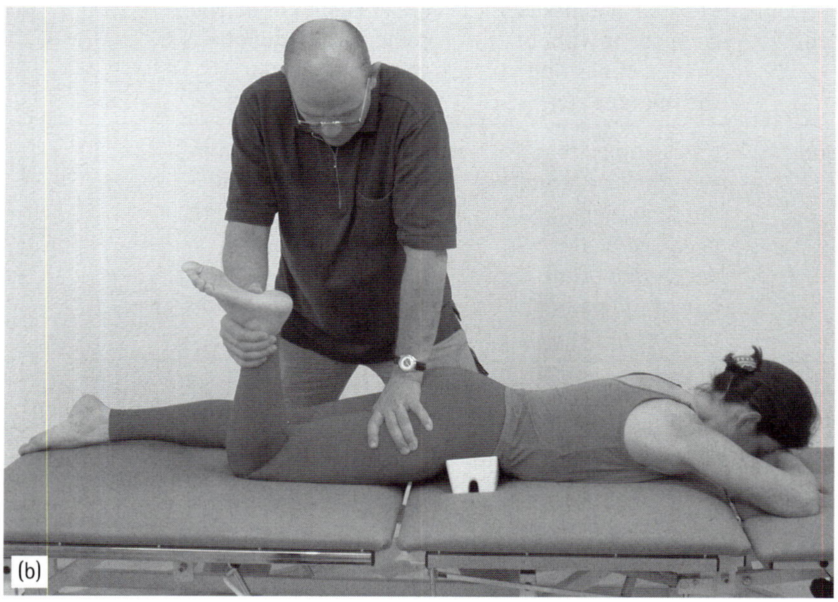

(b)

Figure 9.50a and b Specific provocation and alleviation in the area of the lumbosacral junction with symptomatic turning of the trunk to the right; localization, hip joint – internal rotation (rolling as symptom-provoking mechanism); provocation. **a**, Test start. **b**, Test end.

The change in symptoms can be demonstrated exactly. Although functional demonstration was performed in standing, it is assumed in this example that the same symptoms can be reproduced in prone position by internal rotation of the right leg. If, however, symptoms cannot be reproduced exactly in this position or if other symptoms are reproduced,

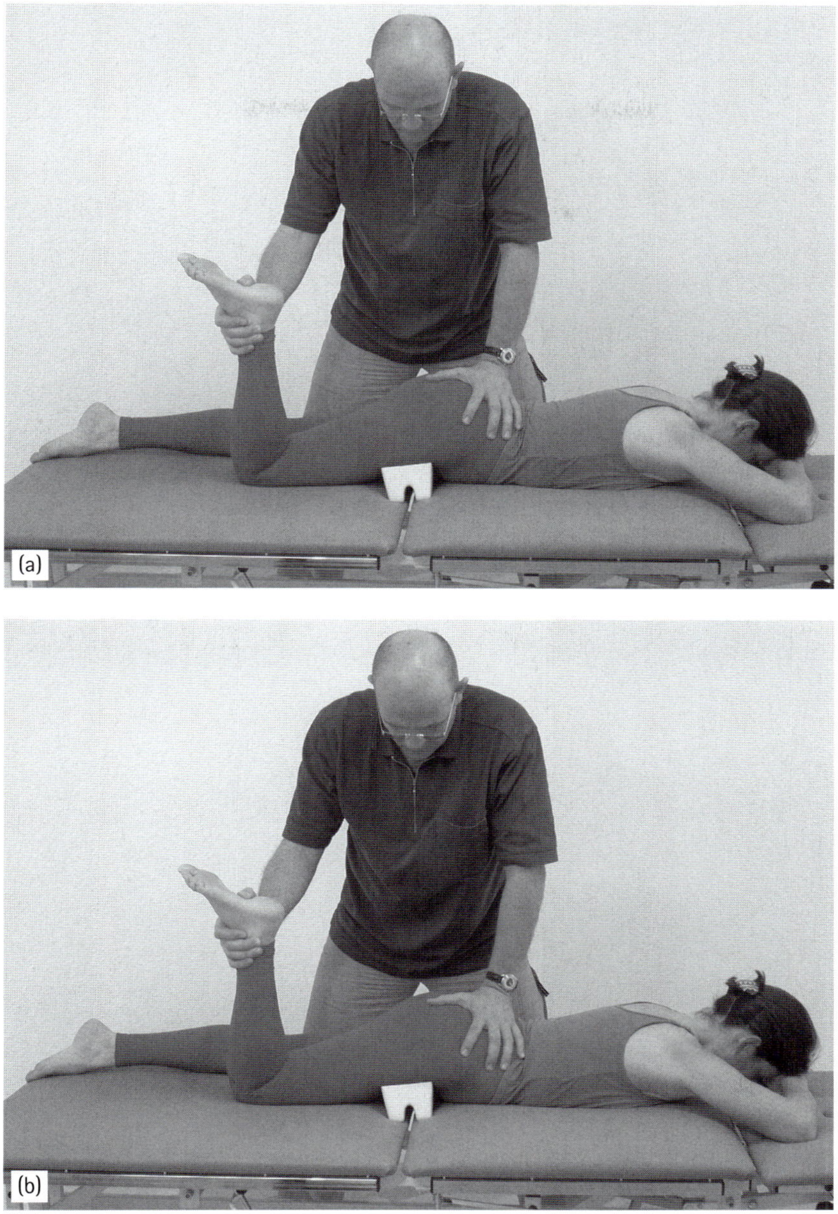

Figure 9.51a and b Specific provocation and alleviation in the area of the lumbosacral junction with symptomatic turning of the trunk to the right; localization, hip joint – internal rotation (rolling as symptom-provoking mechanism); alleviation. a, Test start. b, Test end.

it is questionable whether results found in this way are related to the patient's functional problem:

- provocation of pain (Fig. 9.52a and b, film 112)
- alleviation of pain (Fig. 9.53a and b, film 113).

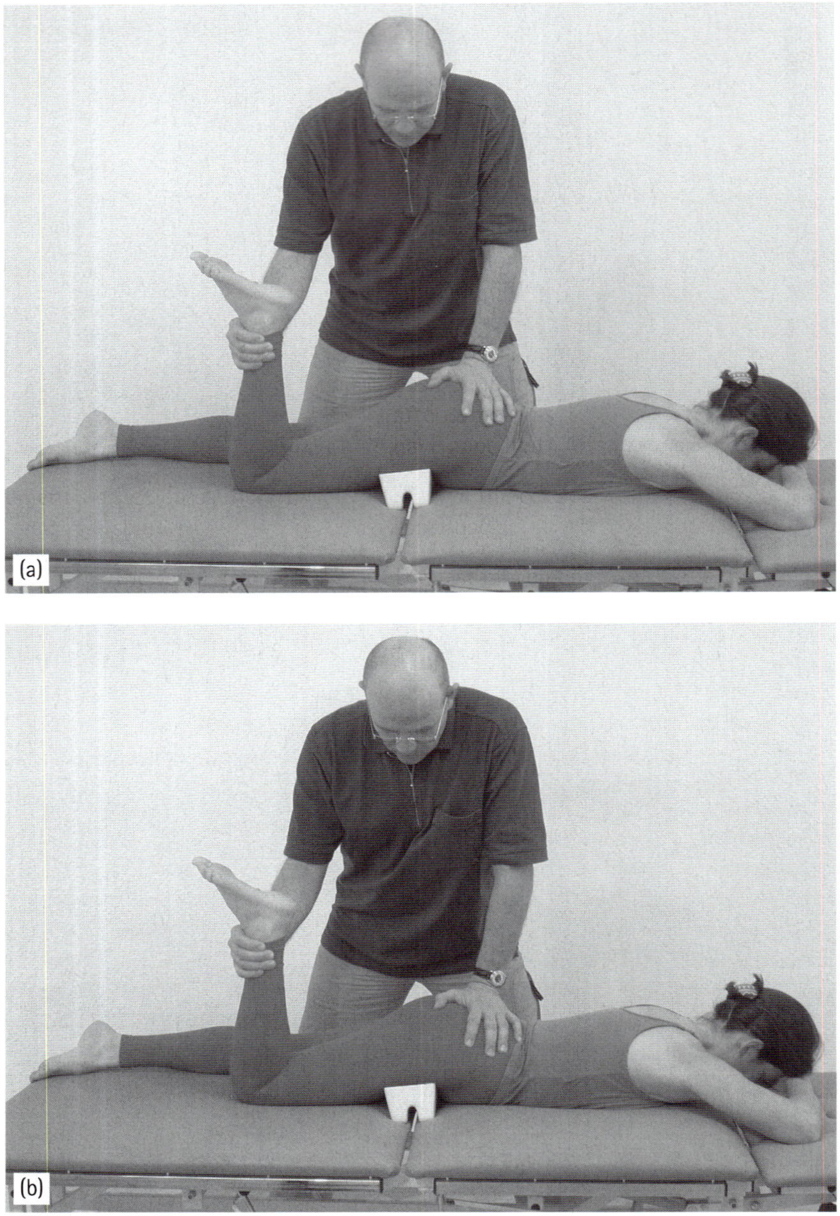

Figure 9.52a and b Specific provocation and alleviation in the area of the lumbosacral junction with symptomatic turning of the trunk to the right; localization, hip joint – internal rotation (gliding as symptom-provoking mechanism); provocation. **a**, Test start. **b**, Test end.

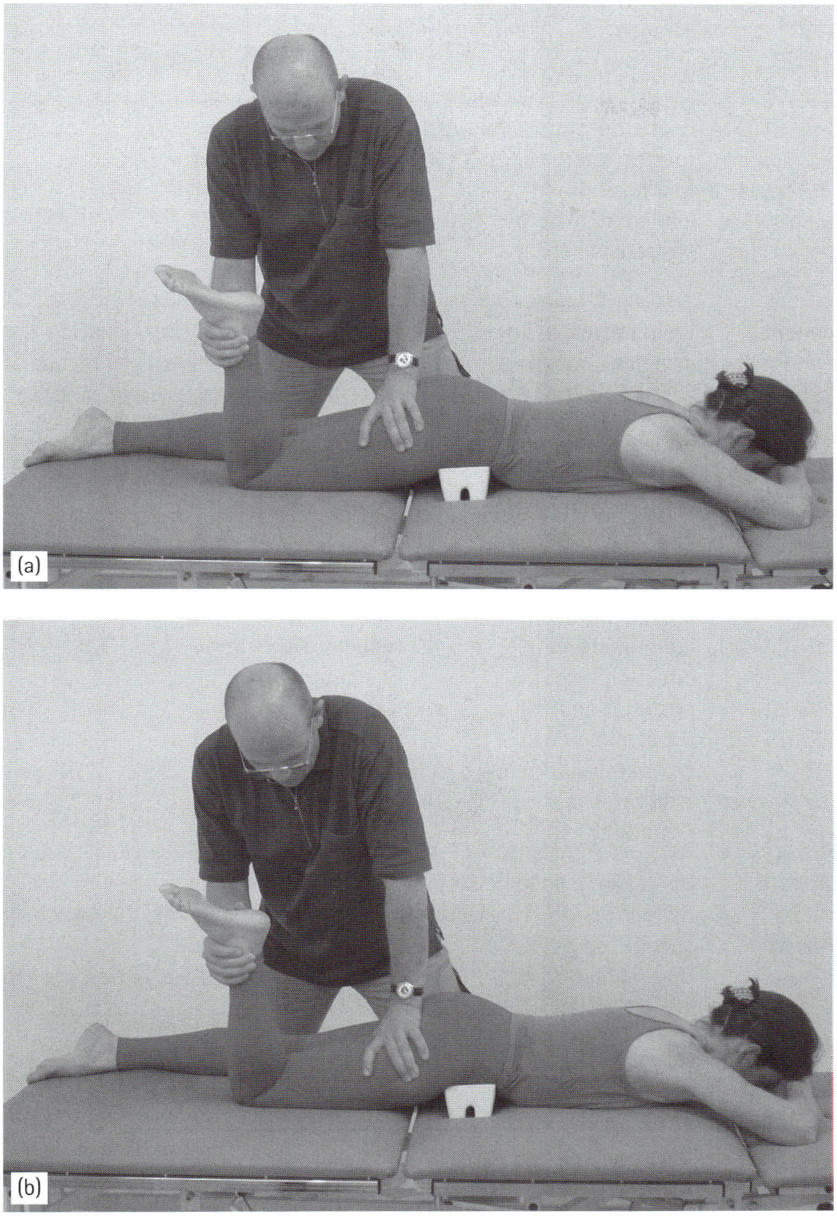

Figure 9.53a and b Specific provocation and alleviation in the area of the lumbosacral junction with symptomatic turning of the trunk to the right; localization, hip joint – internal rotation (gliding as symptom-provoking mechanism); alleviation. **a**, Test start. **b**, Test end.

Assessment			
Goal	**Provocation of pain**	**Alleviation of pain**	**Remarks**
Starting position	Prone, right hip rotated internally to a position immediately before symptoms appear	Prone, right hip rotated internally to a position immediately after symptoms have appeared	
Test movement	Ilium moves in anterior direction, with fixed femur	Femur moves in anterior direction, with fixed ilium	Fixation is done by means of a wedge or sandbag
Neural involvement	Proximal and/or distal component without change of position in the relevant area	Proximal and/or distal component without change of position in the relevant area	
Explanation	Movement of the ilium in anterior direction leads to posterior glide of the femur, which provokes symptomatic structures in the posterior area	This manoeuvre reduces provocation of symptomatic structures in the posterior area of the hip joint	
Additional data to support the hypothesis	General and specific mobility of the hip joint History (e.g., symptom behaviour, type of complaints, 24-hour behaviour) Specific palpation Neurodynamic tests (if specific provocation and alleviation indicate neural involvement) Reproducibility of test results Test treatment Imaging procedures (CT, MRI)		

Differentiation, hip joint – lunge step with left leg – joint vs. iliopsoas muscle

Pain-provoking movement (Fig. 9.54)

- Lunge step with the left leg provokes pain in the right groin.
- Area localization hints at the hip complex. Neural structures have been excluded as symptom-provoking structures.

  The change in symptoms can be demonstrated exactly:

- provocation of pain (Fig. 9.55a and b, film 114)
- alleviation of pain (Fig. 9.56a and b, film 115).

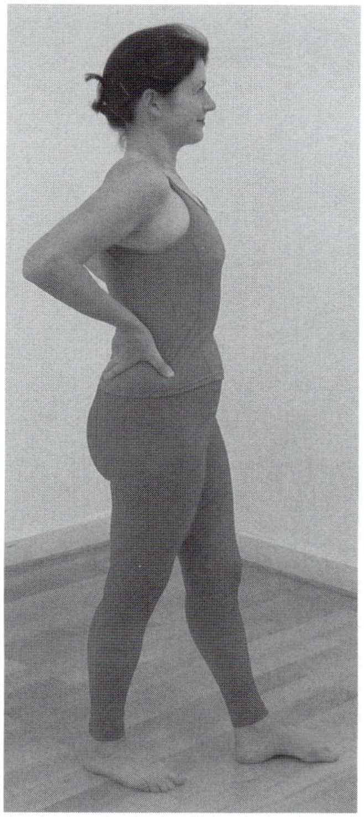

Figure 9.54 Symptom-provoking movement: a lunge step with the left leg provokes pain in the right groin.

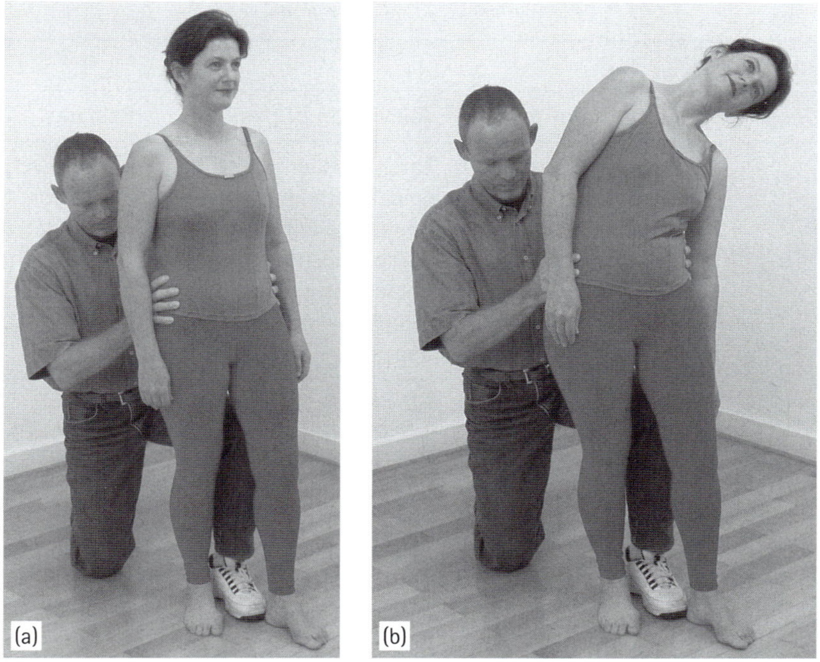

Figure 9.55a and b Specific provocation and alleviation in the area of the lumbosacral junction with symptomatic lunge step with left leg; differentiation, hip joint vs. iliopsoas muscle; provocation.
a, Test start. **b**, Test end.

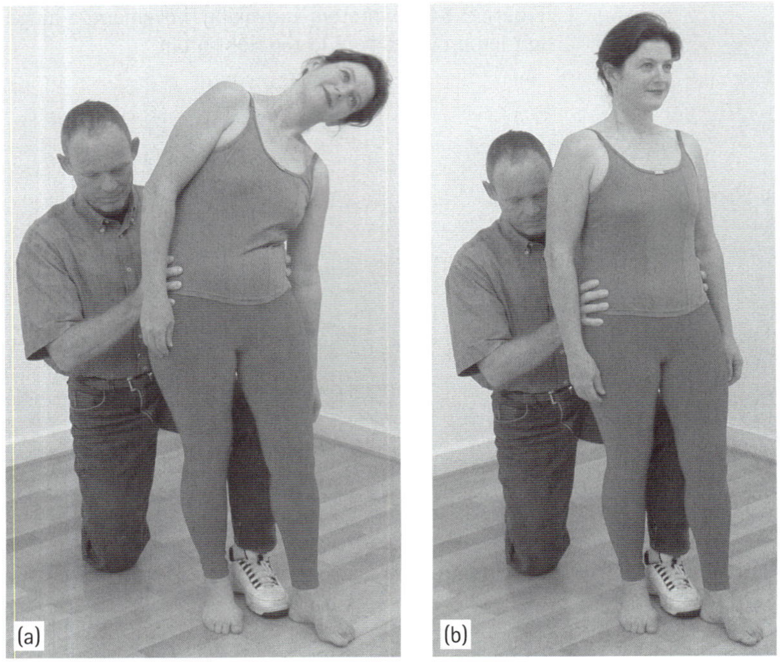

Figure 9.56a and b Specific provocation and alleviation in the area of the lumbosacral junction with symptomatic lunge step with left leg; differentiation, hip joint vs. iliopsoas muscle; alleviation.
a, Test start. b, Test end.

Assessment

Goal	Provocation of pain	Alleviation of pain	Remarks
Starting position	Standing, lunge step with left leg to a position immediately before symptoms appear	Lateral flexion of the spine in standing then, lunge step with left leg to a position immediately after symptoms have appeared	Alternatively, for alleviation, the spine may be lateroflexed to the right after the symptomatic position has been taken
Test movement	Lateral flexion of the spine to the left	Moving the spine back	
Neural involvement	Proximal and/or distal component without change of position in the relevant area	Proximal and/or distal component without change of position in the relevant area	
Explanation	Lateral flexion of the spine to the left elongates the distance between origin and	Lateral flexion of the spine to the right shortens the distance between origin and	

Goal	Provocation of pain	Alleviation of pain	Remarks
	attachment of the iliopsoas muscle. This means an increased mechanical load in the starting position	attachment of the iliopsoas muscle. This means a decreased mechanical load in the starting position	
Additional data to support the hypothesis	General and specific mobility of the hip joint History (e.g., symptom behaviour, type of complaints, 24-hour behaviour) Specific palpation Neurodynamic tests (if specific provocation and alleviation indicate neural involvement) Reproducibility of test results Test treatment Imaging procedures (CT, MRI)		

Localization, hip joint – flexion – movement as symptom-provoking component – rolling

Pain-provoking movement (Fig. 9.57)

- Flexion of the hip joint provokes pain in the right groin.
- Area localization hints at the hip complex.

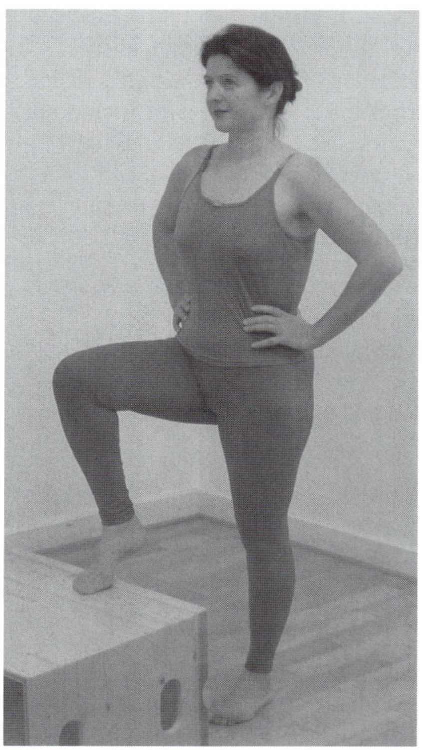

Figure 9.57 Symptom-provoking movement: flexion of the hip joint provokes pain in the right groin.

The change in symptoms can be demonstrated exactly. Although functional demonstration was performed in standing, in this example it is assumed that the same symptoms can be reproduced by flexion from a supine position. If no exact reproduction of symptoms in this position is possible or if other symptoms are reproduced, it is questionable whether the results gained in this way are associated with the patient's functional problem:

- provocation of pain (Fig. 9.58a and b, film 116)
- alleviation of pain (Fig. 9.59a and b, film 117).

Assessment

Goal	Provocation of pain	Alleviation of pain	Remarks
Starting position	Supine, flexion of the right hip joint to a position immediately before symptoms appear	Supine, flexion of the right hip joint to a position immediately after symptoms have appeared	
Test movement	Ilium moves in posterior direction, with fixed femur	Femur moves in posterior direction, with fixed ilium	
Neural involvement	Proximal and/or distal component without change of position in the relevant area	Proximal and/or distal component without change of position in the relevant area	
Explanation	It is assumed that symptomatic structures in the anterior area are provoked by the decentring of the femur due to rolling in anterior direction. The femur is fixed in anterior direction by a belt	Movement of the femur in posterior direction leads to a centring of the hip joint, which takes load off symptomatic structures in the anterior area	If fixation of the ilium with the wedge for provocation is not sufficient, use an additional belt to stabilize the ilium
Additional data to support the hypothesis	General and specific mobility of the hip joint History (e.g., symptom behaviour, type of complaints, 24-hour behaviour) Specific palpation Neurodynamic tests (if specific provocation and alleviation indicate neural involvement) Reproducibility of test results Test treatment Imaging procedures (CT, MRI)		

Localization, hip joint – flexion – movement as symptom-provoking component – gliding

- Provocation of pain (Fig. 9.60a and b, film 118)
- Alleviation of pain (Fig. 9.61a and b, film 119).

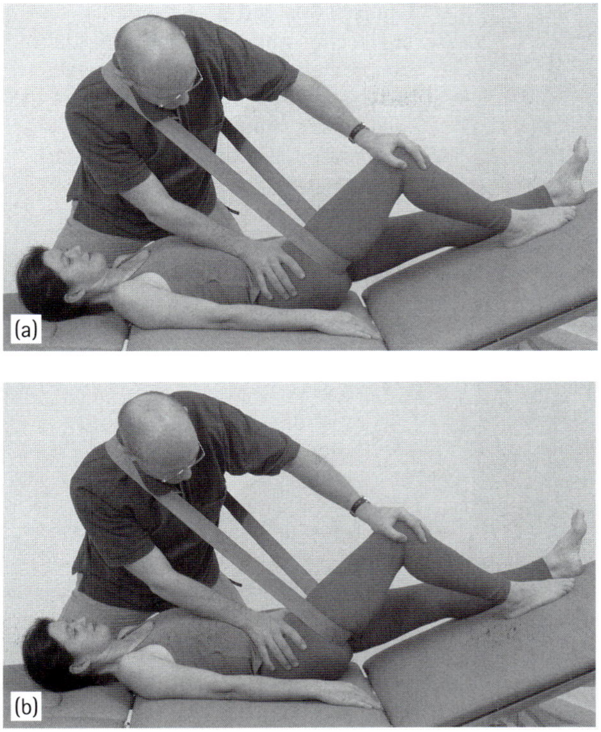

Figure 9.58a and b Specific provocation and alleviation with symptomatic flexion of the hip joint; localization, hip joint – flexion (rolling as symptom-provoking mechanism); provocation. **a**, Test start. **b**, Test end.

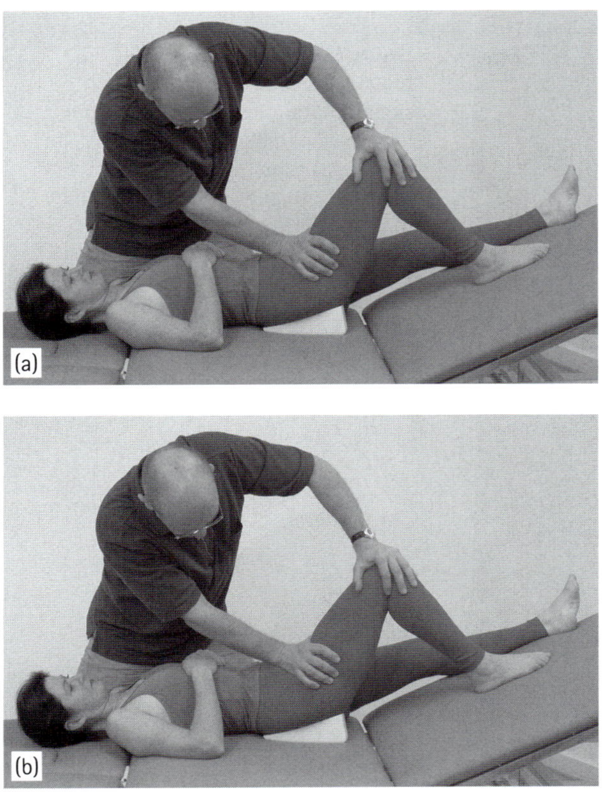

Figure 9.59a and b Specific provocation and alleviation with symptomatic flexion of the hip joint; localization, hip joint – flexion (rolling as symptom-provoking mechanism); alleviation. **a**, Test start. **b**, Test end.

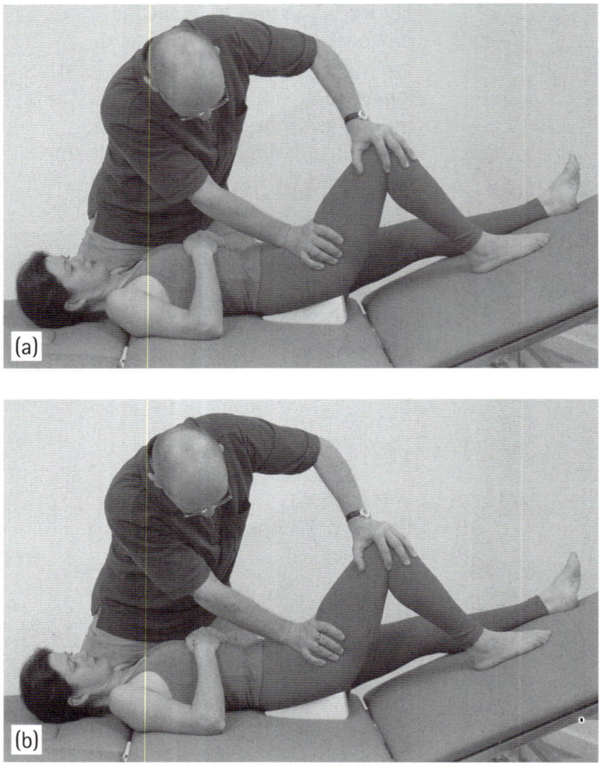

Figure 9.60a and b Specific provocation and alleviation with symptomatic flexion of the hip joint; localization, hip joint – flexion (gliding as symptom-provoking mechanism); provocation. **a**, Test start. **b**, Test end.

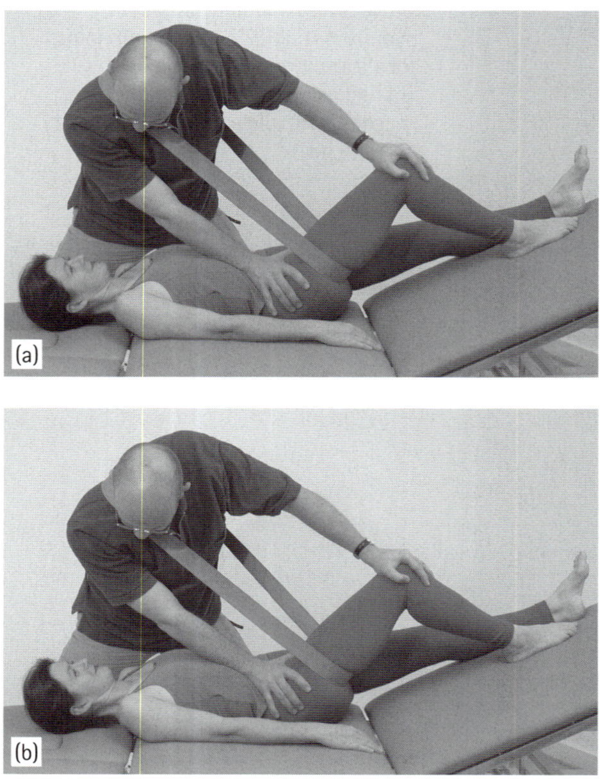

Figure 9.61a and b Specific provocation and alleviation with symptomatic flexion of the hip joint; localization, hip joint – flexion (gliding as symptom-provoking mechanism); alleviation. **a**, Test start. **b**, Test end.

Assessment			
Goal	**Provocation of pain**	**Alleviation of pain**	**Remarks**
Starting position	Supine, flexion of the right hip joint to a position immediately before symptoms appear	Supine, flexion of the right hip joint to a position immediately after symptoms have appeared	
Test movement	Femur moves in posterior direction, with fixed ilium	Ilium moves in posterior direction, with fixed femur	
Neural involvement	Proximal and/or distal component without change of position in the relevant area	Proximal and/or distal component without change of position in the relevant area	
Explanation	It is assumed that symptomatic structures in the posterior area are provoked by the gliding of the femur in posterior direction	Movement of the femur in anterior direction takes load off symptomatic structures in the posterior area of the hip joint. The femur is fixed in anterior direction by a belt	
Additional data to support the hypothesis	General and specific mobility of the hip joint History (e.g., symptom behaviour, type of complaints, 24-hour behaviour) Specific palpation Neurodynamic tests (if specific provocation and alleviation indicate neural involvement) Reproducibility of test results Test treatment Imaging procedures (CT, MRI)		

GENERAL MOVEMENT TESTS

General movement tests identify, quantify, and qualify individual anatomical movements and, in part, movement combinations in the area presumed. The individual manual therapy concepts have respective protocols at their disposal, which more or less have the same goals.

Information gained in this way is used for checking or modifying the relevant hypotheses developed on the basis of anamnesis and area localization and will help in determining further proceedings.

General question: Is there enough information available to bypass general movement tests?	
No	Yes
⇓	⇓
Performance of the general movement tests	• Additional tests • Test treatment

In view of the described clinical presentation and the results of area localization, general movement tests of the following regions seem to be useful.

Lumbar spine/SIJ		
	Active	Passive
Lumbar spine in general	Flexion Extension Rotation (to the right and left) Lateral flexion (to the right and left)	Flexion Extension Rotation (to the right and left) Lateral flexion (to the right and left)
Movement combinations, lumbar spine in general	Symptomatic movements of the lumbar spine	Symptomatic movements of the lumbar spine
SIJ in general		See 'Quick check' section
Hip joint		
	Active	Passive
Hip joint in general	Flexion Extension Internal rotation in extension Internal rotation in flexion External rotation in extension External rotation in flexion Abduction Adduction	Flexion Extension Internal rotation in extension Internal rotation in flexion External rotation in extension External rotation in flexion Abduction Adduction
Movement combinations, hip joint	Symptomatic movements of the hip joint	Symptomatic movements of the hip joint

TREATMENT EXAMPLE, HIP JOINT

SYMPTOMATIC MOVEMENT

Lifting the right leg and placing it on a stool is restricted by 20% as compared with the opposite side and provokes pain in end-range positions (VAS 5/10) in the area of the right groin.

ASSESSMENTS

Area localization

Area localization hints at symptom provocation by the hip complex. There is no contraindication for movement.

Specific provocation and alleviation

The symptomatic movement direction is rolling of the femur in an anterior direction.

Specific mobility
Specific mobility tests show a firm end feel in the posterior direction.

Palpation
Palpation of the dorsal muscles moving the hip joint shows increased tension and increased tenderness as compared with the contralateral side.

HYPOTHESIS
Painfully restricted movement of the right hip joint into flexion is suspected. Symptoms are provoked by rolling of the femur in an anterior direction with simultaneously increased tension of the dorsal structures of the hip complex (Fig. 9.62).

RELAXATION TECHNIQUES

Hold–relax techniques

CO-CONTRACTION AGAINST DISTRACTION (OF THE WEIGHT-BEARING ASPECTS)

Therapy technique (film 120)
Patient's starting position:

- supine (Fig. 9.63a)
- right hip in resting position

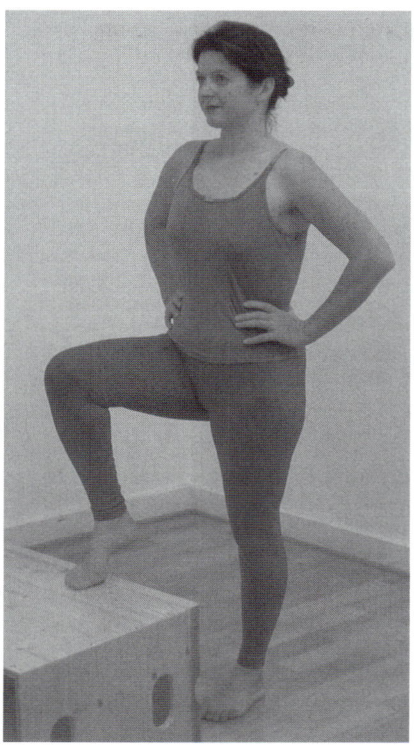

Figure 9.62 Symptom-provoking movement: flexion of the hip joint provokes pain in the right groin.

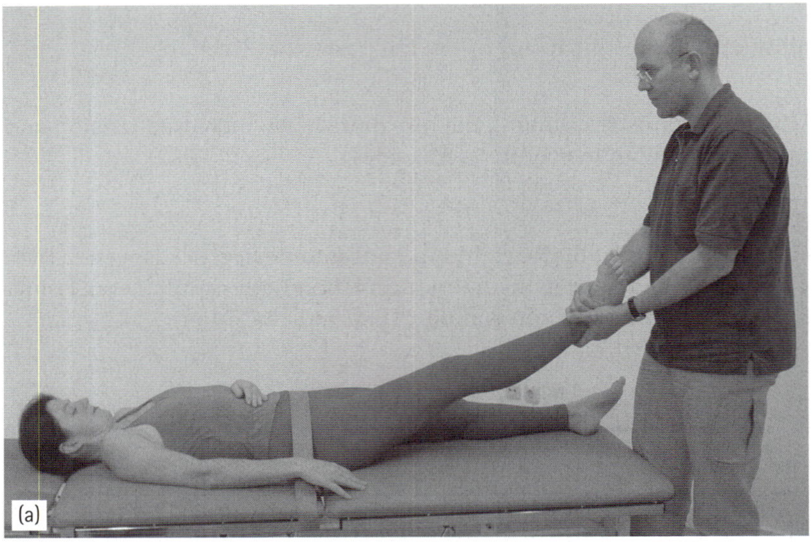

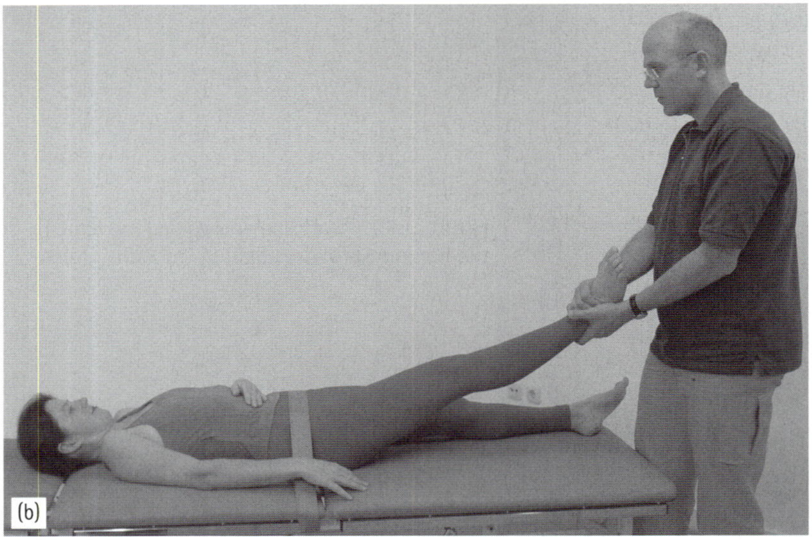

Figure 9.63a and b Hold-relax technique; co-contraction against distraction (weight-bearing aspect); therapy technique. a, Starting position. b, End position.

- knee maximally extended and thus locked
- pelvis fixed against potential co-movements by a belt. Because of the low distraction force, a second belt or a post for further stabilization of the pelvis is not necessary.

Therapist's starting position:

- standing, at the end of the plinth
- grasping patient's lower leg distally.

Movement:

- traction in the hip joint while the patient tries to prevent distraction by muscle contraction (Fig. 9.63b).

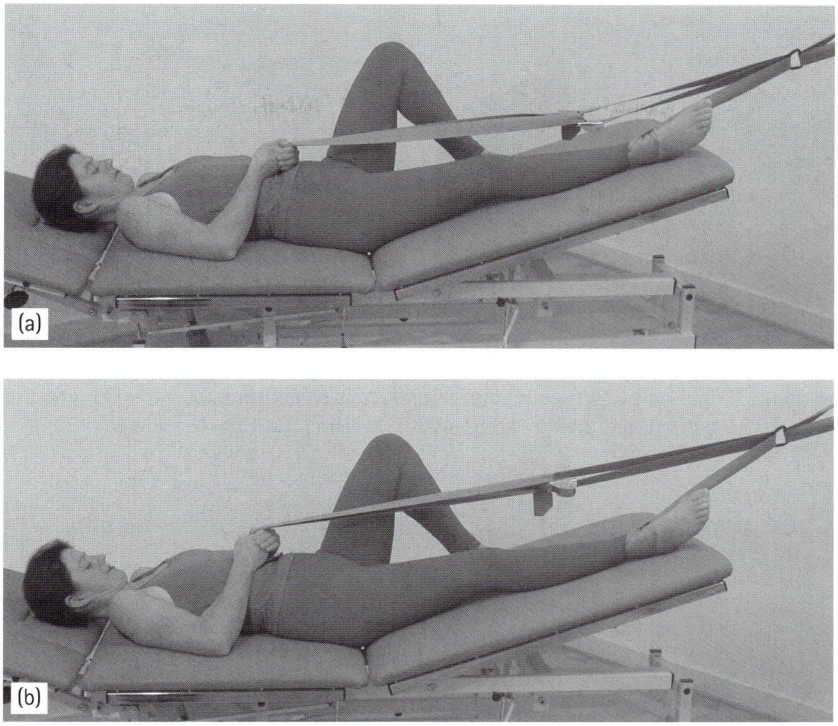

Figure 9.64a and b Hold-relax technique; co-contraction against distraction (weight-bearing aspect); self-exercise. a, Starting position. b, End position.

Self-exercise (film 121)

Patient's starting position:

- supine (Fig. 9.64a)
- a foot cuff or a belt is fixed on the right foot with another belt tied to its lower end
- the belt is put around some firm object and its end is held by the patient's hands
- knee is maximally extended and therefore locked.

Movement:

- pulling the belt while trying to prevent the movement by muscle contraction (Fig. 9.64b).

MOVEMENT-DIRECTED CONTRACTION IN THE DIRECTION OPPOSING THE PAINFUL AND/OR RESTRICTED DIRECTION

Therapy technique (film 122)

Patient's starting position:

- supine, on the plinth (Fig. 9.65a).

Therapist's starting position:

- standing, beside the patient
- patient's leg put over therapist's shoulder.

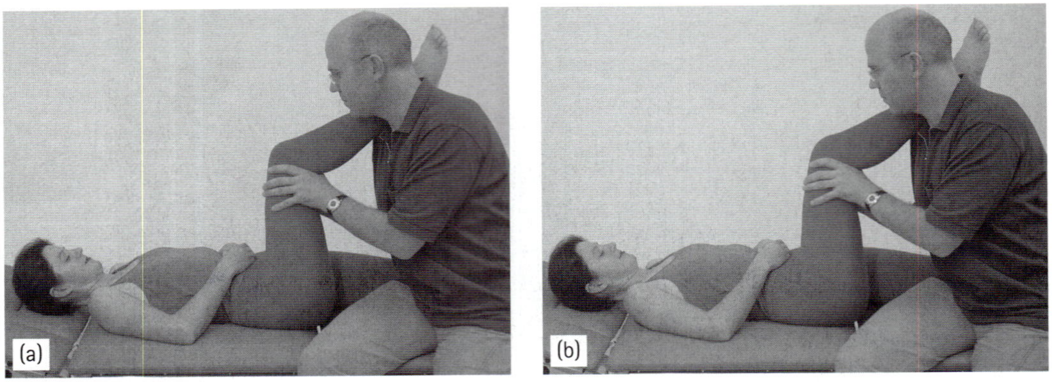

Figure 9.65a and b Hold–relax technique; movement-directed contraction in the direction opposing the painful and/or restricted direction; therapy technique. a, Starting position. b, End position.

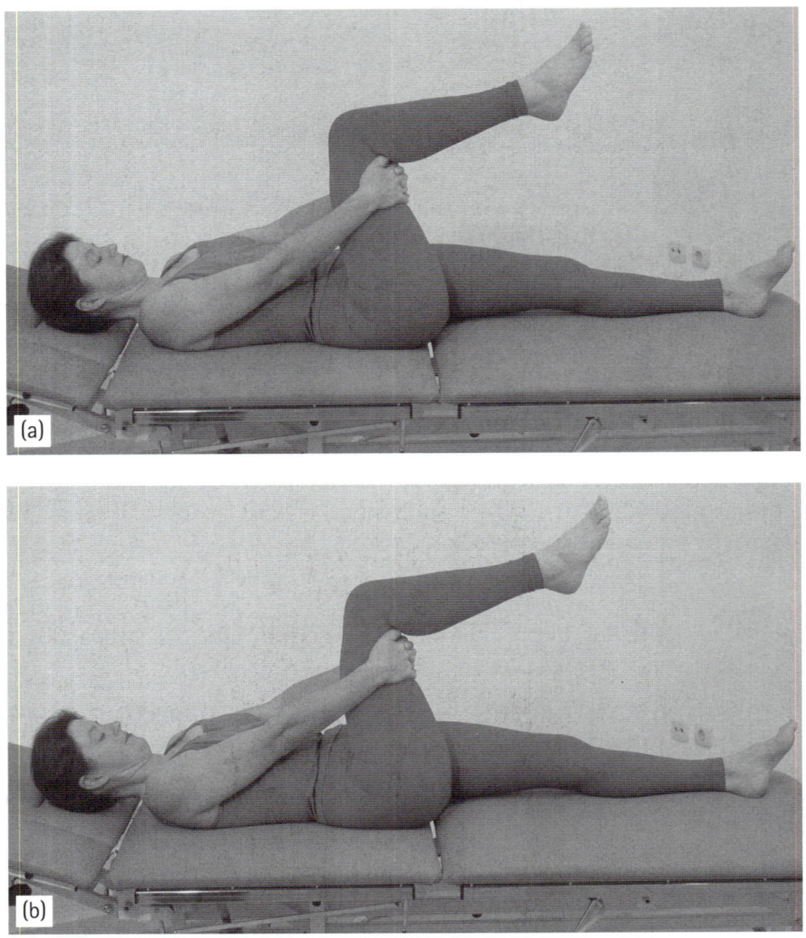

Figure 9.66a and b Hold–relax technique; movement-directed contraction in the direction opposing the painful and/or restricted direction; self-exercise. a, Starting position. b, End position.

Movement:

- flexing patient's hip joint while the patient tries to prevent flexion by muscle contraction (Fig. 9.65b).

Self-exercise (film 123)
Patient's starting position:

- supine (Fig. 9.66a)
- hip flexed
- hands grasping the distal thigh from the back.

Movement:

- flexing the hip joint by pulling with both hands while trying to prevent flexion by muscle contraction (Fig. 9.66b).

MOVEMENT-DIRECTED CONTRACTION IN THE PAINFUL AND/OR RESTRICTED DIRECTION

Therapy technique (film 124)
Patient's starting position:

- supine, on the plinth (Fig. 9.67a).

Therapist's starting position:

- standing, beside the patient
- patient's leg put over therapist's shoulder.

Movement:

- extending patient's hip joint while the patient tries to prevent extension by muscle contraction (Fig. 9.67b).

Self-exercise (film 125)
Patient's starting position:

- supine (Fig. 9.68a)
- hip flexed
- hands grasping the distal thigh at the front.

Movement:

- extending the hip joint by pushing with both hands while trying to prevent extension by muscle contraction (Fig. 9.68b).

Remarks

Goals of the technique
Reduction of tonicity and improvement of the metabolism of the periarticular tissues with a painful movement restriction of the right hip joint in flexion and increased tension in the dorsal structures.

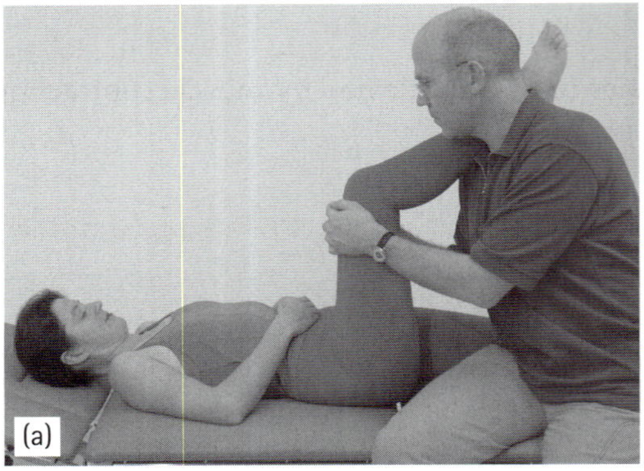

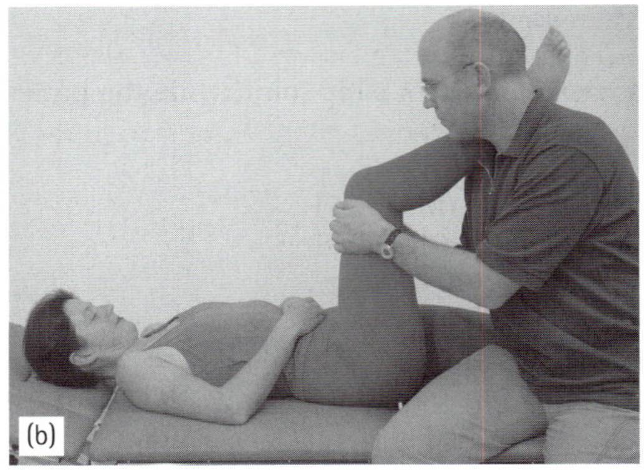

Figure 9.67a and b Hold–relax technique; movement-directed contraction in the painful and/or restricted direction; therapy technique. **a**, Starting position. **b**, End position.

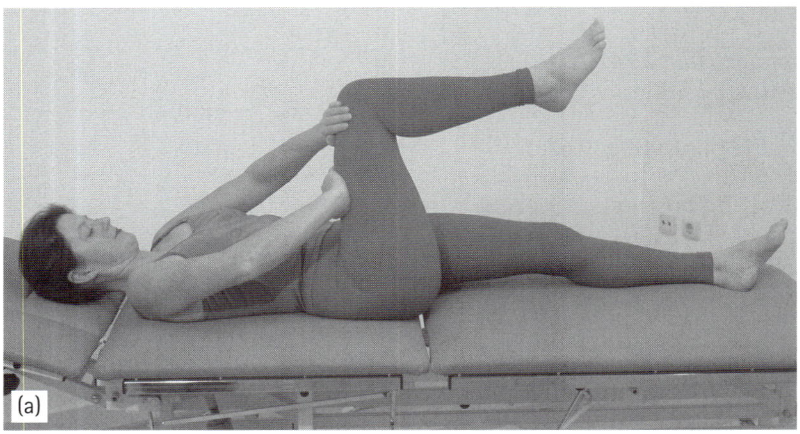

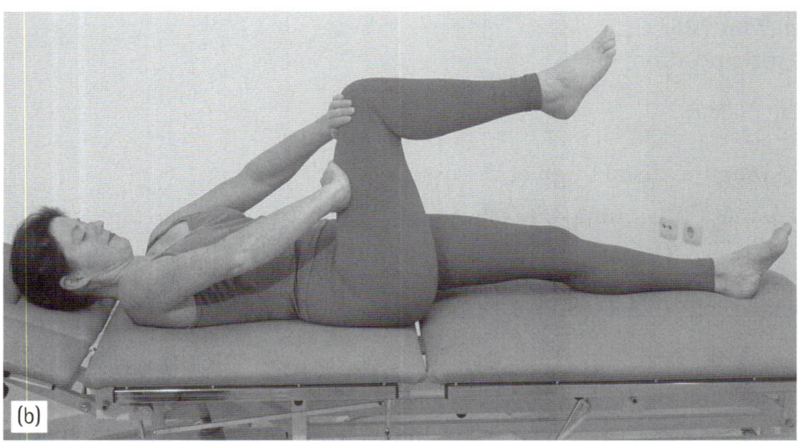

Figure 9.68a and b Hold–relax technique; movement-directed contraction in the painful and/or restricted direction; self-exercise. **a**, Starting position. **b**, End position.

Performance
According to irritability and the desired treatment goal, the joint to be treated is initially pre-positioned. As the self-exercise is performed without 'specific fixation', transferred movement has to be considered when the indication for the exercise is determined.

Dosage (regarding the symptomatic structure)
Both with an acute and with a chronic presentation, contraction should always be pain-free.

Choice of technique
The selection of the technique depends, among other things, on the therapist as well as the patient, on the therapist's clinical experience, but primarily on reassessment. This means that even if all preconditions on the part of therapist and patient seem to be met, it is of no use to continue the technique if reassessment is negative.

Contributing factors
For a satisfactory solution of the patient's current problems it is important to consider the contributing factors and include them in the treatment.

The authors will, however, not go into a description of the various possibilities and their complex contexts as this would exceed the scope of the present book.

Soft tissue techniques

BUTTOCKS MUSCLES

Therapy technique (film 126)
Patient's starting position:

- prone (Fig. 9.69a)
- right knee flexed
- right hip pre-positioned in external rotation.

Therapist's starting position:

- standing, beside the patient at the level of the patient's pelvis
- grasping patient's right distal lower leg with the left hand
- the right hand resting on the patient's buttocks muscles.

Movement:

- passive internal rotation of the right hip with simultaneous manual pressure on the buttocks muscles (Fig. 9.69b)
- releasing pressure, and back to starting position.

Note: If the patient is not able to relax or if performance of the movement seems too difficult, this soft tissue technique can also be performed assistively. Use of the assistive technique results in a simultaneous reciprocal inhibition of the treated muscles, which may facilitate relaxation.

Self-exercise 1 (film 127)
Patient's starting position:

- supine (Fig. 9.70a)
- right hip extended

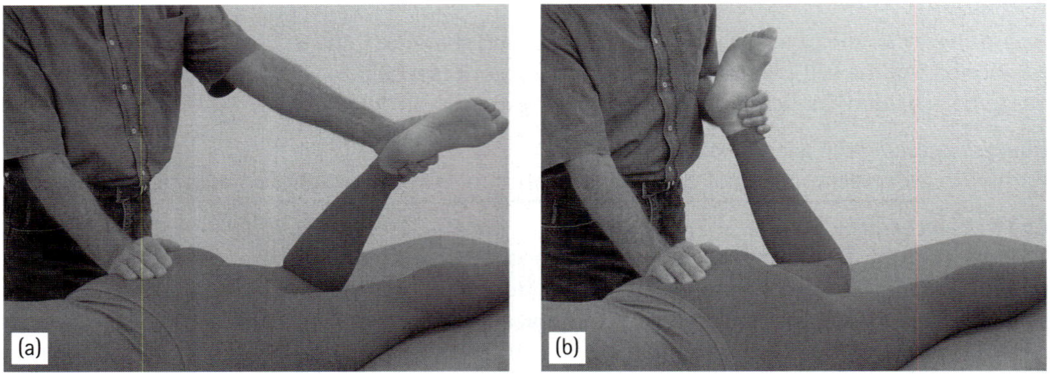

Figure 9.69a and b Soft tissue technique; buttocks muscles; therapy technique. **a**, Starting position. **b**, End position.

- a tennis ball placed under the right buttock in contact with the tense muscles
- right hip pre-positioned in external rotation
- by turning the trunk against the tennis ball, pressure is increased.

Movement:

- internal rotation of the extended right leg while maintaining the adjusted pressure as demonstrated in the film 127. If in this position the pressure is too high, it can be modulated through weight-bearing by the left leg standing on the plinth
- then releasing pressure, and back to starting position.

Self-exercise 2 (film 128)

Patient's starting position:

- supine (Fig. 9.71a)
- both feet standing on the plinth
- a tennis ball placed under the right buttocks to contact the tense muscles
- right hip pre-positioned in external rotation and abduction
- by turning the trunk against the tennis ball, pressure is increased.

Movement:

- adduction of the right leg while maintaining the adjusted pressure, which can be modulated through weight-bearing by the left leg (Fig. 9.71b)
- then releasing pressure, and back to starting position.

Remarks

Goals of the technique

Reduction of tonicity and improvement of the metabolism of the periarticular tissues with a painful movement restriction of the right hip in flexion and increased tension in the dorsal structures.

Performance

As the treatment techniques are performed without 'specific fixation', transferred movement has to be considered when the indication for the technique is determined.

Dosage (regarding the affected symptomatic structure)

Both with an acute and with a chronic presentation, the patient's typical pain in the groin must not be reproduced. Intensity of the pressure exerted on the sensitive dorsal structures of the hip joint depends on the expected training state and load tolerance of the tissue.

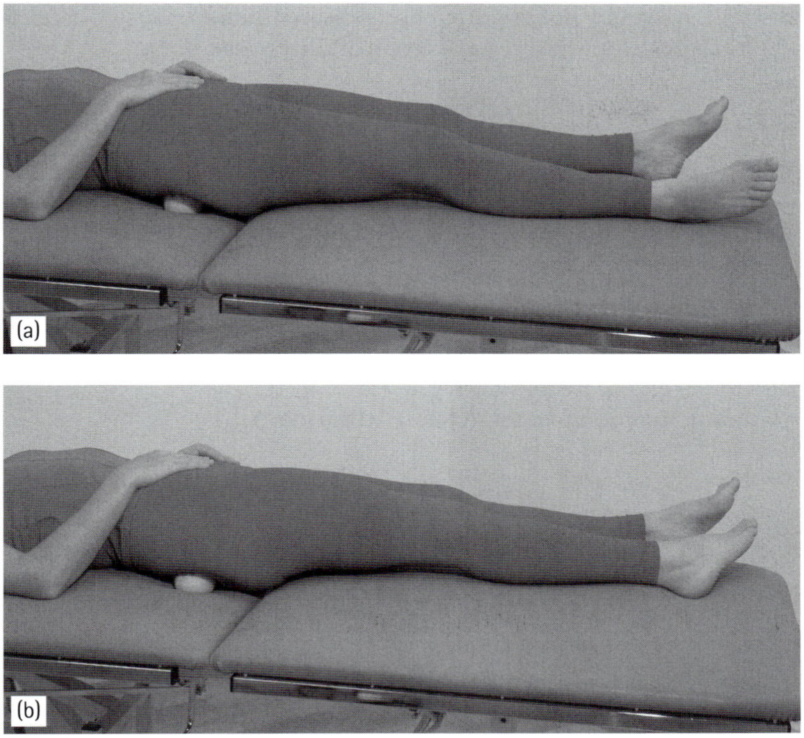

Figure 9.70a and b Soft tissue technique; buttocks muscles; self-exercise 1. **a**, Starting position. **b**, End position.

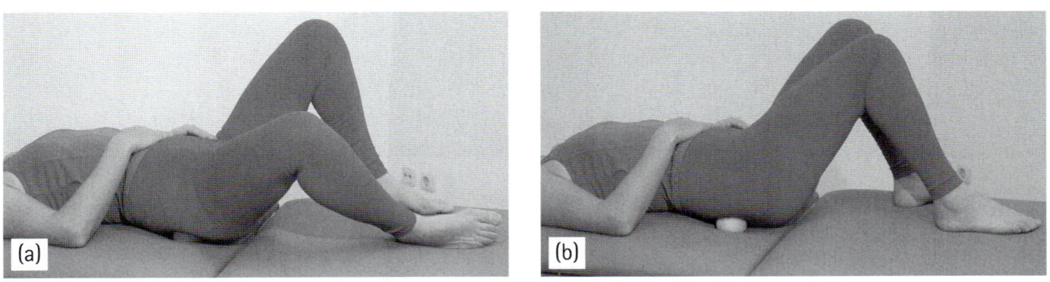

Figure 9.71a and b Soft tissue technique; buttocks muscles; self-exercise 2. **a**, Starting position. **b**, End position.

Choice of technique

The selection of the technique depends, among other things, on the therapist as well as the patient, on the therapist's clinical experience, but primarily on reassessment. This means that even if all preconditions on the part of therapist and patient seem to be met, it is of no use to continue the technique if reassessment is negative.

Contributing factors

For a satisfactory solution of the patient's current problems it is important to consider the contributing factors and include them in the treatment.

The authors will, however, not go into a description of the various possibilities and their complex contexts as this would exceed the scope of the present book.

MOBILIZATION TECHNIQUES

Active procedures

ACTIVE MOBILIZATION PLUS ACCESSORY MOVEMENT

Flexion of the hip with distraction of the weight-bearing aspect

Therapy technique (film 129)

Patient's starting position:

- supine, close to the end of the plinth (Fig. 9.72a)
- a belt surrounding the proximal thigh (close to the joint)
- hip flexed.

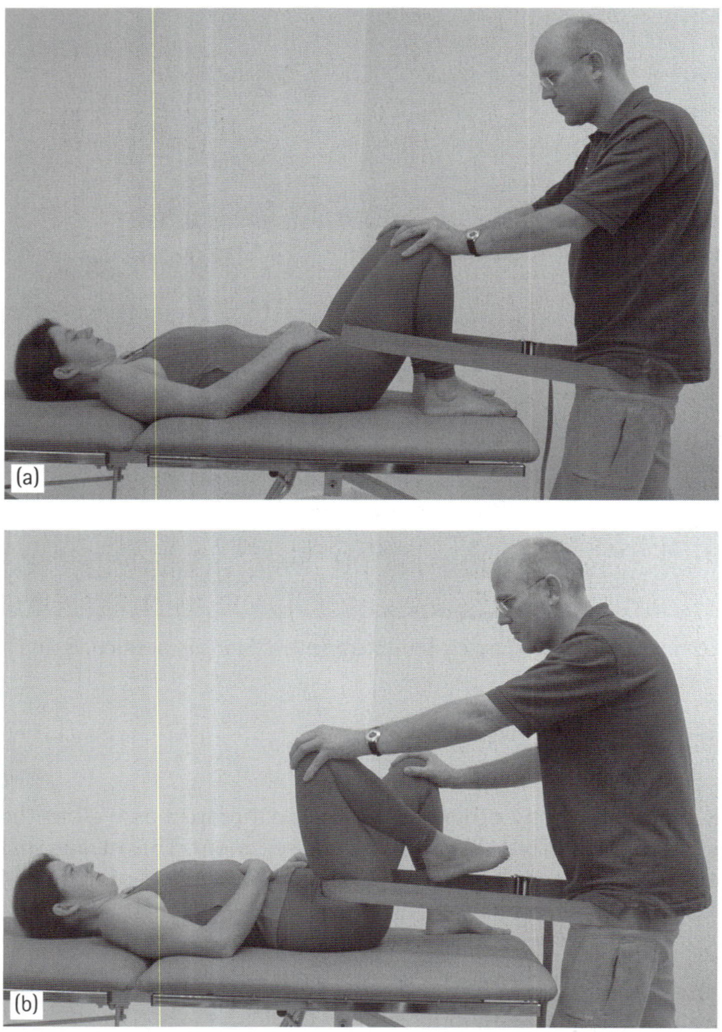

Figure 9.72a and b Active mobilization with accessory movement; flexion of the hip joint with distraction of the weight-bearing aspect; therapy technique. **a**, Starting position. **b**, End position.

Therapist's starting position:

- standing, in front of the patient
- contact with patient's distal femur and distal lower leg
- the belt running around the therapist's pelvis.

Movement:

- pulling the femur in a caudal direction, with subsequent flexion in right hip (Fig. 9.72b)
- guiding leg back into starting position, and releasing traction in caudal direction.

Self-exercise (film 130)

Patient's starting position:

- standing, the symptomatic (right) leg put on a stool, with the foot dorsiflexed (Fig. 9.73a)
- a belt loop surrounding the right femur from the anterior side, as proximally as possible
- patient's left foot is standing in the loop hanging down
- the length of the loop is chosen in such a way that the left leg has to be flexed slightly.

Movement:

- distraction of the weight-bearing aspect of the hip joint by extending the (left) stance leg (Fig. 9.73b)
- then increasing flexion of the right hip joint by plantar flexion of the right foot.

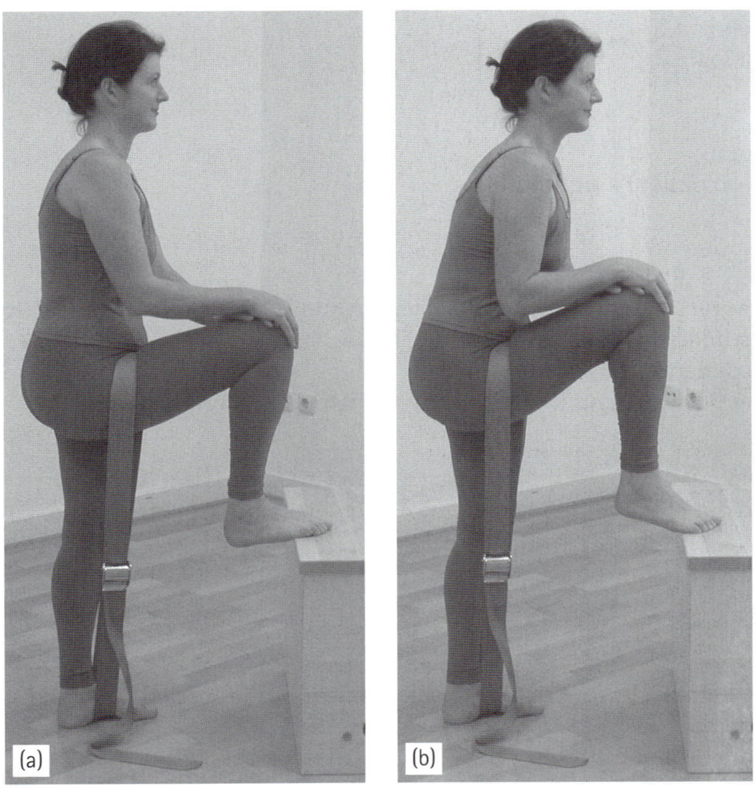

Figure 9.73a and b
Active mobilization with accessory movement; flexion of the hip joint with distraction of the weight-bearing aspect; self-exercise. **a**, Starting position. **b**, End position.

Flexion of the hip with lateral pull – unloaded

Therapy technique (film 131)

Patient's starting position:

- supine (Fig. 9.74a)
- a belt surrounding the pelvis from the left side for fixation.

Therapist's starting position:

- standing, beside the patient
- contact with left hand at patient's pelvis, with right hand at patient's lateral femoral condyle
- a belt running around patient's femur and therapist's pelvis, close to the joint, from the medial side.

Movement:

- pulling the femur in a lateral direction, with subsequent active flexion of the right hip joint (Fig. 9.74b)
- moving leg back into starting position, and then releasing traction in a lateral direction.

Flexion of the hip with lateral pull – loaded

Therapy technique (film 132)

Patient's starting position:

- standing (Fig. 9.75a)
- a belt surrounds the proximal right thigh close to the joint, from the medial side, and runs around the therapist's pelvis
- the weight is on the right leg.

Therapist's starting position:

- standing, beside the patient
- contact with both hands on patient's right ilium
- elbows flexed.

Movement:

- the therapist pulls the femur in a lateral direction by extending both his/her elbows and then has the patient perform a bilateral knee bend (Fig. 9.75b)
- the therapist follows the patient's movement
- moving back into starting position, and then releasing the lateral pull on the femur.

> ***Note:*** The treated leg should not be moved into external rotation in the hip joint. If necessary, the knee should be stabilized manually from the lateral side by the therapist's right hand.

Self-exercise (film 133)

Patient's starting position:

- standing (Fig. 9.76a)
- a belt surrounds the proximal right thigh close to the joint, from the medial side, and is fixed at some fixed object
- right arm supported against some fixed object, the weight on the right leg.

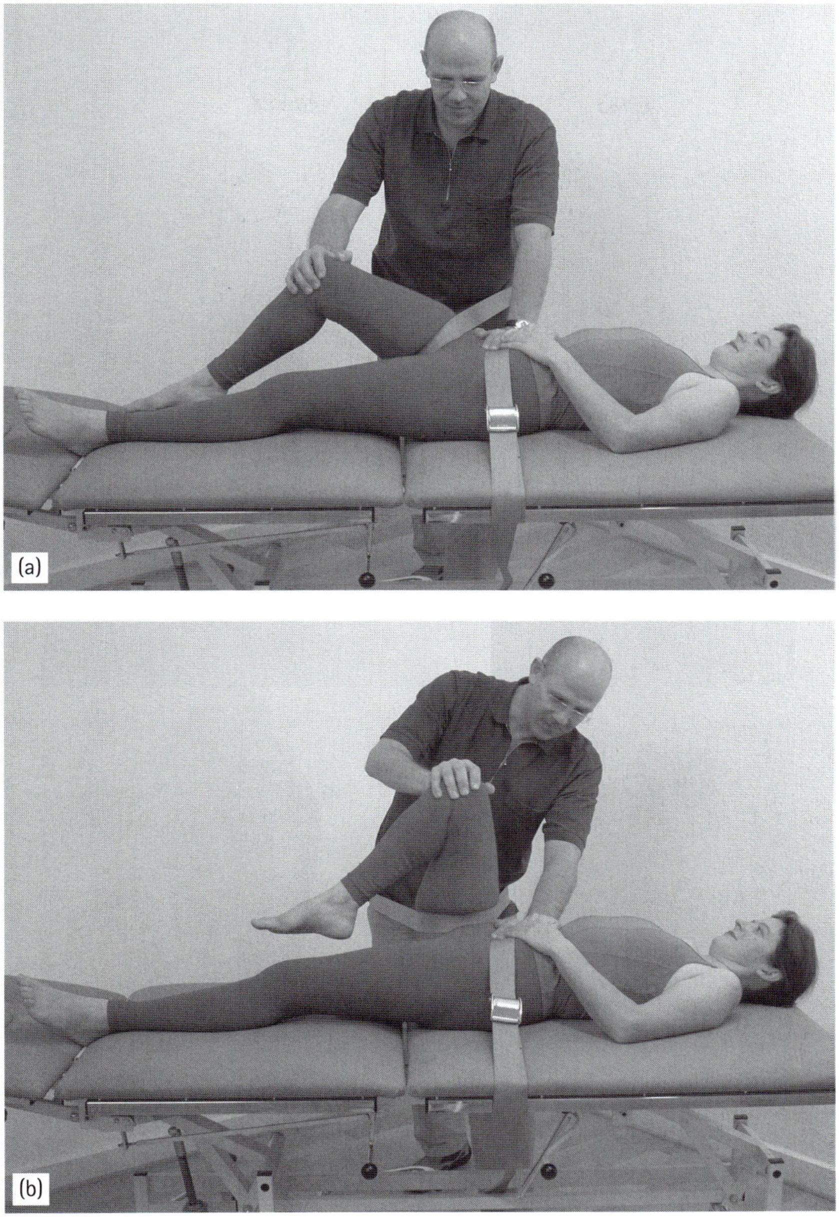

Figure 9.74a and b Active mobilization with accessory movement; flexion of the hip joint with distraction with lateral pull – unloaded; therapy technique. **a**, Starting position. **b**, End position.

Movement:

- by extending the elbow of the supporting arm, the body is shifted and the femur is pulled in a lateral direction (Fig. 9.76b)
- then, bilateral knee bend is performed while maintaining the lateral pull
- moving back into starting position, and then releasing the lateral pull on the femur.

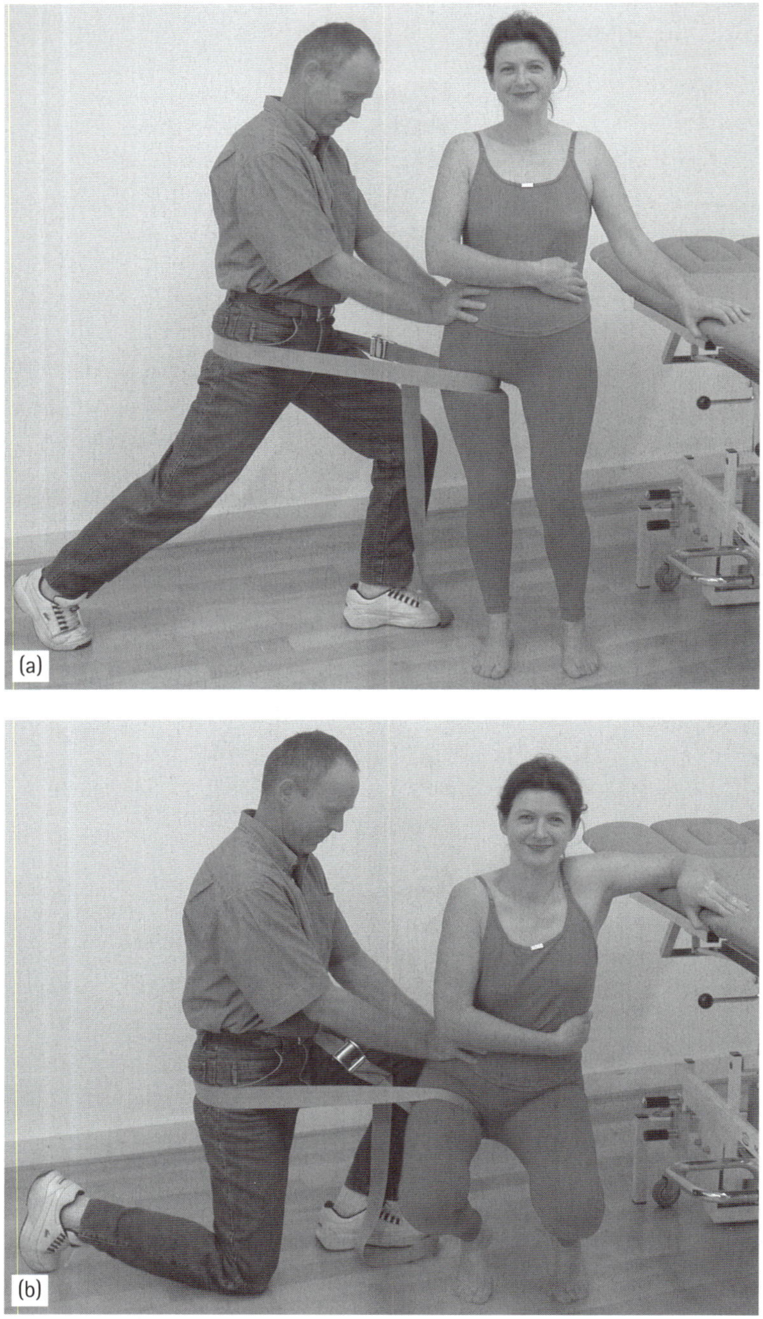

Figure 9.75a and b Active mobilization with accessory movement; flexion of the hip joint with distraction with lateral pull – loaded; therapy technique. **a**, Starting position. **b**, End position.

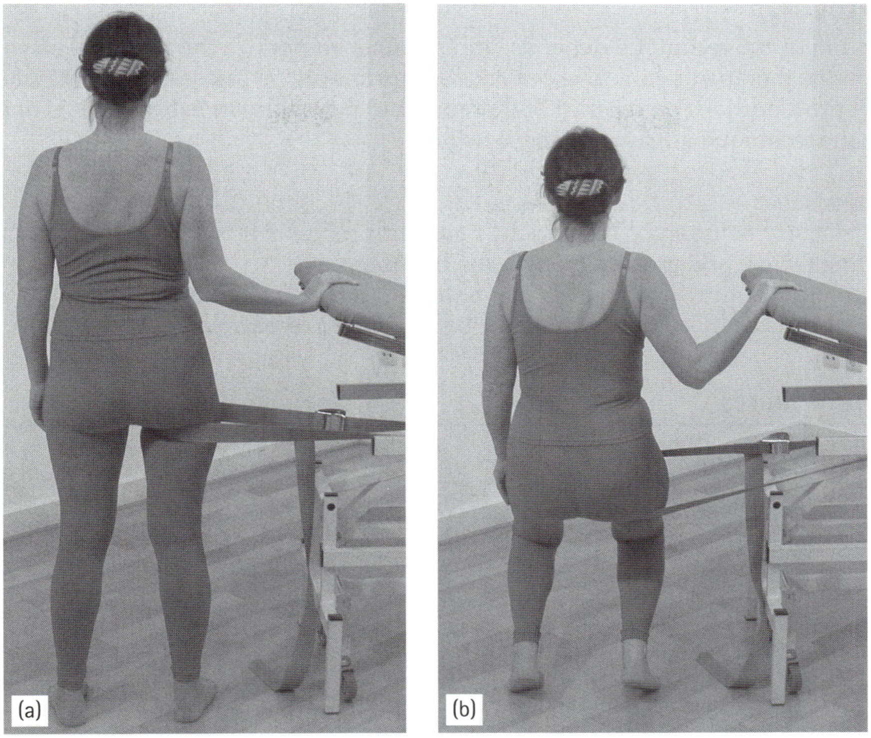

Figure 9.76a and b Active mobilization with accessory movement; flexion of the hip joint with distraction with lateral pull – loaded; self-exercise. **a**, Starting position. **b**, End position.

Note: When teaching the exercise, it should be mentioned that no external rotation in the hip joint must occur during knee bend. If this is not possible, use a circular belt around both distal femurs to avoid excessive rotation.

Remarks

Goals of the technique

With painfully restricted flexion of the right hip and increased tension of the dorsal structures, these techniques serve to:

- reduce tonicity and improve the metabolism of the affected tissues
- restore pain-free function (change input to the respective centres of the central nervous system).

Performance

With respect to the lateral pull and the distraction of the weight-bearing part, attention has to be paid to the treatment plane (Kaltenborn 1999).

Dosage

Both with an acute and with a chronic presentation, this technique should be pain-free and should not provoke the patient's symptoms in the right groin.

Choice of technique

The selection of the technique depends, among other things, on the therapist as well as the patient, on the therapist's clinical experience, but primarily on reassessment. This means that even if all preconditions on the part of therapist and patient seem to be met, it is of no use to continue the technique if reassessment is negative.

Contributing factors

For a satisfactory solution of the patient's current problems it is important to consider the contributing factors and include them in the treatment.

The authors will, however, not go into a description of the various possibilities and their complex contexts as this would exceed the scope of the present book.

Passive procedures

TRANSLATORY MOVEMENTS

Distraction of the weight-bearing aspect, in flexion

Therapy technique (film 134)

Patient's starting position:

- supine (Fig. 9.77a)
- a circular belt fixes the pelvis against the plinth
- a second belt, running in a craniocaudal direction and contacting the sciatic tuberosity of that side, fixes the pelvis against co-movement in a caudal direction
- the hip joint is pre-positioned in flexion, shortly before symptoms appear
- another belt runs around the anterior aspect of the patient's proximal thigh, close to the joint, and around the posterior aspect of the therapist's pelvis.

Therapist's starting position:

- standing, at the foot end of the plinth
- belt running around the therapist.

Movement:

- distraction in the hip joint (at a right angle to the treatment plane of the weight-bearing aspect) (Fig. 9.77b).

Self-exercise (here: treatment of the left leg) (film 135)

Patient's starting position:

- supine (Fig. 9.78a)
- one leg flexed in the hip joint shortly before symptoms appear, the foot placed against some fixed object
- a belt loop surrounds the proximal thigh of that leg as close to the joint as possible
- the other foot is placed in the belt loop
- the length of the belt loop is chosen in such a way that this leg is just slightly flexed.

Movement:

- the leg with the foot in the loop is extended (Fig. 9.78b)
- this results in distraction of the weight-bearing aspect of the flexed hip joint of the leg to be treated.

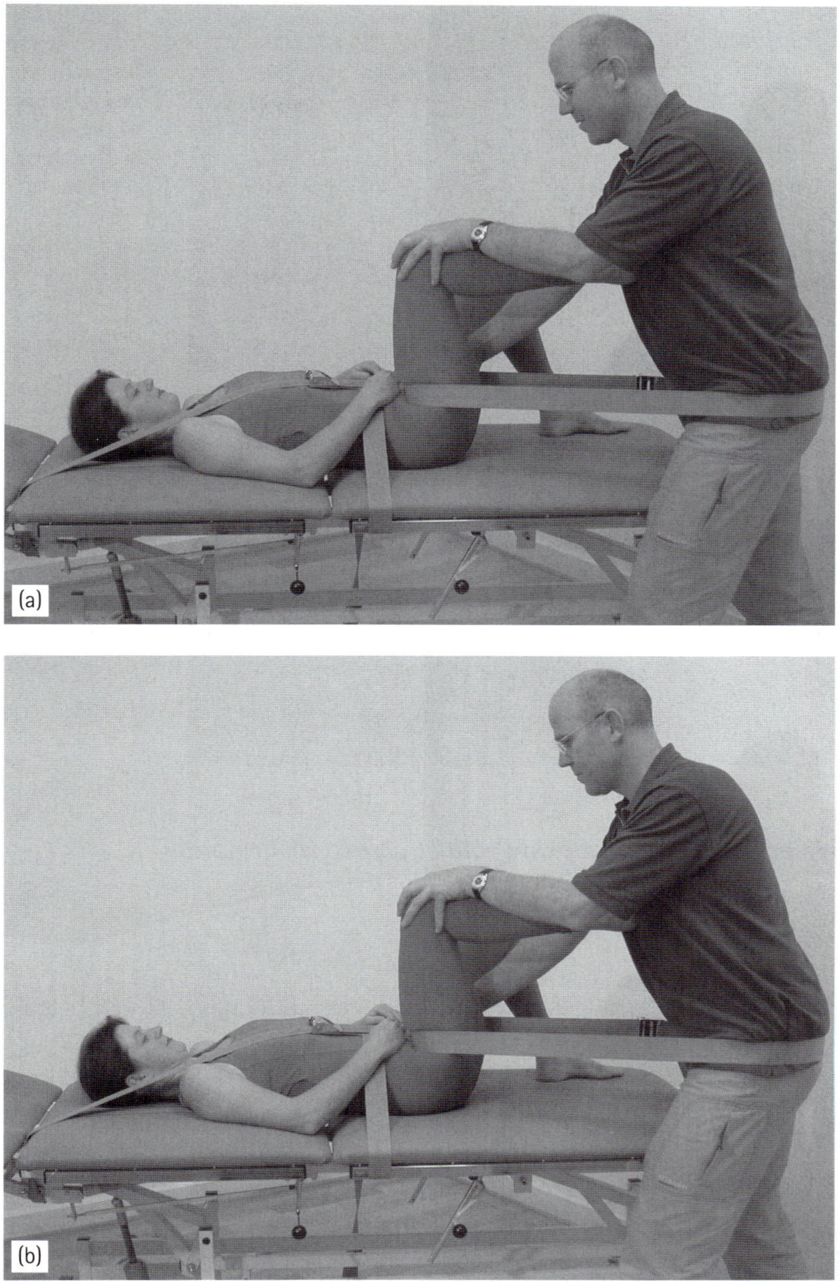

Figure 9.77a and b Translatory movement; distraction of the weight-bearing aspect of the flexed hip joint; therapy technique. a, Starting position. b, End position.

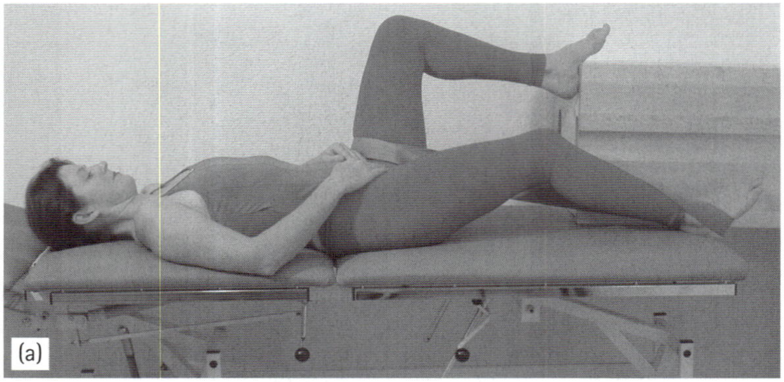

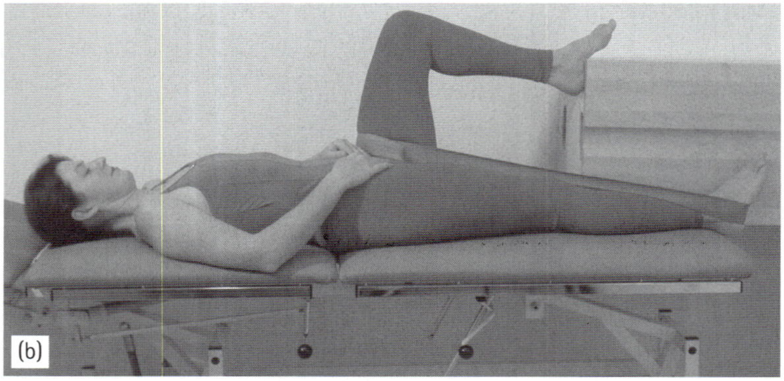

Figure 9.78a and b
Translatory movement; distraction of the weight-bearing aspect of the flexed hip joint; self-exercise. **a**, Starting position. **b**, End position.

Dorsal glide of the femur, in flexion/adduction/external rotation

Therapy technique (film 136)

Patient's starting position:

- supine (Fig. 9.79a)
- hip joint pre-positioned in flexion/adduction/external rotation, shortly before symptoms appear
- pelvis on the right side stably supported by a wedge or sandbag
- additional fixation of the pelvis by a belt, if necessary.

Therapist's starting position:

- standing, at the left side of the plinth
- stabilizing patient's left ilium, and contacting patient's knee.

Movement:

- pushing the femur in posterior-lateral direction (Fig. 9.79b).

Self-exercise (film 137)

Patient's starting position:

- quadruped position (Fig. 9.80a)
- the body is moved backwards and to the right side until the right hip is pre-positioned in flexion/adduction/external rotation, shortly before symptoms appear.

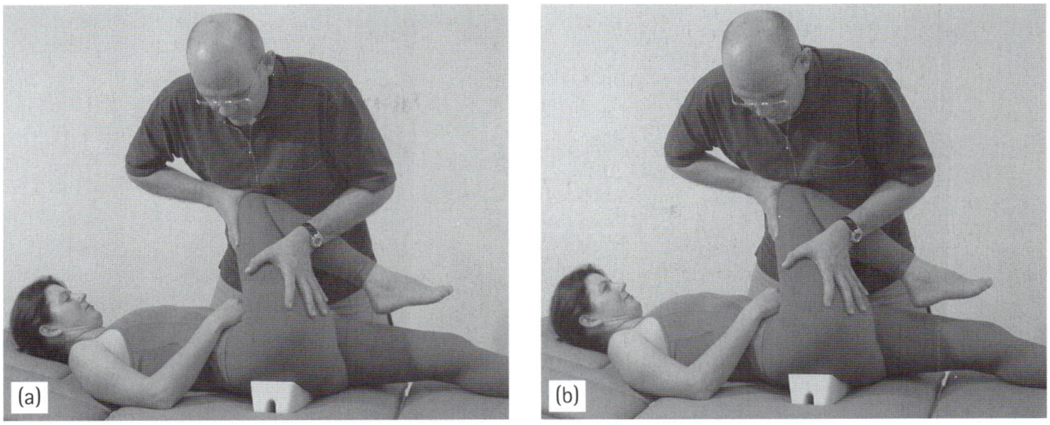

Figure 9.79a and b Translatory movement; dorsal glide of the femur in flexion/adduction/external rotation; therapy technique. a, Starting position. b, End position.

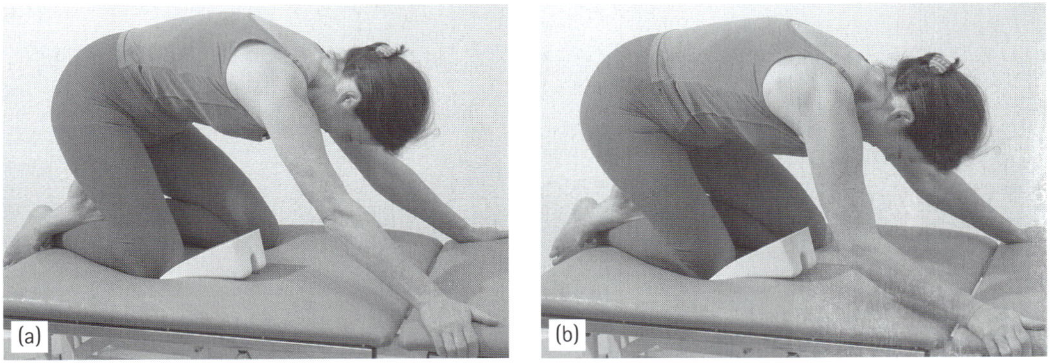

Figure 9.80a and b Translatory movement; dorsal glide of the femur in flexion/adduction/external rotation; self-exercise. a, Starting position. b, End position.

Movement:

- shifting weight on the right knee (Fig. 9.80b)
- additionally, both hands are firmly pushed against the supporting surface and pulled towards the right knee, without moving on the supporting surface
- due to weight-bearing and pull via the arms, the femur is pushed into a posterior or posterior-lateral direction. The right knee is stabilized by a wedge or sandbag.

ANGULAR MOVEMENTS

Flexion/adduction/external rotation

Therapy technique (film 138)

Patient's starting position:

- supine (Fig. 9.81a)
- hip joint pre-positioned in flexion/adduction/external rotation, shortly before symptoms appear.

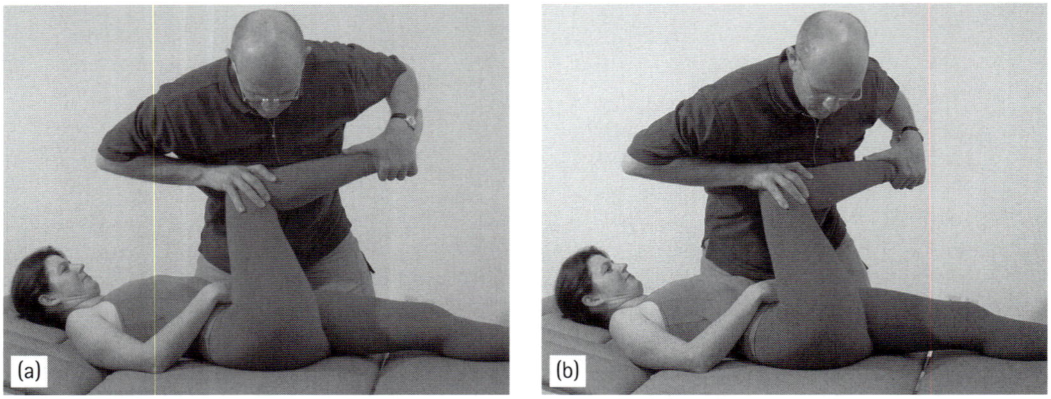

Figure 9.81a and b Passive angular movement; flexion/adduction/external rotation; therapy technique. a, Starting position. b, End position.

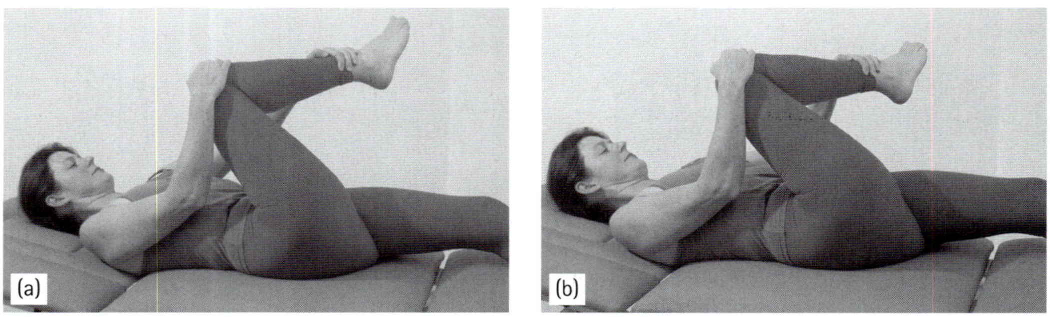

Figure 9.82a and b Passive angular movement; flexion/adduction/external rotation; self-exercise. a, Starting position. b, End position.

Therapist's starting position:

- standing, at the patient's side.

Movement:

- increasing external rotation in the right hip while flexion and adduction remain unchanged (Fig. 9.81b)
- in doing so, a constant pressure in a posterior direction is exerted to prevent continuing movement of the pelvis.

Self-exercise (film 139)

Patient's starting position:

- supine (Fig. 9.82a)
- right knee flexed, right hip pre-positioned in flexion/adduction/external rotation in a position shortly before symptoms appear
- care has to be taken that adduction does not go beyond the point where the pelvis would be lifted from the supporting surface.

Movement:

- increasing external rotation in right hip while flexion and adduction remain unchanged (Fig. 9.82b).

Remarks

Goals of the technique

With painfully restricted flexion of the right hip and increased tension of the dorsal structures, these techniques serve to mobilize non-symptomatic tissue.

Performance

The patient's typical symptoms should not be reproduced by the demonstrated techniques.

Dosage

As in this example symptom provocation by movement of the femur in an anterior direction is assumed, the symptomatic structures are probably not directly stressed by the demonstrated techniques. The patient's typical pain in the right groin with flexion should not appear. Dosage is determined by the expected training state of the tissue and, above all, by reassessment.

Choice of technique

The selection of the technique depends, among other things, on the therapist as well as the patient, on the therapist's clinical experience, but primarily on reassessment. This means that even if all preconditions on the part of therapist and patient seem to be met, it is of no use to continue the technique if reassessment is negative.

Contributing factors

For a satisfactory solution of the patient's current problems it is important to consider the contributing factors and include them in the treatment.

The authors will, however, not go into a description of the various possibilities and their complex contexts as this would exceed the scope of the present book.

Chapter 10

Anteromedial knee

CHAPTER CONTENTS

AREA LOCALIZATION

IDENTIFICATION OF THE POTENTIALLY AFFECTED AREA BY DEMONSTRATION OF A SYMPTOMATIC FUNCTIONAL MOVEMENT/POSITION

Based on the information gained from the anamnesis so far, the therapist ascertains more details about potentially affected sections. This is done by means of area localization, which represents the beginning of the physical examination. Information gained in this way is used to check or modify the relevant hypotheses developed on the basis of the anamnesis and will determine further proceedings.

Area localization is explained by means of one example. In this example, the patient feels pain in the area of the anteromedial knee complex. Clinical experience and known clinical patterns suggest primarily the following areas as potential sources of the current complaints:

- knee complex
- lumbar spine
- neural structures
- hip complex (the assumed symptomatic movements make it seem improbable that the hip complex might be the symptom-provoking area; it is hence not tested further).

General question: Is there enough information available to bypass area localization?	
No	Yes
⇓	⇓
Performance of area localization	• General movement tests • Additional tests • Test treatment

Example 1: Extension

Symptom area: anteromedial knee
Symptom provocation: extension of the knee (Fig. 10.1)

With this presentation, clinical experience suggests primarily the knee complex, lumbar spine, and neural structures as symptom-provoking areas.

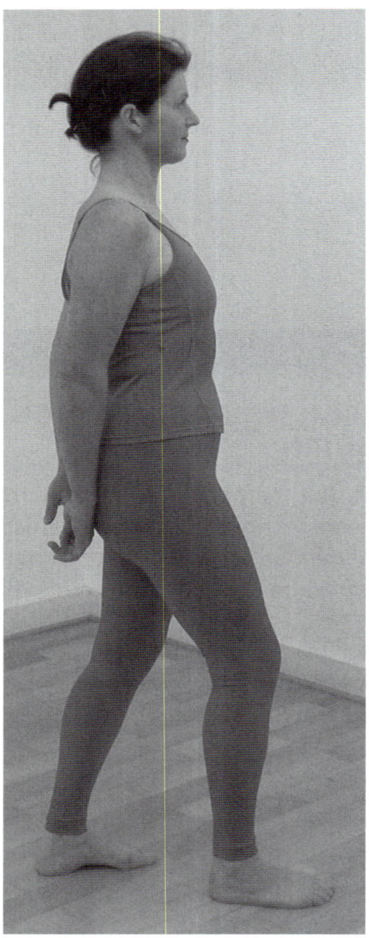

Figure 10.1 Symptom-provoking movement: extension of the knee joint provokes pain in the anteromedial side of the knee.

Below, examples illustrate how to differentiate between these areas. To this end, area localization is first attempted by means of active movements alone. If this is not possible, tests will be performed by means of assistive/passive movements.

Hypothesis 1: The symptom-provoking area is the lumbar spine
Differentiation: lumbar spine vs. knee complex.

The change in symptoms can be demonstrated exactly:

- provocation of pain (Fig. 10.2a and b, film 140)
- alleviation of pain (Fig. 10.3a and b, film 141).

The result of area localization has to be verified by further specific tests; otherwise the result remains in doubt.

Assessment

Goal	Provocation of pain	Alleviation of pain	Remarks
Starting position	Standing, extension of the knee to a position immediately before symptoms appear. The pelvis is fixed by the therapist	Standing, pelvis fixed by the therapist, lumbar spine pre-positioned in flexion, extension of the knee to a position immediately after symptoms have appeared	
Test movement	Flexion of the lumbar spine	Guiding the lumbar spine back	
Explanation	If by any movement of the lumbar spine (here, as an example, flexion) the typical symptoms are reproduced, an isolated lesion of the knee complex is at least questionable	If by any movement of the lumbar spine (here, as an example, guiding back from flexion) the typical symptoms are alleviated, an isolated lesion of the knee complex is at least questionable	
Additional data to support the hypothesis	General and specific mobility of lumbar spine and knee complex History (e.g., symptom behaviour, type of complaints, 24-hour behaviour) Palpation Reproducibility of test results Test treatment Imaging procedures (CT, MRI)		

Hypothesis 2: The symptom-provoking area is the neural structures
Differentiation: neural involvement vs. knee complex.

The change in symptoms can be demonstrated exactly:

- provocation of pain (Fig. 10.4a and b, film 142)
- alleviation of pain (Fig. 10.5a and b, film 143).

The result of area localization has to be verified by further specific tests; otherwise the result will remain in doubt.

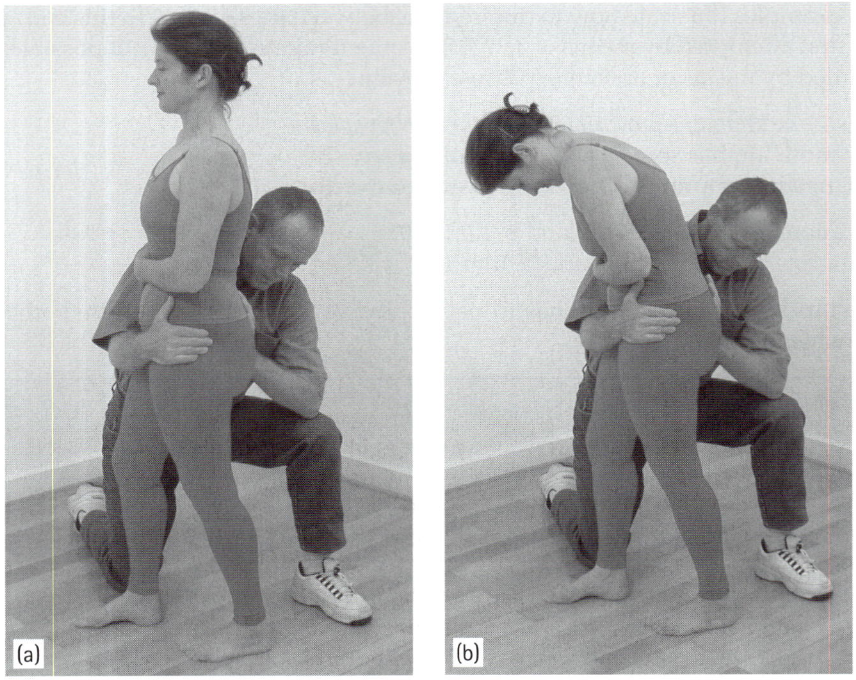

Figure 10.2a and b Area localization with symptomatic extension of the knee joint; differentiation between lumbar spine and knee complex; provocation. **a**, Starting position. **b**, End position.

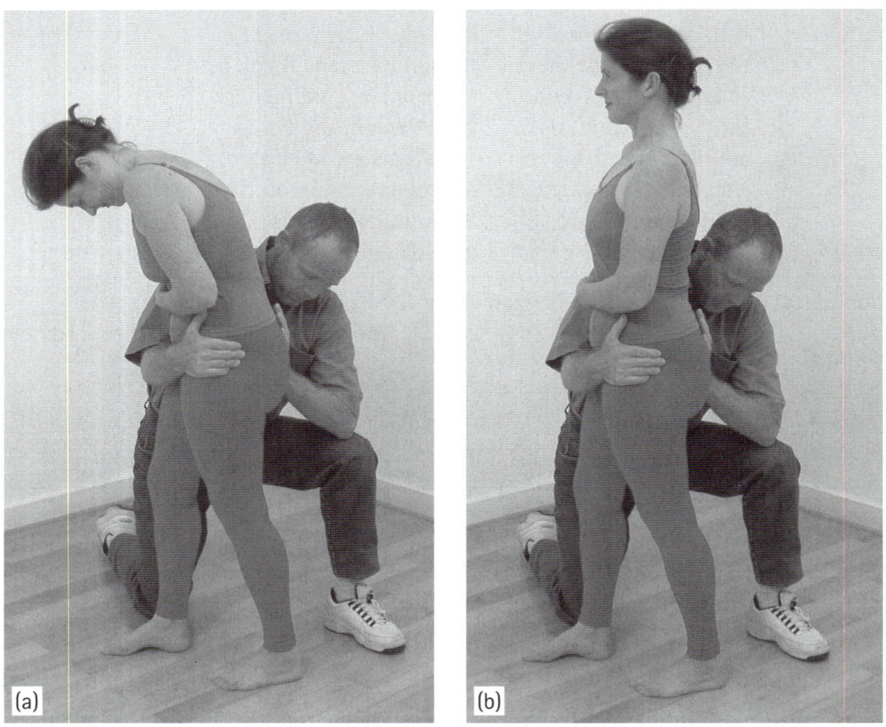

Figure 10.3a and b Area localization with symptomatic extension of the knee joint; differentiation between lumbar spine and knee complex; alleviation. **a**, Starting position. **b**, End position.

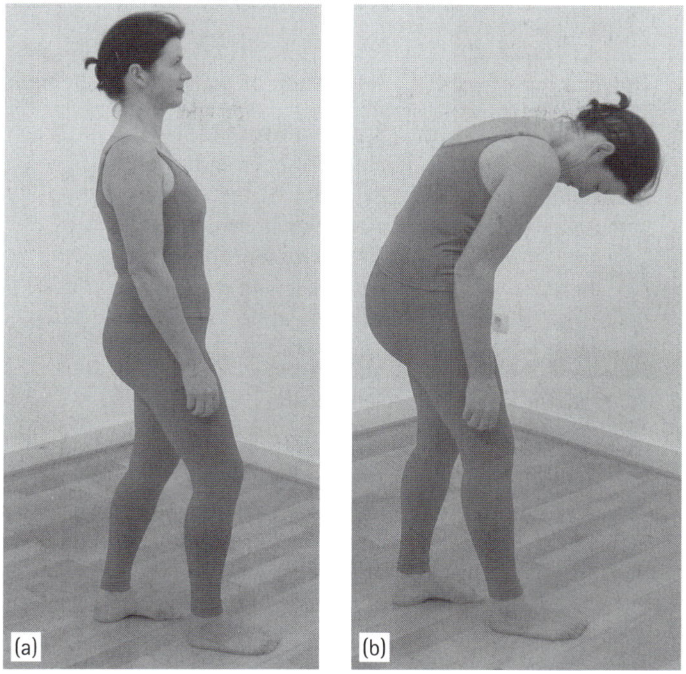

Figure 10.4a and b Area localization with symptomatic extension of the knee joint; differentiation between neural structures and knee complex; provocation. **a**, Starting position. **b**, End position.

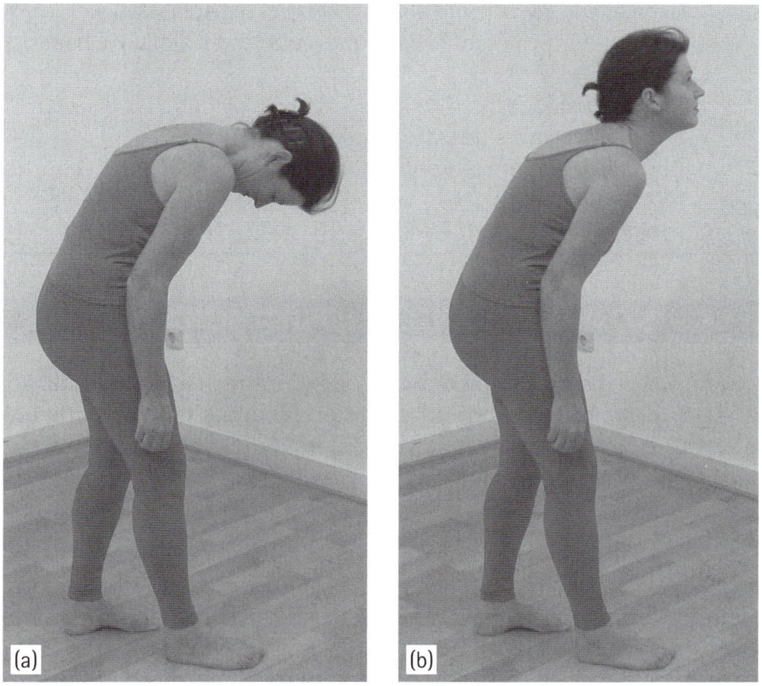

Figure 10.5a and b Area localization with symptomatic extension of the knee joint; differentiation between neural structures and knee complex; alleviation. **a**, Starting position. **b**, End position.

Assessment			
Goal	**Provocation of pain**	**Alleviation of pain**	**Remarks**
Starting position	Standing, extension of the knee to a position immediately before symptoms appear	Standing with the spine pre-positioned in flexion, extension of the knee to a position immediately after symptoms have appeared, with whole spine adjusted in flexion before	
Test movement	Flexion of the cervical spine, then flexion of the remaining spine	Moving the cervical spine back	
Explanation	The test movement produces mechanical stress on the neural structures and the structures associated with them	The test movement reduces mechanical stress on the neural structures and the structures associated with them	If the typical pain is provoked or alleviated by these manoeuvres without moving the knee complex, this suggests at least an involvement of the neural structures
Additional data to support the hypothesis	Further movements of proximal and distal components to increase neural tension, not directly involved in extension of the knee (e.g., upper extremity) General and specific mobility of the affected area History (e.g., symptom behaviour, type of complaints, 24-hour behaviour) Palpation Neurodynamic tests Nerve provocation tests (e.g., bow string sign) Reproducibility of test results Test treatment Imaging procedures (CT, MRI)		

QUICK CHECK – SYMPTOMS, ANTEROMEDIAL KNEE

If neither the area nor a symptom-provoking or symptom-reducing action is known, the quick check is used to try to load individual potential areas with specific biomechanically provocative movement combinations. The chosen movement combinations correspond with the straining and often symptom-provoking movements of the individual sections.

LUMBAR SPINE

Movement (film 226)

- Extension/lateral flexion to the right, and rotation to the same as well as to the opposite side, with overpressure (Fig. 10.6a and b)
- Extension/lateral flexion to the left, and rotation to the same as well as to the opposite side, with overpressure (Fig. 10.7a and b).

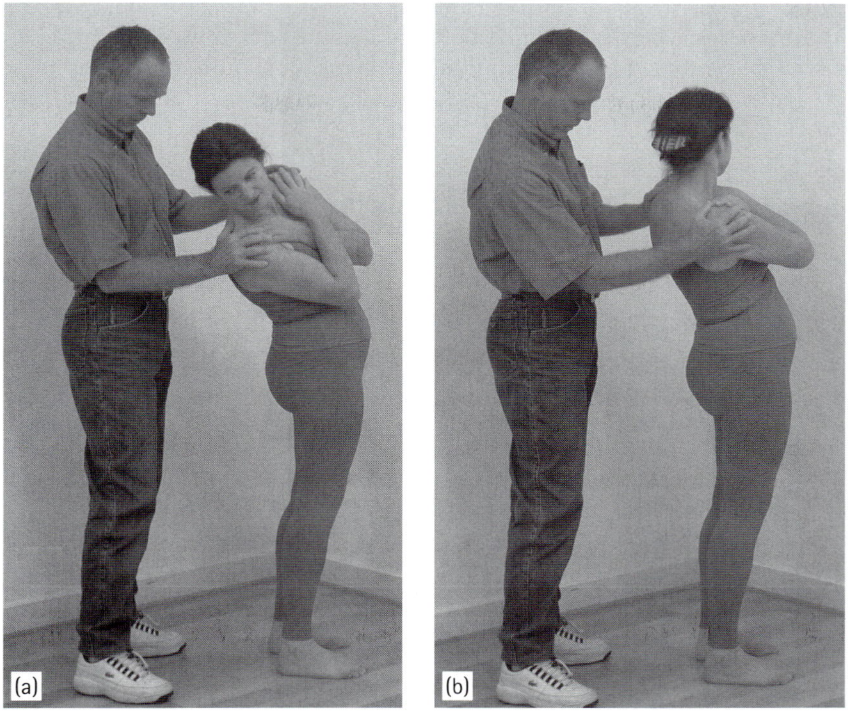

Figure 10.6a and b Quick check lumbar spine; extension, lateral flexion to the right. **a**, Rotation to the same side. **b**, Rotation to the opposite side.

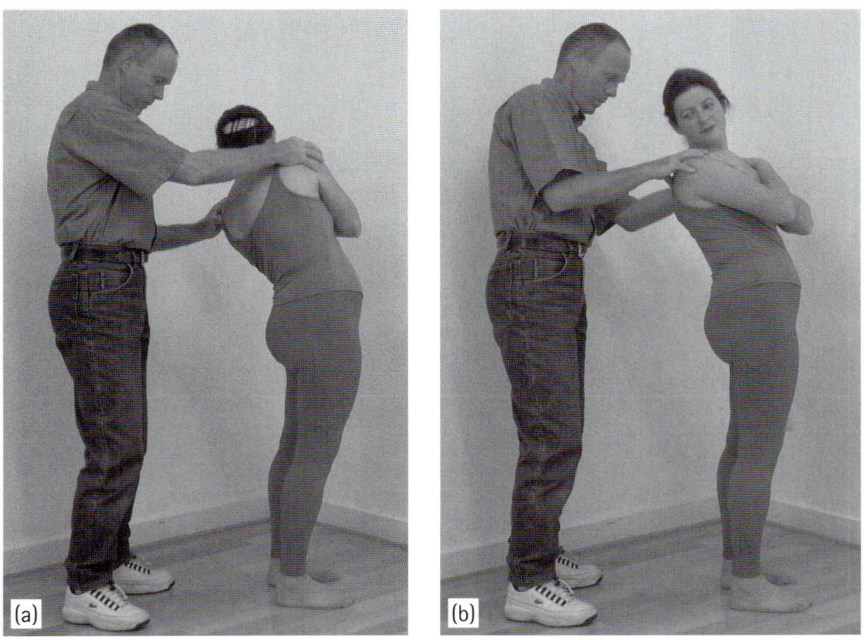

Figure 10.7a and b Quick check lumbar spine; extension, lateral flexion to the left. **a**, Rotation to the same side. **b**, Rotation to the opposite side.

Note: If the anamnesis suggests that flexion of the spine contributes to symptom provocation, the described movement combinations in extension should, of course, be performed in flexion.

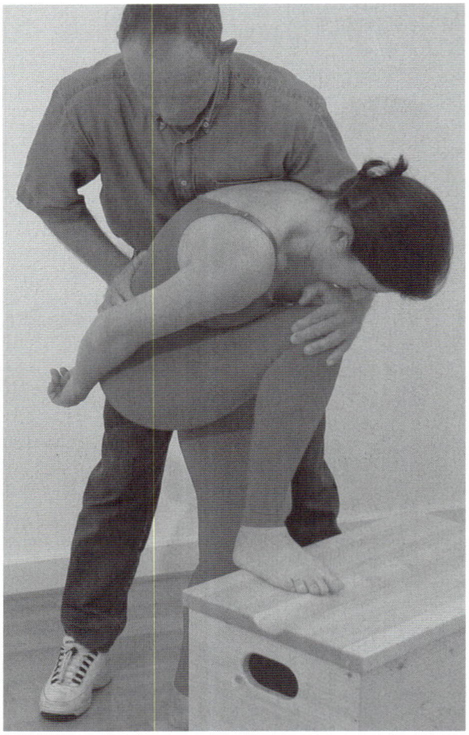

Figure 10.8 Quick check hip; flexion/adduction/internal rotation.

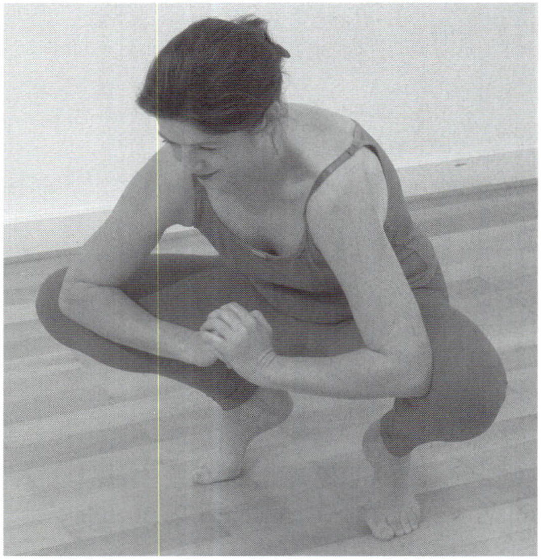

Figure 10.9 Quick check hip; flexion/abduction/external rotation.

HIP

Movement (film 228)

- Flexion/adduction/internal rotation, with overpressure (Fig. 10.8)
- Flexion/abduction, with overpressure (Fig. 10.9).

KNEE COMPLEX

Movement (film 229)

- Flexion/abduction/internal rotation in the knee, with overpressure (Fig. 10.10)
- Flexion/adduction/external rotation in the knee, with overpressure (Fig. 10.11)

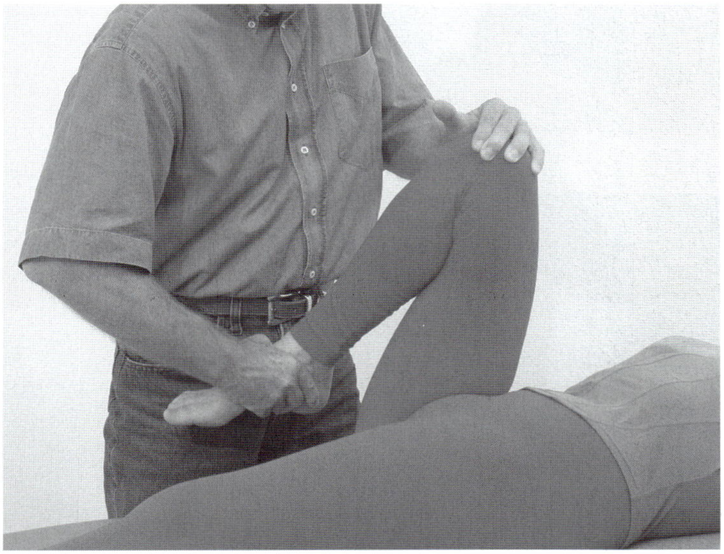

Figure 10.10 Quick check knee; flexion/abduction/internal rotation.

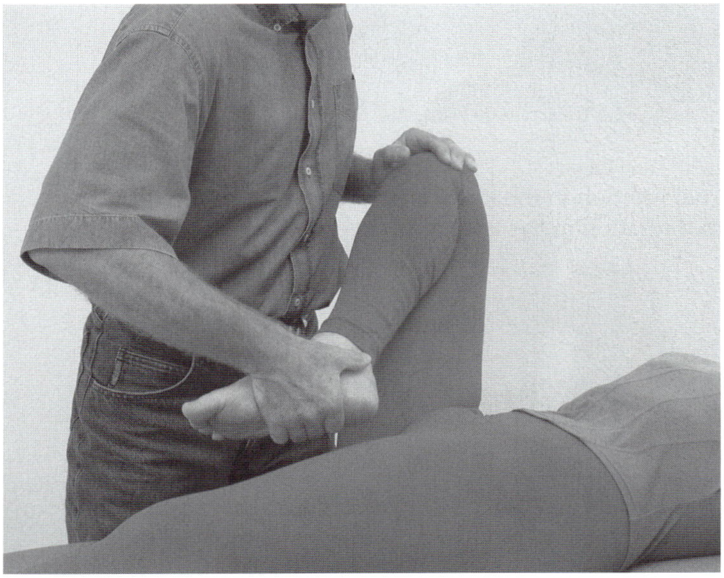

Figure 10.11 Quick check knee; flexion/adduction/external rotation.

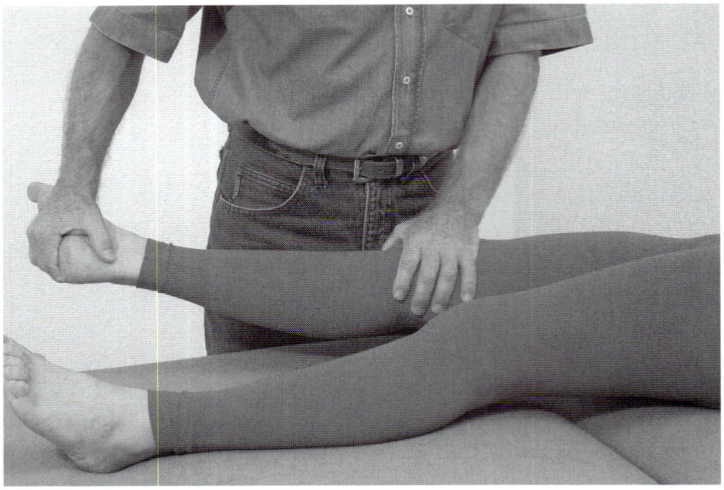

Figure 10.12 Quick check knee; extension/adduction/external rotation.

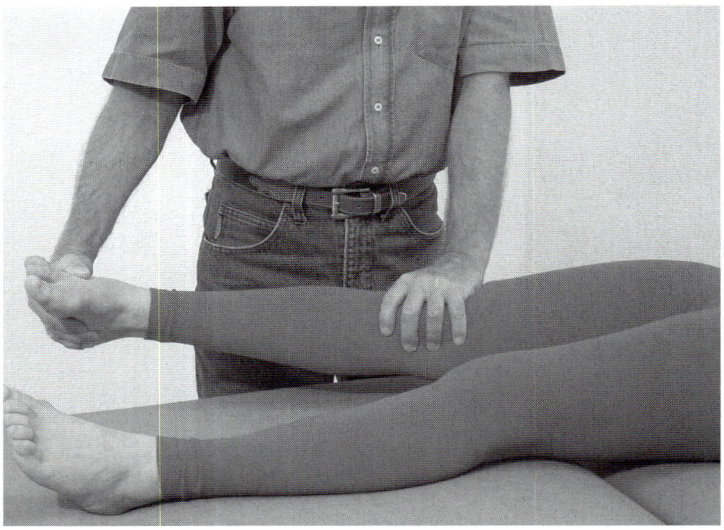

Figure 10.13 Quick check knee; extension/abduction/internal rotation.

- Extension/adduction/external rotation in the knee, with overpressure (Fig. 10.12)
- Extension/abduction/internal rotation in the knee, with overpressure (Fig. 10.13).

NEURAL STRUCTURES

Tension tests

- Slump test (Fig. 10.14, film 241)
- Prone knee bend (test of the femoral nerve) (Fig. 10.15).

Note: Even an area that proves negative in the quick check may possibly be symptom-provoking (another movement combination, or passive overpressure may be required).

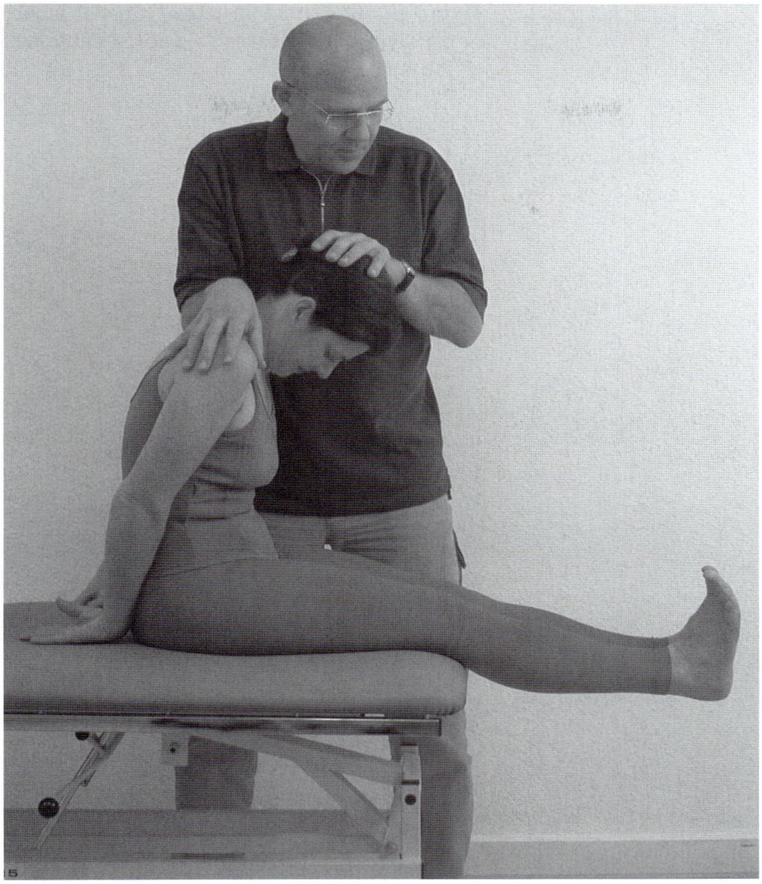

Figure 10.14 Quick check neurodynamics; slump test.

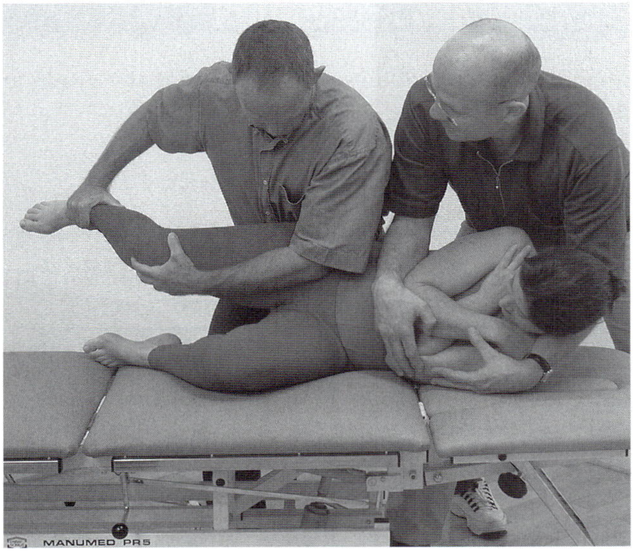

Figure 10.15 Quick check neurodynamics; prone knee bend (PKB) test.

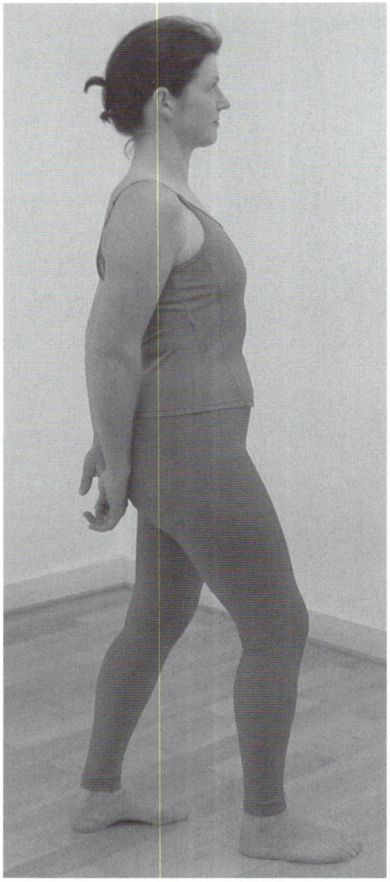

Figure 10.16 Symptom-provoking movement: extension of the knee joint provokes pain at the anteromedial aspect of the knee.

SPECIFIC PROVOCATION AND ALLEVIATION

Specific provocation and alleviation allows one to differentiate within an articular complex and to identify the symptom-provoking movement direction(s).

SPECIFIC PROVOCATION AND ALLEVIATION, KNEE JOINT (SYMPTOMS, ANTEROMEDIAL)

Differentiation, knee joint – extension – intra-articular vs. extra-articular (symptom provocation by an intra-articular component)

Pain-provoking movement (Fig. 10.16)

- Extension of the knee joint provokes pain in the anteromedial aspect of the knee.
- Area localization hints at the knee complex.

The change in symptoms can be demonstrated exactly:

- provocation of pain (Fig. 10.17a and b, film 144)
- alleviation of pain (Fig. 10.18a and b, film 145).

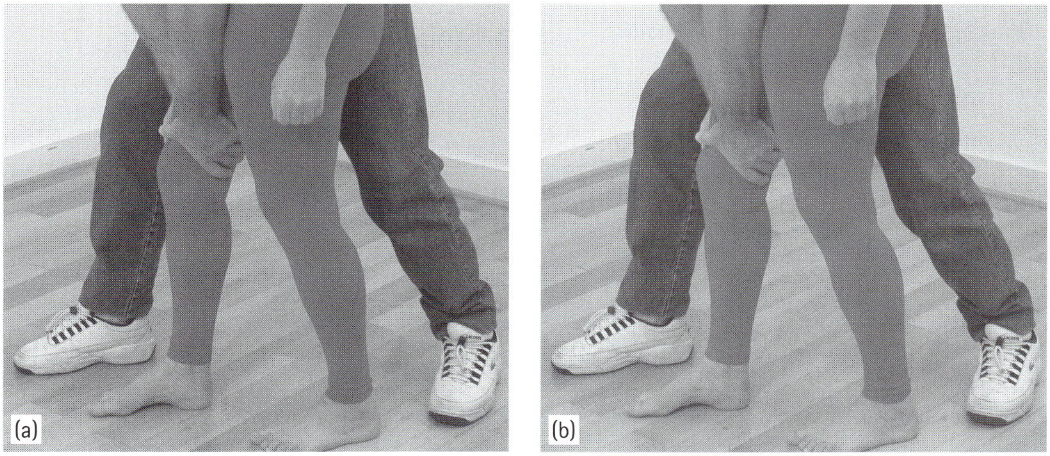

Figure 10.17a and b Specific provocation and alleviation in the area of the knee joint with symptomatic extension of the knee; differentiation, intra-articular vs. extra-articular (symptom provocation by an intra-articular mechanism); provocation. **a**, Test start. **b**, Test end.

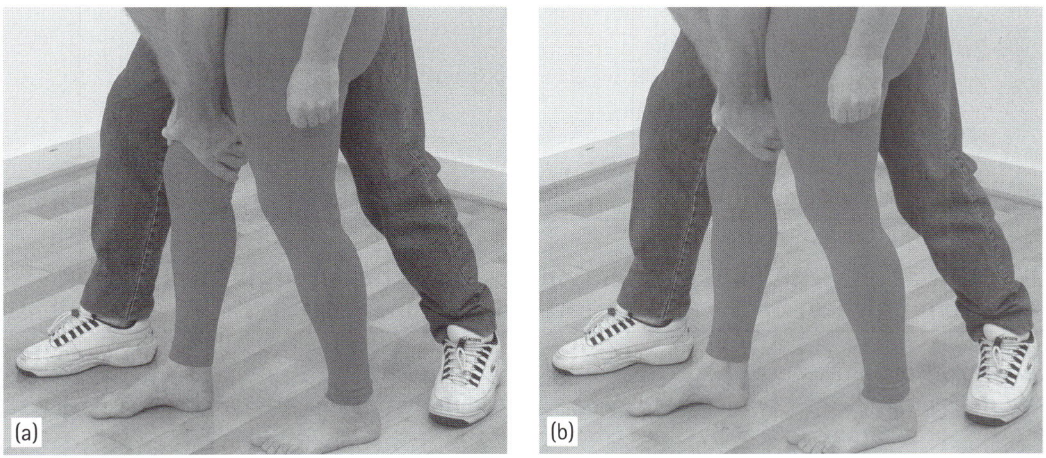

Figure 10.18a and b Specific provocation and alleviation in the area of the knee joint with symptomatic extension of the knee; differentiation, intra-articular vs. extra-articular (symptom provocation by an intra-articular mechanism); alleviation. **a**, Test start. **b**, Test end.

Assessment

Goal	Provocation of pain	Alleviation of pain	Remarks
Starting position	Extension to a position immediately after symptoms have appeared	Extension to a position immediately after symptoms have appeared	Because with pre-positioning to a position before symptoms appear non-symptomatic parts of the affected joint may be compressed,

Goal	Provocation of pain	Alleviation of pain	Remarks
			a symptomatic position is also chosen for provocation
Test movement	Femur moves in distal direction (compression)	Femur moves in proximal direction (traction)	
Neural involvement	Proximal and/or distal component without change of position in the relevant area	Proximal and/or distal component without change of position in the relevant area	
Explanation	This manoeuvre increases the intra-articular compression forces in the knee joint	This manoeuvre reduces the intra-articular compression forces in the knee joint	
Additional data to support the hypothesis	General and specific mobility of the knee joint History (e.g., symptom behaviour, type of complaints, 24-hour behaviour) Specific palpation Nerve mobility tests (if specific provocation and alleviation indicate neural involvement) Reproducibility of test results Test treatment Imaging procedures (CT, MRI)		

Differentiation, knee joint – extension – extra-articular vs. intra-articular (symptom provocation by an extra-articular component)

Pain-provoking movement

- Extension of the knee joint provokes pain in the anteromedial aspect of the knee.
- Area localization hints at the knee complex.

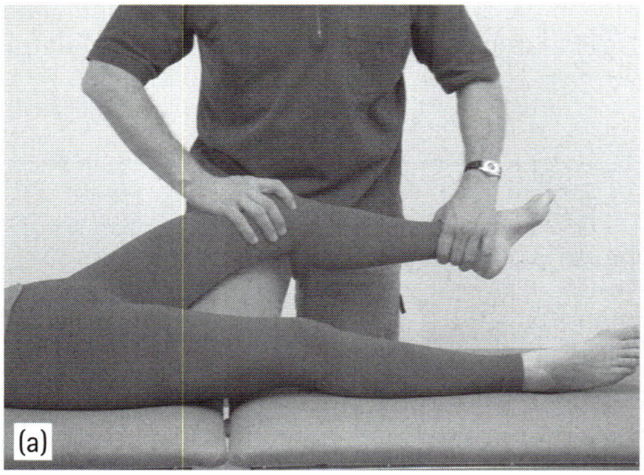

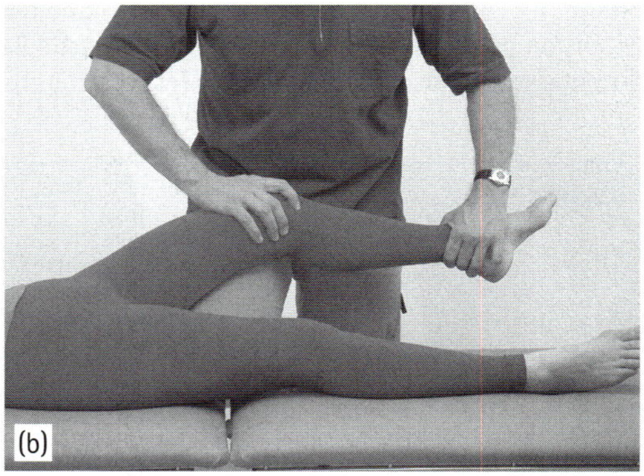

Figure 10.19a and b Specific provocation in the area of the knee joint with symptomatic extension of the knee; differentiation, extra-articular vs. intra-articular (symptom provocation by an extra-articular mechanism). a, Test start. b, Test end.

The change in symptoms can be demonstrated exactly:

- provocation of pain (Fig. 10.19a and b, film 146).

Assessment			
Goal	**Provocation of pain**	**Alleviation of pain**	**Remarks**
Starting position	Extension to a position immediately after symptoms have appeared	None	The lying position is chosen because it is much easier to perform the test whilst lying as well as standing. To use this altered position, it is important that the specific symptoms of the patient are possible to provoke in this non-weightbearing position
Test movement	Tibia moves in distal direction (traction)		
Neural involvement	Proximal and/or distal component without change of position in the relevant area		
Explanation	This manoeuvre increases the extra-articular tractive forces in the knee joint		Alleviation is usually not possible, as approximation of the joint surfaces seems too little for relaxation of extra-articular structures
Additional data to support the hypothesis	General and specific mobility of the knee joint History (e.g., symptom behaviour, type of complaints, 24-hour behaviour) Specific palpation Nerve mobility tests (if specific provocation and alleviation indicate neural involvement) Reproducibility of test results Test treatment Imaging procedures (CT, MRI)		

Localization, knee joint – extension – movement as symptom-provoking component

Pain-provoking movement

- Extension of the right knee joint provokes pain in the anteromedial aspect of the right knee.
- Area localization hints at the knee complex.

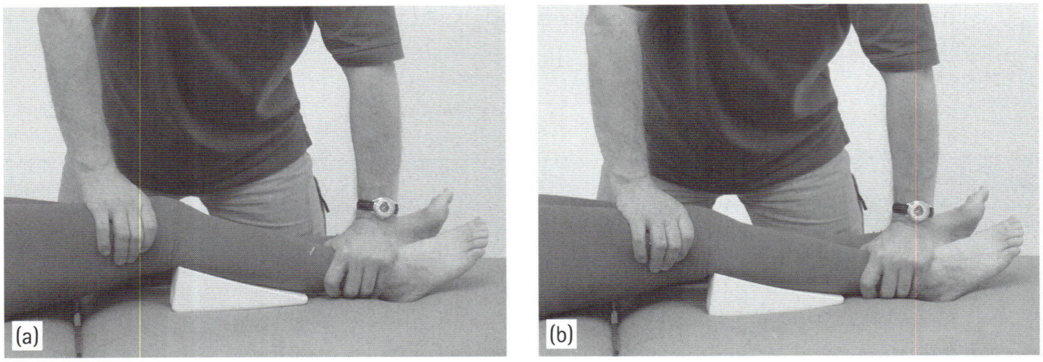

Figure 10.20a and b Specific provocation and alleviation in the area of the knee joint with symptomatic extension of the knee; localization (symptom provocation by movement); provocation. **a**, Test start. **b**, Test end.

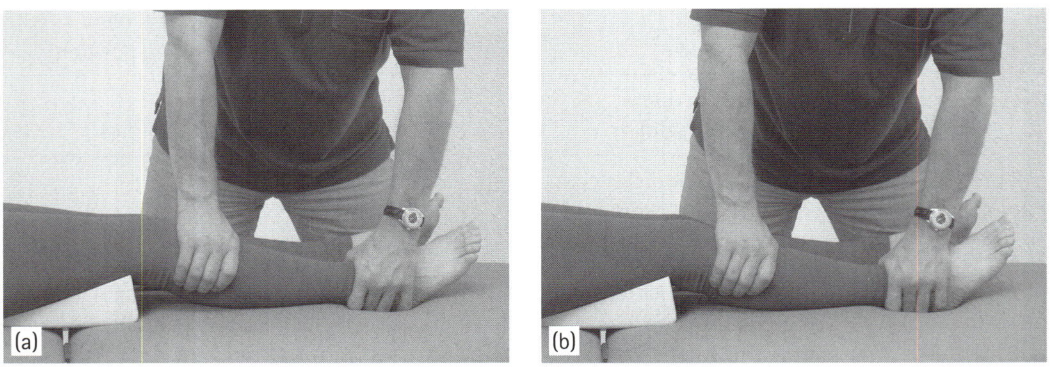

Figure 10.21a and b Specific provocation and alleviation in the area of the knee joint with symptomatic extension of the knee; localization (symptom provocation by movement); alleviation. **a**, Test start. **b**, Test end.

The change in symptoms can be demonstrated exactly:

- provocation of pain (Fig. 10.20a and b, film 147)
- alleviation of pain (Fig. 10.21a and b, film 148).

Assessment

Goal	Provocation of pain	Alleviation of pain	Remarks
Starting position	Extension to a position immediately before symptoms appear. Tibia proximally completely supported by a wedge	Extension to a position immediately after symptoms have appeared. Femur distally completely supported by a wedge	

Goal	Provocation of pain	Alleviation of pain	Remarks
Test movement	Femur moves in posterior direction, with fixed tibia (results in a movement of the tibia in anterior direction)	Tibia moves in posterior direction with fixed femur	Fixation is achieved by means of a wedge or sandbag
Neural involvement	Proximal and/or distal component without change of position in the relevant area	Proximal and/or distal component without change of position in the relevant area	
Explanation	If symptoms are caused by movement of the tibia in anterior direction, this manoeuvre (tibia moves in anterior direction) results in an increase in symptoms (both with an intra-articular and with an extra-articular dysfunction)	If symptoms are caused by movement of the tibia in anterior direction, this manoeuvre (tibia moves in posterior direction) results in reduction of symptoms (both with an intra-articular and with an extra-articular dysfunction)	This differentiation test aims at identifying the symptomatic movement direction. Due to the complexity of the movement apparatus or possible adaptations of biomechanics to the pathology, other movement directions might have to be considered as well and be tested appropriately (e.g., in medial or lateral direction)
Additional data to support the hypothesis	General and specific mobility of the knee joint History (e.g., symptom behaviour, type of complaints, 24-hour behaviour) Specific palpation Neurodynamic tests (if specific provocation and alleviation indicate neural involvement) Reproducibility of test results Test treatment Imaging procedures (CT, MRI)		

GENERAL MOVEMENT TESTS

General movement tests identify, quantify, and qualify individual anatomical movements and, in part, movement combinations in the area presumed. The individual manual therapy concepts have respective protocols at their disposal, which more or less have the same goals.

Information gained in this way is used for checking or modifying the relevant hypotheses developed on the basis of anamnesis and area localization and will help in deciding how to proceed.

General question: Is there enough information available to bypass general movement tests?	
No	Yes
⇓	⇓
Performance of the general movement tests	● Additional tests ● Test treatment

In view of the described clinical presentation and the results of area localization, general movement tests of the following regions seem to be useful.

Lumbar spine		
	Active	**Passive**
Lumbar spine in general	Flexion Extension Rotation (to the right and left) Lateral flexion (to the right and left)	Flexion Extension Rotation (to the right and left) Lateral flexion (to the right and left)
Movement combinations, lumbar spine in general	Symptomatic movements of the lumbar spine	Symptomatic movements of the lumbar spine
Hip joint		
	Active	**Passive**
Hip joint in general	Flexion Extension Internal rotation in extension Internal rotation in flexion External rotation in extension External rotation in flexion Abduction Adduction	Flexion Extension Internal rotation in extension Internal rotation in flexion External rotation in extension External rotation in flexion Abduction Adduction
Movement combinations, hip joint	Symptomatic movements of the hip joint	Symptomatic movements of the hip joint
Knee		
	Active	**Passive**
Knee in general	Flexion Extension Internal rotation of the lower leg with flexed knee External rotation of the lower leg with flexed knee	Flexion Extension Internal rotation of the lower leg External rotation of the lower leg Abduction Adduction

TREATMENT EXAMPLE, KNEE JOINT

SYMPTOMATIC MOVEMENT

Extension of the right knee is restricted by 10° as compared with the opposite side and provokes pain in end-range positions (VAS 3/10) in the area of the anteromedial knee, right side.

ASSESSMENTS

Area localization

Area localization hints at symptom provocation by the knee complex. There is no contraindication for movement.

Specific provocation and alleviation

The symptomatic movement direction is gliding of the tibia in an anterior direction. Symptoms are provoked by an intra-articular mechanism (compression).

Specific mobility

Specific mobility tests show a firm end feel with restricted gliding of the tibia in an anterior direction.

Palpation

Palpation of the periarticular structures shows tissue changes as compared with the non-affected side. The patient's specific pain cannot be reproduced by palpation. Palpation of the muscles moving the knee shows increased tension as compared with the opposite side.

HYPOTHESIS

It is suspected that movement of the right knee joint into extension is painfully restricted by an intra-articular mechanism (compression) with simultaneously restricted translatory mobility of the tibia in an anterior direction with increased tension of the muscles moving the knee (Fig. 10.22).

RELAXATION TECHNIQUES

Hold–relax techniques

CO-CONTRACTION AGAINST DISTRACTION

Therapy technique (film 149)

Patient's starting position:

- prone (Fig. 10.23a)
- right knee extended (to a position before symptoms appear)
- thigh fixed by two belts posteriorly and distally.

Therapist's starting position:

- standing, at the foot end of the plinth
- grasping patient's lower leg distally.

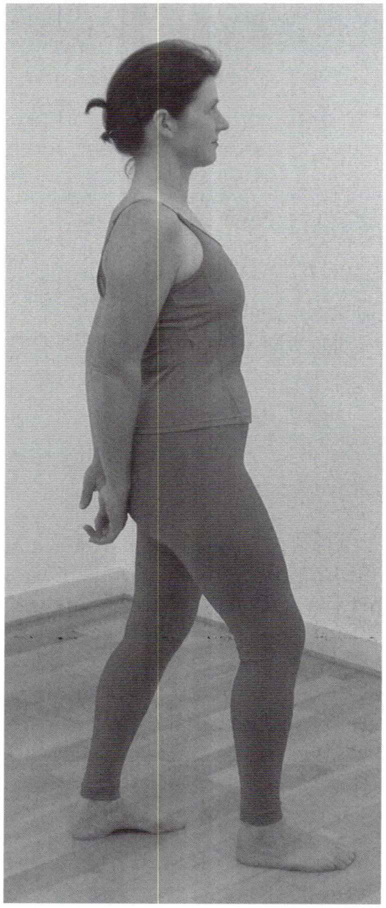

Figure 10.22 Symptom-provoking movement: extension of the knee joint provokes pain in the anteromedial aspect of the knee.

Movement:

- traction in the knee joint while the patient tries to prevent distraction by muscle contraction (Fig. 10.23b).

Self-exercise (film 150)

Patient's starting position:

- sitting (Fig. 10.24a)
- right lower leg/foot fixed
- right knee joint extended (to a position before symptoms appear).

Movement:

- traction in knee joint by pulling the ipsilateral side of the pelvis back while the patient tries to prevent distraction by muscle contraction (Fig. 10.24b).

Note: If performance of this movement is too difficult for the patient, the same exercise arrangement as in film 121 can be used. In doing so, care has to be taken to adjust the knee in a symptom-free position first.

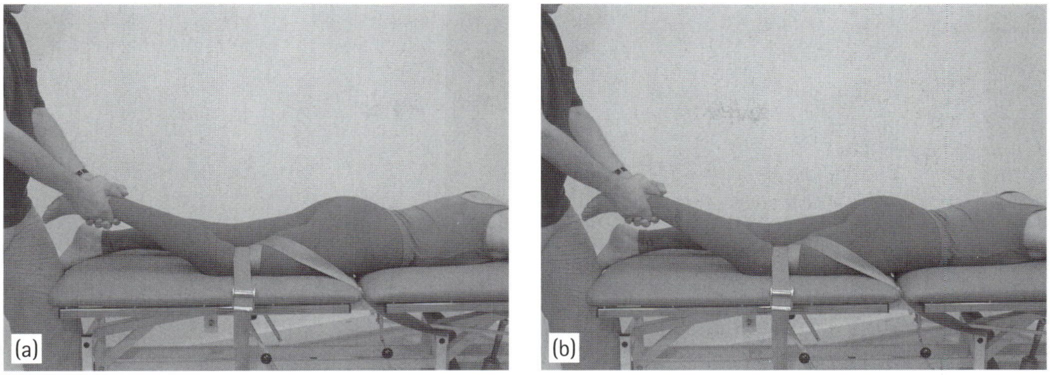

Figure 10.23a and b Hold-relax technique; co-contraction against distraction; therapy technique. a, Starting position. b, End position.

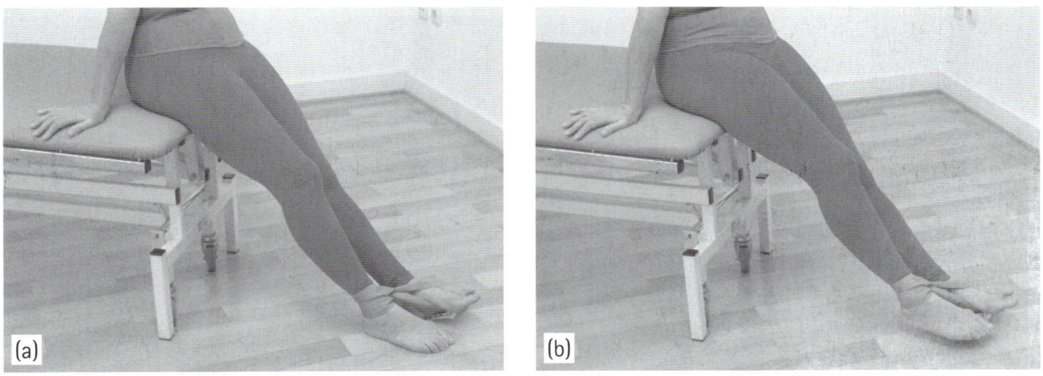

Figure 10.24a and b Hold-relax technique; co-contraction against distraction; self-exercise. a, Starting position. b, End position.

MOVEMENT-DIRECTED CONTRACTION IN THE DIRECTION OPPOSING THE PAINFUL AND/OR RESTRICTED DIRECTION

Therapy technique (film 151)

Patient's starting position:

- sitting on the plinth with the femur fixed by a belt (Fig. 10.25a).

Therapist's starting position:

- standing, in front of the patient
- fixing patient's thigh and grasping lower leg distally.

Movement:

- extension in the knee joint while the patient tries to prevent extension by muscle contraction (Fig. 10.25b).

Self-exercise (film 152)

Patient's starting position:

- sitting (Fig. 10.26a)
- fixation of right lower leg by left foot.

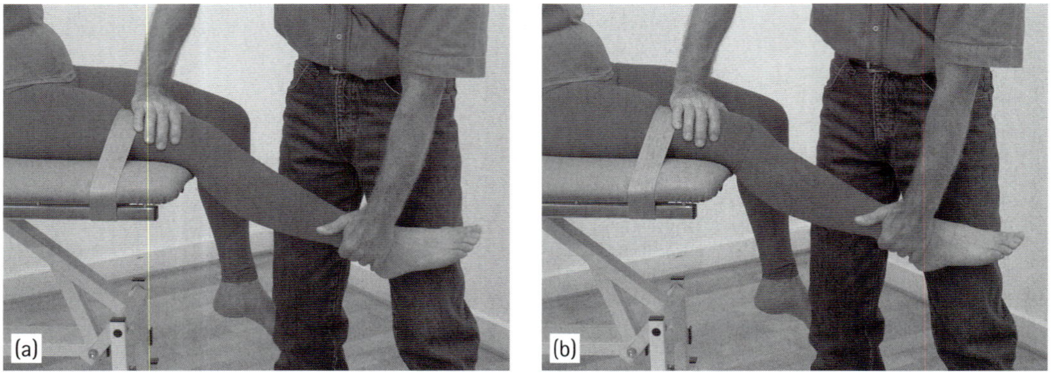

Figure 10.25a and b Hold-relax technique; movement-directed contraction in the direction opposing the painful and/or restricted direction; therapy technique. **a**, Starting position. **b**, End position.

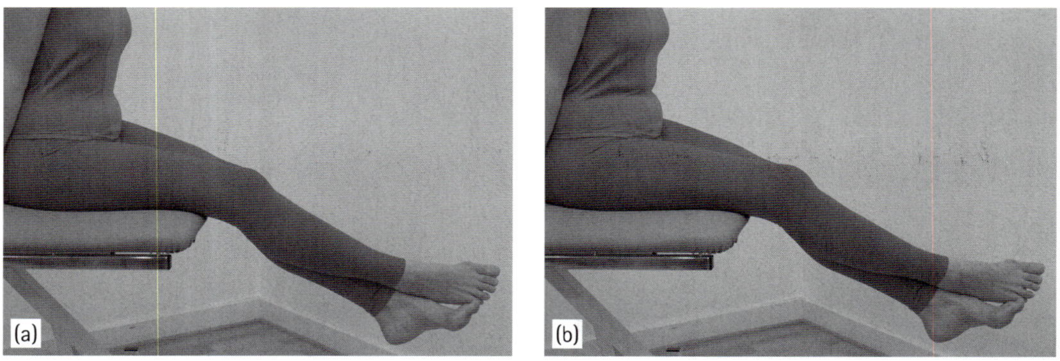

Figure 10.26a and b Hold-relax technique; movement-directed contraction in the direction opposing the painful and/or restricted direction; self-exercise. **a**, Starting position. **b**, End position.

Movement:

- flexion of right knee against the fixation (Fig. 10.26b).

MOVEMENT-DIRECTED CONTRACTION IN THE PAINFUL AND/OR RESTRICTED DIRECTION

Therapy technique (film 153)

Patient's starting position:

- sitting on the plinth with the femur fixed by a belt (Fig. 10.27a).

Therapist's starting position:

- standing, in front of the patient
- fixing patient's thigh and grasping lower leg distally.

Movement:

- flexion in the knee joint while the patient tries to prevent flexion by muscle contraction (Fig. 10.27b).

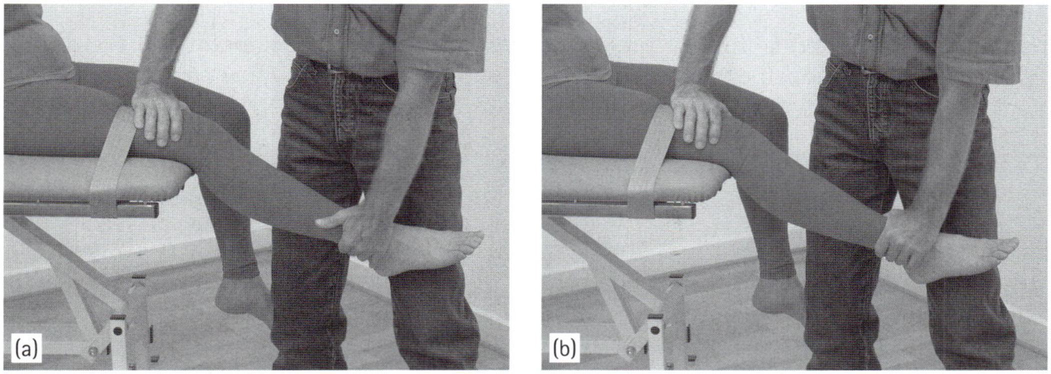

Figure 10.27a and b Hold-relax technique; movement-directed contraction in the painful and/or restricted direction; therapy technique. a, Starting position. b, End position.

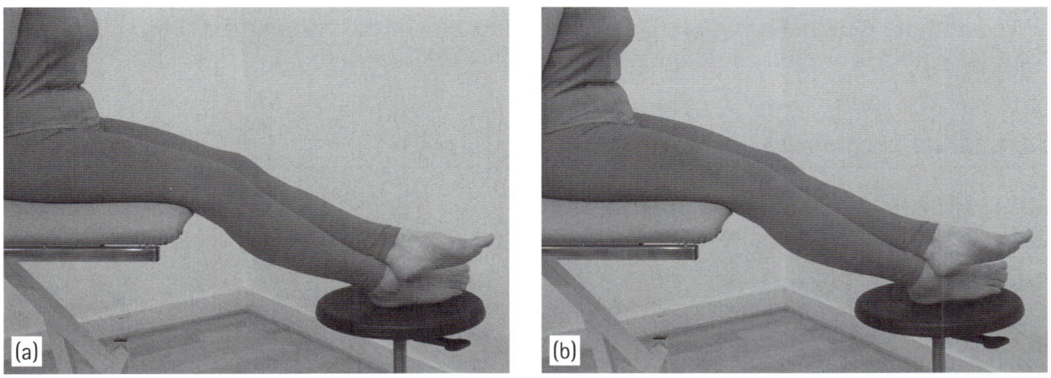

Figure 10.28a and b Hold-relax technique; movement-directed contraction in the painful and/or restricted direction; self-exercise. a, Starting position. b, End position.

Self-exercise (film 154)

Patient's starting position:

- sitting (Fig. 10.28a)
- a stool is put under the right foot to maintain the angular position in the knee
- the left foot is put over the right one for fixation.

Movement:

- extension of the knee against the fixation (Fig. 10.28b).

Remarks

Goals of the technique

Reduction of tonicity and improvement of the metabolism of the periarticular tissues when extension of the right knee is painfully restricted by an intra-articular mechanism (compression) and, simultaneously, translatory mobility of the tibia in an anterior direction is restricted and tension in the muscles moving the knee is increased.

Performance

The joint to be treated is initially pre-positioned depending on irritability and the desired treatment goal. As the self-exercise is performed without 'specific fixation', transferred movement has to be considered when the indication for the exercise is determined.

Dosage (regarding the affected symptomatic structure)

Both with an acute and with a chronic presentation, contraction should always be pain-free.

Choice of technique

The selection of the technique depends, among other things, on the therapist as well as the patient, on the therapist's clinical experience, but primarily on reassessment. This means that even if all preconditions on the part of therapist and patient seem to be met, it is of no use to continue the technique if reassessment is negative.

Contributing factors

For a satisfactory solution of the patient's current problems it is important to consider the contributing factors and include them in the treatment.

The authors will, however, not go into a description of the various possibilities and their complex contexts as this would exceed the scope of the present book.

Soft tissue techniques

HAMSTRINGS

Therapy technique (film 155)

Patient's starting position:

- prone (Fig. 10.29a).

Therapist's starting position:

- standing, beside the patient at the level of the patient's thigh.

Movement:

- passive extension of the knee with simultaneous manual pressure on the hamstrings (Fig. 10.29b)
- releasing pressure, and back to starting position.

> ***Note:*** If the patient is not able to relax or if performance of the movement seems too difficult, this soft tissue technique can also be performed assistively. Use of the assistive technique results in a simultaneous reciprocal inhibition of the treated muscles, which may facilitate relaxation.

Self-exercise (film 156)

Patient's starting position:

- sitting, knee in flexed position (Fig. 10.30a)
- grasping the thigh with both hands so that fingers rest on the hamstrings.

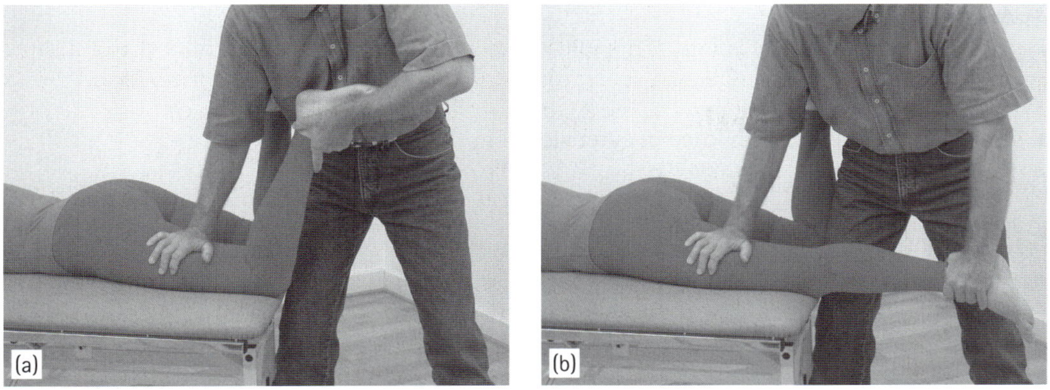

Figure 10.29a and b Soft tissue technique; hamstrings; therapy technique. **a**, Starting position. **b**, End position.

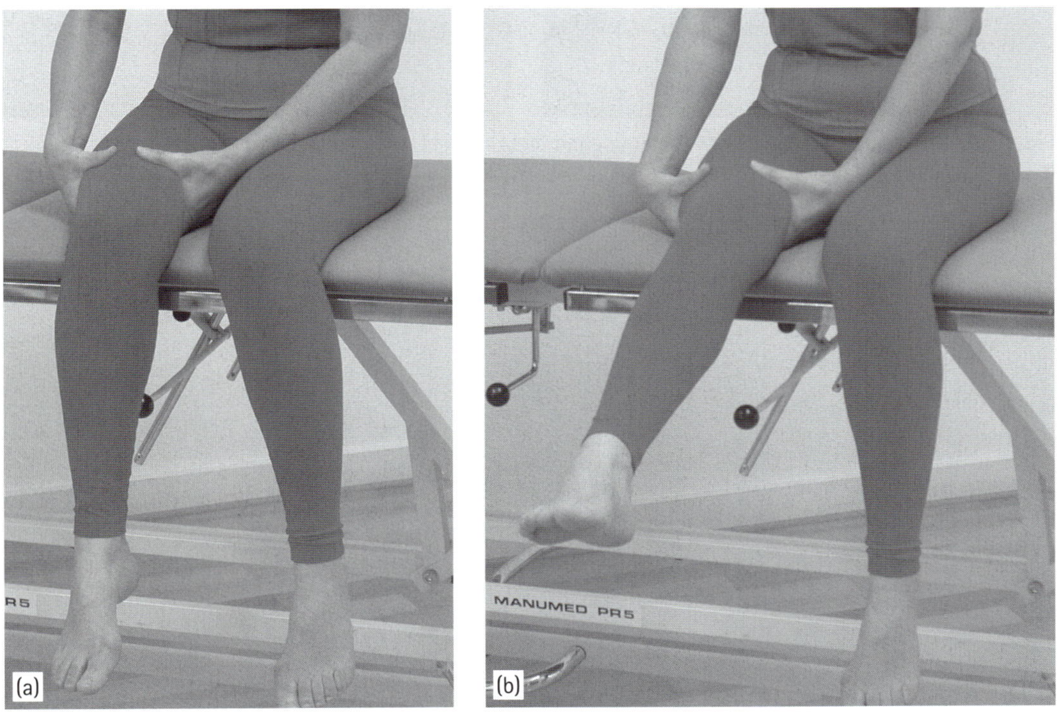

Figure 10.30a and b Soft tissue technique; hamstrings; self-exercise. **a**, Starting position. **b**, End position.

Movement:

- pressure with the fingers on the hamstrings (Fig. 10.30b)
- active extension of the knee
- releasing pressure, and back to starting position.

QUADRICEPS MUSCLE

Therapy technique (film 157)

Patient's starting position:

- sitting on the plinth, with knee in extension (Fig. 10.31a).

Therapist's starting position:

- standing, in front of the patient.

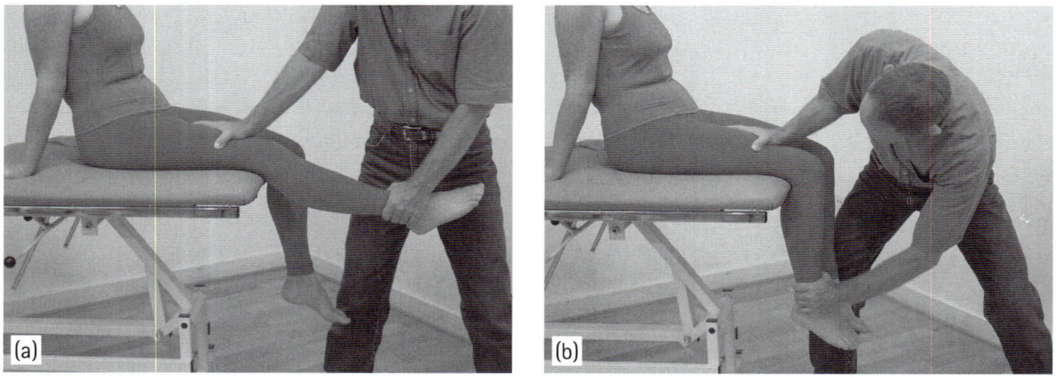

Figure 10.31a and b Soft tissue technique; quadriceps muscle; therapy technique. **a**, Starting position. **b**, End position.

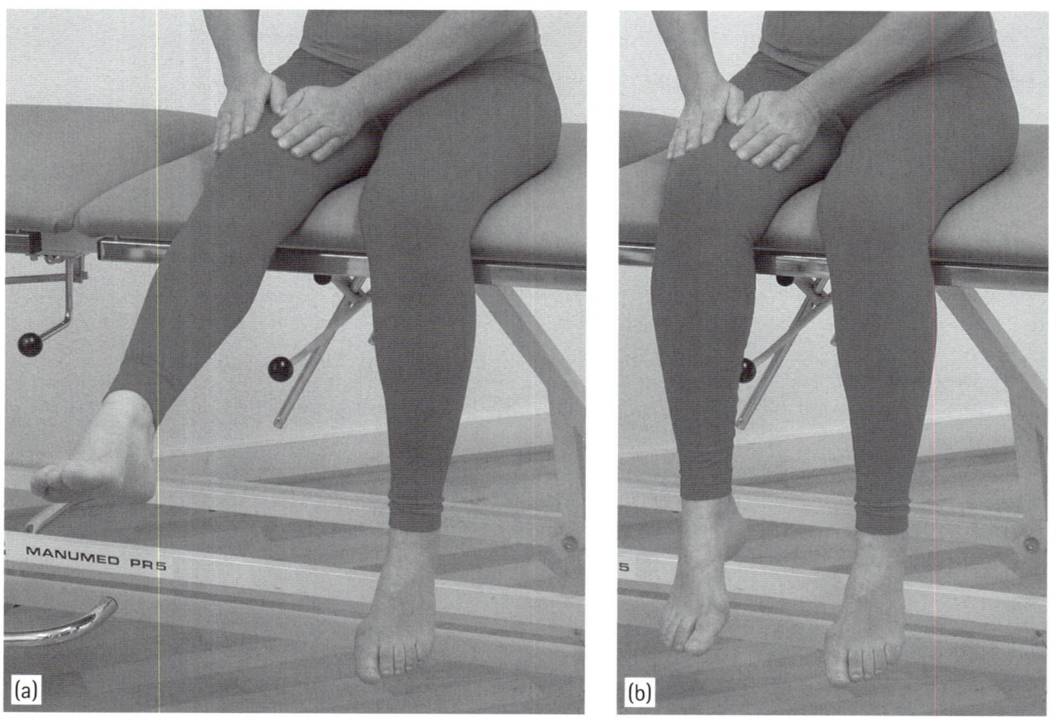

Figure 10.32a and b Soft tissue technique; quadriceps muscle; self-exercise. **a**, Starting position. **b**, End position.

Movement:

- passive flexion of the knee with simultaneous manual pressure on the quadriceps muscle (Fig. 10.31b)
- releasing pressure, and back to starting position.

Note: If the patient is not able to relax or if performance of the movement seems too difficult, this soft tissue technique can also be performed assistively. Use of the assistive technique results in a simultaneous reciprocal inhibition of the treated muscles, which may facilitate relaxation.

Self-exercise (film 158)

Patient's starting position:

- sitting with knee in extension (Fig. 10.32a)
- both hands are placed on the quadriceps muscle.

Movement:

- pressure with the hands on the quadriceps muscle (Fig. 10.32b)
- flexion of the right knee
- releasing pressure of the hands, and back to starting position.

Remarks

Goals of the technique

Reduction of tonicity and improvement of the metabolism of the treated tissues when extension of the right knee is painfully restricted by an intra-articular mechanism (compression) and, simultaneously, translatory mobility of the tibia in anterior direction is restricted and tension in the muscles moving the knee is increased.

Performance

Treatment is performed in the pain-free range of movement. As the treatment techniques are performed without 'specific fixation', transferred movement has to be considered when the indication for the technique is determined.

Dosage (regarding the affected symptomatic structure)

Both with an acute and with a chronic presentation, contraction should always be pain-free.

Choice of technique

The selection of the technique depends, among other things, on the therapist as well as the patient, on the therapist's clinical experience, but primarily on reassessment. This means that even if all preconditions on the part of therapist and patient seem to be met, it is of no use to continue the technique if reassessment is negative.

Contributing factors

For a satisfactory solution of the patient's current problems it is important to consider the contributing factors and include them in the treatment.

The authors will, however, not go into a description of the various possibilities and their complex contexts as this would exceed the scope of the present book.

MOBILIZATION TECHNIQUES

Active procedures

ACTIVE MOBILIZATION

Extension (roll-gliding) via the femur

Therapy technique (film 159)

Patient's starting position:

- supine (Fig. 10.33a)
- a belt surrounds the lower leg proximally to stabilize towards the posterior direction.

Therapist's starting position:

- standing, at the patient's side
- contact with patient's distal lower leg, patient's knee pre-positioned in extension in a position shortly before symptoms appear.

Movement:

- the patient is asked to extend the knee by pressing against the belt with the right leg (Fig. 10.33b)
- pressure of the leg against the belt moves the femur in a posterior direction against the fixed tibia (roll-gliding in extension).

Self-exercise (film 160)

Patient's starting position:

- sitting (Fig. 10.34a)
- the right lower leg resting on a chair with extended knee, in a position shortly before symptoms appear
- the proximal lower leg is supported by a wedge close to the knee, and the distal lower leg is fixed by a belt.

Movement:

- extension of the right knee (Fig. 10.34b)
- the pressure of the leg against the wedge (chair) moves the femur in a posterior direction against the fixed tibia (roll-gliding in extension).

Remarks

Goals of the technique

Improvement of the restriction of knee extension when extension of the right knee is painfully restricted by an intra-articular mechanism (compression) and, simultaneously, translatory mobility of the tibia in anterior direction is restricted and tension in the muscles moving the knee is increased.

Performance

The joint to be treated is first pre-positioned in accordance with irritability or the desired treatment goal.

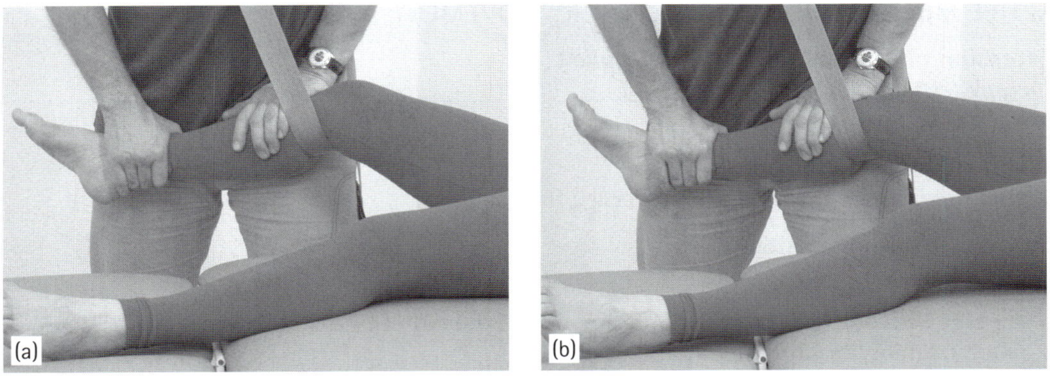

Figure 10.33a and b Active mobilization; extension (roll-gliding); therapy technique. **a**, Starting position. **b**, End position.

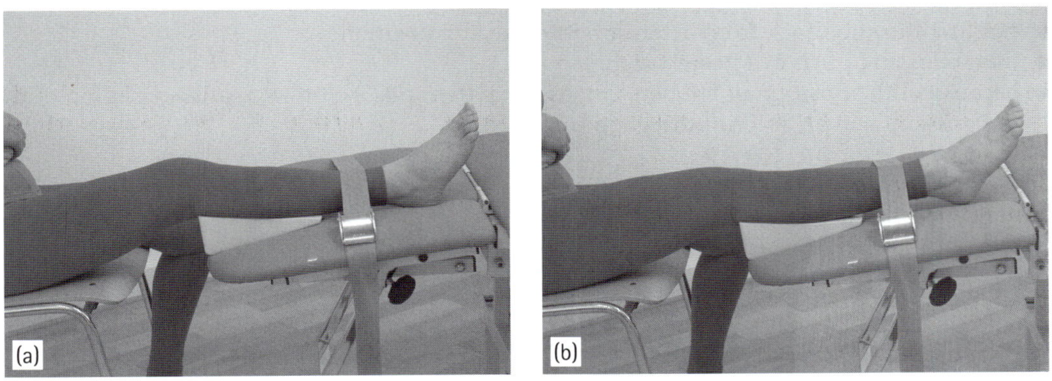

Figure 10.34a and b Active mobilization; extension (roll-gliding); self-exercise. **a**, Starting position. **b**, End position.

Dosage

The patient's typical pain in the anteromedial area of the knee should not appear. The patient should rather feel a pulling sensation in the posterior area of the knee. If the typical pain is not reproduced, it can be assumed that the symptomatic structure/area is not stressed.

Choice of technique

The selection of the technique depends, among other things, on the therapist as well as the patient, on the therapist's clinical experience, but primarily on reassessment. This means that even if all preconditions on the part of therapist and patient seem to be met, it is of no use to continue the technique if reassessment is negative.

Contributing factors

For a satisfactory solution of the patient's current problems it is important to consider the contributing factors and include them in the treatment.

The authors will, however, not go into a description of the various possibilities and their complex contexts as this would exceed the scope of the present book.

ACTIVE MOBILIZATION PLUS ACCESSORY MOVEMENT

Extension of the knee with anterior glide

Therapy technique (film 161)

Patient's starting position:

- standing (Fig. 10.35a)
- a belt surrounds the proximal lower leg from behind.

Therapist's starting position:

- kneeling, in front of the patient
- contact with both hands at the anterior side of the patient's distal femur
- a belt running around the therapist's pelvis
- length of the belt adjusted so that the therapist's elbows are slightly flexed.

Movement:

- pushing the patient's femur in a posterior direction by extension of both the therapist's elbows, and subsequently having the patient actively extend the right knee
- guiding the knee back from extension into starting position
- then releasing push in a posterior direction
- because of the position of the belt, extension of therapist's elbows results in gliding of the patient's tibia in an anterior direction (Fig. 10.35b).

Self-exercise (film 162)

Patient's starting position:

- standing (Fig. 10.36a)
- a belt surrounds the tibia from the posterior side
- a second, circular belt surrounds the distal femur from the anterior side and, at the same time from the posterior side, the other leg, which is placed backwards.

Movement:

- due to knee extension of the backward leg, the femur is pushed, via the belt, in a posterior direction against the tibia fixed in an anterior direction (Fig. 10.36b)

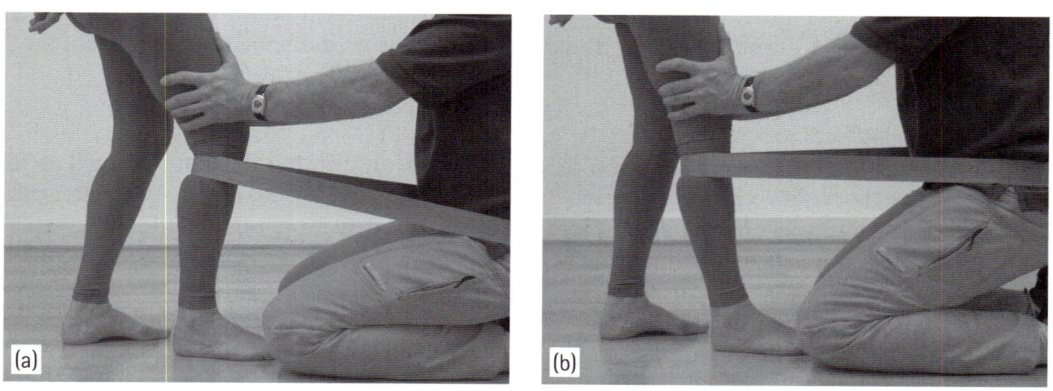

Figure 10.35a and b Active mobilization with accessory movement; extension with anterior glide; therapy technique. a, Starting position. b, End position.

- in this position, the right knee is extended and moved back
- then releasing the posterior push via the belt.

Extension of the knee with lateral glide

Therapy technique (film 163)

Patient's starting position:

- standing (Fig. 10.37a)
- a belt medially surrounds the lower leg.

Therapist's starting position:

- kneeling, beside the patient
- contact with both hands on the lateral side of the patient's distal femur
- belt running around the therapist's trunk
- the length of the belt is adjusted so that the therapist's elbows are slightly flexed.

Movement:

- pushing the femur in a medial direction by extension of both the therapist's elbows, and subsequently having the patient actively extend the right knee (Fig. 10.37b)
- guiding knee back from extension into starting position

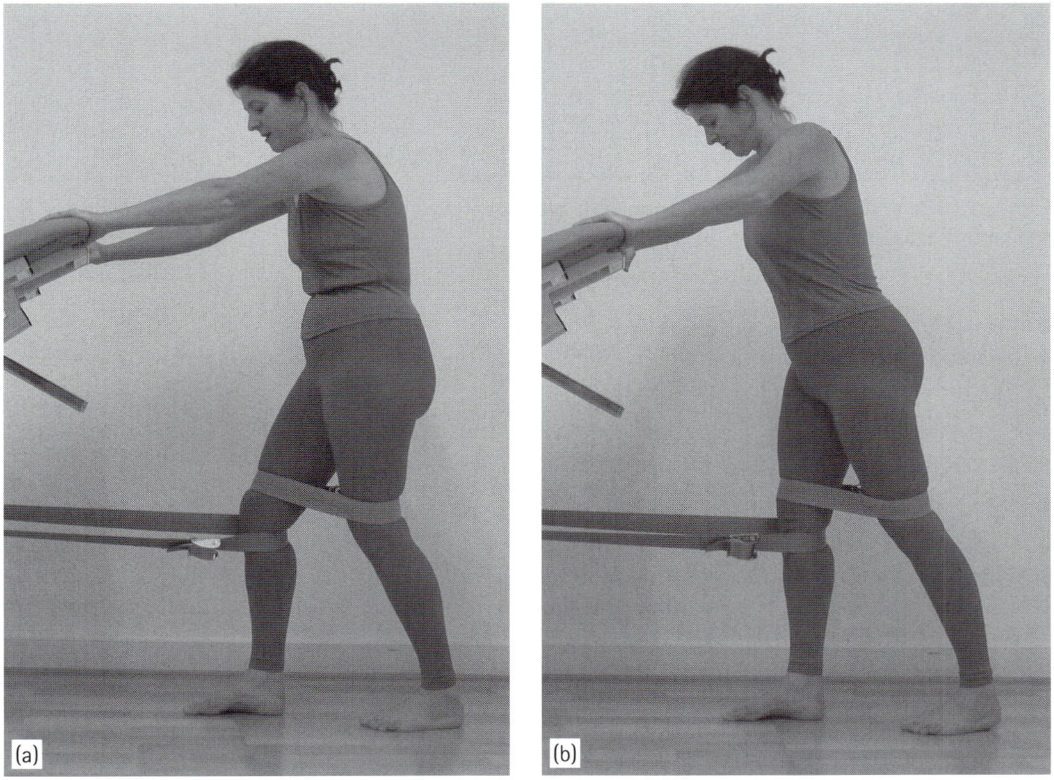

Figure 10.36a and b Active mobilization with accessory movement; extension with anterior glide; self-exercise. **a**, Starting position. **b**, End position.

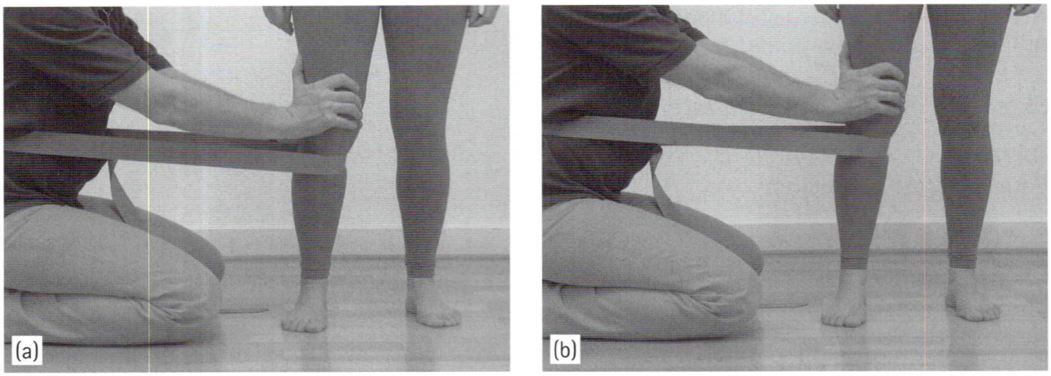

Figure 10.37a and b Active mobilization with accessory movement; extension with lateral glide; therapy technique. a, Starting position. b, End position.

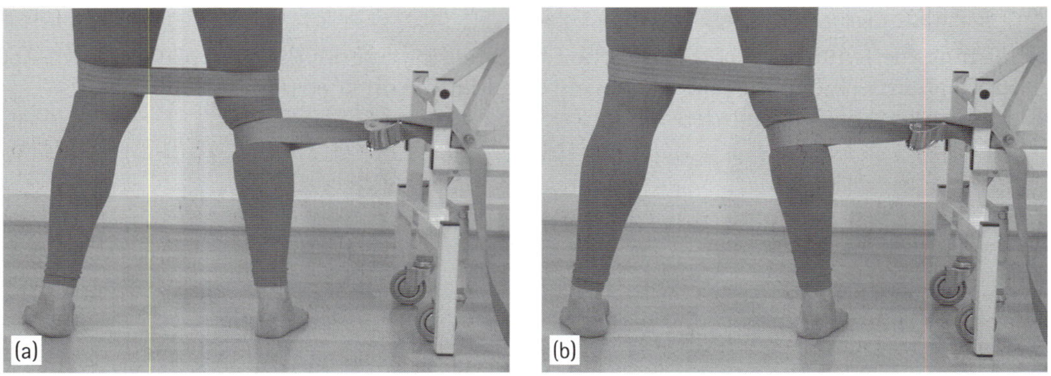

Figure 10.38a and b Active mobilization with accessory movement; extension with lateral glide; self-exercise. a, Starting position. b, End position.

- then releasing push in a medial direction
- because of the position of the belt, extension of the therapist's elbows results in gliding of the patient's tibia in a lateral direction.

Self-exercise (film 164)

Patient's starting position:

- standing (Fig. 10.38a)
- a belt surrounds the tibia from the medial side
- a second, circular belt surrounds the distal femur from the lateral side and, at the same time, the other leg, which is placed laterally.

Movement:

- due to abduction of the left leg, the femur is pushed, via the belt, medially against the tibia, which is fixed in a lateral direction by the tightened belt (Fig. 10.38b)
- in this position, the right knee is extended and moved back
- then releasing the medial push via the belt by easing the abduction of the left leg.

Remarks

Goals of the technique

With painfully restricted extension of the right knee due to an intra-articular mechanism (compression) and simultaneously restricted translatory mobility of the tibia in an anterior direction with increased tension of the muscles moving the knee, these techniques serve to:

- improve restricted extension of the knee
- reduce tonicity and improve the metabolism of the affected tissues
- restore pain-free function (change input to the respective centres of the central nervous system).

Performance

In active mobilization with gliding in an anterior or lateral direction, the push is performed in relation to the treatment plane (parallel to the tibial plateau).

Dosage

Both with an acute (predominantly peripheral pain mechanisms) and with a chronic presentation (predominantly central pain mechanisms), this technique should not provoke the patient's symptoms. Dosage depends on the expected training state of the tissue and, above all, on reassessment.

Choice of technique

The selection of the technique depends, among other things, on the therapist as well as the patient, on the therapist's clinical experience, but primarily on reassessment. This means that even if all preconditions on the part of therapist and patient seem to be met, it is of no use to continue the technique if reassessment is negative.

Contributing factors

For a satisfactory solution of the patient's current problems it is important to consider the contributing factors and include them in the treatment.

The authors will, however, not go into a description of the various possibilities and their complex contexts as this would exceed the scope of the present book.

Passive procedures

TRANSLATORY MOVEMENTS

Traction

Therapy technique (film 165)

Patient's starting position:

- prone (Fig. 10.39a)
- distal femur supported on a pad and fixed by a belt, a second belt is circular around the distal femur to stabilize in distal direction
- distal lower leg surrounded by both hands of the therapist and supported by a belt loop.

Therapist's starting position:

- standing, at the foot end of the plinth
- a belt, which is linked to the foot loop, goes around the therapist.

Movement:

- distraction in the submaximally pre-positioned knee joint (right-angled to treatment plane) (Fig. 10.39b).

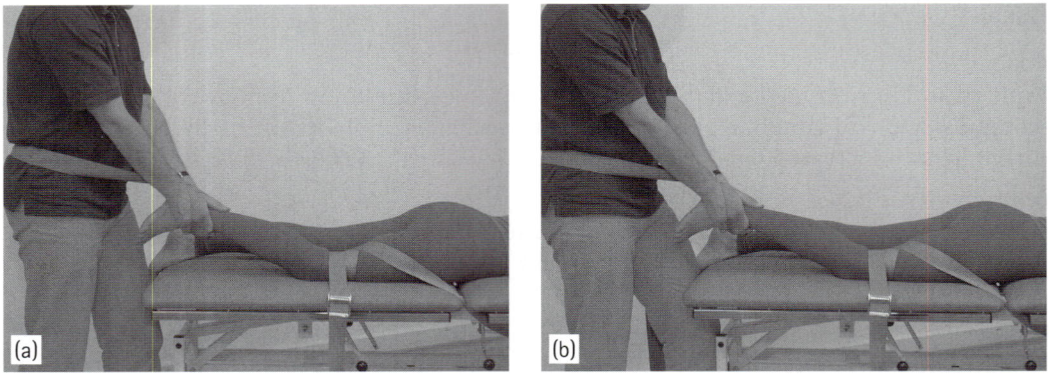

Figure 10.39a and b Translatory movement; traction; therapy technique. **a**, Starting position. **b**, End position.

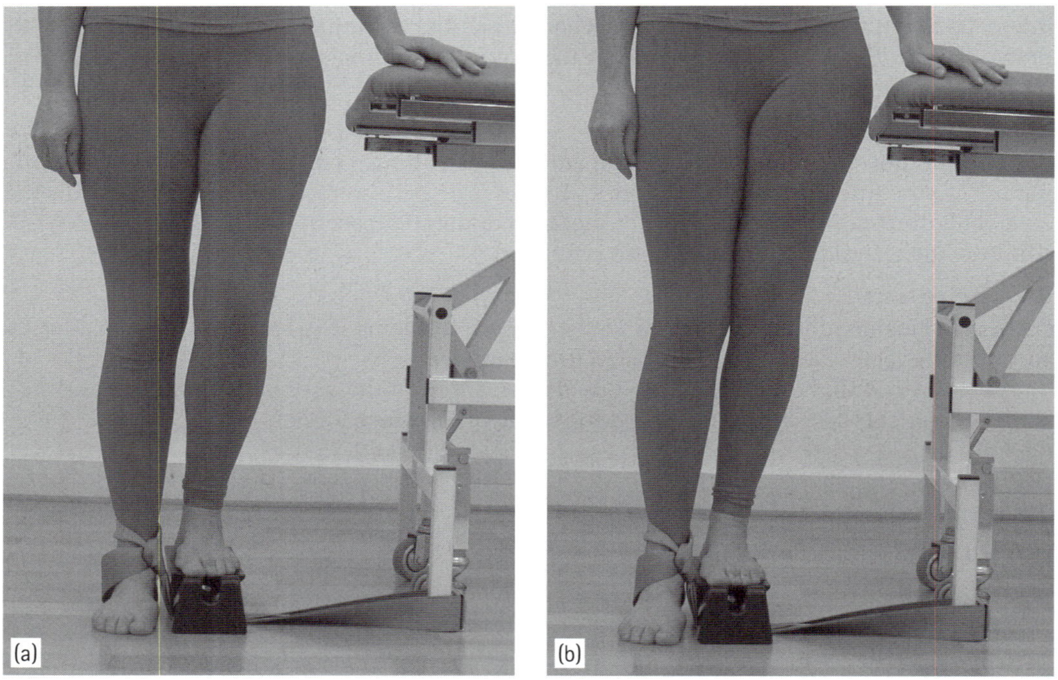

Figure 10.40a and b Translatory movement; traction; self-exercise. **a**, Starting position. **b**, End position.

Self-exercise (film 166)

Patient's starting position:

- standing (Fig. 10.40a)
- a belt loop is surrounding the right foot
- the belt passes underneath a base of 5–10 cm height (2–4 inches), which is situated at the left of the right foot and on which the patient places the left foot
- then, the right knee joint is pre-positioned in a position shortly before symptoms appear
- to maintain equilibrium, the patient holds on to a stable piece of furniture.

Movement:

- the body is pushed up by extension of the left leg (Fig. 10.40b)
- meanwhile, the right leg hangs as loose as possible so that traction in the right knee occurs.

Remarks (on traction)

Goals of the technique
With extension of the right knee painfully restricted by an intra-articular mechanism (compression) and simultaneously restricted translatory mobility of the tibia in an anterior direction associated with increased tension of the muscles moving the knee, these techniques serve to improve mobility by mobilization of non-symptomatic tissue.

Performance
The higher the tissue resistance to be overcome by mobilization, the more important fixation becomes to avoid pre-positioned movement.

Dosage
As, in this example, an intra-articular mechanism is assumed, the technique will probably not directly stress the symptomatic structures. The patient's typical pain with extension should not appear. Dosage is determined by the expected training state of the tissue and, above all, by reassessment.

Choice of technique
The selection of the technique depends, among other things, on the therapist as well as the patient, on the therapist's clinical experience, but primarily on reassessment. This means that even if all preconditions on the part of therapist and patient seem to be met, it is of no use to continue the technique if reassessment is negative.

Contributing factors
For a satisfactory solution of the patient's current problems it is important to consider the contributing factors and include them in the treatment.

The authors will, however, not go into a description of the various possibilities and their complex contexts as this would exceed the scope of the present book.

Femoral glide in posterior direction

Therapy technique (film 167)
Patient's starting position:

- supine (Fig. 10.41a)
- tibia supported by a wedge, knee pre-positioned in a position shortly before symptoms appear
- the distal lower leg is fixed by one of the therapist's hands or by a belt, according to the therapist's preference.

Therapist's starting position:

- standing, beside the patient
- contact with the patient's distal femur.

Movement:

- central push of the femur in a posterior direction (Fig. 10.41b)
- it is also possible to push the medial and/or lateral part of the femur separately in a posterior direction.

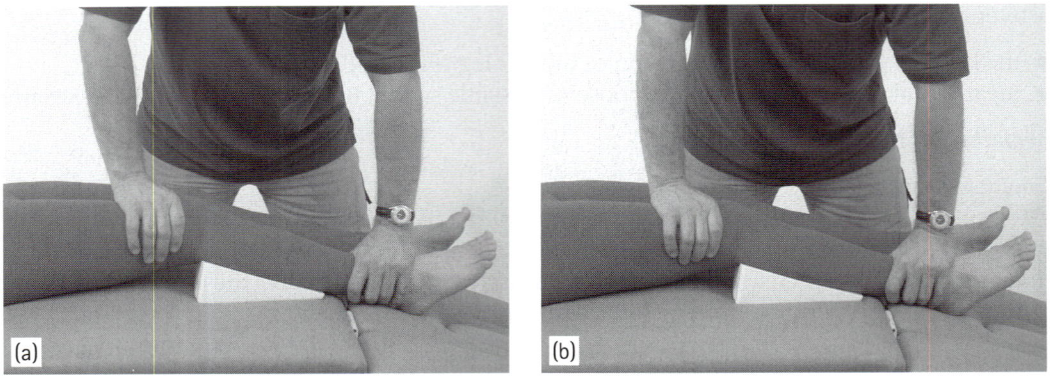

Figure 10.41a and b Translatory movement; posterior glide of the femur; therapy technique. **a**, Starting position. **b**, End position.

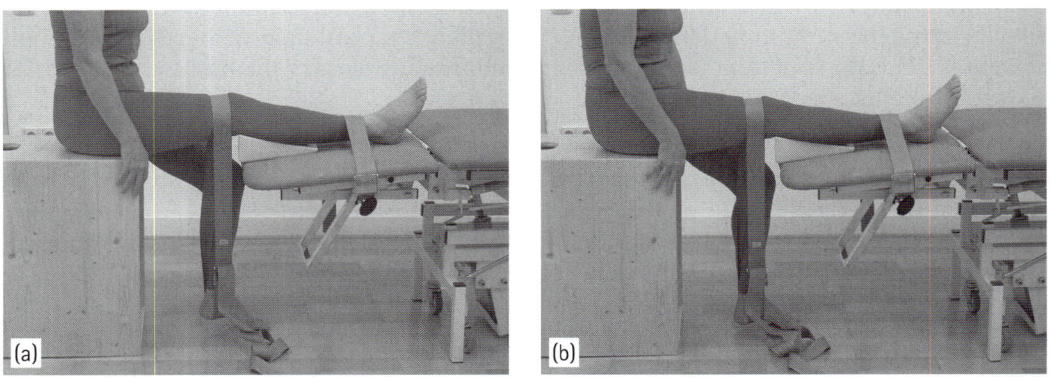

Figure 10.42a and b Translatory movement; posterior glide of the femur; self-exercise. **a**, Starting position. **b**, End position.

Self-exercise (film 168)

Patient's starting position:

- sitting (Fig. 10.42a)
- the right leg, extended to a position shortly before symptoms appear, is supported on a chair, or another appropriate piece of furniture, the seat of which ends at the proximal edge of the tibia
- a wedge is placed under the tibia, close to the knee joint
- the distal lower leg is fixed by a belt
- a belt loop surrounds the distal femur (quite close to the joint) from the anterior side
- the left heel is placed into the loop, and the belt length is adjusted so that the tip of the left foot touches the floor.

Movement:

- lowering the left heel results, via the belt, in a posterior glide of the femur against the fixed tibia (Fig. 10.42b).

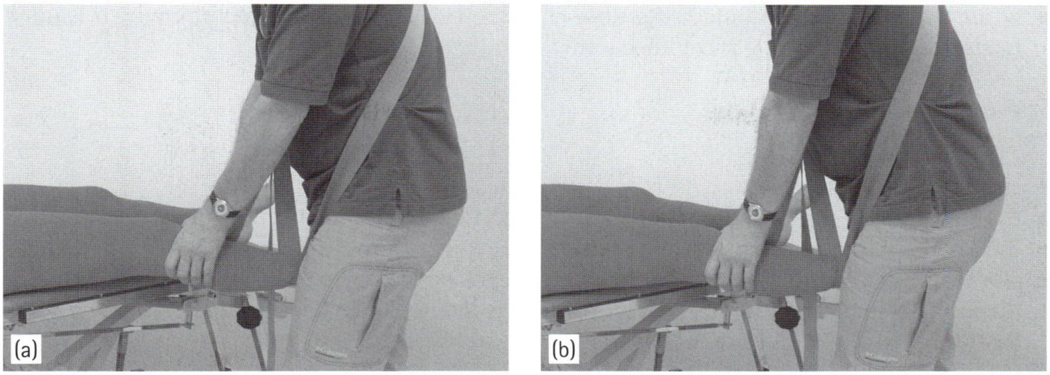

Figure 10.43a and b Passive angular movement; posterior gapping with simultaneous distraction; therapy technique. a, Starting position. b, End position.

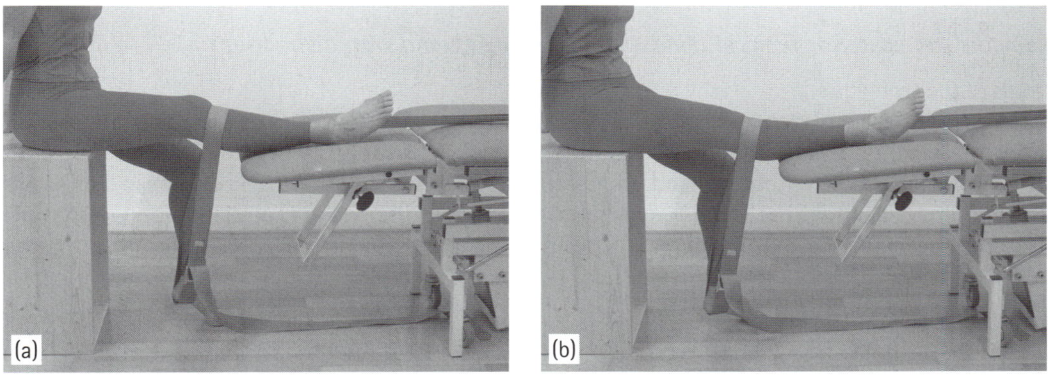

Figure 10.44a and b Passive angular movement; posterior gapping with simultaneous distraction; self-exercise. a, Starting position. b, End position.

ANGULAR MOVEMENTS

Posterior gapping with simultaneous distraction

Therapy technique (film 169)

Patient's starting position:

- supine, at the right side of the plinth (Fig. 10.43a)
- the right leg protruding laterally beyond the plinth.

Therapist's starting position:

- standing, at the right side of the plinth
- a belt surrounds the therapist and the patient's distal lower leg
- the patient's right foot is secured between the therapist's thighs
- both the therapist's hands are placed proximally on the patient's tibia, from the front.

Movement:

- movement backwards of therapist's body results in a pull in the direction of distraction (Fig. 10.43b)

- while this pull is maintained, the tibia is pushed in a posterior direction, which leads to posterior gapping of the right knee joint.

Self-exercise (film 170)

Patient's starting position:

- sitting (Fig. 10.44a)
- the lower leg is supported on a chair and fixed in a distal direction by a foot cuff or a belt
- the knee is extended to a position shortly before symptoms appear
- a belt loop surrounds the proximal tibia (quite close to the joint) from the anterior side
- the left heel is placed into the belt loop, and the length of the belt is adjusted in such a way that the tip of the left foot touches the floor.

Movement:

- moving the right half of the pelvis back results in distraction in the right knee (Fig. 10.44b)
- lowering the left heel (pull on the belt) results in posterior gapping in the right knee.

Remarks (on posterior femoral glide and posterior gapping with distraction)

Goals of the technique

With painfully restricted extension of the right knee due to an intra-articular mechanism (compression) and simultaneously restricted translatory mobility of the tibia in an anterior direction, associated with increased tension of the muscles moving the knee, these techniques serve to improve mobility. The demonstrated techniques attempt to mobilize non-symptomatic tissue. For this reason, symptom provocation in symptomatic tissue (pain in the anteromedial area of the knee) is not desirable.

Performance

The more tissue resistance has to be overcome by mobilization, the more important is fixation to prevent uncontrolled continuation of the movement.

Dosage

As, in this example, an intra-articular mechanism of symptom provocation is assumed, and as the primary goal of the technique is mobilization of non-symptomatic tissue, direct load on symptomatic structures due to the technique is undesirable. To control this, it is assumed that the patient's typical pain should not appear with extension.

Only pull at the posterior side of the right knee must be felt. If this cannot be achieved with the demonstrated techniques, their continuation is not recommended. If application without reproduction of the typical pain is possible, dosage is determined by the expected training state of the tissue and, above all, by reassessment.

Choice of technique

The selection of the technique depends, among other things, on the therapist as well as the patient, on the therapist's clinical experience, but primarily on reassessment. This means that even if all preconditions on the part of therapist and patient seem to be met, it is of no use to continue the technique if reassessment is negative.

Contributing factors

For a satisfactory solution of the patient's current problems it is important to consider the contributing factors and include them in the treatment.

The authors will, however, not go into a description of the various possibilities and their complex contexts as this would exceed the scope of the present book.

Chapter 11

Anterolateral knee

CHAPTER CONTENTS

AREA LOCALIZATION

IDENTIFICATION OF THE POTENTIALLY AFFECTED AREA BY DEMONSTRATION OF A SYMPTOMATIC FUNCTIONAL MOVEMENT/POSITION

Based on the information gained from the anamnesis so far, the therapist ascertains more details about potentially affected sections. This is done by means of area localization, which represents the beginning of the physical examination. Information gained in this way is used to check or modify the relevant hypotheses developed on the basis of the anamnesis and will determine further proceedings.

Area localization is explained by means of an example in which the patient feels pain in the area of the anterolateral knee complex. Clinical experience and known clinical patterns suggest primarily the following sections as potential sources of current complaints:

- knee complex
- lumbar spine
- neural structures.

General question: Is there enough information available to skip area localization?	
No	Yes
⇓	⇓
Performance of area localization	• General movement tests • Additional tests • Test treatment

Example 1: Squatting

Symptom area: anterolateral aspect of the knee
Symptom provocation: squatting (Fig. 11.1)

With this presentation, clinical experience suggests primarily the knee complex, lumbar spine, and neural structures as symptom-provoking areas.

Below, examples illustrate how to differentiate between these areas. To this end, area localization is first attempted by means of active movements alone. If this is not possible, tests will be performed by means of assistive/passive movements.

Hypothesis 1: The symptom-provoking area is the lumbar spine
Differentiation: lumbar spine vs. knee complex.

The change in symptoms can be demonstrated exactly:

- provocation of pain (Fig. 11.2a and b, film 171)
- alleviation of pain (Fig. 11.3a and b, film 172).

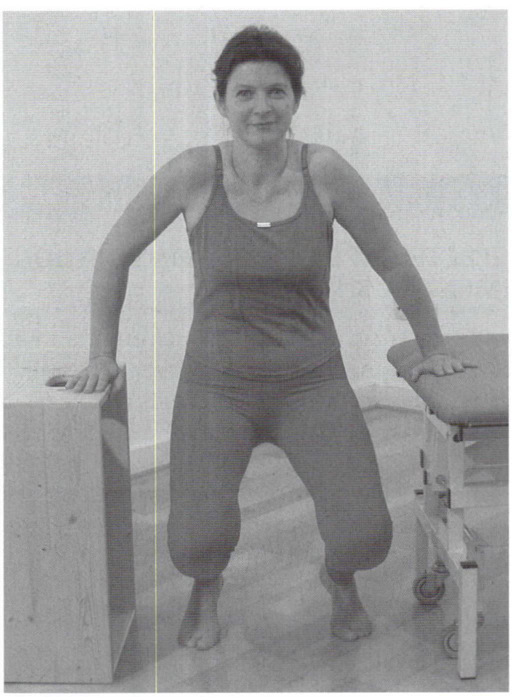

Figure 11.1 Symptom-provoking movement: flexion of the knee (squatting) provokes pain in the anterolateral side of the knee.

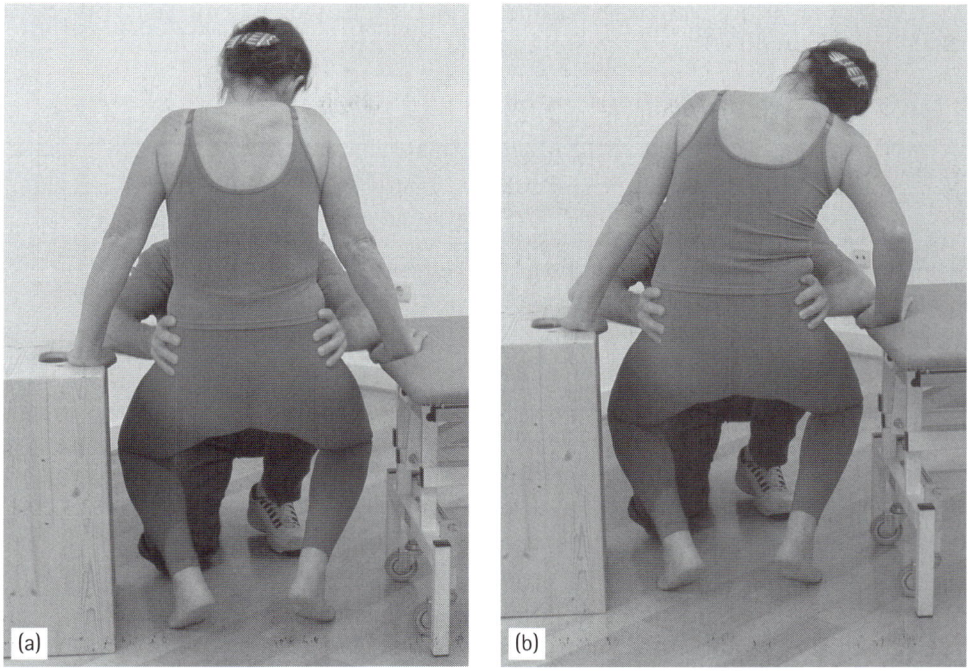

Figure 11.2a and b Area localization with symptomatic flexion of the knee (squatting); differentiation between lumbar spine and knee complex; provocation. **a**, Starting position. **b**, End position.

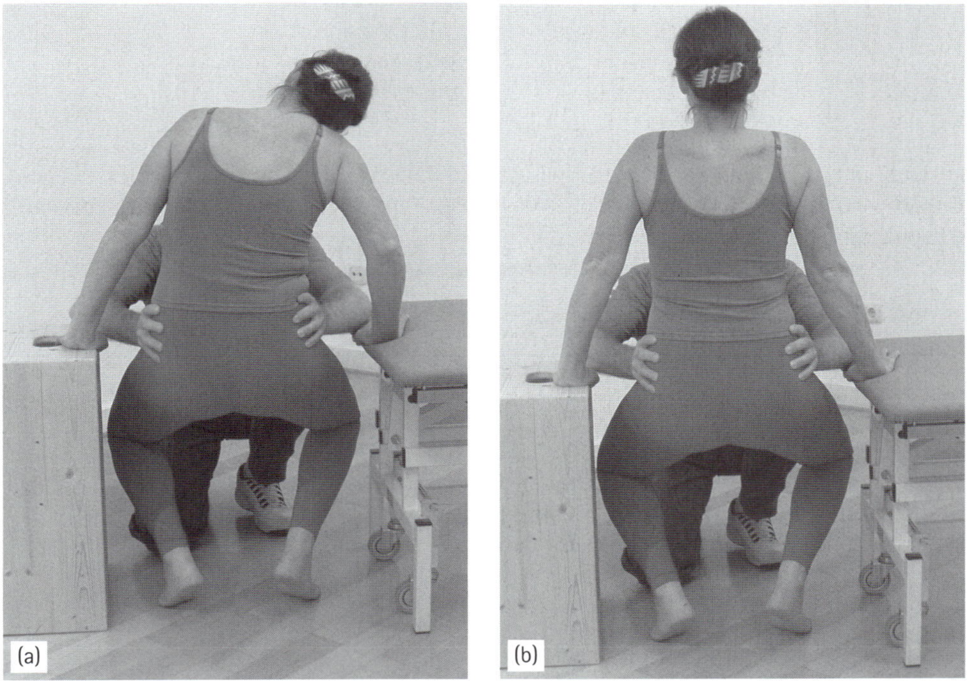

Figure 11.3a and b Area localization with symptomatic flexion of the knee (squatting); differentiation between lumbar spine and knee complex; alleviation. **a**, Starting position. **b**, End position.

The result of area localization should be verified by further specific tests; otherwise the result will remain in doubt.

Assessment			
Goal	**Provocation of pain**	**Alleviation of pain**	**Remarks**
Starting position	Squatting in a position immediately before symptoms appear	With the lumbar spine pre-positioned in lateral flexion to the affected side, squatting in a position immediately after symptoms have appeared	
Test movement	Lateral flexion of the lumbar spine to the affected side	Moving the lumbar spine back	
Explanation	If by any movement of the lumbar spine (here, as an example, lateral flexion to the right) the typical symptoms are reproduced, an isolated lesion of the knee complex is doubtful	If by any movement of the lumbar spine (here, as an example, moving back from lateral flexion) the typical symptoms are alleviated, an isolated lesion of the knee complex is doubtful	
Additional data to support the hypothesis	General and specific mobility of lumbar spine and knee complex History (e.g., symptom behaviour, type of complaints, 24-hour behaviour) Palpation Reproducibility of test results Test treatment Imaging procedures (CT, MRI)		

Hypothesis 2: The symptom-provoking area is the neural structures

Differentiation: neural involvement vs. knee complex.

The change in symptoms can be demonstrated exactly:

- provocation of pain (Fig. 11.4a and b, film 173)
- alleviation of pain (Fig. 11.5a and b, film 174).

The result of area localization should be verified by further specific tests; otherwise the result will remain in doubt.

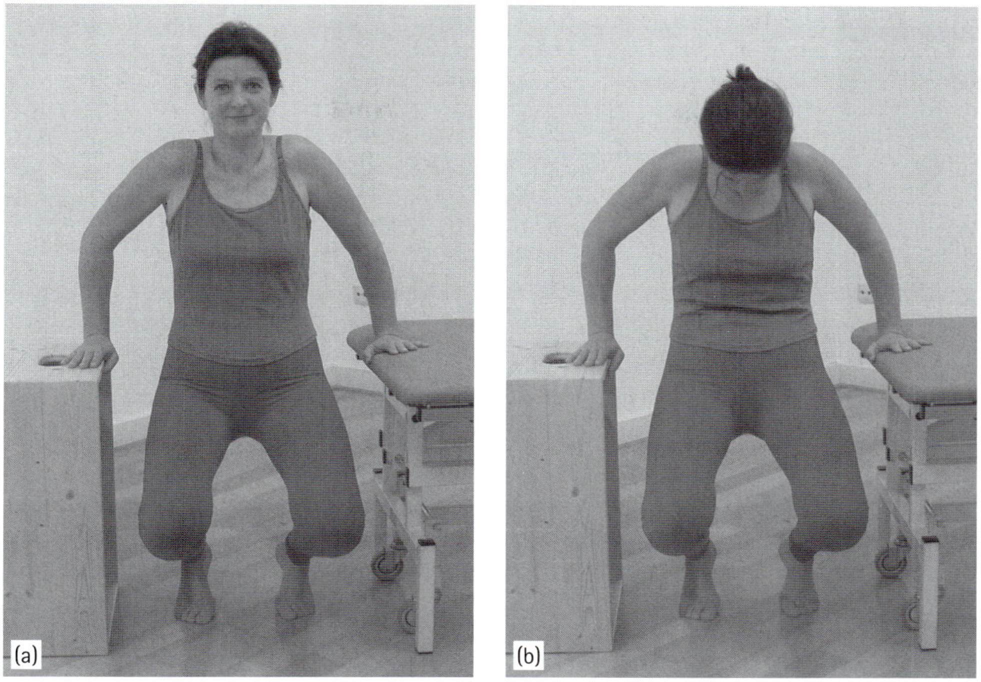

Figure 11.4a and b Area localization with symptomatic flexion of the knee (squatting); differentiation between neural structures and knee complex; provocation. **a**, Starting position. **b**, End position.

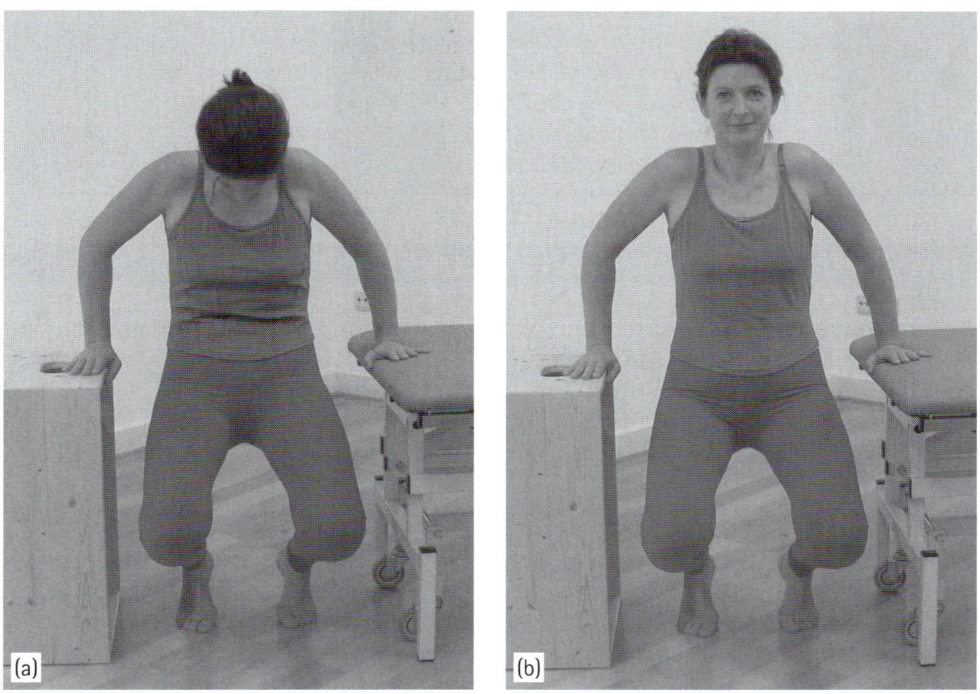

Figure 11.5a and b Area localization with symptomatic flexion of the knee (squatting); differentiation between neural structures and knee complex; alleviation. **a**, Starting position. **b**, End position.

Assessment			
Goal	**Provocation of pain**	**Alleviation of pain**	**Remarks**
Starting position	Squatting in a position immediately before symptoms appear	With the lumbar spine pre-positioned in flexion, squatting in a position immediately after symptoms have appeared, with cervical spine adjusted in flexion before	
Test movement	Flexion of the cervical spine	Moving the cervical spine back	
Explanation	The test movement produces mechanical stress on the neural structures and the structures associated with them	The test movement reduces mechanical stress on the neural structures and the structures associated with them	If the typical pain is provoked or alleviated by these manoeuvres without moving the knee complex, this suggests at least an involvement of the neural structures
Additional data to support the hypothesis	Further movements of proximal and distal components to increase neural tension not directly involved in extension of the knee (e.g., upper extremity) General and specific mobility of the affected area History (e.g., symptom behaviour, type of complaints, 24-hour behaviour) Palpation Neurodynamic tests; Nerve provocation tests (e.g., bow string sign) Reproducibility of test results Test treatment Imaging procedures (CT, MRI)		

QUICK CHECK – SYMPTOMS, ANTEROLATERAL KNEE

If neither the area nor a symptom-provoking or symptom-reducing action is known, the quick check is used to try to load individual potential areas with specific biomechanically provocative movement combinations. The chosen movement combinations correspond with the straining and often symptom-provoking movements of the individual sections.

LUMBAR SPINE

Movement (film 226)

- Extension/lateral flexion to the right, and rotation to the same as well as to the opposite side, with overpressure (Fig. 11.6a and b)
- Extension/lateral flexion to the left, and rotation to the same as well as to the opposite side, with overpressure (Fig. 11.7a and b).

Note: If the anamnesis suggests that flexion of the spine contributes to symptom provocation, the described movement combinations in extension should, of course, be performed in flexion.

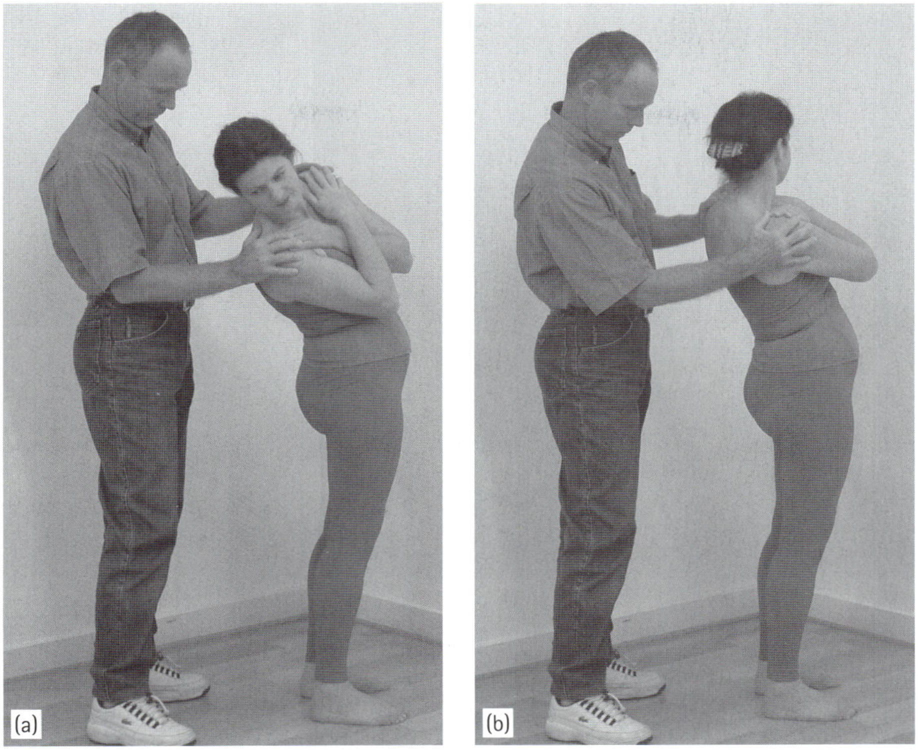

Figure 11.6a and b Quick check lumbar spine; extension, lateral flexion to the right. **a**, Rotation to the same side. **b**, Rotation to the opposite side.

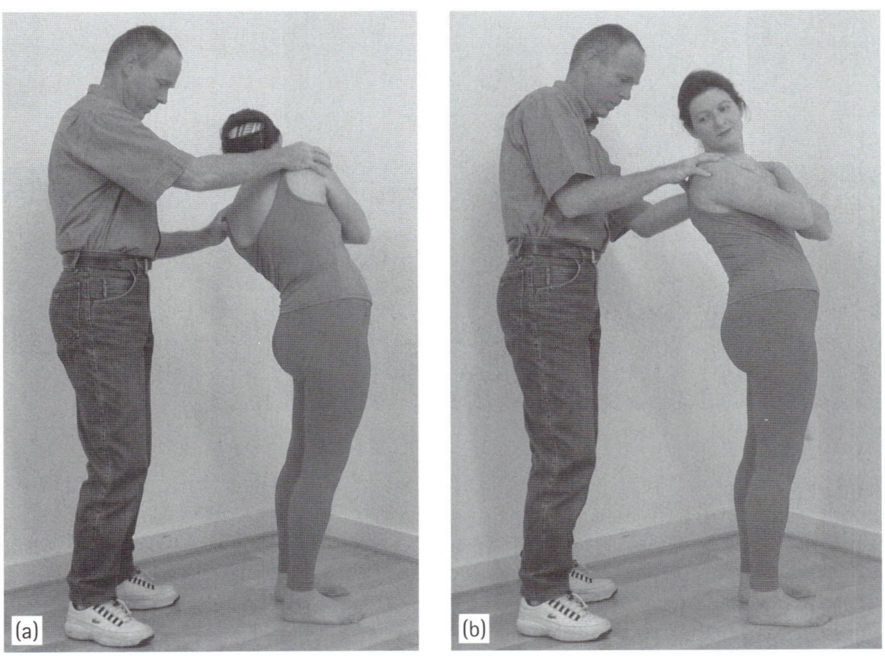

Figure 11.7a and b Quick check lumbar spine; extension, lateral flexion to the left. **a**, Rotation to the same side. **b**, Rotation to the opposite side.

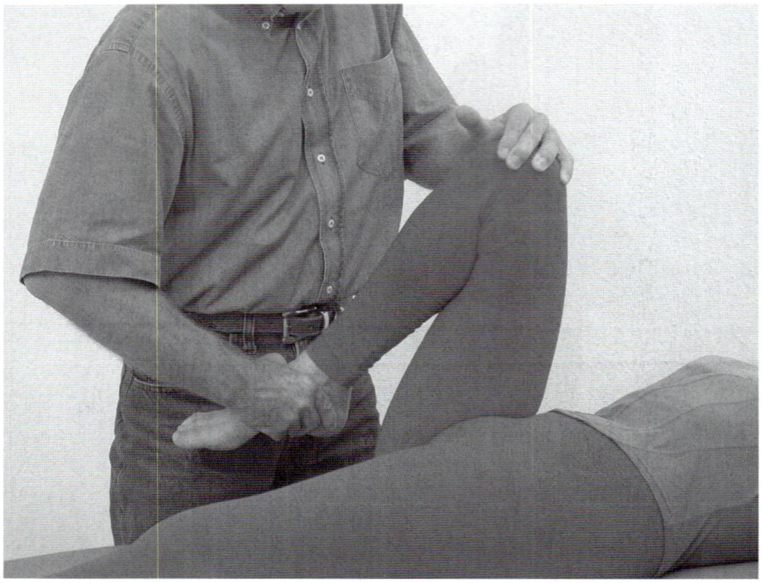

Figure 11.8 Quick check knee; flexion/abduction/internal rotation.

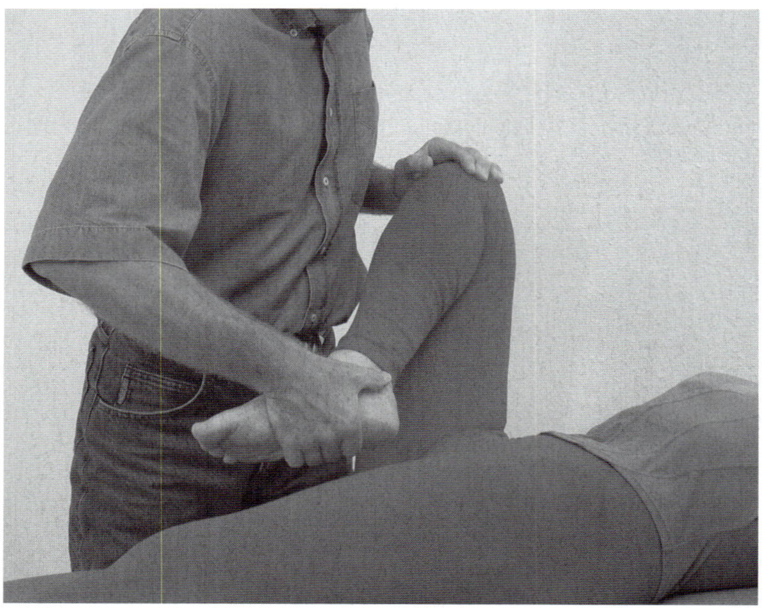

Figure 11.9 Quick check knee; flexion/adduction/external rotation.

KNEE COMPLEX

Movement (film 229)

- Flexion/abduction/internal rotation in the knee, with overpressure (Fig. 11.8)
- Flexion/adduction/external rotation in the knee, with overpressure (Fig. 11.9)
- Extension/adduction/external rotation in the knee, with overpressure (Fig. 11.10)
- Extension/abduction/internal rotation in the knee, with overpressure (Fig. 11.11).

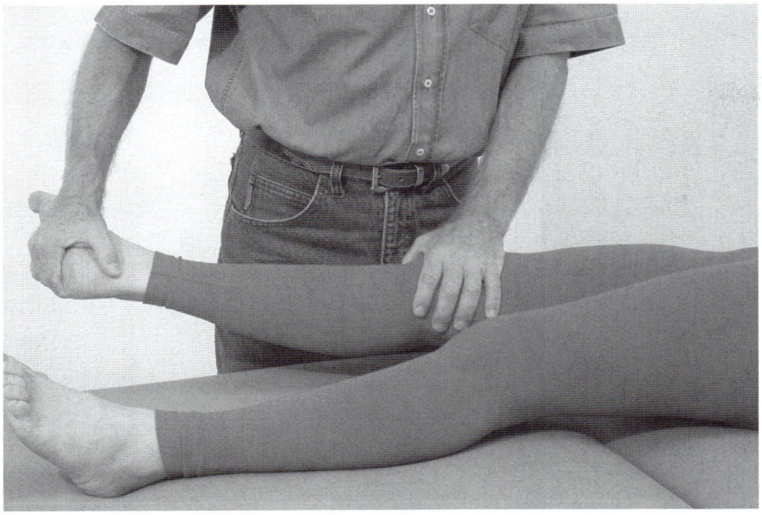

Figure 11.10 Quick check knee; extension/adduction/external rotation.

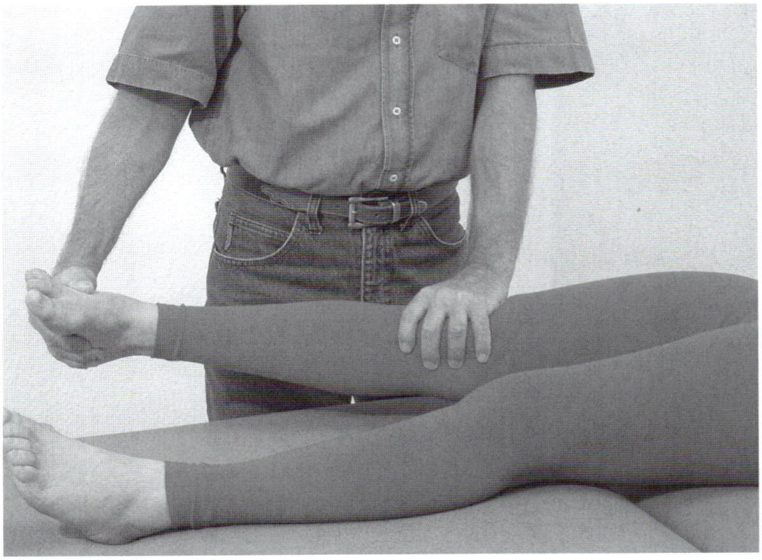

Figure 11.11 Quick check knee; extension/abduction/internal rotation.

NEURAL STRUCTURES

Tension tests

- Slump test (Fig. 11.12, film 616)
- Straight leg raise (SLR; Fig. 11.13, film 618)
- Prone knee bend (PKB; Fig. 11.14, film 241).

Note: Even an area that proves negative in the quick check may possibly be symptom-provoking (another movement combination, or passive overpressure may be required).

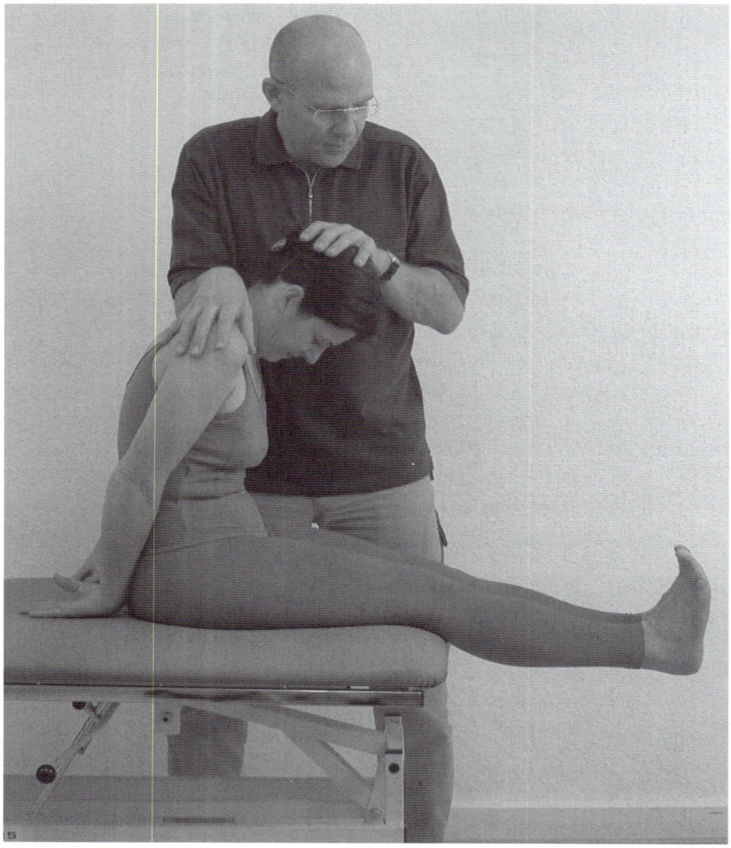

Figure 11.12 Quick check neurodynamics; slump test.

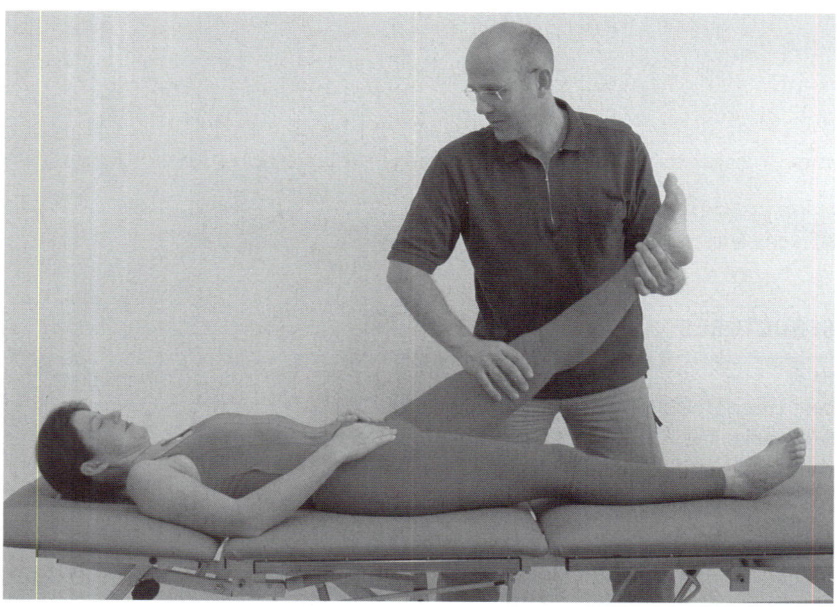

Figure 11.13 Quick check neurodynamics; straight leg raise (SLR) test.

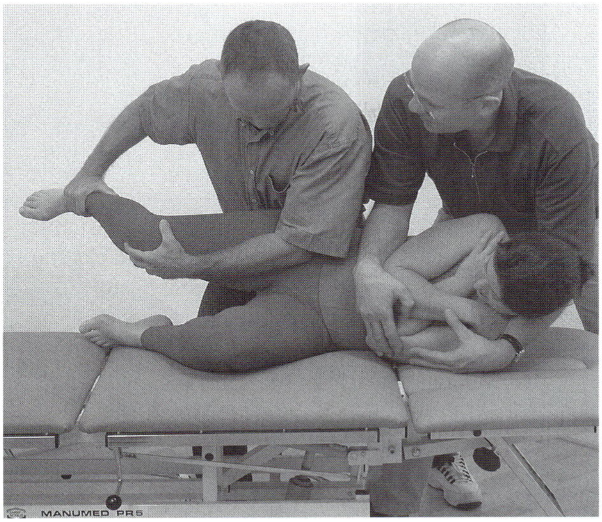

Figure 11.14 Quick check neurodynamics; prone knee bend (PKB) test.

SPECIFIC PROVOCATION AND ALLEVIATION

Specific provocation and alleviation allows one to differentiate within an articular complex and to identify the symptom-provoking movement direction(s).

SPECIFIC PROVOCATION AND ALLEVIATION, KNEE COMPLEX (SYMPTOMS, ANTEROLATERAL)

Localization, knee joint – flexion – movement as symptom-provoking component

Pain-provoking movement (Fig. 11.15)

- Flexion of the right knee joint provokes pain in the anterolateral aspect of the right knee.
- Area localization hints at the knee complex.

The change in symptoms can be demonstrated exactly:

- provocation of pain (Fig. 11.16a and b, film 175)
- alleviation of pain (Fig. 11.17a and b, film 176).

Assessment

Goal	Provocation of pain	Alleviation of pain	Remarks
Starting position	Flexion to a position immediately before symptoms appear	Flexion to a position immediately after symptoms have appeared	
Test movement	Tibia moves in posterior direction	Tibia moves in anterior direction	

Goal	Provocation of pain	Alleviation of pain	Remarks
Neural involvement	Proximal and/or distal component without change of position in the relevant area	Proximal and/or distal component without change of position in the relevant area	
Explanation	If symptoms are caused by movement of the tibia in posterior direction, this manoeuvre (tibia moves in posterior direction) will result in increased symptoms both with an intra-articular and with an extra-articular dysfunction	If symptoms are caused by movement of the tibia in posterior direction, this manoeuvre (tibia moves in anterior direction) will result in reduced symptoms both with an intra-articular and with an extra-articular dysfunction	If movements cannot be performed exactly or if proportions make it impossible to move the entire tibia, the medial and the lateral part of the tibia may be moved separately
Additional data to support the hypothesis	General and specific mobility of the knee joint History (e.g., symptom behaviour, type of complaints, 24-hour behaviour) Specific palpation Neurodynamic tests (if specific provocation and alleviation indicate neural involvement) Reproducibility of test results Test treatment Imaging procedures (CT, MRI)		

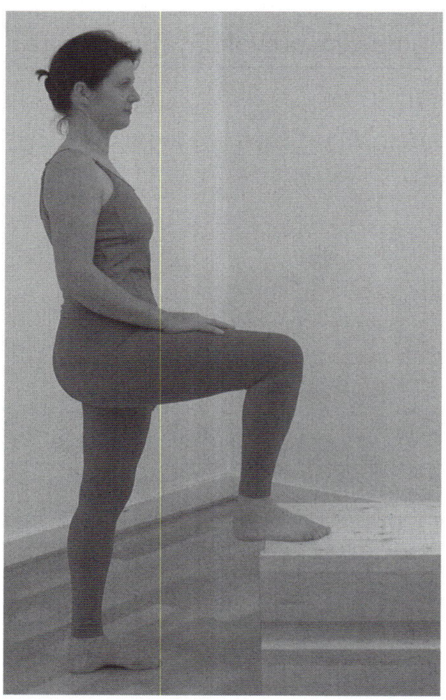

Figure 11.15 Symptom-provoking movement: flexion of the knee joint provokes pain in the anterolateral aspect of the knee.

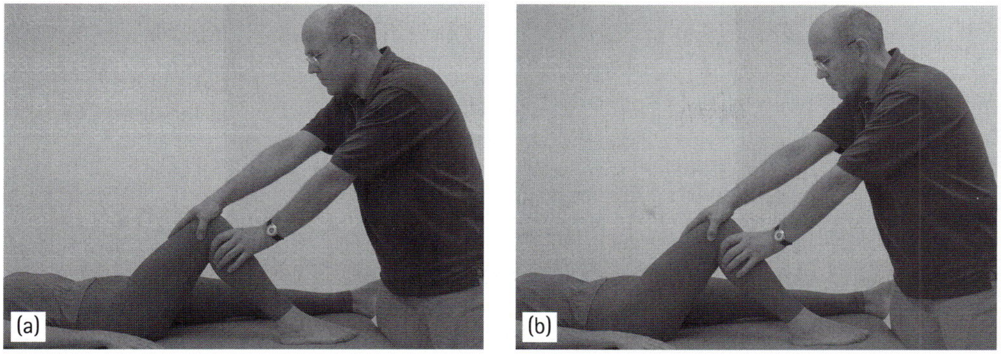

Figure 11.16a and b Specific provocation and alleviation in the area of the knee joint with symptomatic flexion; localization (symptom provocation by movement); provocation. **a**, Test start. **b**, Test end.

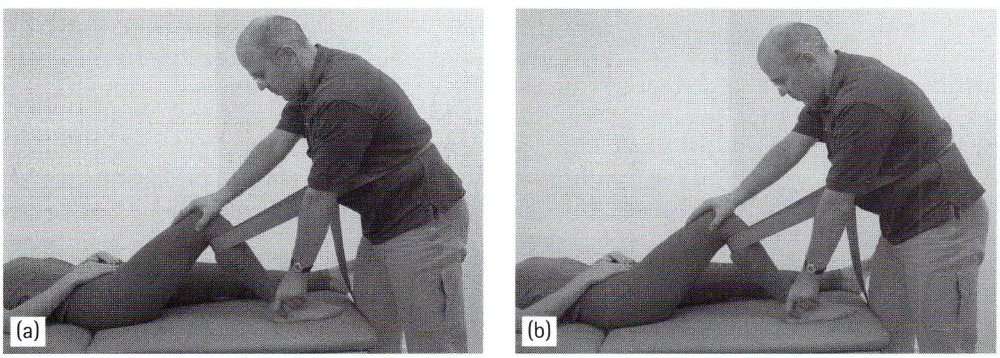

Figure 11.17a and b Specific provocation and alleviation in the area of the knee joint with symptomatic flexion; localization (symptom provocation by movement); alleviation. **a**, Test start. **b**, Test end.

Localization, patellofemoral joint – flexion – intra-articular vs. extra-articular (symptom provocation by an intra-articular component)

- Flexion of the right knee joint provokes pain in the anterolateral aspect of the right knee.
- Area localization hints at the knee complex.

The change in symptoms can be demonstrated exactly:

- provocation of pain (Fig. 11.18a and b, film 177).

Assessment

Goal	Provocation of pain	Alleviation of pain	Remarks
Starting position	Flexion to a position immediately after symptoms have appeared	None	Alleviation is usually not possible, as in this situation the tension of the soft tissues at the anterior side of the knee joint does

Goal	Provocation of pain	Alleviation of pain	Remarks
			not allow a separation of femur and patella
Test movement	Patella moves in posterior direction (compression)	None	
Neural involvement	Proximal and/or distal component without change of position in the relevant area		
Explanation	This manoeuvre increases the intra-articular compression forces in the patellofemoral joint		
Additional data to support the hypothesis	General and specific mobility of the patellofemoral joint History (e.g., symptom behaviour, type of complaints, 24-hour behaviour) Specific palpation Neurodynamic tests (if specific provocation and alleviation indicate neural involvement) Reproducibility of test results Test treatment Imaging procedures (CT, MRI)		

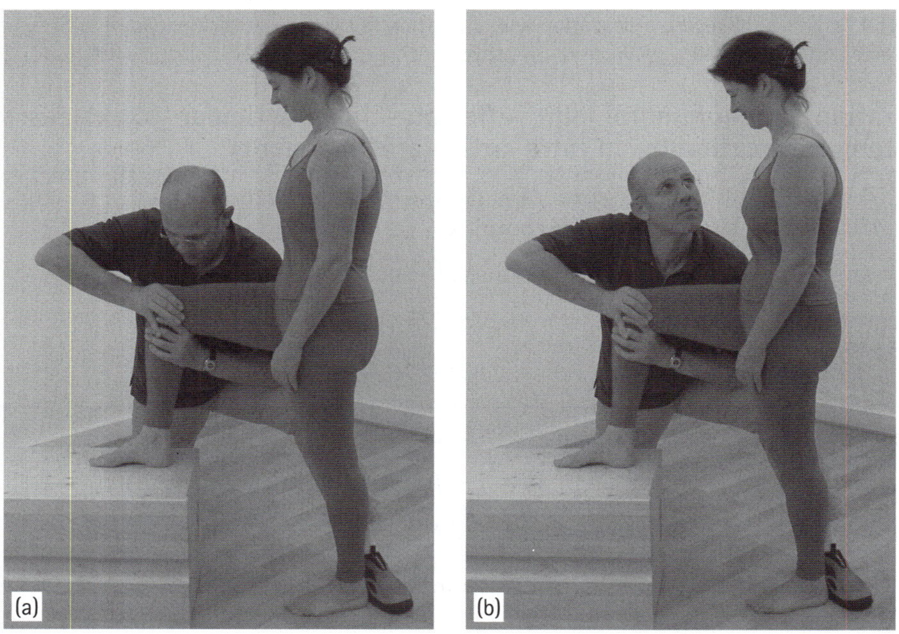

Figure 11.18a and b Specific provocation in the area of the knee joint with symptomatic flexion; differentiation, patellofemoral joint, intra-articular vs. extra-articular (symptom provocation by an intra-articular mechanism). **a**, Test start. **b**, Test end.

Localization, patellofemoral joint – flexion – movement as symptom-provoking component

- Flexion of the right knee joint provokes pain in the anterolateral aspect of the right knee.
- Area localization hints at the knee complex.

The change in symptoms can be demonstrated exactly:

- provocation of pain (Fig. 11.19a and b, film 179)
- alleviation of pain (Fig. 11.20a and b, film 180).

Assessment

Goal	Provocation of pain	Alleviation of pain	Remarks
Starting position	Flexion to a position immediately before symptoms appear	Flexion to a position immediately after symptoms have appeared	
Test movement	Patella moves in lateral direction	Patella moves in medial direction	
Neural involvement	Proximal and/or distal component without change of position in the relevant area	Proximal and/or distal component without change of position in the relevant area	
Explanation	If symptoms are caused by movement of the patella in lateral direction, this manoeuvre (patella moves in lateral direction) results in an increase in symptoms	If symptoms are alleviated by movement of the patella in medial direction, this manoeuvre (patella in medial direction) results in reduction of symptoms	
Additional data to support the hypothesis	General and specific mobility of the patellofemoral joint History (e.g., symptom behaviour, type of complaints, 24-hour behaviour) Specific palpation Neurodynamic tests (if specific provocation and alleviation indicate neural involvement) Reproducibility of test results Test treatment Imaging procedures (CT, MRI)		

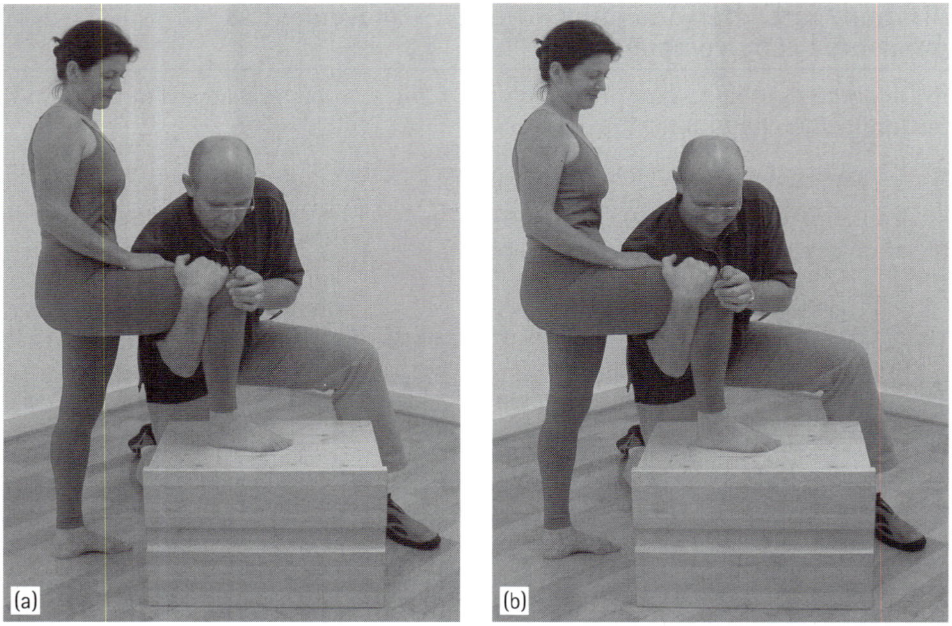

Figure 11.19a and b Specific provocation and alleviation in the area of the knee joint with symptomatic flexion; localization, patellofemoral joint (symptom provocation by movement); provocation. **a**, Test start. **b**, Test end.

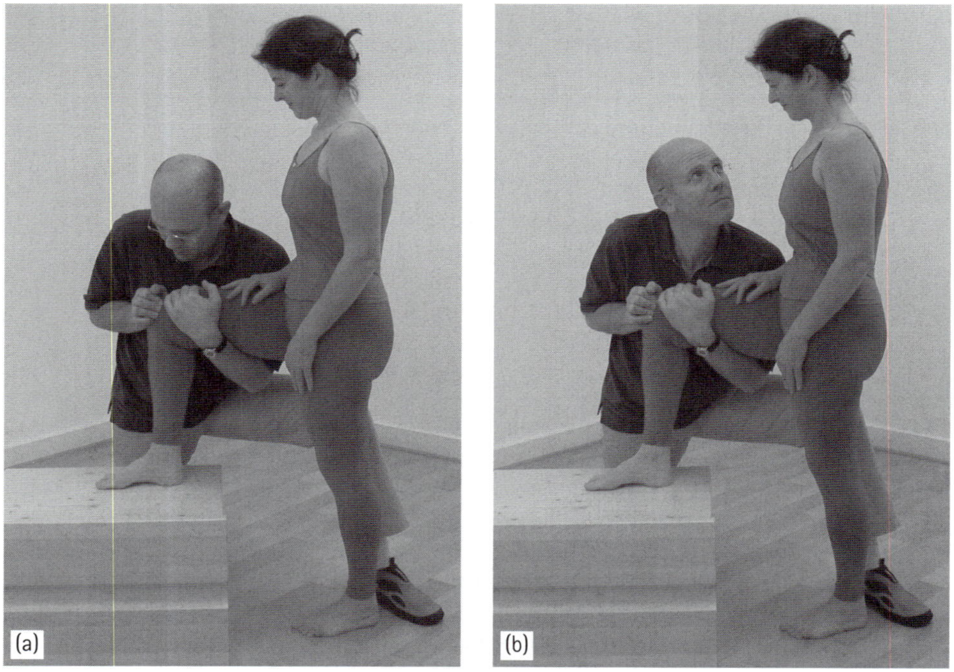

Figure 11.20a and b Specific provocation and alleviation in the area of the knee joint with symptomatic flexion; localization, patellofemoral joint (symptom provocation by movement); alleviation. **a**, Test start. **b**, Test end.

GENERAL MOVEMENT TESTS

General movement tests identify, quantify, and qualify individual anatomical movements and, in part, movement combinations in the area presumed. The individual manual therapy concepts have respective protocols at their disposal, which more or less have the same goals.

Information gained in this way is used for checking or modifying the relevant hypotheses developed on the basis of anamnesis and area localization and will help in deciding how to proceed.

General question: Is there enough information available to skip general movement tests?	
No	Yes
⇓	⇓
Performance of the general movement tests	• Additional tests • Test treatment

In view of the described clinical presentation and the results of area localization, general movement tests of the following regions seem to be useful.

Lumbar spine		
	Active	Passive
Lumbar spine in general	Flexion Extension Rotation (to the right and left) Lateral flexion (to the right and left)	Flexion Extension Rotation (to the right and left) Lateral flexion (to the right and left)
Movement combinations, lumbar spine in general	Symptomatic movements of the lumbar spine	Symptomatic movements of the lumbar spine
Hip		
	Active	Passive
Hip joint in general	Flexion Extension Internal rotation in extension Internal rotation in flexion External rotation in extension External rotation in flexion Abduction Adduction	Flexion Extension Internal rotation in extension Internal rotation in flexion External rotation in extension External rotation in flexion Abduction Adduction

	Active	Passive
Movement combinations, hip joint	Symptomatic movements of the hip joint	Symptomatic movements of the hip joint
Knee		
	Active	Passive
Knee in general	Flexion Extension Internal rotation of the lower leg with flexed knee External rotation of the lower leg with flexed knee	Flexion Extension Internal rotation of the lower leg External rotation of the lower leg Abduction Adduction

TREATMENT EXAMPLE, PATELLOFEMORAL JOINT

SYMPTOMATIC MOVEMENT

Flexion of the right knee with squatting provokes pain at an angle of 100° (VAS 4/10) in the area of the anterolateral aspect of the right knee.

ASSESSMENTS

Area localization

Area localization hints at symptom provocation by the knee complex. There is no contraindication for movement.

Specific provocation and alleviation

Specific provocation and alleviation hints at the patellofemoral joint. The symptomatic movement direction is movement of the patella in lateral direction. Symptoms are provoked by an intra-articular mechanism (compression of the patella against the femur).

Specific mobility

Specific mobility tests show restricted mobility of the patella in a medial direction.

Palpation

Palpation of the periarticular structures shows tissue changes as compared with the non-affected side. The patient's specific pain cannot be reproduced by palpation. Palpation of the muscles moving the patella shows increased tension as compared with the opposite side.

HYPOTHESIS

Painful dysfunction of the right patellofemoral joint by an intra-articular mechanism (compression) with simultaneously restricted mobility of the patella in a medial direction and increased tension of the muscles moving the patella is suspected (Fig. 11.21).

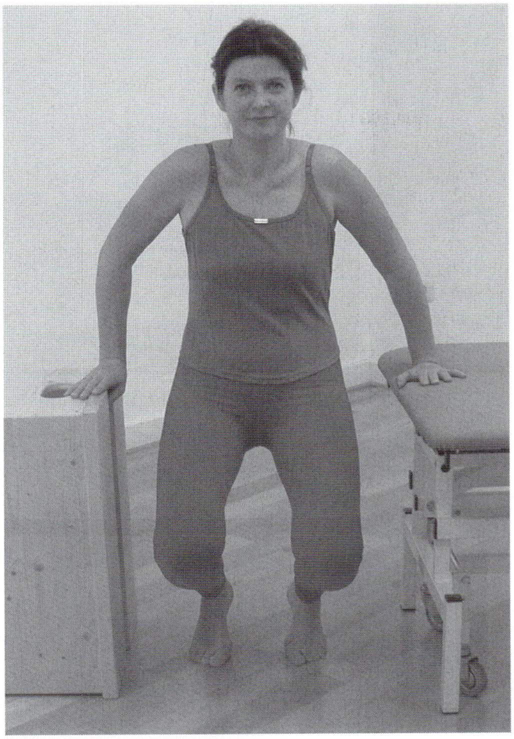

Figure 11.21 Symptom-provoking movement: flexion of the knee joint provokes pain in the anterolateral aspect of the knee.

RELAXATION TECHNIQUES

Hold–relax techniques

CONTRACTION OF THE MUSCLES DECENTRING THE PATELLA, LATERAL SIDE

Therapy technique (film 181)

Patient's starting position:

- lying on the left side (Fig. 11.22a)
- left hip flexed
- right leg extended in hip joint and flexed in knee joint.

Therapist's starting position:

- standing, behind the patient
- stabilizing the adjusted position of the right leg.

Movement:

- adduction in hip joint while the patient tries to prevent adduction by muscle contraction (Fig. 11.22b).

Self-exercise (film 182)

Patient's starting position:

- lying on the left side (Fig. 11.23a)
- right leg extended in hip joint, flexed in knee joint

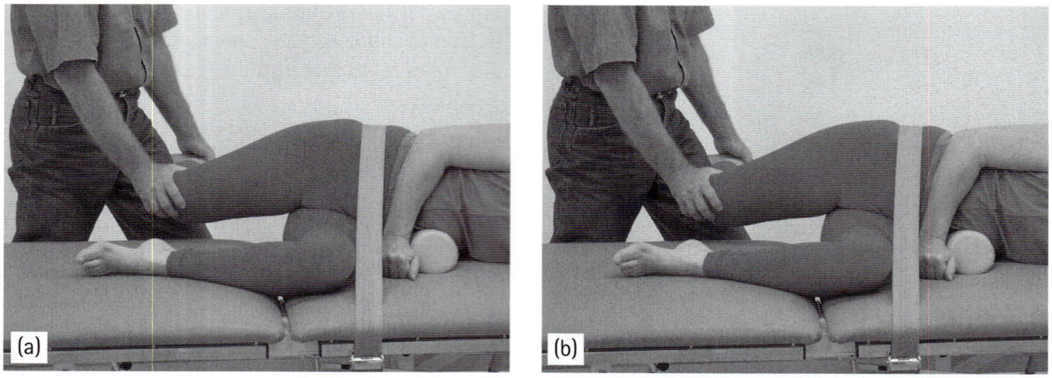

Figure 11.22a and b Hold-relax technique; contraction of the muscles on the lateral side decentring the patella; therapy technique. **a**, Starting position. **b**, End position.

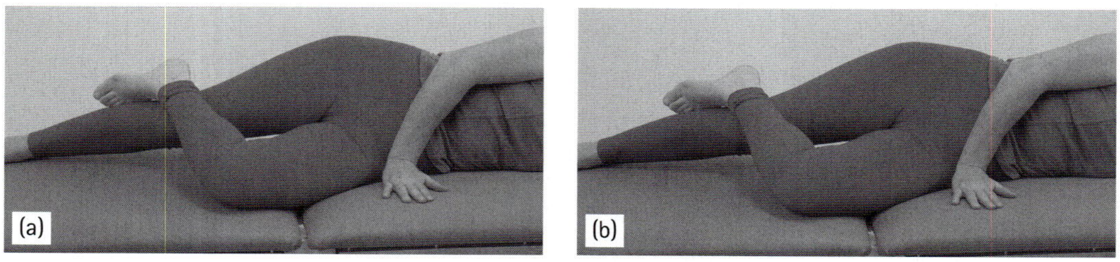

Figure 11.23a and b Hold-relax technique; contraction of the muscles on the lateral side decentring the patella; self-exercise. **a**, Starting position. **b**, End position.

- left leg flexed in hip and knee
- distal left lower leg and foot contact distal thigh.

Movement:

- via pressure of left lower leg, the patient tries to move the right hip further into adduction while opposing this movement with the abductors. In doing so, the left side of the pelvis should be pulled backwards and simultaneously slightly in a cranial direction (Fig. 11.23b).

CONTRACTION OF THE MUSCLES DECENTRING THE PATELLA, ANTERIOR SIDE

Therapy technique (film 183)

Patient's starting position:

- prone, on the left side of the plinth (Fig. 11.24a)
- left leg, with flexed hip and knee, placed on the floor
- right leg extended on the plinth
- hip extension of right leg reinforced, if need be, by adjusting the foot part of the plinth in a higher position.

Therapist's starting position:

- standing, beside the patient
- fixing the patient's pelvis and grasping the patient's lower leg distally.

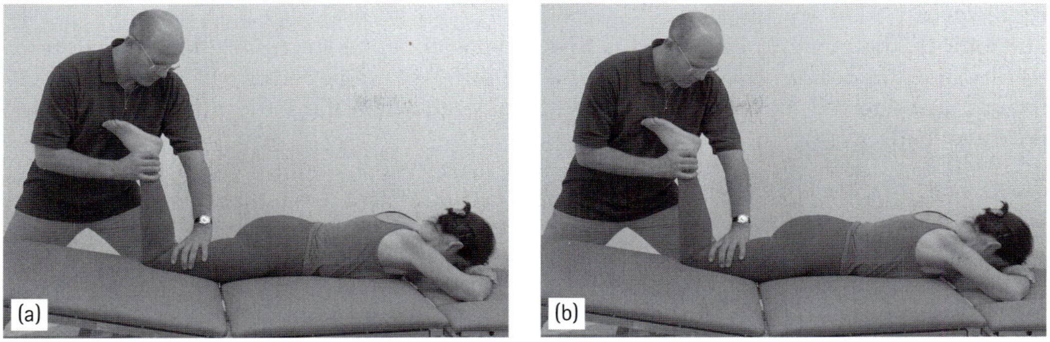

Figure 11.24a and b Hold-relax technique; contraction of the muscles on the anterior side decentring the patella; therapy technique. **a**, Starting position. **b**, End position.

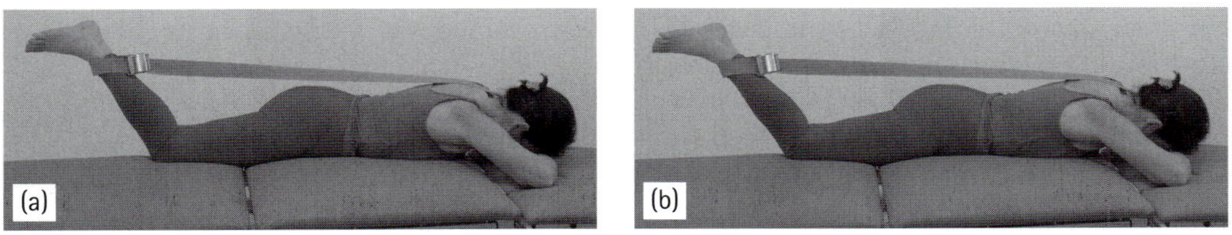

Figure 11.25a and b Hold-relax technique; contraction of the muscles on the anterior side decentring the patella; self-exercise. **a**, Starting position. **b**, End position.

Movement:

- the patient's knee is pre-positioned in flexion, in a position before symptoms appear
- then the therapist tries to move the knee further into flexion while the patient tries to prevent flexion by muscle contraction (Fig. 11.24b).

Self-exercise (film 184)

Patient's starting position:

- prone, on the left side of the plinth (Fig. 11.25a)
- left leg with flexed hip and knee placed on the floor
- right leg extended on the plinth, with a belt around the distal lower leg
- knee pre-positioned in flexion in a position before symptoms appear.

Movement:

- the patient tries to move the knee further into flexion by pulling the belt while at the same time trying to prevent flexion by muscle contraction (Fig. 11.25b).

Remarks

Goals of the technique

Reduction of tonicity and improvement of the metabolism of the periarticular tissues with a painfully restricted movement of the right patellofemoral joint due to an intra-articular mechanism (compression) and simultaneously restricted mobility of the patella in a medial direction with increased tension in the muscles moving the patella.

Performance

The joint that is going to be treated is first pre-positioned as necessary depending on irritability and the desired treatment goal. As the self-exercise is performed without 'specific fixation', transferred movement has to be considered when the indication for the exercise is determined.

Dosage (regarding the affected symptomatic structure)

Both with an acute and with a chronic presentation, contraction should always be pain-free.

Choice of technique

The selection of the technique depends, among other things, on the therapist as well as the patient, on the therapist's clinical experience, but primarily on reassessment. This means that even if all preconditions on the part of therapist and patient seem to be met, it is of no use to continue the technique if reassessment is negative.

Contributing factors

For a satisfactory solution of the patient's current problems it is important to consider the contributing factors and include them in the treatment.

The authors will, however, not go into a description of the various possibilities and their complex contexts as this would exceed the scope of the present book.

Soft tissue techniques

LATERAL MUSCLES DECENTRING THE PATELLA

Therapy technique (film 185)

Patient's starting position:

- lying on the left side (Fig. 11.26a)
- right hip extended and abducted, right knee flexed.

Therapist's starting position:

- standing, behind the patient.

Movement:

- passive adduction of right hip with simultaneous manual pressure on the lateral muscles decentring the patella (Fig. 11.26b)
- releasing pressure, and back to starting position.

Self-exercise (film 186)

Patient's starting position:

- standing, right knee supported on a chair (Fig. 11.27a)
- right hip extended, abducted, and externally rotated.

Movement:

- adduction of right hip by shifting the pelvis to the right (adduction in right hip), with simultaneous manual pressure through a tennis ball on the lateral muscles decentring the patella (Fig. 11.27b)
- releasing pressure, and back to starting position.

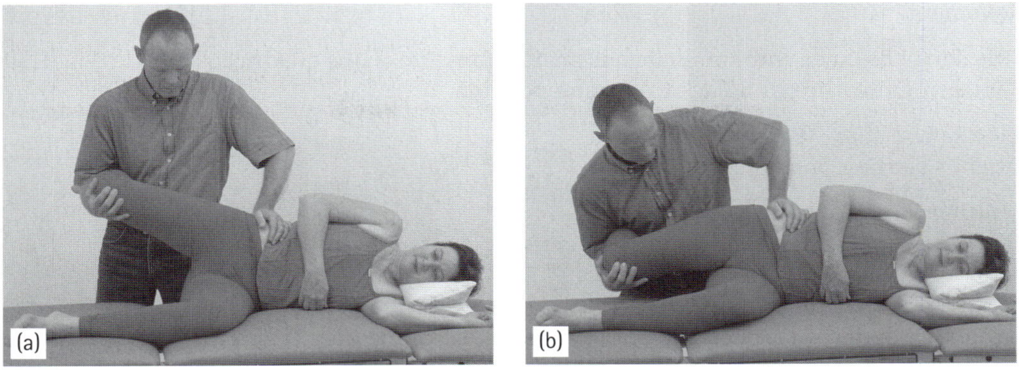

Figure 11.26a and b Soft tissue technique; lateral muscles decentring the patella; therapy technique. a, Starting position. b, End position.

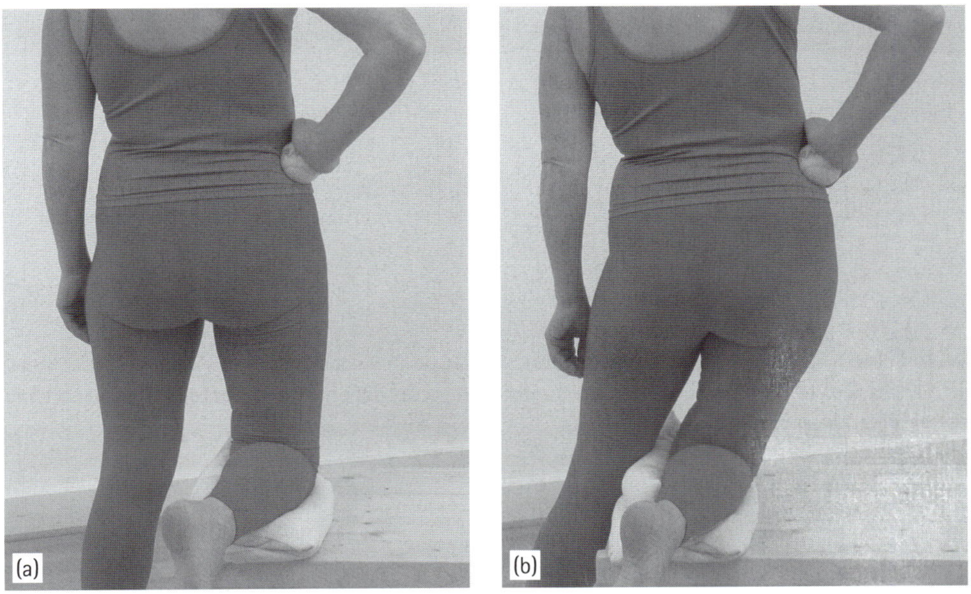

Figure 11.27a and b Soft tissue technique; lateral muscles decentring the patella; self-exercise. a, Starting position. b, End position.

ANTERIOR MUSCLES DECENTRING THE PATELLA

Therapy technique (film 187)

Patient's starting position:

- supine, at the foot end of the plinth (Fig. 11.28a)
- left foot placed on the edge of the plinth
- right knee extended.

Therapist's starting position:

- standing, in front of the patient
- fixing patient's distal right lower leg, and contacting anterior side of patient's thigh with the other hand.

Movement:

- flexion of the knee with simultaneous manual pressure on the quadriceps muscle (Fig. 11.28b)
- releasing pressure, and back to starting position.

Self-exercise (film 188)
Patient's starting position:

- sitting (Fig. 11.29a)
- both hands placed on the quadriceps muscle.

Movement:

- pressure on the quadriceps muscle, active flexion of the knee (Fig. 11.29b)
- releasing pressure, and back to starting position.

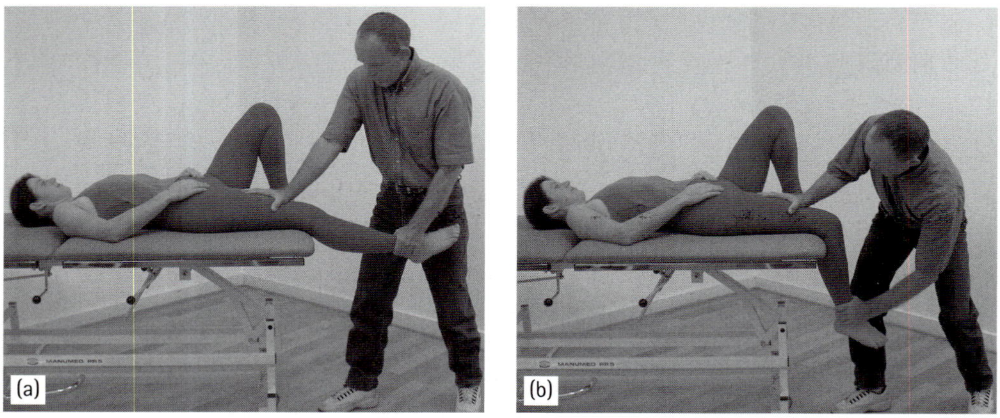

Figure 11.28a and b Soft tissue technique; anterior muscles decentring the patella; therapy technique. a, Starting position. b, End position.

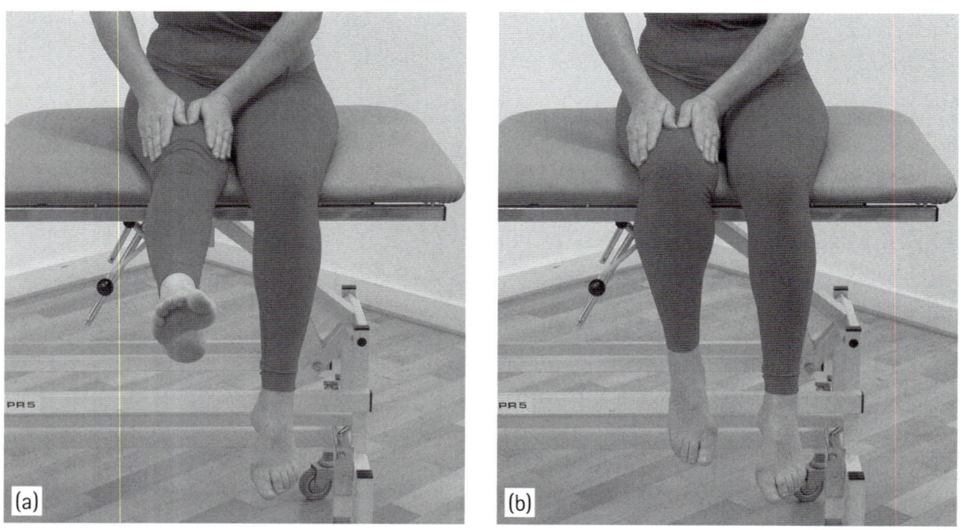

Figure 11.29a and b Soft tissue technique; anterior muscles decentring the patella; self-exercise. a, Starting position. b, End position.

Remarks

Goals of the technique

Reduction of tonicity and improvement of the metabolism of the periarticular tissues with a painfully restricted movement of the right patellofemoral joint by an intra-articular mechanism (compression) and simultaneously restricted mobility of the patella in medial direction with increased tension in the muscles moving the patella.

Performance

Treatment is performed within pain-free movement range. As treatment techniques are performed without 'specific fixation', transferred movement has to be considered when the indication for the technique is determined.

Dosage

Both with an acute and with a chronic presentation, the treatment technique should always be pain-free.

Choice of technique

The selection of the technique depends, among other things, on the therapist as well as the patient, on the therapist's clinical experience, but primarily on reassessment. This means that even if all preconditions on the part of therapist and patient seem to be met, it is of no use to continue the technique if reassessment is negative.

Contributing factors

For a satisfactory solution of the patient's current problems it is important to consider the contributing factors and include them in the treatment.

The authors will, however, not go into a description of the various possibilities and their complex contexts as this would exceed the scope of the present book.

MOBILIZATION TECHNIQUES

Active procedures

ACTIVE MOBILIZATION PLUS ACCESSORY MOVEMENT

Flexion of the knee with gliding of the patella in a mediodistal direction

Therapy technique (film 189)

Patient's starting position:

- lying on the left side (Fig. 11.30a)
- left hip and knee flexed
- right hip extended and adducted, right knee slightly flexed and supported stably by a wedge or sandbag.

Therapist's starting position:

- standing, behind the patient
- fixing patient's distal right lower leg to control the rotated position of the right hip
- left hand contacting patient's patella, from the proximal-lateral side (using a tissue to avoid sliding of the patella).

Movement:

- pushing the patella in a mediodistal direction (Fig. 11.30b)

- having patient actively flex right knee while maintaining the push, and then move back to starting position
- then releasing the push on the patella.

Self-exercise (film 190)

Patient's starting position:

- sitting on the table (Fig. 11.31a)
- the right knee is extended
- the left hand is stabilizing the right femur medially, and the right hand is in contact with the patella laterally.

Movement:

- while pushing the patella in a mediodistal direction, move the knee from extension into flexion and then back to the starting position (Fig. 11.31b).

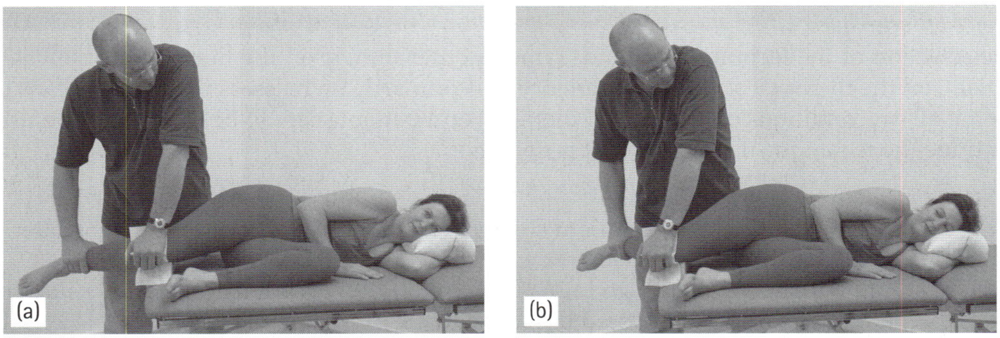

Figure 11.30a and b Active mobilization with accessory movement; flexion with mediodistal gliding of the patella; therapy technique. **a**, Starting position. **b**, End position.

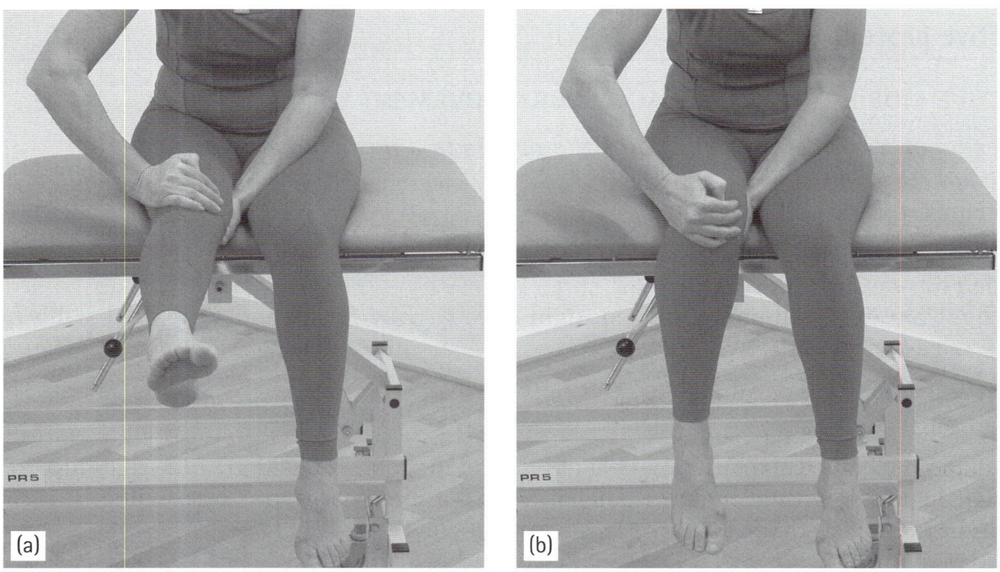

Figure 11.31a and b Active mobilization with accessory movement; flexion with mediodistal gliding of the patella; self-exercise. **a**, Starting position. **b**, End position.

Remarks

Goals of the technique

With a painfully restricted movement of the right patellofemoral joint due to an intra-articular mechanism (compression) and simultaneously restricted mobility of the patella in a medial direction with increased tension in the muscles moving the patella, these techniques serve to:

- reduce tonicity and improve the metabolism of the affected tissues
- restore pain-free function (change the input to the respective centres of the central nervous system (CNS)).

Performance

Fixation of the distal right lower leg prevents internal rotation of the right hip induced by pushing the patella in a medial direction.

Dosage

Both with an acute and with a chronic presentation, the treatment technique should always be pain-free. Dosage depends on the expected training state of the tissue and, above all, on reassessment.

Choice of technique

The selection of the technique depends, among other things, on the therapist as well as the patient, on the therapist's clinical experience, but primarily on reassessment. This means that even if all preconditions on the part of therapist and patient seem to be met, it is of no use to continue the technique if reassessment is negative.

Contributing factors

For a satisfactory solution of the patient's current problems it is important to consider the contributing factors and include them in the treatment.

The authors will, however, not go into a description of the various possibilities and their complex contexts as this would exceed the scope of the present book.

Passive procedures

TRANSLATORY MOVEMENTS

Gliding of the patella in mediodistal direction

Therapy technique (film 196 – 4)

Patient's starting position:

- lying on the left side (Fig. 11.32a)
- left hip and knee flexed
- right hip extended and adducted, right knee slightly flexed and stably supported on a wedge or sandbag.

Therapist's starting position:

- standing, behind the patient
- fixing patient's distal right lower leg to control rotated position of right hip
- contacting patella with left hand, from the proximal-lateral side.

Movement:

- pushing patella in a mediodistal direction (Fig. 11.32b).

Self-exercise (film 192)

Patient's starting position:

- sitting on the plinth, right foot placed on a stool so that the right knee is flexed (Fig. 11.33a)
- stabilizing right knee with left hand from the medial side
- contacting lateral patellar edge with right hand, from the proximal-lateral side.

Movement:

- pushing the patella in a mediodistal direction (Fig. 11.33b).

Remarks

Goals of the technique

With a painfully restricted movement of the right patellofemoral joint due to an intra-articular mechanism (compression) and simultaneously restricted mobility of the patella in a medial

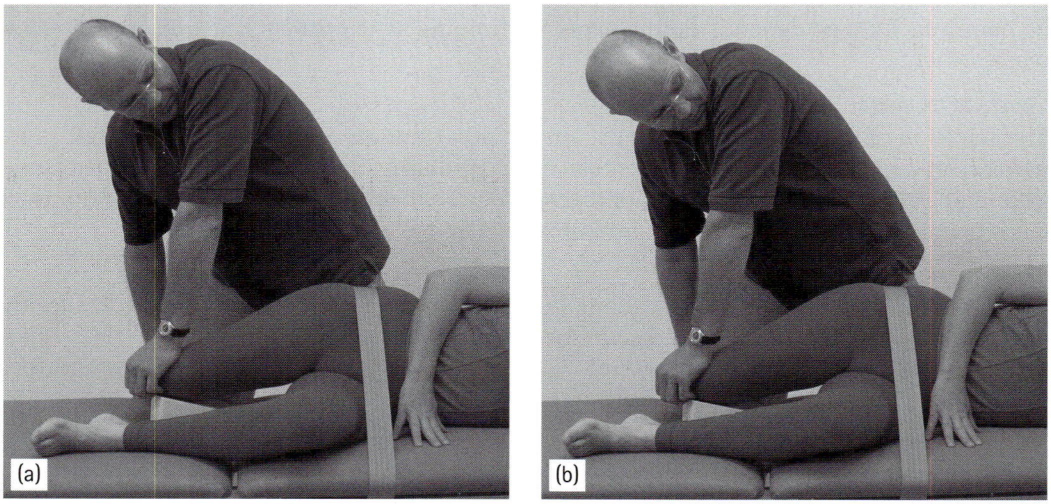

Figure 11.32a and b Translatory movement; gliding of the patella in a mediodistal direction; therapy technique. **a**, Starting position. **b**, End position.

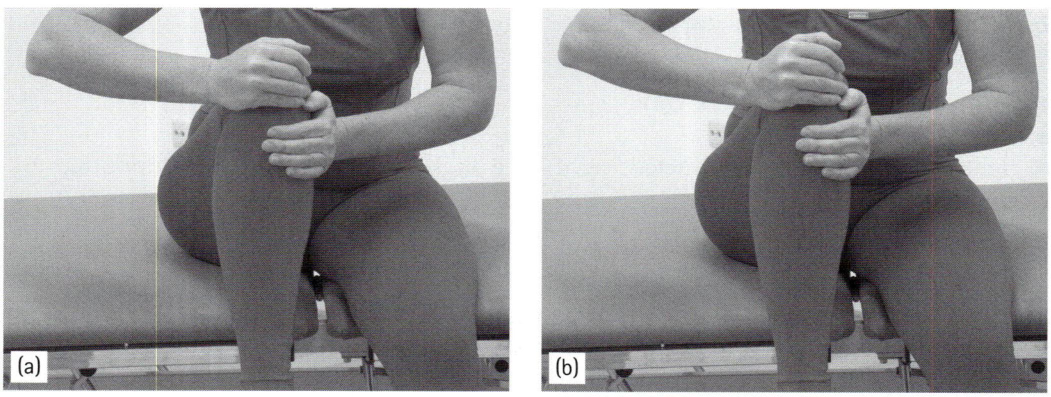

Figure 11.33a and b Translatory movement; gliding of the patella in a mediodistal direction; self-exercise. **a**, Starting position. **b**, End position.

direction, these techniques serve to improve mobility by mobilization of non-symptomatic tissue.

Performance

The higher the resistance to be overcome by mobilization, the more important fixation becomes to avoid transferred movement.

Dosage

As in this example an intra-articular mechanism is assumed, it is improbable that symptomatic structures will be directly loaded by the technique, because the specific provocation and alleviation shows that the movement of the patella in a lateral direction is responsible for the symptoms. The patient's typical pain with flexion should not appear. Dosage is determined by the expected training state of the tissue and, above all, by reassessment.

Choice of technique

The selection of the technique depends, among other things, on the therapist as well as the patient, on the therapist's clinical experience, but primarily on reassessment. This means that even if all preconditions on the part of therapist and patient seem to be met, it is of no use to continue the technique if reassessment is negative.

Contributing factors

For a satisfactory solution of the patient's current problems it is important to consider the contributing factors and include them in the treatment.

The authors will, however, not go into a description of the various possibilities and their complex contexts as this would exceed the scope of the present book.

Compression of the patella in flexion

Therapy technique (film 193)

Patient's starting position:

- supine (Fig. 11.34a)
- knee pre-positioned in the same angular position in which symptoms appear under load.

Therapist's starting position:

- standing, beside the patient
- stabilizing the patient's femur and pelvis with right hand
- contacting the patient's patella with left hand.

Movement:

- intermittent compression in the symptom-provoking direction (Fig. 11.34b).

Self-exercise (film 194)

Patient's starting position:

- sitting on the edge of the plinth (Fig. 11.35a)
- the affected knee in the same angular position in which symptoms appear under load
- contacting the patella with one hand over the other.

Movement:

- intermittent compression in the symptom-provoking direction (Fig. 11.35b).

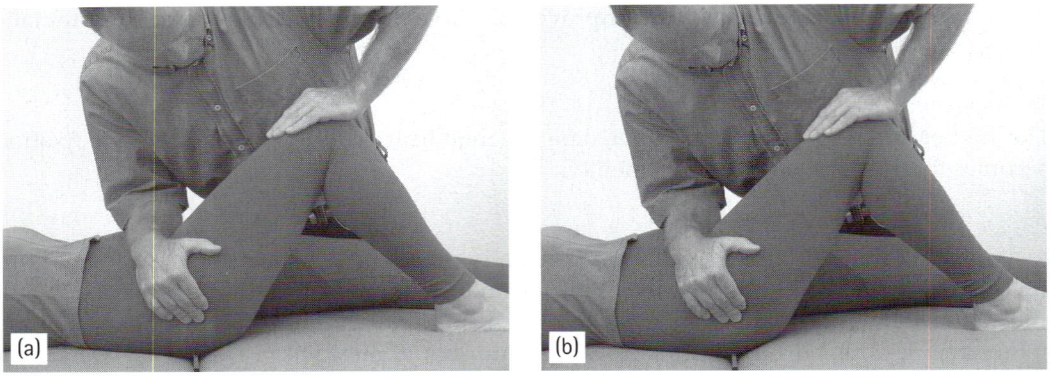

Figure 11.34a and b Translatory movement; compression of the patella in flexion; therapy technique. a, Starting position. b, End position.

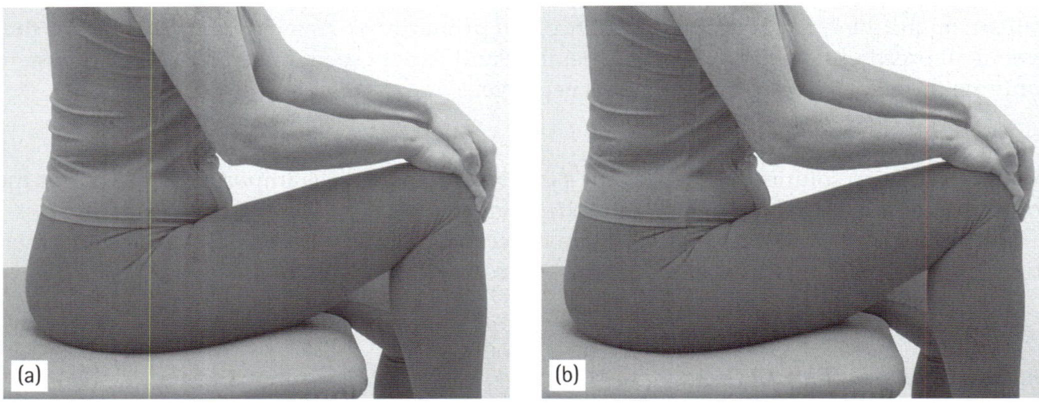

Figure 11.35a and b Translatory movement; compression of the patella in flexion; self-exercise. a, Starting position. b, End position.

ANGULAR MOVEMENTS

Compression in the patellofemoral joint with passive flexion of the knee joint

Therapy technique (film 195)

Patient's starting position:

- sitting, at the end of the plinth (Fig. 11.36a)
- the affected knee extended.

Therapist's starting position:

- standing, in front of the patient
- fixing the patient's distal right lower leg
- contacting the patient's patella.

Movement:

- compressing the patella in the symptom-provoking direction (Fig. 11.36b)
- the knee is passively flexed while the pressure is maintained
- releasing pressure, and back to starting position.

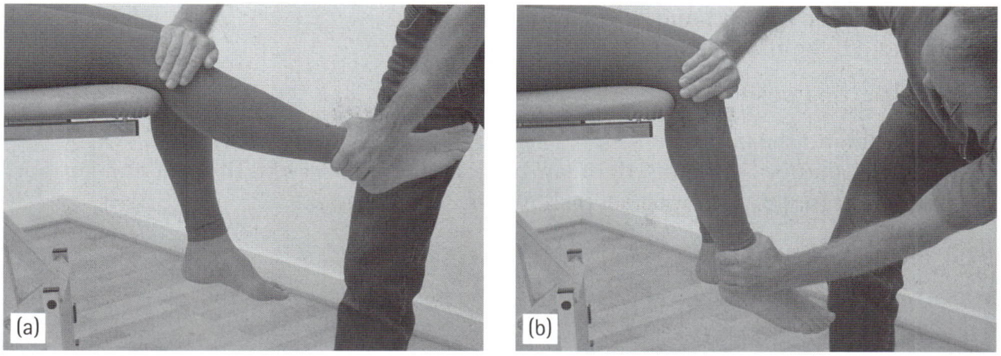

Figure 11.36a and b Passive angular movement; compression in patellofemoral joint with passive knee flexion; therapy technique. a, Starting position. b, End position.

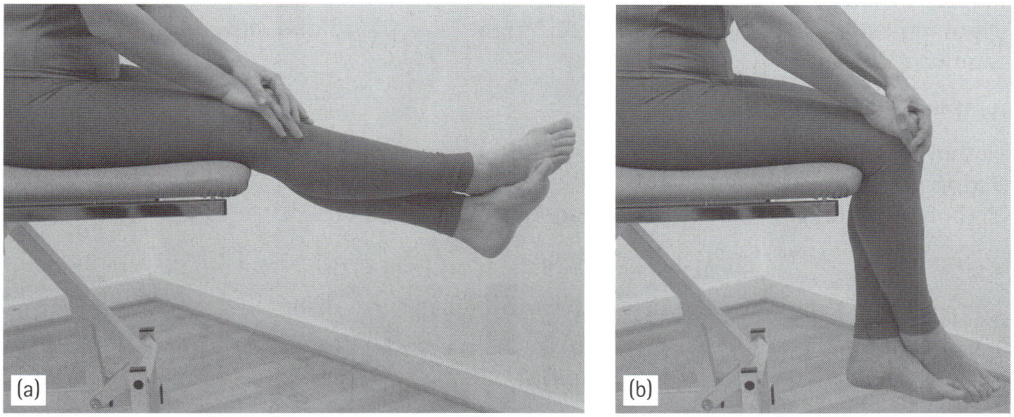

Figure 11.37a and b Passive angular movement; compression in patellofemoral joint with passive knee flexion; self-exercise. a, Starting position. b, End position.

Self-exercise (film 196)

Patient's starting position:

- sitting, the right leg crossed over the left leg (Fig. 11.37a)
- extension of the left knee induces passive extension of the right knee
- contacting the patella with both hands, from the front.

Movement:

- compressing the patella in the symptom-provoking direction (Fig. 11.37b)
- passive flexion of the right knee by lowering the left lower leg
- releasing pressure, and back to starting position.

Mobilization of structures on the lateral side of the thigh

Therapy technique (film 196 – 2)

Patient's starting position:

- lying on the right side (Fig. 11.38a)
- left leg resting on the plinth, flexed in hip and knee, right leg extended and externally rotated in hip, flexed by 90° in knee

- left knee grasped by left hand
- pelvis and left leg fixed by a belt.

Therapist's starting position:

- standing, behind the patient
- fixing the position of patient's right leg by grasping patient's right knee and supporting patient's right foot by therapist's left shoulder.

Movement:

- adduction of right hip joint (Fig. 11.38b).

Alternative therapy technique (film 196 – 3)
Patient's starting position:

- lying on the left side (Fig. 11.39a)
- left leg flexed in hip and knee
- right leg extended and adducted in hip, right knee flexed and supported by a wedge or sandbag.

Therapist's starting position:

- standing, behind the patient
- fixing patient's pelvis with left hand
- right hand contacting structures at patient's lateral distal thigh.

Movement:

- pressure and simultaneous push with the right hand in a distal direction (Fig. 11.39b).

Self-exercise (film 196 – 1)
Patient's starting position:

- lying on the left side (Fig. 11.40a)
- left leg flexed in hip and knee, right leg slightly flexed and adducted in hip joint
- right knee slightly flexed
- left lower leg crossed over right leg so that it rests on the distal thigh, directly proximal to the knee.

Movement:

- pressure with left lower leg against right thigh, with simultaneous rolling of the pelvis in a posterior direction (Fig. 11.40b).

Remarks

Goals of the technique (compression techniques)
With painfully restricted movement of the right patellofemoral joint due to an intra-articular mechanism and simultaneously restricted mobility of the patella in medial direction with increased tension of the muscles moving the patella, these techniques serve to:

- restore normal function of the symptomatic tissue by application of the symptom-provoking stimulus dosed according to the current load tolerance
- restore symptom-free function by changing the input to the respective centres of the CNS.

While intermittent compression is applied with acute presentations, compression techniques with simultaneous passive angular movement presuppose higher load tolerance.

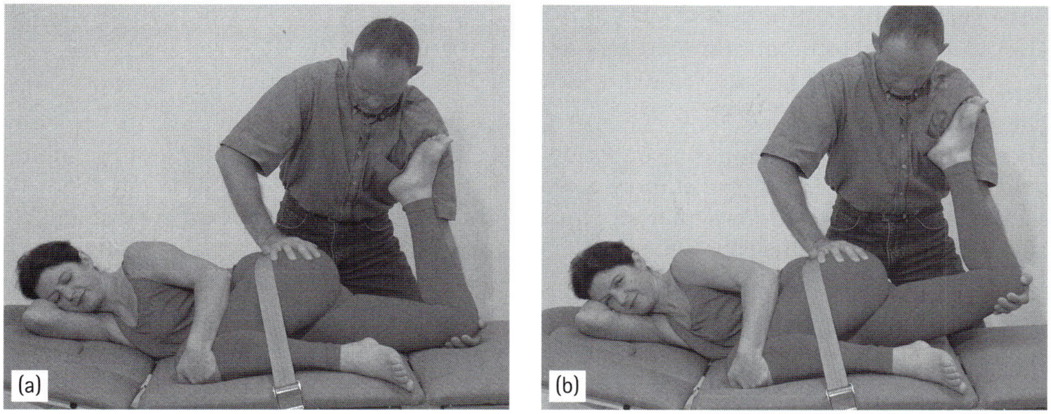

Figure 11.38a and b Passive angular movement; mobilization of the lateral structures of the thigh; therapy technique. **a**, Starting position. **b**, End position.

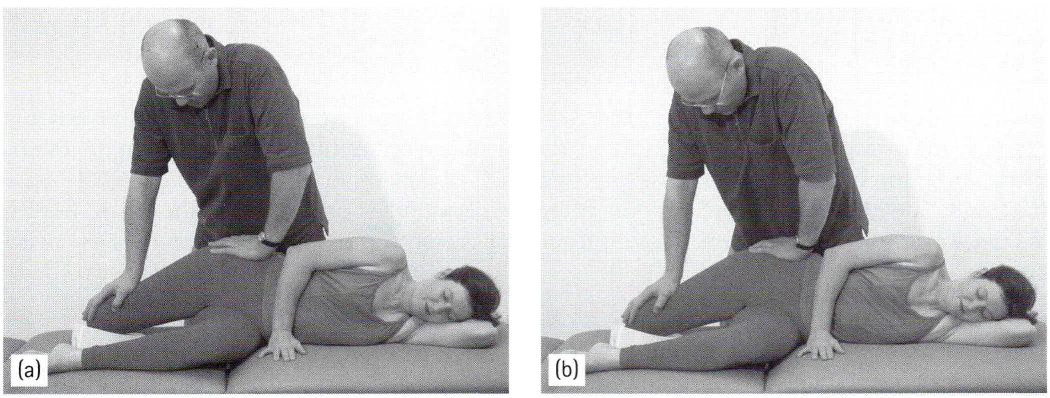

Figure 11.39a and b Passive angular movement; mobilization of the lateral structures of the thigh – alternative therapy technique. **a**, Starting position. **b**, End position.

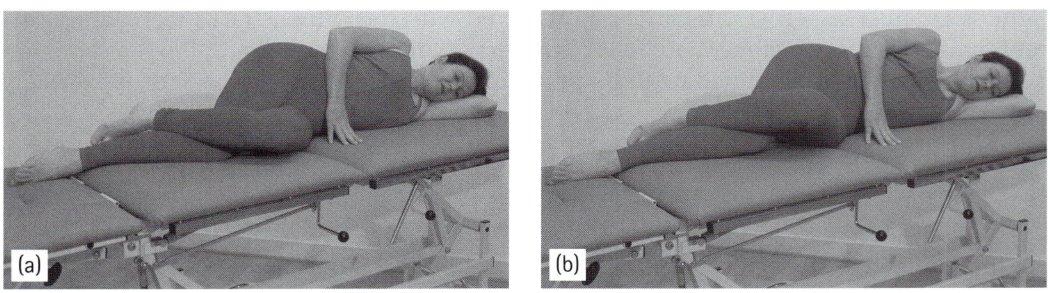

Figure 11.40a and b Passive angular movement; mobilization of the lateral structures of the thigh; self-exercise. **a**, Starting position. **b**, End position.

Performance
The compression techniques should generally be performed without provoking pain.

Dosage
The demonstrated compression techniques involve direct load on the symptomatic structure. Therefore, their dosage should be determined by the current state of healing of the injured structure. Since, however, the authors are not aware of any reliable information about the course of healing of intra-articular structures in humans, careful reassessment remains the only way of checking the chosen dosage.

Choice of technique
The selection of the technique depends, among other things, on the therapist as well as the patient, on the therapist's clinical experience, but primarily on reassessment. This means that even if all preconditions on the part of therapist and patient seem to be met, it is of no use to continue the technique if reassessment is negative.

Contributing factors
For a satisfactory solution of the patient's current problems it is important to consider the contributing factors and include them in the treatment.

The authors will, however, not go into a description of the various possibilities and their complex contexts as this would exceed the scope of the present book.

Remarks

Goals of the technique (mobilization techniques)
With painfully restricted flexion of the right patello-femoral joint due to an intra-articular mechanism (compression) and simultaneously restricted mobility of the patella in the medial direction, these techniques serve to improve the mobility of structures on the lateral side of the thigh. The demonstrated techniques attempt to mobilize non-symptomatic tissue. For this reason, symptom provocation in symptomatic tissue (pain in the anterolateral area of the knee) is not desirable.

Performance
The more tissue resistance has to be overcome by mobilization, the more important is fixation to prevent uncontrolled continuation of the movement.

Dosage
As, in this example, an intra-articular mechanism of symptom provocation is assumed and, as the primary goal of the technique is mobilization of non-symptomatic tissue, direct load on symptomatic structures due to the technique is undesirable. To control this, it is assumed that the patient's typical pain should not appear with extension. Only pull at the lateral side of the right thigh must be felt. If this cannot be achieved with the demonstrated techniques, their continuation is not recommended. If application without reproduction of the typical pain is possible, dosage is determined by the expected training state of the tissue and, above all, by reassessment.

Choice of technique
See the comment above under remarks for 'Goals of the technique' (compression techniques).

Contributing factors
See the comment above under remarks for 'Goals of the technique' (compression techniques).

Chapter 12

Medial malleolus

CHAPTER CONTENTS

AREA LOCALIZATION

IDENTIFICATION OF THE POTENTIALLY AFFECTED AREA BY DEMONSTRATION OF A SYMPTOMATIC FUNCTIONAL MOVEMENT/POSITION

Based on the information gained from the anamnesis so far, the therapist ascertains more details about potentially affected sections. This is done by means of area localization, which represents the beginning of the physical examination. Information gained in this way is used to check or modify the relevant hypotheses developed on the basis of the anamnesis and will determine further proceedings.

Area localization is explained by means of two examples. In both, the patient feels pain in the area of the medial malleolus. Clinical experience and known clinical patterns suggest primarily the following areas as potential origins of the current complaints:

- foot complex
- lumbar spine
- neural structures.

General question: Is there enough information available to skip area localization?	
No	Yes
⇓	⇓
Performance of area localization	• General movement tests • Additional tests • Test treatment

Example 1: Loading in the stance phase

Symptom area: medial malleolus
Symptom provocation: loading (stance phase) of the right leg (Fig. 12.1)

With this presentation, clinical experience suggests primarily the foot complex, lumbar spine, and neural structures as symptom-provoking areas.

Below, examples illustrate how to differentiate between these areas. To this end, area localization is first attempted by means of active movements alone. If this is not possible, tests will be performed by means of assistive/passive movements.

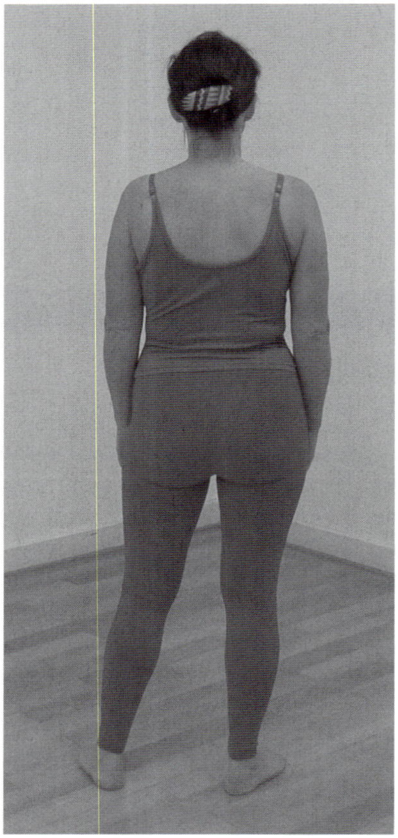

Figure 12.1 Symptom-provoking movement: loading (stance phase) of the right foot provokes pain in the area of the right medial malleolus.

Hypothesis 1: The symptom-provoking area is the lumbar spine

Differentiation: lumbar spine vs. foot complex.

The change in symptoms can be demonstrated exactly:

- provocation of pain (Fig. 12.2a and b, film 197)
- alleviation of pain (Fig. 12.3a and b, film 198).

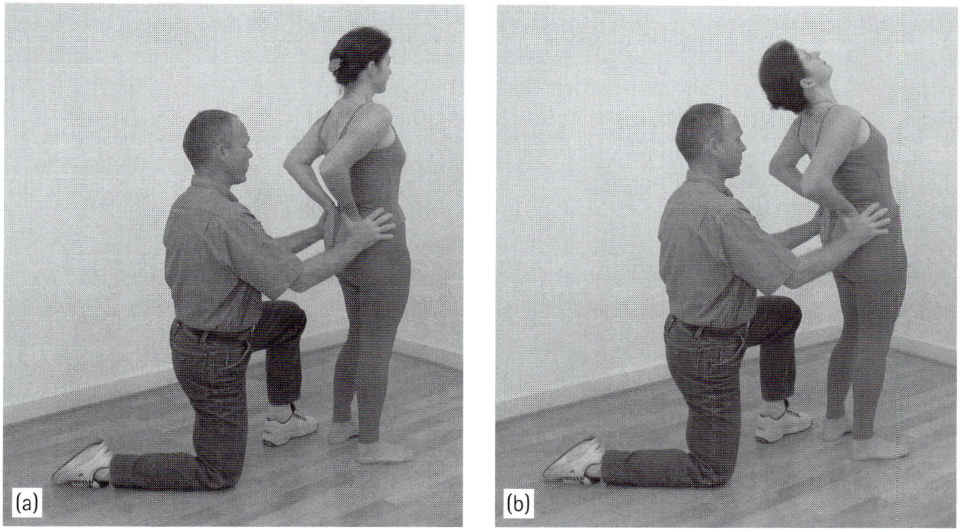

Figure 12.2a and b Area localization with symptomatic loading of the right foot; differentiation between lumbar spine and foot complex; provocation. **a**, Starting position. **b**, End position.

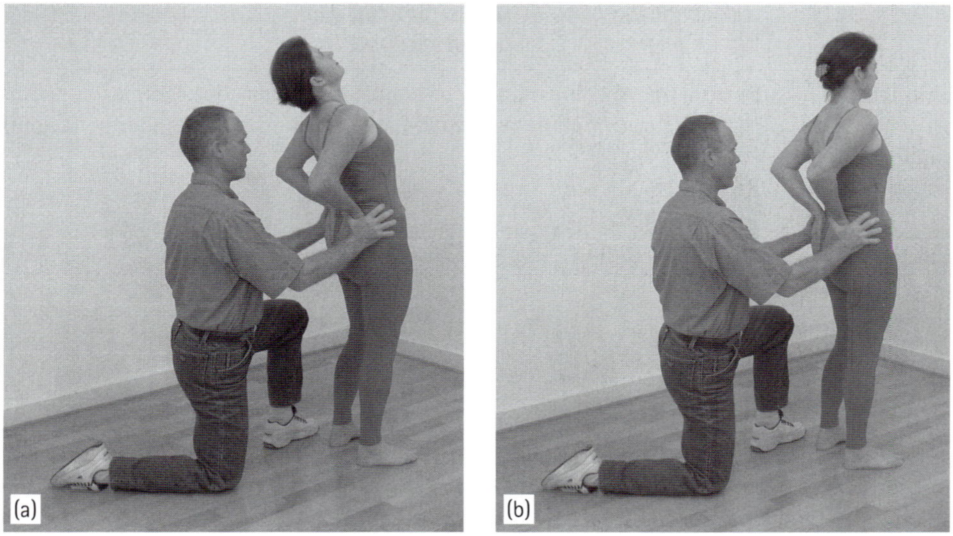

Figure 12.3a and b Area localization with symptomatic loading of the right foot; differentiation between lumbar spine and foot complex; alleviation. **a**, Starting position. **b**, End position.

The result of area localization should be verified by further specific tests; otherwise the result remains in doubt.

Assessment			
Goal	**Provocation of pain**	**Alleviation of pain**	**Remarks**
Starting position	Loading the right leg (stance phase) to an extent immediately before symptoms appear	With the lumbar spine pre-positioned in extension, load the right leg (stance phase) to an extent immediately after symptoms have appeared	
Test movement	Extension of the lumbar spine	Moving the lumbar spine back	
Explanation	If by any movement of the lumbar spine (here, as an example, extension) the typical symptoms are reproduced, an isolated lesion of the foot complex is questionable	If by any movement of the lumbar spine (here, as an example, moving back from extension) the typical symptoms are alleviated, an isolated lesion of the foot complex is questionable	
Additional data to support the hypothesis	General and specific mobility of lumbar spine and foot complex History (e.g., symptom behaviour, type of complaints, 24-hour behaviour) Palpation Reproducibility of test results Test treatment Imaging procedures (CT, MRI)		

Hypothesis 2: The symptom-provoking area is the neural structures
Differentiation: neural involvement vs. foot complex.

The change in symptoms can be demonstrated exactly:

- provocation of pain (Fig. 12.4a and b, film 199)
- alleviation of pain (Fig. 12.5a and b, film 200).

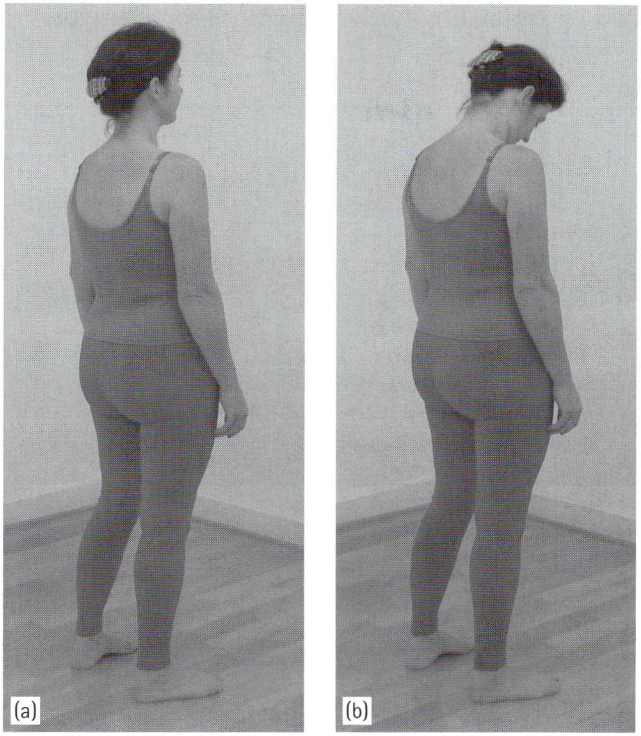

Figure 12.4a and b Area localization with symptomatic loading of the right foot; differentiation between neural structures and foot complex; provocation. **a**, Starting position. **b**, End position.

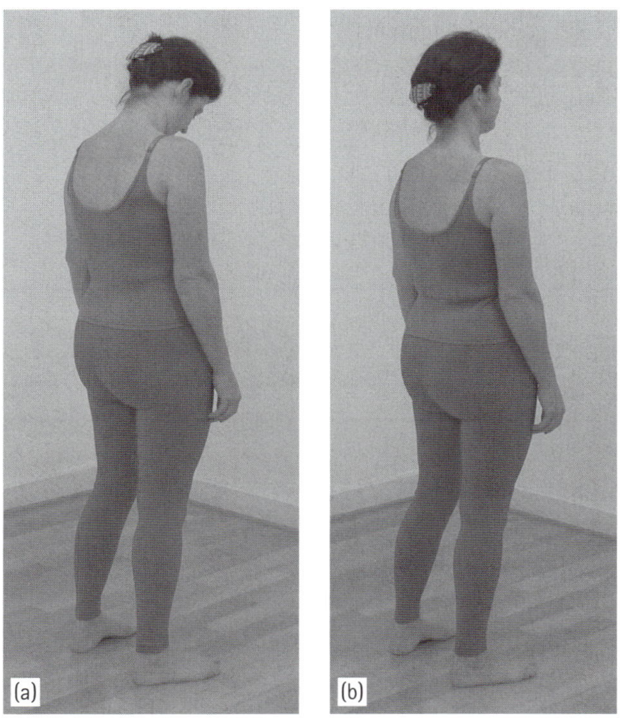

Figure 12.5a and b Area localization with symptomatic loading of the right foot; differentiation between neural structures and foot complex; alleviation. **a**, Starting position. **b**, End position.

The result of area localization should be verified by further specific tests; otherwise the result remains in doubt.

Assessment			
Goal	**Provocation of pain**	**Alleviation of pain**	**Remarks**
Starting position	Loading the right leg (stance phase) to an extent immediately before symptoms appear	With the cervical spine pre-positioned in flexion, load the right leg (stance phase) to an extent immediately after symptoms have appeared	
Test movement	Flexion of the cervical spine	Moving the cervical spine back	
Explanation	The test movement produces mechanical stress on the neural structures and the structures associated with them	The test movement reduces mechanical stress on the neural structures and the structures associated with them	If the typical pain is provoked or alleviated by these manoeuvres without moving the foot complex, this suggests at least an involvement of the neural structures
Additional data to support the hypothesis	Further movements of proximal and distal components to increase neural tension, which do not increase load on the symptomatic area (e.g., upper extremity) General and specific mobility of the affected area History (e.g., symptom behaviour, type of complaints, 24-hour behaviour) Palpation Neurodynamic tests Nerve provocation tests (e.g., bow string sign) Reproducibility of test results Test treatment Imaging procedures (CT, MRI)		

Example 2: Dorsal flexion

Symptom area: medial malleolus
Symptom provocation: dorsal flexion of the right foot (Fig. 12.6)

With this presentation, clinical experience suggests primarily the foot complex, lumbar spine, and neural structures as symptom-provoking areas.

Below, examples illustrate how to differentiate between these areas. To this end, area localization is first attempted by means of active movements alone. If this is not possible, tests will be performed by means of assistive/passive movements.

Hypothesis 1: The symptom-provoking area is the lumbar spine
Differentiation: lumbar spine vs. foot complex.

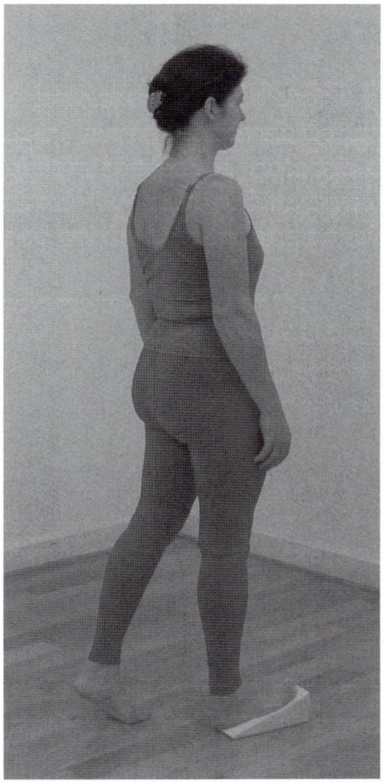

Figure 12.6 Symptom-provoking movement: dorsal flexion of the right foot provokes pain in the area of the right medial malleolus.

The change in symptoms can be demonstrated exactly:

- provocation of pain (Fig. 12.7a and b, film 201)
- alleviation of pain (Fig. 12.8a and b, film 202).

The result of area localization should be verified by further specific tests; otherwise the result remains in doubt.

Assessment

Goal	Provocation of pain	Alleviation of pain	Remarks
Starting position	Dorsal flexion of the foot to a position immediately before symptoms appear	With the lumbar spine pre-positioned in extension, dorsal flexion of the foot to a position immediately after symptoms have appeared	
Test movement	Extension of the lumbar spine	Moving the lumbar spine back	
Explanation	If by any movement of the lumbar spine (here, as an example, extension) the typical symptoms are reproduced, an isolated	If by any movement of the lumbar spine (here, as an example, moving back from extension) the typical symptoms are alleviated, an isolated	The hypothesis of neural involvement is of high probability here and has to be checked further

Goal	Provocation of pain	Alleviation of pain	Remarks
	lesion of the foot complex is questionable	lesion of the foot complex is questionable	
Additional data to support the hypothesis	General and specific mobility of lumbar spine and foot complex History (e.g., symptom behaviour, type of complaints, 24-hour behaviour) Palpation Reproducibility of test results Neurodynamic tests Test treatment Imaging procedures (CT, MRI)		

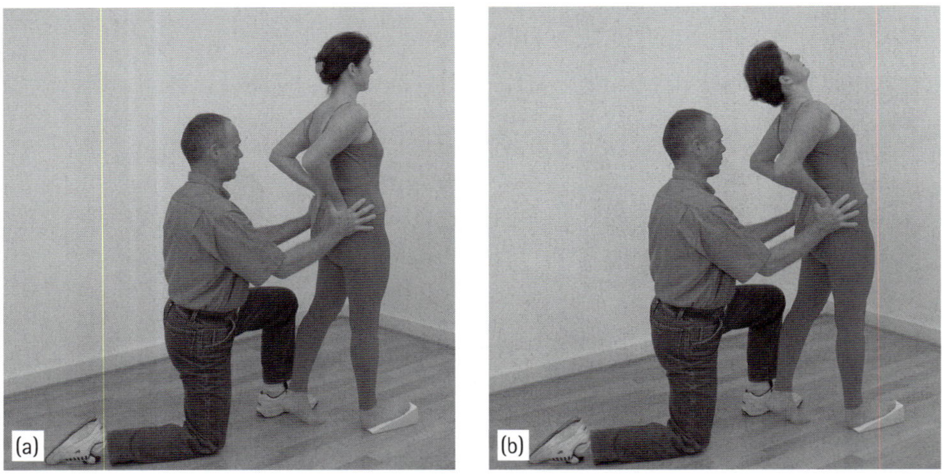

Figure 12.7a and b Area localization with symptomatic dorsal flexion of the right foot; differentiation between lumbar spine and foot complex; provocation. **a**, Starting position. **b**, End position.

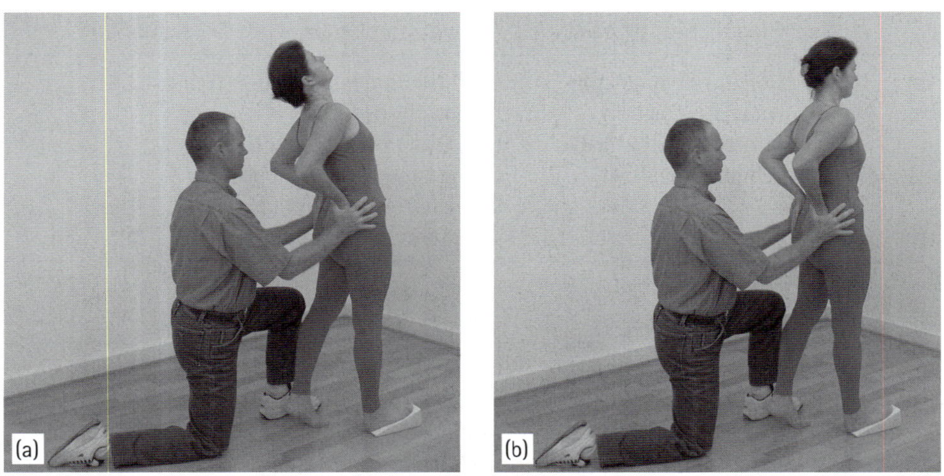

Figure 12.8a and b Area localization with symptomatic dorsal flexion of the right foot; differentiation between lumbar spine and foot complex; alleviation. **a**, Starting position. **b**, End position.

Hypothesis 2: The symptom-provoking area is the neural structures

Differentiation: neural involvement vs. foot complex.

The change in symptoms can be demonstrated exactly:

- provocation of pain (Fig. 12.9a and b, film 203)
- alleviation of pain (Fig. 12.10a and b, film 204).

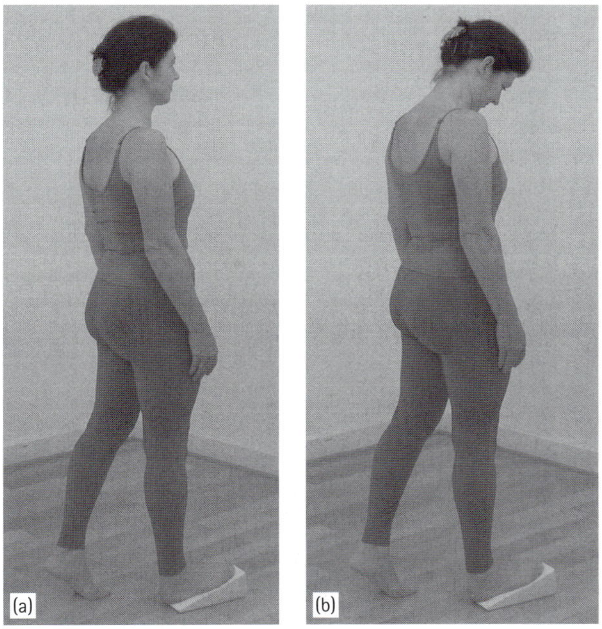

Figure 12.9a and b Area localization with symptomatic dorsal flexion of the right foot; differentiation between neural structures and foot complex; provocation. **a**, Starting position. **b**, End position.

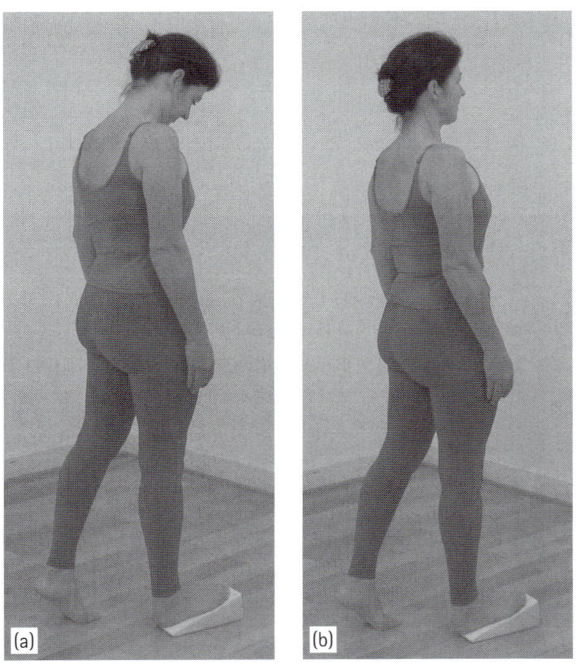

Figure 12.10a and b Area localization with symptomatic dorsal flexion of the right foot; differentiation between neural structures and foot complex; alleviation. **a**, Starting position. **b**, End position.

The result of area localization should be verified by further specific tests; otherwise the result remains in doubt.

Assessment			
Goal	**Provocation of pain**	**Alleviation of pain**	**Remarks**
Starting position	Dorsal flexion of the foot to a position immediately before symptoms appear	With the cervical spine pre-positioned in flexion, dorsal flexion of the foot to a position immediately after symptoms have appeared	
Test movement	Flexion of the cervical spine	Moving the cervical spine back	
Explanation	The test movement produces mechanical stress on the neural structures and the structures associated with them	The test movement reduces mechanical stress on the neural structures and the structures associated with them	If the typical pain is provoked or alleviated by these manoeuvres without moving the foot complex, this suggests at least an involvement of the neural structures
Additional data to support the hypothesis	Further movements of proximal and distal components to increase neural tension, which do not increase load on the symptomatic area (e.g., upper extremity) General and specific mobility of the affected area History (e.g., symptom behaviour, type of complaints, 24-hour behaviour) Palpation Neurodynamic tests Nerve provocation tests (e.g., bow string sign) Reproducibility of test results Test treatment Imaging procedures (CT, MRI)		

QUICK CHECK – SYMPTOMS, MEDIAL MALLEOLUS

If neither the area nor a symptom-provoking or symptom-reducing action is known, the quick check is used to try to load individual potential areas with specific biomechanically provocative movement combinations. The chosen movement combinations correspond with the straining and often symptom-provoking movements of the individual sections.

LUMBAR SPINE

Movement (film 226)

- Extension/lateral flexion to the right, and rotation to the same as well as to the opposite side, with overpressure (Fig. 12.11a and b)
- Extension/lateral flexion to the left, and rotation to the same as well as to the opposite side, with overpressure (Fig. 12.12a and b).

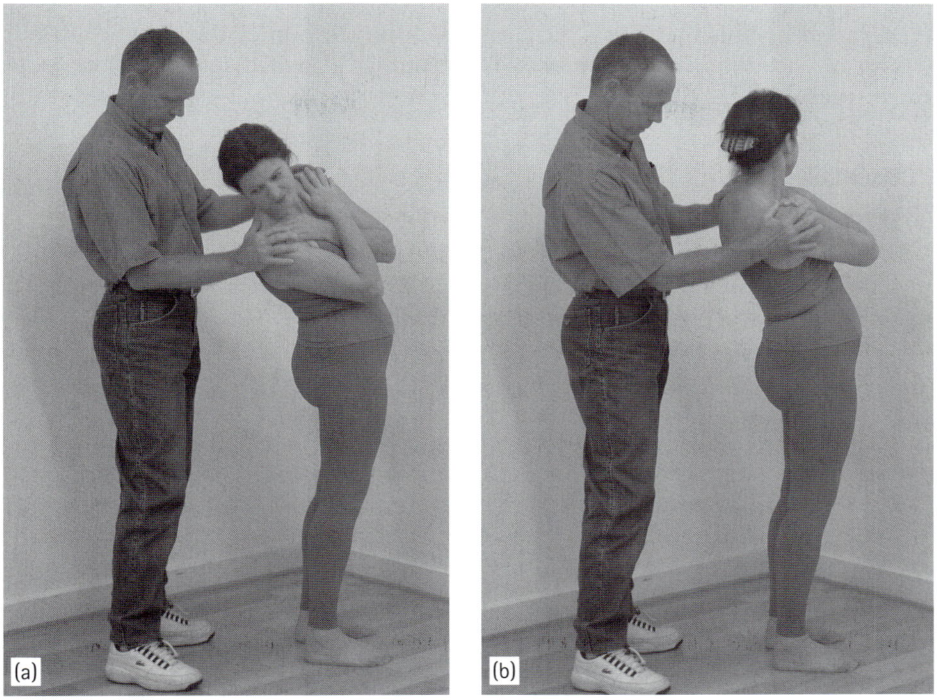

Figure 12.11a and b Quick check lumbar spine; extension, lateral flexion to the right. a, Rotation to the same side. b, Rotation to the opposite side.

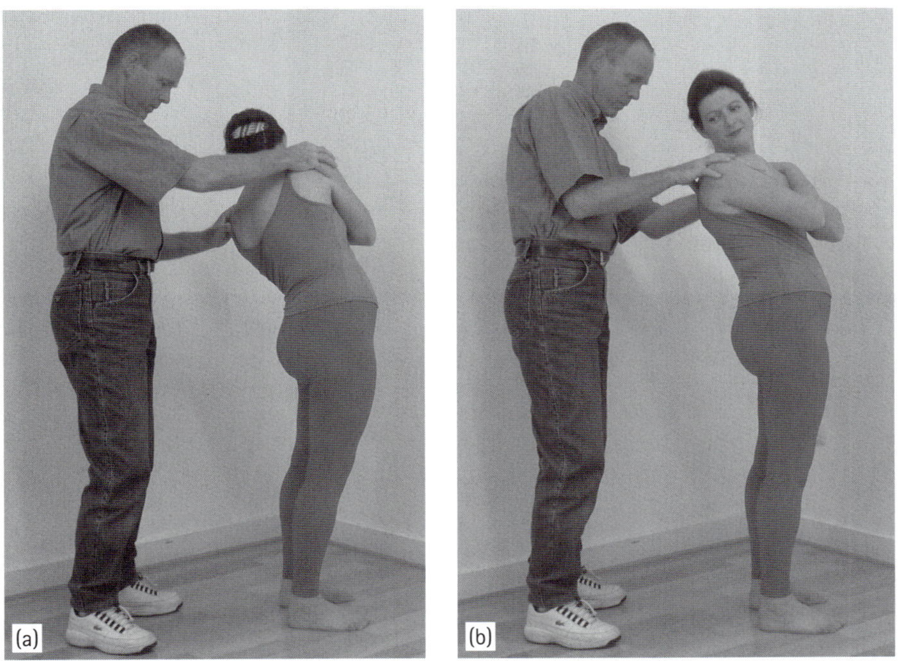

Figure 12.12a and b Quick check lumbar spine; extension, lateral flexion to the left. a, Rotation to the same side. b, Rotation to the opposite side.

Note: If, based on the anamnesis, it is assumed that flexion of the spine contributes to symptom provocation, the movement combinations described for extension should, of course, be performed in flexion.

FOOT COMPLEX

Movement (film 230)

- Plantar flexion/abduction/pronation (Fig. 12.13a)
- Dorsal flexion/adduction/supination (Fig. 12.13b)
- Dorsal flexion/abduction/pronation (Fig. 12.14a)
- Plantar flexion/adduction/supination (Fig. 12.14b).

NEURAL STRUCTURES

Tension tests

- Slump test (Fig. 12.15, film 616)
- Straight leg raise (SLR; Fig. 12.16, film 618).

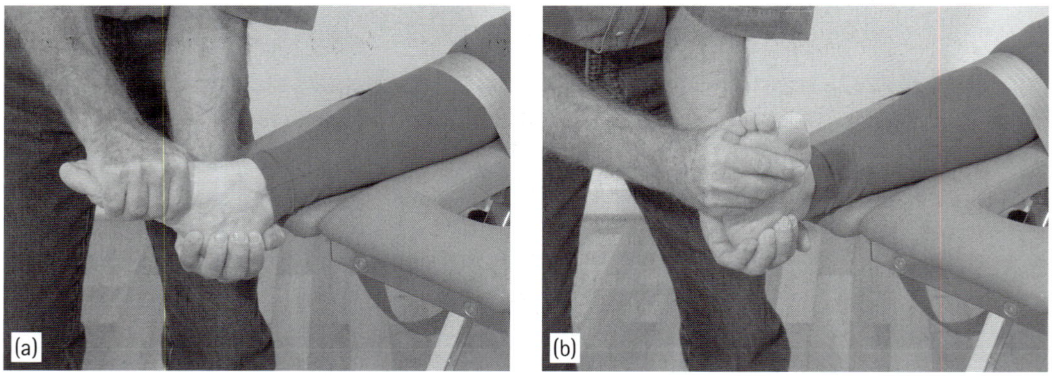

Figure 12.13a and b Quick check foot complex. a, Plantar flexion/abduction/pronation. b, Dorsal flexion/adduction/supination.

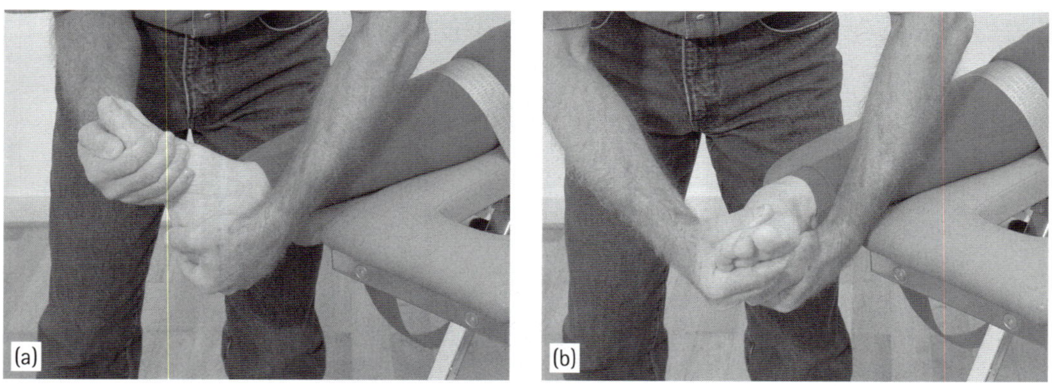

Figure 12.14a and b Quick check foot complex. a, Dorsal flexion/abduction/pronation. b, Plantar flexion/adduction/supination.

Note: Even an area that proves negative in the quick check may possibly be symptom-provoking (another movement combination, or passive overpressure may be required).

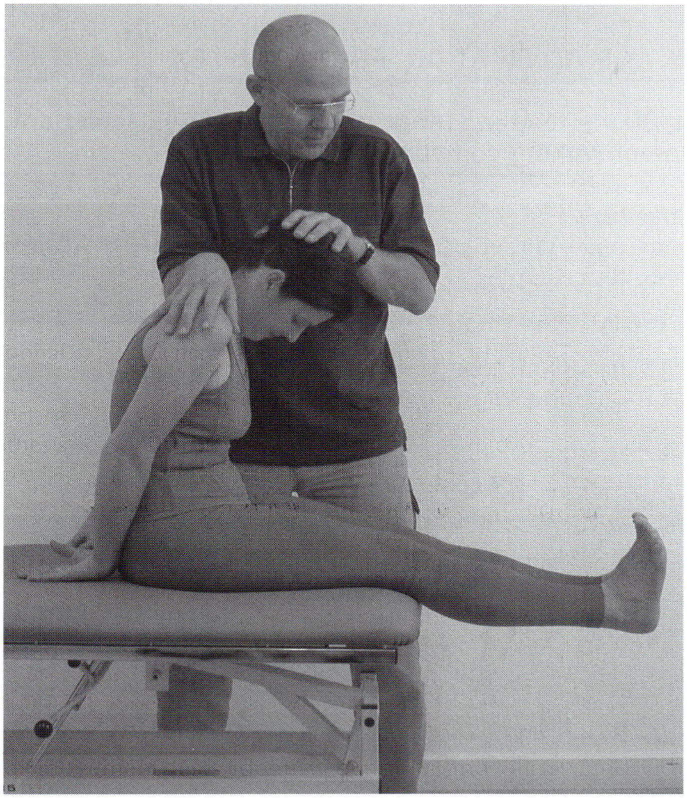

Figure 12.15 Quick check neurodynamics; slump test.

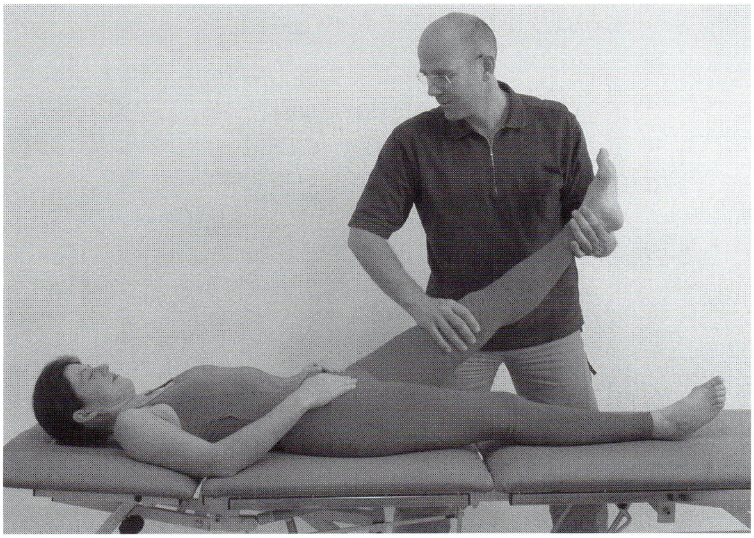

Figure 12.16 Quick check neurodynamics; straight leg raise (SLR) test.

SPECIFIC PROVOCATION AND ALLEVIATION

Specific provocation and alleviation allows one to differentiate within an articular complex and to identify the symptom-provoking movement direction(s).

SPECIFIC PROVOCATION AND ALLEVIATION, FOOT COMPLEX

Differentiation, foot complex – load in stance phase – upper vs. lower ankle (compression as symptom-provoking component)

Pain-provoking movement (Fig. 12.17)

- Loading the right leg (stance phase) provokes pain in the area of the medial malleolus.
- Area localization hints at the foot complex.

The change in symptoms can be demonstrated exactly:

- provocation of pain (Fig. 12.18a–d, film 205)
- alleviation of pain (Fig. 12.19a–d, film 206).

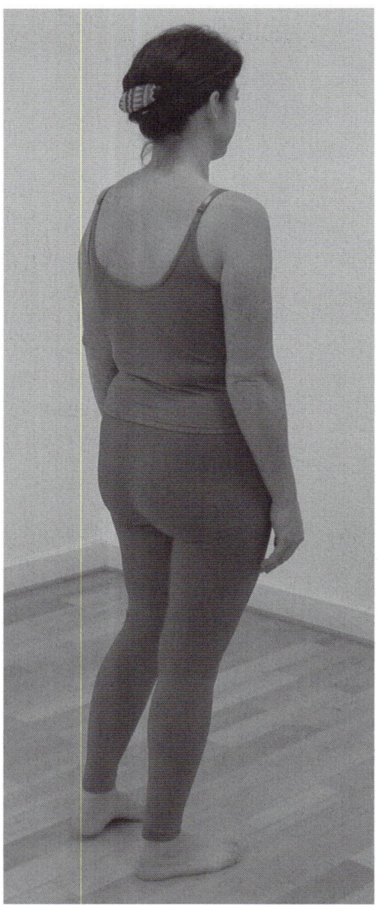

Figure 12.17 Symptom-provoking movement: loading (stance phase) of the right foot provokes pain in the area of the right medial malleolus.

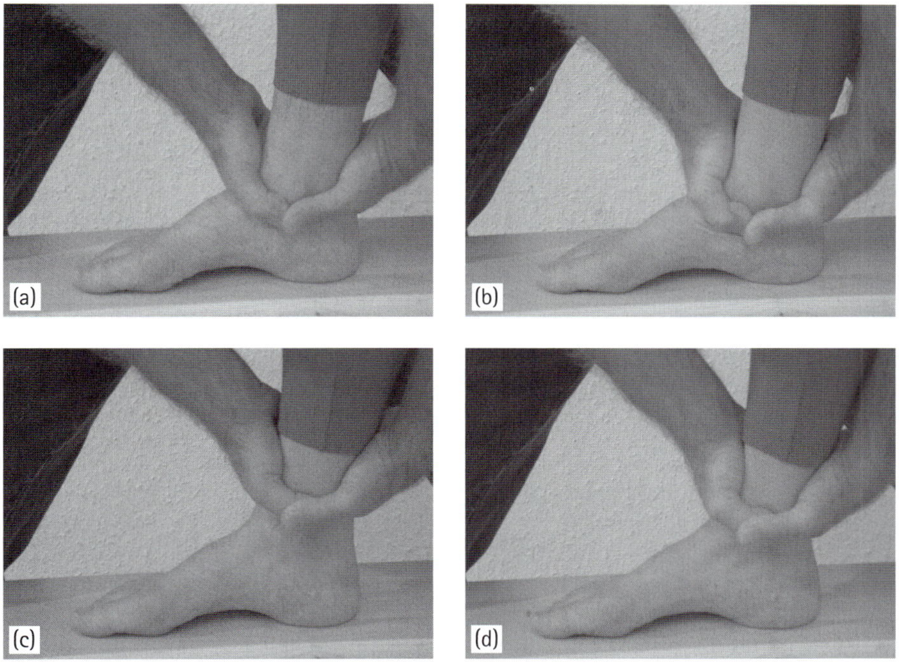

Figure 12.18a–d Specific provocation and alleviation, foot complex, with loading in the stance phase; differentiation, upper vs. lower ankle (compression as symptom-provoking mechanism). First step: contact talus; provocation. **a**, Test start. **b**, Test end. Second step: contact lower leg; provocation. **c**, Test start. **d**, Test end.

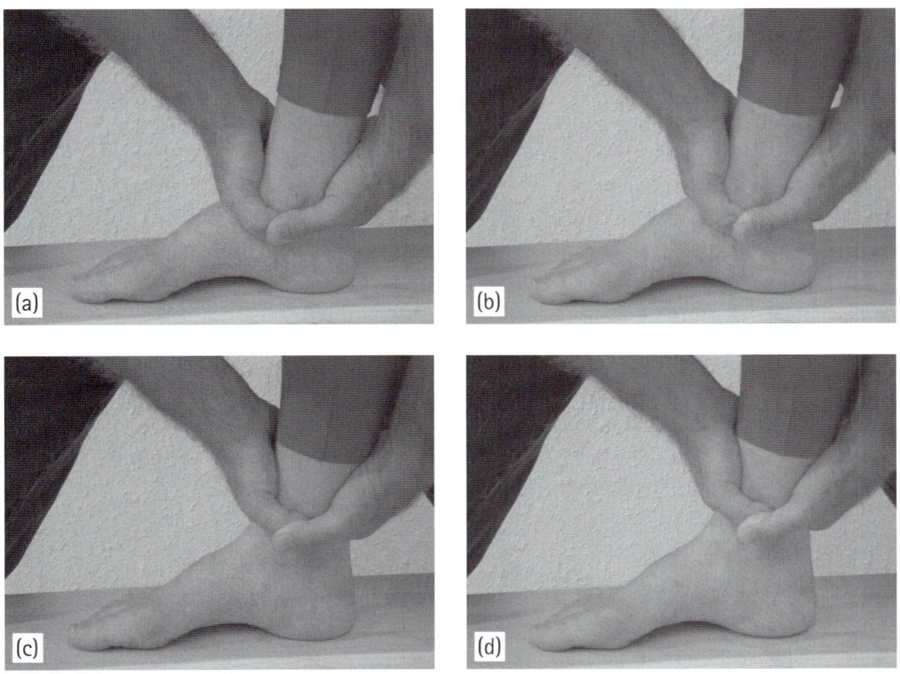

Figure 12.19a–d Specific provocation and alleviation, foot complex, with loading in the stance phase; differentiation, upper vs. lower ankle (compression as symptom-provoking mechanism). First step: contact talus; alleviation. **a**, Test start. **b**, Test end. Second step: contact lower leg; alleviation. **c**, Test start. **d**, Test end.

Assessment			
Goal	**Provocation of pain**	**Alleviation of pain**	**Remarks**
Starting position	Loading (stance phase) to an extent immediately after symptoms have appeared	Loading (stance phase) to an extent immediately after symptoms have appeared	Because with pre-positioning to a position before symptoms appear non-symptomatic parts of the affected joint may be compressed, a symptomatic position is also chosen for provocation
Test movement	Compression: talus – calcaneus lower leg – talus	Traction: talus – calcaneus lower leg – talus	Traction and compression are performed at a right angle to the treatment plane (Kaltenborn 1999)
Neural involvement	Proximal and/or distal component without change of position in the relevant area	Proximal and/or distal component without change of position in the relevant area	
Explanation	This manoeuvre increases the intra-articular compression forces in: ● lower ankle ● upper ankle	This manoeuvre reduces the intra-articular compression forces in: ● lower ankle ● upper ankle	
Additional data necessary to support the hypothesis	General and specific mobility of the foot complex History (e.g., symptom behaviour, type of complaints, 24-hour behaviour) Specific palpation Nerve mobility tests (if specific provocation and alleviation indicate neural involvement) Reproducibility of test results Test treatment Imaging procedures (CT, MRI)		

Localization, lower ankle – dorsal flexion

Pain-provoking movement (Fig. 12.20)

- Dorsal flexion of the right foot provokes pain at the medial malleolus.
- Area localization hints at the foot complex.
- Specific provocation and alleviation hints at the lower ankle.

The change in symptoms can be demonstrated exactly:

- provocation of pain (Fig. 12.21a–d, film 207)
- alleviation of pain (Fig. 12.22a and b, film 208).

The following procedure aims at ascertaining which of the two joints (upper or lower ankle) causes the symptoms. Because of the complexity of the biomechanics of the lower ankle it is difficult to move in a symptom-provoking direction in one of the two joints while alleviating symptoms in the other one. For that reason, the first step of differentiation is checking the possible principal movement directions in the lower ankle. If thereby the symptoms are not changed, this supports the hypothesis that the source of the symptoms is the upper ankle. This hypothesis has to be checked with further tests, though.

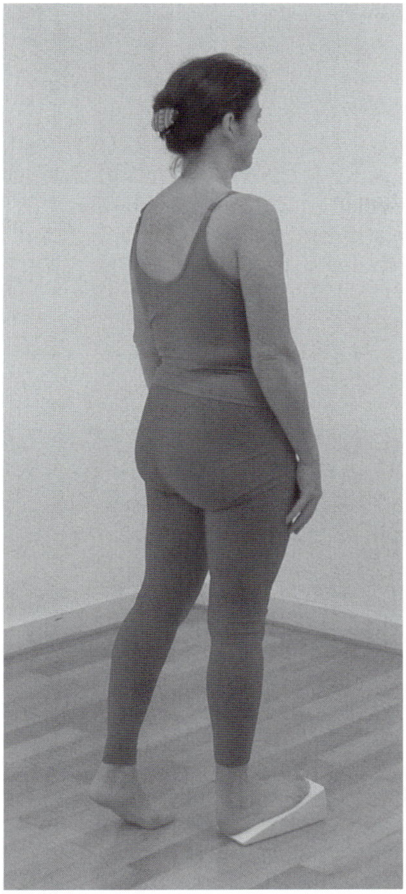

Figure 12.20 Symptom-provoking movement: dorsal flexion of the right foot provokes pain in the area of the right medial malleolus.

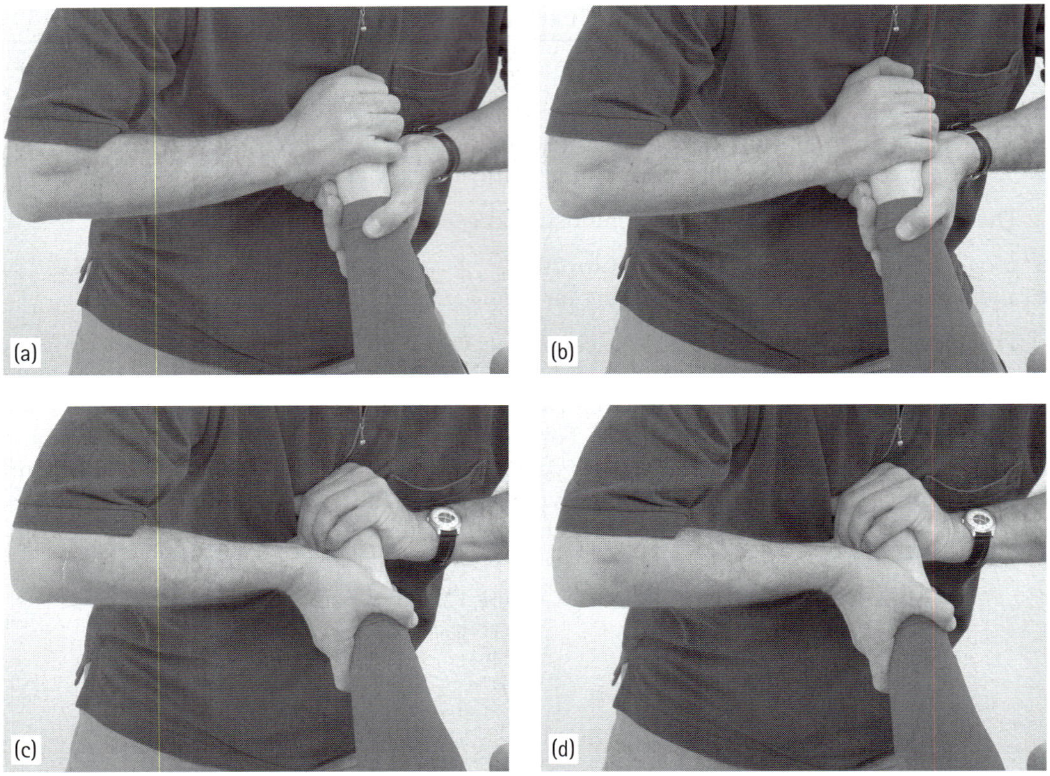

Figure 12.21a–d Specific provocation and alleviation, foot complex, with symptomatic dorsal flexion; localization, lower ankle. First step: calcaneus in lateral direction; provocation. **a**, Test start. **b**, Test end. Second step: calcaneus in medial direction; provocation. **c**, Test start. **d**, Test end.

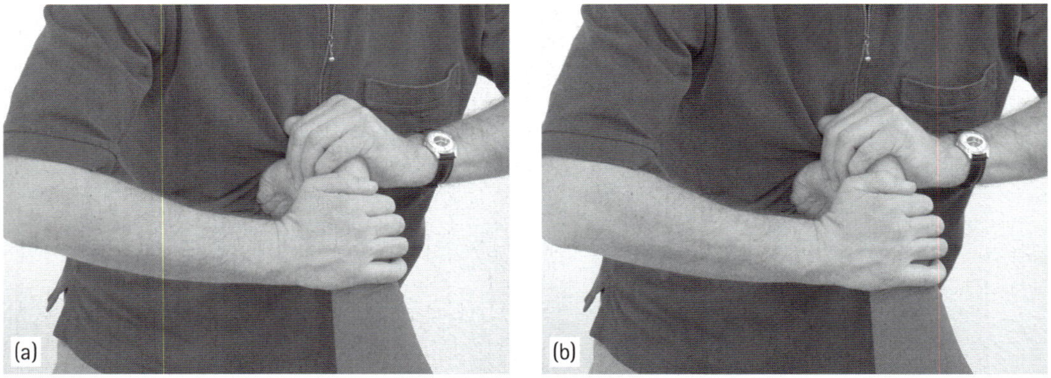

Figure 12.22a and b Specific provocation and alleviation, foot complex, with symptomatic dorsal flexion; localization, lower ankle; calcaneus in lateral direction; alleviation. **a**, Test start. **b**, Test end.

Assessment			
Goal	**Provocation of pain**	**Alleviation of pain**	**Remarks**
Starting position	Dorsal flexion to a position immediately before symptoms appear	Dorsal flexion to a position immediately after symptoms have appeared	
Test movement	Push of the calcaneus in medial direction, with fixed talus	Push of the calcaneus in lateral direction, with fixed talus	To make sure that the source of symptoms is located in the lower ankle, the calcaneus has to be moved for provocation in both lateral and medial directions. If one direction of push provokes the symptoms and the reverse direction alleviates them, it can be assumed that the lower ankle is responsible for the symptoms
Neural involvement	Proximal and/or distal component without change of position in the relevant area	Proximal and/or distal component without change of position in the relevant area	
Explanation	If the symptoms are caused by movement of the calcaneus in medial direction, medial push of the calcaneus with fixed talus will increase the symptoms	If the symptoms are caused by movement of the calcaneus in lateral direction, this manoeuvre will alleviate the symptoms	
Additional data to support the hypothesis	General and specific mobility of the ankle History (e.g., symptom behaviour, type of complaints, 24-hour behaviour) Specific palpation Neurodynamic tests (if specific provocation and alleviation indicate neural involvement) Reproducibility of test results Test treatment Imaging procedures (CT, MRI)		

Localization, upper ankle – dorsal flexion – movement as symptom-provoking component – direction of rolling

Pain-provoking movement

- Dorsal flexion of the right foot provokes pain at the medial malleolus.
- Area localization hints at the foot complex.
- Specific provocation and alleviation hints at the upper ankle (no change with provocation and alleviation, lower ankle).

The change in symptoms can be demonstrated exactly:

- provocation of pain (Fig. 12.23a and b, film 209)
- alleviation of pain (Fig. 12.24a and b, film 210).

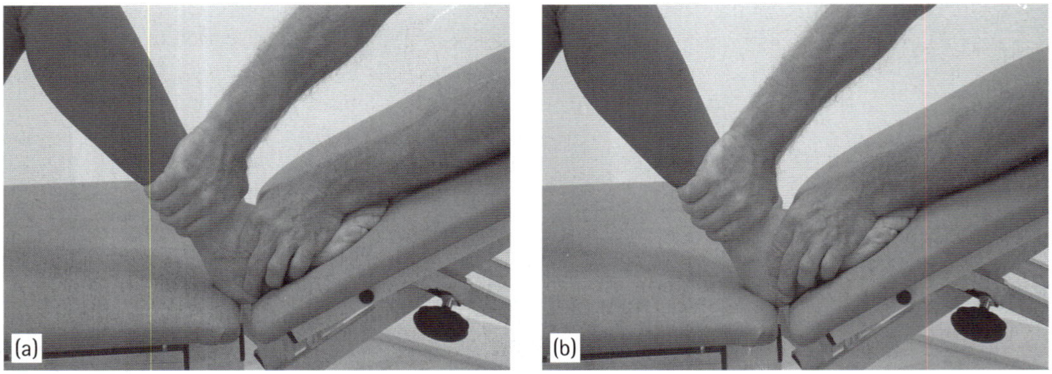

Figure 12.23a and b Specific provocation and alleviation, foot complex, with symptomatic dorsal flexion; localization, upper ankle – dorsal flexion (rolling as symptom-provoking mechanism); provocation. **a**, Test start. **b**, Test end.

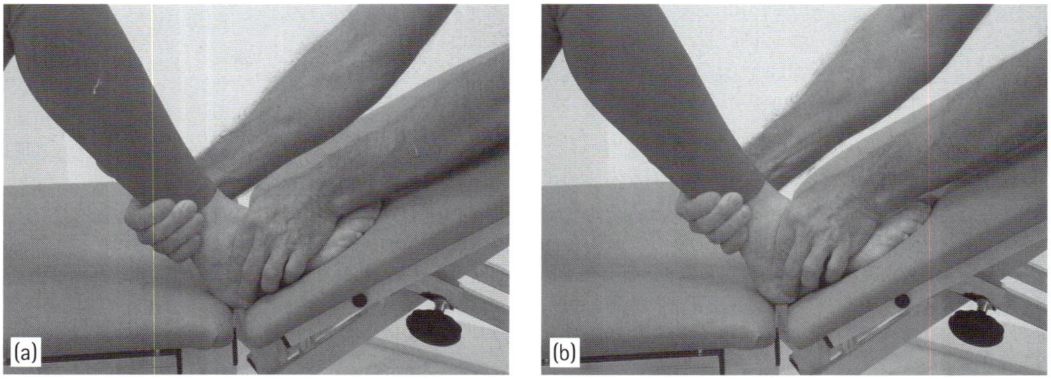

Figure 12.24a and b Specific provocation and alleviation, foot complex, with symptomatic dorsal flexion; localization, upper ankle – dorsal flexion (rolling as symptom-provoking mechanism); alleviation. **a**, Test start. **b**, Test end.

Assessment

Goal	Provocation of pain	Alleviation of pain	Remarks
Starting position	Dorsal flexion to a position immediately before symptoms appear	Dorsal flexion to a position immediately after symptoms have appeared	
Test movement	Push of lower leg in posterior direction, with fixed talus	Pull of lower leg in anterior direction, with fixed talus	
Neural involvement	Proximal and/or distal component without change of position in the relevant area	Proximal and/or distal component without change of position in the relevant area	
Explanation	If symptoms are caused by movement of the talus in anterior direction (anterior rolling), this manoeuvre (talus in anterior direction) results in an increase in symptoms, both with intra-articular and with extra-articular dysfunction	If symptoms are caused by movement of the talus in anterior direction (anterior rolling), this manoeuvre (talus in posterior direction) results in a reduction of symptoms, both with intra-articular and with extra-articular dysfunction	
Additional data to support the hypothesis	General and specific mobility of the upper ankle History (e.g., symptom behaviour, type of complaints, 24-hour behaviour) Specific palpation Neurodynamic tests (if specific provocation and alleviation indicate neural involvement) Reproducibility of test results Test treatment Imaging procedures (CT, MRI)		

Localization, upper ankle – dorsal flexion – movement as symptom-provoking component – direction of gliding

Pain-provoking movement

- Dorsal flexion of the right foot provokes pain at the medial malleolus.
- Area localization hints at the foot complex.
- Specific provocation and alleviation hints at the upper ankle.

The change in symptoms can be demonstrated exactly:

- provocation of pain (Fig. 12.25a and b, film 211)
- alleviation of pain (Fig. 12.26a and b, film 212).

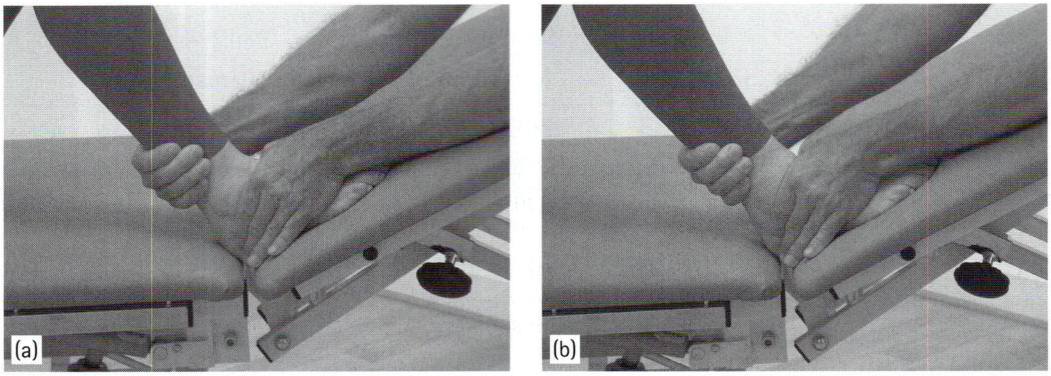

Figure 12.25a and b Specific provocation and alleviation, foot complex, with symptomatic dorsal flexion; localization, upper ankle – dorsal flexion (gliding as symptom-provoking mechanism); provocation. **a**, Test start. **b**, Test end.

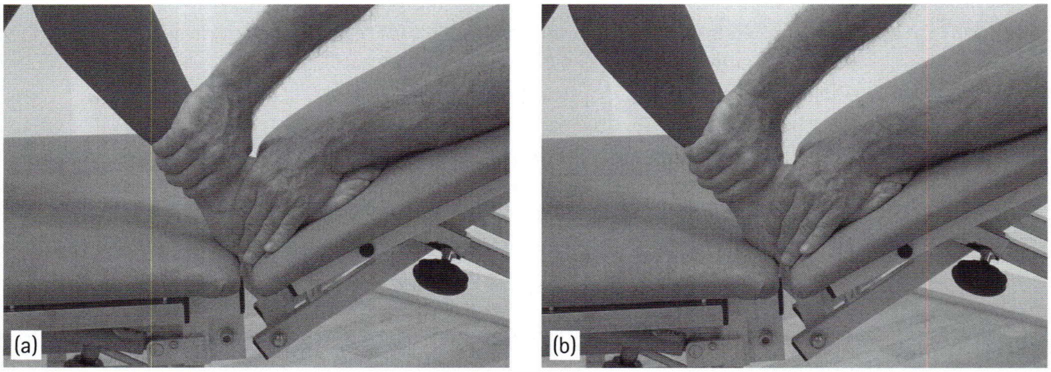

Figure 12.26a and b Specific provocation and alleviation, foot complex, with symptomatic dorsal flexion; localization, upper ankle – dorsal flexion (gliding as symptom-provoking mechanism); alleviation. **a**, Test start. **b**, Test end.

Assessment

Goal	Provocation of pain	Alleviation of pain	Remarks
Starting position	Dorsal flexion to a position immediately before symptoms appear	Dorsal flexion to a position immediately after symptoms have appeared	
Test movement	Pushing lower leg in anterior direction, with fixed talus	Pushing lower leg in posterior direction	
Neural involvement	Proximal and/or distal component without change of	Proximal and/or distal component without change of	

Goal	Provocation of pain	Alleviation of pain	Remarks
	position in the relevant area	position in the relevant area	
Explanation	If symptoms are caused by movement of the talus in posterior direction (posterior gliding), this manoeuvre (talus in posterior direction) results in an increase in symptoms	If symptoms are caused by movement of the talus in posterior direction (posterior gliding), this manoeuvre (talus in anterior direction) results in a reduction of symptoms	
Additional data to support the hypothesis	General and specific mobility of the upper ankle History (e.g., symptom behaviour, type of complaints, 24-hour behaviour) Specific palpation Neurodynamic tests (if specific provocation and alleviation indicate neural involvement) Reproducibility of test results Test treatment Imaging procedures (CT, MRI)		

GENERAL MOVEMENT TESTS

General movement tests identify, quantify, and qualify individual anatomical movements and, in part, movement combinations in the area concerned. The individual manual therapy concepts have respective protocols at their disposal, which more or less have the same goals.

Information gained in this way is used for checking or modifying the relevant hypotheses developed on the basis of anamnesis and area localization and will help in determining how to proceed.

General question: Is there enough information available to skip general movement tests?	
No	Yes
⇓	⇓
Performance of the general movement tests	• Additional tests • test treatment

In view of the described clinical presentation and the results of area localization, general movement tests of the following regions seem to be useful.

LUMBAR SPINE

	Active	Passive
Lumbar spine in general	Flexion Extension Rotation (to the right and left) Lateral flexion (to the right and left)	Flexion Extension Rotation (to the right and left) Lateral flexion (to the right and left)
Movement combinations, lumbar spine in general	Symptomatic movements of the lumbar spine	Symptomatic movements of the lumbar spine
Foot		
	Active	**Passive**
Foot in general	Flexion Extension Inversion Eversion	Flexion Extension Inversion Eversion

TREATMENT EXAMPLE, FOOT COMPLEX

SYMPTOMATIC MOVEMENT

Dorsal flexion of the right foot is restricted by 20% as compared with the contralateral side and provokes pain in end-range positions (VAS 4/10) in the area of the medial malleolus.

ASSESSMENTS

Area localization

Area localization hints at symptom provocation by the foot complex. There is neural involvement. But symptom provocation via the foot complex is possible without neural pretensioning, too, with pain intensity then amounting to 3/10. For that reason, it is clear that in the current presentation both the foot complex and the neural structures are involved. There is no contraindication for movement.

Specific provocation and alleviation

- Specific provocation and alleviation hints at symptom provocation by the upper ankle with neural involvement and indicates an extra-articular mechanism (traction of upper ankle in symptomatic position increases the symptoms).
- Pushing the talus in a posterior direction provokes the symptoms.
- Pushing the lower leg in a posterior direction alleviates the symptoms.

Specific mobility

Specific mobility tests show restricted dorsal glide of the talus in the upper ankle as compared with the contralateral side and reveal a firm end feel.

Neurodynamics

Lifting the extended right leg (SLR) shows different quality of movement (resistance behaviour during movement) as well as a changed sensory response (area and type of sensation) as compared with the left side.

Palpation

Palpation shows tissue changes over the medial malleolus (swelling and increased tenderness). The patient's typical symptoms cannot be reproduced by palpation.

Palpation of the spine, which had been performed because of the altered neurodynamics and the relations between the symptomatic tissue and the sacral plexus, showed local tissue changes at level L4 and changed movement resistance as compared with the opposite side.

HYPOTHESIS

Painfully restricted dorsal flexion of the upper ankle due to an extra-articular mechanism with restricted posterior glide of the talus and simultaneous neural involvement is suspected (Fig. 12.27).

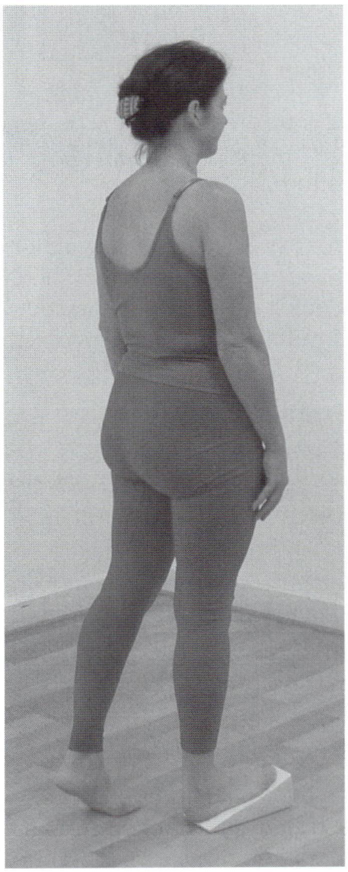

Figure 12.27 Symptom-provoking movement: dorsal flexion of the right foot provokes pain in the area of the right medial malleolus.

RELAXATION TECHNIQUES

Soft tissue techniques

TISSUE AROUND THE MEDIAL MALLEOLUS

Therapy technique (film 213)
Patient's starting position:

- prone, feet beyond the plinth, the knee slightly flexed (lower leg supported) (Fig. 12.28a)
- patient's forefoot contacting therapist's thigh
- a change in knee flexion will induce changes in neural tension.

Therapist's starting position:

- standing, at the foot end of the plinth.

Movement:

- passive dorsal flexion of the upper ankle by forward movement of therapist's thigh with simultaneous pressure on the tissue around the medial malleolus (Fig. 12.28b)
- releasing pressure, and guiding back to starting position.

Self-exercise (film 214)
Patient's starting position:

- sitting, with legs crossed (Fig. 12.29a).

Movement:

- active dorsal flexion of the upper ankle with simultaneous pressure on the tissue around the medial malleolus (Fig. 12.29b)
- releasing pressure, and moving back to starting position.

Remarks

Goals of the technique
With a painfully restricted dorsal flexion of the upper ankle due to an extra-articular mechanism and restricted posterior glide of the talus with simultaneous neural involvement, these techniques serve to:

- reduce tonicity and improve the metabolism of the treated soft tissues
- mobilize the tender periarticular tissue, with dosage adjusted as necessary
- restore pain-free function by changing the input to the respective centres of the central nervous system (CNS).

Performance
Treatment is done within the pain-free range of movement. As the treatment techniques are performed without specific fixation, transferred movement has to be considered when the indication for the technique is determined.

Dosage (regarding the affected symptomatic structure)
Both with an acute and with a chronic presentation, the treatment technique should always be pain-free.

Choice of technique
The selection of the technique depends, among other things, on the therapist as well as the patient, on the therapist's clinical experience, but primarily on reassessment. This means that

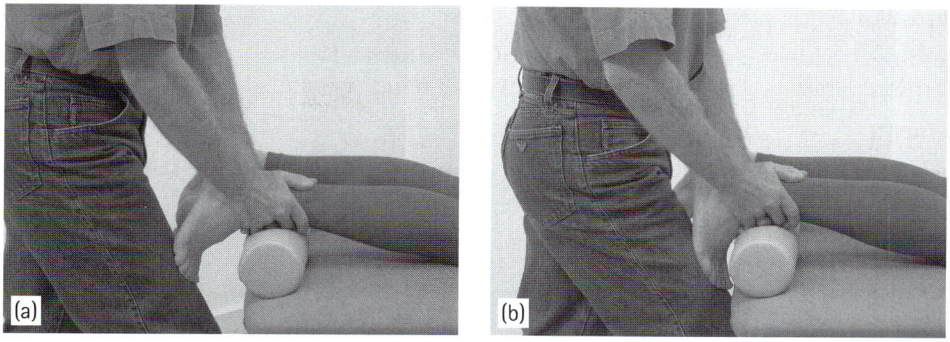

Figure 12.28a and b Soft tissue technique; tissue around medial malleolus; therapy technique. **a**, Starting position. **b**, End position.

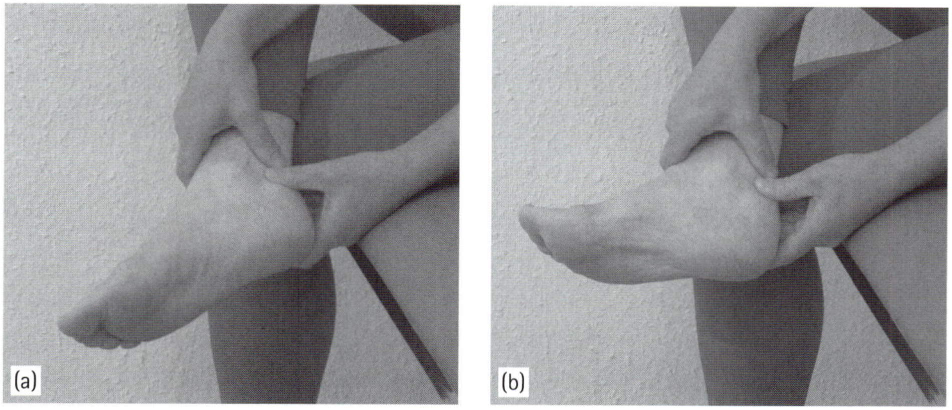

Figure 12.29a and b Soft tissue technique; tissue around medial malleolus; self-exercise. **a**, Starting position. **b**, End position.

even if all preconditions on the part of therapist and patient seem to be met, it is of no use to continue the technique if reassessment is negative.

Contributing factors

For a satisfactory solution of the patient's current problems it is important to consider the contributing factors and include them in the treatment.

The authors will, however, not go into a description of the various possibilities and their complex contexts as this would exceed the scope of the present book.

MOBILIZATION TECHNIQUES

Active procedures

ACTIVE MOBILIZATION PLUS ACCESSORY MOVEMENT

Dorsal flexion with anterior glide of the talus in the upper ankle

Therapy technique (film 215)

Patient's starting position:

- supine, the right foot resting on the plinth (Fig. 12.30a).

Therapist's starting position:

- standing, beside the patient at the level of the patient's foot
- grasping patient's distal lower leg with the left hand, patient's foot with the right hand.

Movement:

- pushing the lower leg in a posterior direction (anterior glide of the talus) parallel to the treatment plane (Kaltenborn 1999)
- then active dorsal flexion in upper ankle (Fig. 12.30b)
- moving back to starting position
- releasing the posterior push on the lower leg.

Self-exercise (film 216)

Patient's starting position:

- sitting, the right heel placed on a stool (Fig. 12.31a)
- a belt running around the right distal lower leg

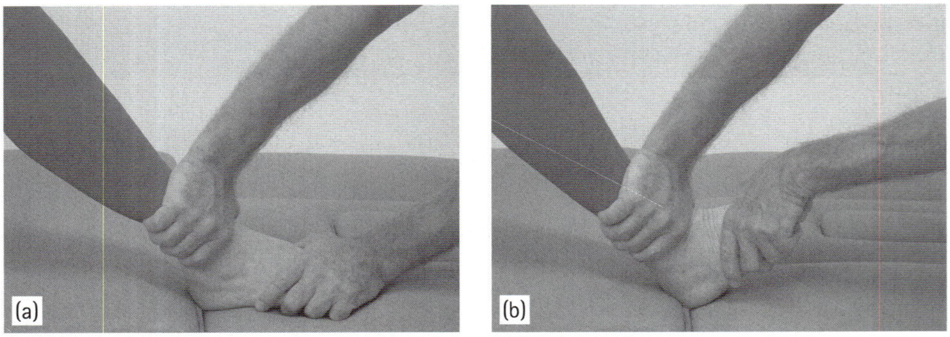

Figure 12.30a and b Active mobilization with accessory movement; dorsal flexion with anterior gliding of the talus in the upper ankle; therapy technique. a, Starting position. b, End position.

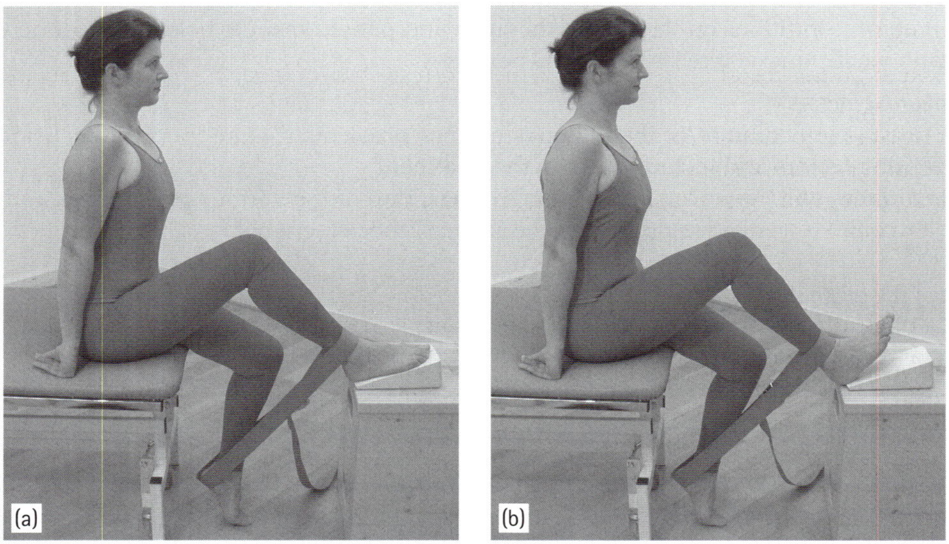

Figure 12.31a and b Active mobilization with accessory movement; dorsal flexion with anterior gliding of the talus in the upper ankle; self-exercise. a, Starting position. b, End position.

- heel of the left foot placed in the belt loop
- forefoot resting on the floor.

Movement:

- pressing left heel against the belt (anterior glide of the talus), dorsal flexion of the right upper ankle (Fig. 12.31b)
- moving back to starting position, and releasing pressure.

Neural mobilization with unilateral pressure in posterior–anterior direction (L4)

Therapy technique (film 217)

Patient's starting position:

- lying on the left side (Fig. 12.32a)
- hips and knees flexed, feet in resting position
- to achieve more neural pretension, the spine may be pre-positioned in flexion.

Therapist's starting position:

- standing, behind the patient
- contacting patient's costal process of L4.

Movement:

- pressure on the costal process of L4 in a posterior–anterior direction (Fig. 12.32b)
- foot of the affected side moves into dorsal flexion
- knee moves into extension
- then moving the leg back, and releasing pressure.

Self-exercise (film 218)

Patient's starting position:

- lying on the left side (Fig. 12.33a)
- hips and knees flexed, feet in resting position
- to achieve more neural pretension, the spine may be pre-positioned in flexion.

Movement:

- pressure on the costal process of L4 in a posterior–anterior direction (position marked by tape) (Fig. 12.33b)
- foot moves into dorsal flexion
- knee moves into extension
- then moving the leg back, and releasing pressure.

Remarks

Goals of the technique

With a painfully restricted dorsal flexion of the upper ankle due to an extra-articular mechanism and restricted posterior glide of the talus with simultaneous neural involvement and local tissue changes at the level of L4 as well as changed movement resistance as compared with the contralateral side, these techniques serve to:

- reduce tonicity and improve the metabolism of the affected tissues
- restore pain-free function by changing the input to the respective centres of the CNS (movement into dorsal flexion with simultaneously changed afferent input to the CNS – talus moved in anterior direction and push on L4 while the patient moves into dorsal flexion without pain).

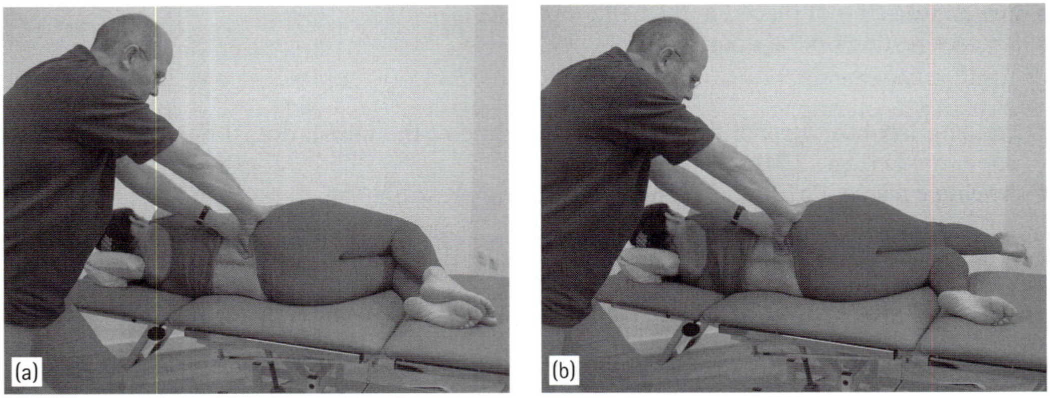

Figure 12.32a and b Active mobilization with accessory movement; neural mobilization with unilateral pressure in a posterior-anterior direction (L4); therapy technique. **a**, Starting position. **b**, End position.

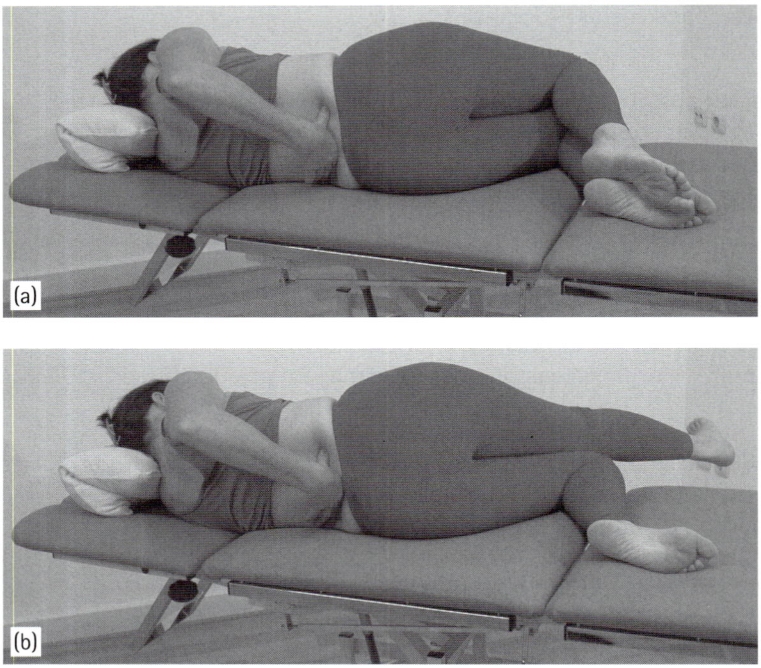

Figure 12.33a and b Active mobilization with accessory movement; neural mobilization with unilateral pressure in a posterior-anterior direction (L4); self-exercise. **a**, Starting position. **b**, End position.

Performance

The patient's typical symptoms should not be reproduced by the demonstrated techniques.

Dosage

Both with an acute and with a chronic presentation, the patient's symptoms should not be provoked by these techniques. Dosage depends on the expected training state of the tissue and, above all, on reassessment.

Choice of technique

The selection of the technique depends, among other things, on the therapist as well as the patient, on the therapist's clinical experience, but primarily on reassessment. This means that even if all preconditions on the part of therapist and patient seem to be met, it is of no use to continue the technique if reassessment is negative.

Contributing factors

For a satisfactory solution of the patient's current problems it is important to consider the contributing factors and include them in the treatment.

The authors will, however, not go into a description of the various possibilities and their complex contexts as this would exceed the scope of the present book.

Passive procedures

TRANSLATORY MOVEMENTS

Traction in the upper ankle

Therapy technique (film 219)

Patient's starting position:

- supine (Fig. 12.34a)
- lower leg fixed on the plinth by a belt
- to increase neural tension, the patient may be positioned in long-sitting
- the foot is pre-positioned in a position shortly before symptoms appear.

Therapist's starting position:

- standing, at the end of the plinth
- grasping patient's right foot from the medial side so that little finger and hypothenar are resting on patient's talus
- left hand placed on the right hand from the lateral side, with the same grip; in this way the foot is grasped securely
- a belt loop runs crossed over the therapist's hands and then around the therapist's pelvis.

Movement:

- traction in upper ankle right-angled to the treatment plane (Fig. 12.34b).

Self-exercise (film 220)

Patient's starting position:

- supine, on a smooth surface, the talus surrounded by a loop; the end of the loop is linked to a firm object in such a way that the right foot is close to this object (Fig. 12.35a)
- the left foot is placed on a stool left of the firm object
- a belt surrounds the top of the right foot and leads to the patient's hands. Pulling the belt will induce more or less dorsal flexion of the foot.

Movement:

- by pressing the left leg against the stool, the body will be pushed away from the fixed talus (traction in upper ankle) (Fig. 12.35b).

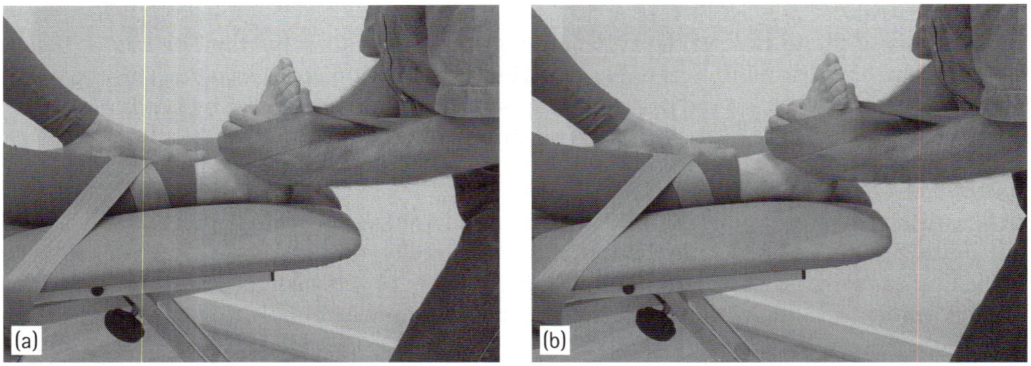

Figure 12.34a and b Translatory movement; traction in the upper ankle; therapy technique. a, Starting position. b, End position.

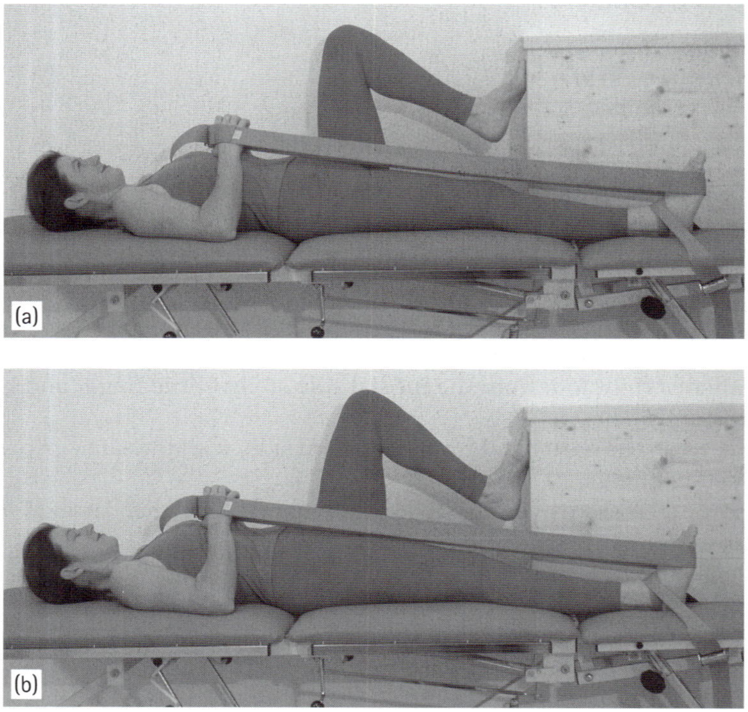

Figure 12.35a and b Translatory movement; traction in the upper ankle; self-exercise. a, Starting position. b, End position.

Dorsal glide in the upper ankle

Therapy technique (film 221)

Patient's starting position:

- stride position, the right leg placed behind, the foot on a wedge (high end under the heel) (Fig. 12.36a)
- dorsal flexion of the upper ankle is pre-positioned by changing the size of the stride up to a position shortly before symptoms appear.

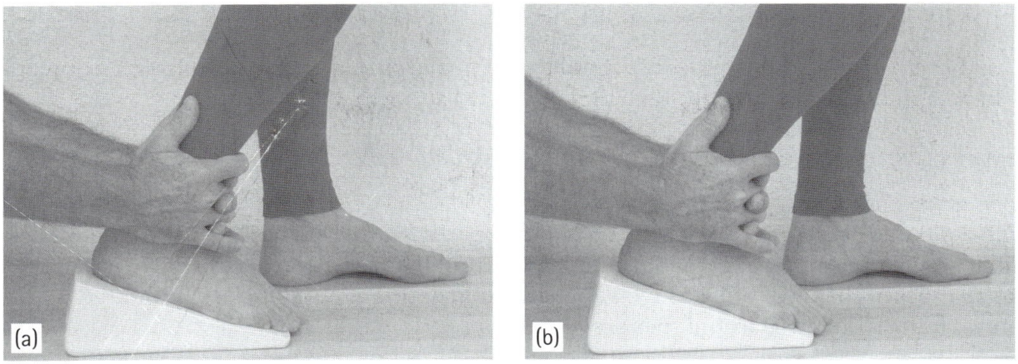

Figure 12.36a and b Translatory movement; dorsal glide in the upper ankle; therapy technique. **a**, Starting position. **b**, End position.

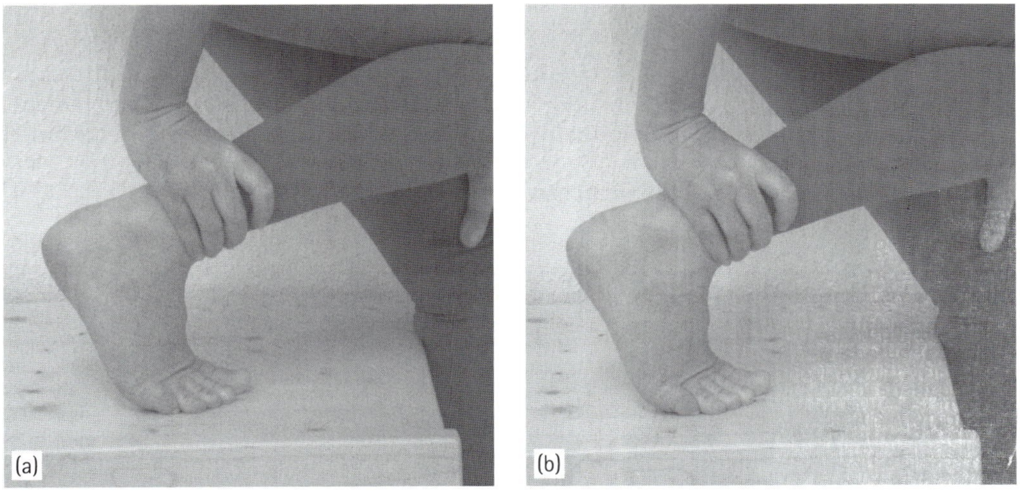

Figure 12.37a and b Translatory movement; dorsal glide in the upper ankle; self-exercise. **a**, Starting position. **b**, End position.

Therapist's starting position:

- kneeling, behind the patient's right leg
- contacting patient's distal right lower leg with the right hand, from behind (contact with the thenar at the posterior side of the malleolus).

Movement:

- making the talus glide in the upper ankle in a posterior direction by pushing the lower leg in an anterior direction (Fig. 12.36b).

Self-exercise (film 222)

Patient's starting position:

- sitting on a low stool (Fig. 12.37a)
- the tip of the right foot placed beside the stool
- foot pre-positioned in dorsal flexion to a position shortly before symptoms appear
- contacting the distal right lower leg with the right hand, from behind.

Movement:

- making the talus glide in the upper ankle in a posterior direction by pushing the lower leg in an anterior direction (Fig. 12.37b).

Remarks (regarding treatment of a symptomatic structure/direction)

Goals of the technique

With a painfully restricted dorsal flexion of the upper ankle due to an extra-articular mechanism and restricted posterior glide of the talus with simultaneous neural involvement and local tissue changes at the level of L4 as well as changed movement resistance as compared with the contralateral side, these techniques serve to:

- restore normal function of the symptomatic tissue by application of the symptom-provoking stimulus dosed according to the current load tolerance
- restore symptom-free function by changing the input to the respective centres of the CNS.

Performance

The joint that is to be treated is first adjusted according to irritability and the desired treatment goal. By the specific fixation of this technique, transferred movement is prevented as far as possible. This should be considered when the indication is determined.

Dosage (regarding the affected symptomatic structure)

Acute presentation (predominantly peripheral pain mechanisms)

Phase	Limitation of movement due to pain and resistance	Concept	Movement grade
Inflammation phase	No pain	Kaltenborn–Evjenth	Up to the beginning of II
	No resistance	Maitland	Up to II
Proliferation phase	Up to P1	Kaltenborn–Evjenth	Up to the 1st third of II
	Slowly progressing up to low resistance	Maitland	Up to III^{-}
Remodelling/ organization phase	Slowly progressing up to maximum resistance	Kaltenborn–Evjenth	Up to III
	(Note: duration of turnover!)	Maitland	Up to IV^{++} or III^{++}

Note: The chances of a disturbed (delayed) course of healing and their consequences for the loading capacity of the tissue (e.g., diabetes, old age, partial or general immobilization) have to be considered.

- *Traction:* Specific provocation and alleviation showed a reproduction of the patient's typical pain with this technique (extra-articular mechanism).
- *Posterior glide:* Examination of specific mobility showed restricted posterior glide. With regard to mobilization in the restricted direction it has to be considered, however, that the symptomatic tissue might be loaded. This would show in a reproduction of the typical symptoms. In that case, the same rules would hold for dosage of treatment as with the above-described traction technique. If, on the other hand, typical symptoms are not reproduced with the gliding technique, dosage is determined by the expected training state of the tissue.

Chronic presentation (predominantly central pain mechanisms): Since here it is assumed that pain no longer represents a protection mechanism, the therapist has to consider the expected training state of the treated tissue as well as the patient's personal expectations. If there is any doubt, treatment will always be started with very low force, and progression will be made conditional on reassessment. Hence with a chronic presentation, pain is not always the limiting factor regarding dosage of treatment.

Choice of technique

The selection of the technique depends, among other things, on the therapist as well as the patient, on the therapist's clinical experience, but primarily on reassessment. This means that even if all preconditions on the part of therapist and patient seem to be met, it is of no use to continue the technique if reassessment is negative.

Contributing factors

For a satisfactory solution of the patient's current problems it is important to consider the contributing factors and include them in the treatment.

The authors will, however, not go into a description of the various possibilities and their complex contexts as this would exceed the scope of the present book.

ACCESSORY MOVEMENTS

Unilateral push of L4 in posterior-anterior direction

Therapy technique (film 223)

Patient's starting position:

- prone (Fig. 12.38a).

Therapist's starting position:

- standing, at the patient's right side
- contacting patient's costal process of L4 with the hypothenar, reinforced by the other hand.

Movement:

- unilateral push on the costal process of L4 in a posterior-anterior direction (Fig. 12.38b).

Self-exercise (film 224)

Patient's starting position:

- supine, feet placed on the supporting surface (Fig. 12.39a)
- contact with right costal process of L4 by placing a tennis ball underneath.

Movement:

- rolling the body to the right against the tennis ball (Fig. 12.39b).

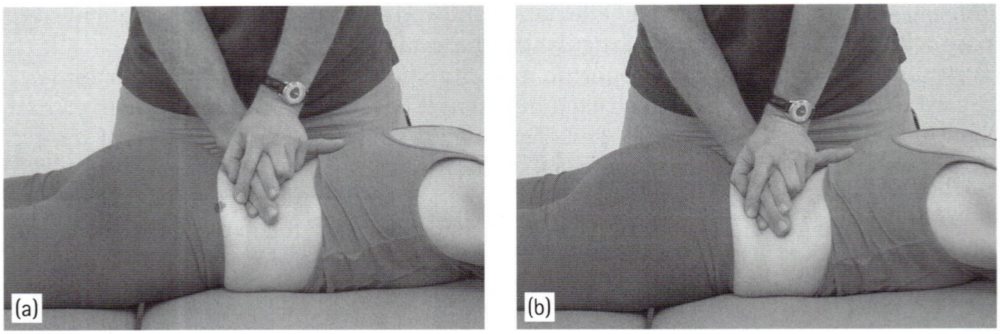

Figure 12.38a and b Accessory movement; unilateral push in a posterior-anterior direction (L4); therapy technique. **a**, Starting position. **b**, End position.

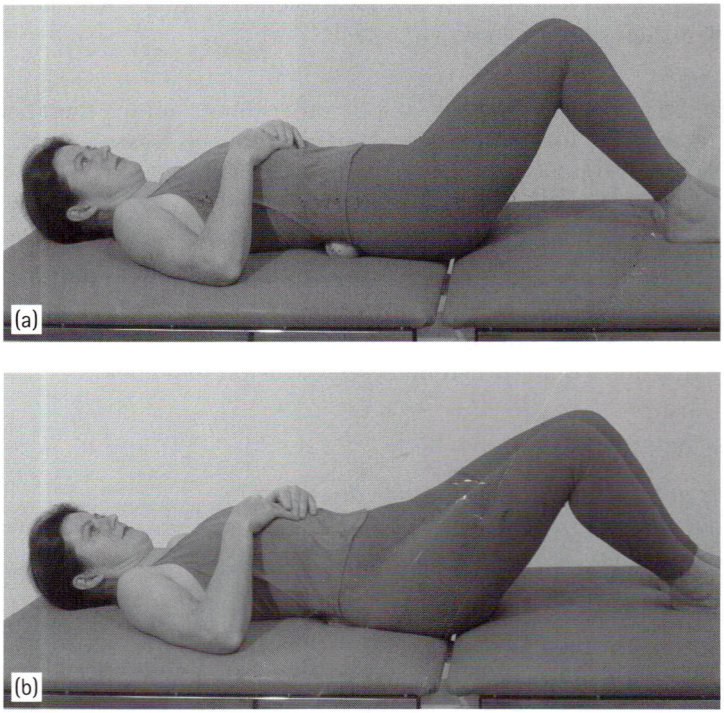

Figure 12.39a and b Accessory movement; unilateral push in a posterior-anterior direction (L4); self-exercise. **a**, Starting position. **b**, End position.

Remarks

Goals of the technique

With a painfully restricted dorsal flexion of the upper ankle due to an extra-articular mechanism and restricted posterior glide of the talus with simultaneous neural involvement and local tissue changes at the level of L4 as well as changed movement resistance as compared with the contralateral side, this technique serves to:

- restore symptom-free function by changing the input to the respective centres of the CNS
- reduce tenderness of the tissue in the symptomatic area (Vicenzino et al. 1998).

Performance

As the technique is performed without specific fixation, transferred movement has to be considered when the indication for the technique is determined.

Dosage

The dosage of the technique applied in the study of Vicenzino et al. (1998), which led to the described reduction of tenderness and improvement of function in the symptomatic area, was of grade III (Maitland 1994). This corresponds with the authors' experience.

Choice of technique

The selection of the technique depends, among other things, on the therapist as well as the patient, on the therapist's clinical experience, but primarily on reassessment. This means that even if all preconditions on the part of therapist and patient seem to be met, it is of no use to continue the technique if reassessment is negative.

Contributing factors

For a satisfactory solution of the patient's current problems it is important to consider the contributing factors and include them in the treatment.

The authors will, however, not go into a description of the various possibilities and their complex contexts as this would exceed the scope of the present book.

References and further reading

Beattie P. The relationship between symptoms and abnormal magnetic resonance images of lumbar intervertebral discs. Physical Therapy 1996; 6.

Butler D. Integrating pain awareness into physiotherapy-wise action for the future. In: Gifford L, ed. Topical Issues in Pain. Kestrel: NOI; 1998.

Butler D. Mobilisation of the Nervous System. Melbourne: Churchill Livingstone; 1994.

Cohen M. Arthralgia and myalgia. In: Campell J, ed. Pain 1996 – An Updated Review. Seattle: IASP; 1996.

Cohen, M. The clinical challenge of secondary hyperalgesia. In: Shacklock M, ed. Moving in on Pain. Chatswood: Butterworth-Heinemann; 1995.

Currier D, Nelson R. Dynamics of Human Biologic Tissues. Philadelphia: F.A. Davis; 1992.

Cyriax J. Textbook of Orthopaedic Medicine Diagnosis of Soft Tissue Lesions. London: Baillière Tindall; 1982.

de Bono E. Laterales Denken. Düsseldorf: ECON; 1992.

Dubner R, Basbaum A. Spinal dorsal horn plasticity following tissue or nerve injury. In: Wall P, Melzack R, eds. Textbook of Pain. Edinburgh: Churchill Livingstone; 1994.

Edwards B. Combined movements of the cervical spine in examination and treatment. In: Grant R, ed. Physical Therapy of the Cervical and the Thoracic Spine. Melbourne: Churchill Livingstone; 1992.

Evjenth O, Gloeck C. Die Symptomlokalisation an der Wirbelsäule und den Extremitätegelenken. Kursunterlagen; 1996.

Evjenth O, Hamberg J. Muscle Stretching in Manual Therapy. Oslo: Alfta Rehab; 1984.

Fortin JD, Dwyer A, West S, Pier J. Sacroiliac joint pain referral patterns upon application of a new injection/arthrography technique. I: Asymptomatic volunteers. Spine 19 (13): 1994a; 1475–82.

Fortin JD, Dwyer A, Aprill C, Ponthieux B, Pier J. Sacroiliac joint pain referral patterns. II: Clinical evaluation. Spine 19(13): 1994b; 1483–9.

Frankel V, Nordin M. Basic Biomechanics of the Musculoskeletal System. Philadelphia: Lea & Febiger; 1989.

Frisch H. Programmierte Untersuchung des Bewegungsapparates. Heidelberg: Springer; 1995.

Gifford L. Personal communication. 1999.

Gifford L. Tissue and input related mechanisms. In: Gifford L, ed. Topical Issues in Pain. Kestrel: NOI; 1998.

Gifford L, Butler D. The integration of pain sciences into clinical practice. Journal of Hand Therapy 1997; 10.

Greenman P. Principles of Manual Medicine. Baltimore: Williams & Wilkins; 1996.

Grice A. A Biomedical Approach to Cervical and Dorsal Adjusting. Modern Developments in Principles and Practice of Chiropractic. New York: Appleton-Century-Crofts; 1979.

Haldeman S. Principles and Practice of Chiropractic, 3rd edn. New York: McGraw-Hill Medical, 2005.

Harding V, Simmonds M, Watson P. Physical therapy for chronic pain. Pain–Clinical Updates, 1998; 3.

Harkins SW, Kwentus J, Price DD. Pain and the elderly. In: Al BE, ed. Advances in Pain Research and Therapy. New York: Raven Press; 1984.

Hengeveld E. Clinical Reasoning in Manueller Therapie – eine klinische Fallstudie. Manuelle Therapie 1998; 1.

Hides JA. Multifidus muscle recovery is not automatic after resolution of acute first-episode low back pain. Spine 1996; 21(23): 2763–9.

Jones M. Clinical Reasoning: Fundament der klinischen Praxis und Brücke zwischen den Ansätzen der Manuellen Therapie, Teil 1. Manuelle Therapie 1997a; 1.

Jones M. Fundament der klinischen Praxis und Brücke zwischen den Ansätzen der Manuellen Therapie Teil 2. Manuelle Therapie 1997b; 2.

Jones M. Clinical reasoning and pain. Manual Therapy 1995; 1.

Kaltenborn F. Manuelle Therapie nach Kaltenborn. Teil 1. Extremitäten. Oslo: Norlis Bokhandel; 1999.

Kaltenborn F. Wirbelsäule – Manuelle Untersuchung und Mobilisation. Oslo: Norlis Bokhandel; 1992.

Kannus P, Jozsa L, Renström P, et al. The effects of training, immobilisation and remobilisation on musculoskeletal tissue. Scand J Med Sci Sports 1992; 2.

Keefe FJ, Beaupre PM, Weiner DK, Siegler IC. Pain in older adults: a cognitive and behavioural perspective. In: Ferrell BR, Ferrell BA, eds. Pain in the Elderly. Seattle: IASP; 1996.

Kendall F, Kendall-McCreary E. Muskeln – Funktionen und Tests. Stuttgart: G. Fischer; 1988.

Korr I. The Neurobiologic Mechanisms in Manipulative Therapy. New York: Plenum; 1978.

Lederman E. Fundamentals of Manual Therapy. Edinburgh: Churchill Livingstone; 1997.

Leroux JL, Thomas E, Bonnel F, Blotman F. Diagnostic value of clinical tests for shoulder impingement syndrome. Revue du Rhumatisme (Engl. ed.) 1995; 6.

Lewis T. Pain. New York: Macmillan; 1942.

Lewis T. Experiments relating to cutaneous hyperalgesia and its spread through somatic fibres. Clinical Science 1935; 2.

Lewit K. Manuelle Medizin im Rahmen der medizinischen Rehabilitation. Berlin: Urban & Schwarzenberg; 1987.

Maitland GD. Manipulation der peripheren Gelenke. Heidelberg: Springer; 1996.

Maitland GD. Manipulation der Wirbelsäule. Heidelberg: Springer; 1994.

McKenzie R. Treat your own back. Spinal Publications New Zealand Ltd; 1998.

Merskey H, Bogduk N. Pain Therms. Classification of Chronic Pain. Seattle: IASP; 1994.

Meyer R, Campell J, Raja S. Peripheral neural mechanisms of nociception. In: Wall P, Melzach R, eds. Textbook of Pain. Edinburgh: Churchill Livingstone; 1994.

Milgrom C, Schaffler M, Gilbert S, van Holsbeeck M. Rotator cuff changes in asymptomatic adults. Journal of Bone and Joint Surgery 1995; 77-B:2.

Mulligan BR. Manual Therapy – 'NAGS', 'SNAGS', 'MWMS' etc. Wellington: Plane View Services Ltd; 1999.

Mumenthaler M. Neurologische Differentialdiagnostik – Syndrome und Leitsymptome. Stuttgart: Thieme; 1988.

Noyes F, Grood E. The strength of the anterior cruciate ligament in humans and rhesus monkeys: age related and species related changes. Journal of Bone and Joint Surgery 1976; 58 A.

Panjabi M. The stabilising system of the spine. Part 1: Function, dysfunction, adaptation and enhancement. Journal of Spinal Disorders 1992a; 5.

Panjabi M. The stabilising system of the spine. Part 2: Neutral zone and stability hypothesis. Journal of Spinal Disorders 1992b; 5.

Pearcy MJ, Tibrewal SB. Axial rotation and lateral bending in the normal lumbar spine measured by three-dimensional radiography. Spine 1984; 9(6): 582–7.

Pfund R, Jones M, Magarey M, Simmons N. Manueller Test zur Differenzierung von Strukturen im subakromialen Raum, Teil 1. Manuelle Therapie 1998a; 2.

Pfund R, Jones M, Magarey M, Simmons N. Manueller Test zur Differenzierung von Strukturen im subakromialen Raum, Teil 2. Manuelle Therapie 1998b; 4.

Rahlmann J. Mechanisms of intervertebral joint fixation: A literature review. Journal of Manipulative and Physiological Therapeutics 1987; 4.

Röthig OP, Becker H, Carl K (eds) Sportwissenschaftliches Lexikon. Schorndorf: Hofmann; 1983.

Sandoz R. Some physical mechanisms and effects of spinal adjustment. Annals of the Swiss Chiropractic Association 1976; 6.

Schomacher J. ICIDH-2 – Internationale Klassifikation der Schäden, Aktivitäten und Partizipationen. Manuelle Therapie 1999; 2.

Ure BM, Tiling T, Kirchner R, Rixen D. Zuverlässigkeit der klinischen Untersuchung der Schulter im Vergleich zur Arthroskopie. Eine prospektive Studie. Unfallchirurg 1993; 7.

van den Berg F. Angewandte Physiologie. Vol. 1. Das Bindegewebe des Bewegungsapparates verstehen und beeinflussen. Stuttgart: Thieme; 1998.

Vicenzino B, Collins D, Benson H, Wright A. An investigation of the interrelationship between manipulative therapy-induced hypoalgesia and sympathoexcitation. Journal of Manipulative and Physiological Therapeutics 1998 Sep; 21(7): 448–53.

Waddell G. The Back Pain Revolution. Edinburgh: Churchill-Livingstone, 1998.

Ward R, Sprafka S. Glossary of osteopathic terminology. Journal of the American Osteopathic Association 1981; 8.

Wiemann K, Klee A, Stratmann M. Filamentäre Quellen der Muskel-Ruhe-Spannung und die Behandlung muskulärer Dysbalancen. Deutsche Zeitschrift für Sportmedizin 1998; 4.

Winkel D, Vleeming A, Fisher S, Meijer O, Vroege C. Nichtoperative Orthopädie der Weichteile des Bewegungsapparates. Stuttgart: G. Fischer; 1985.

Zahnd F, Baumgartner W. Intervertebrale Bewegungen bei passiven bilateralen und unilateralen posterior-anterioren Manipulationen – ein Pilotversuch. Manuelle Therapie 2000; 4.

Zahnd F, Mühlemann D. Einführung in Manuelle Techniken – Oberflächen- und Röntgenanatomie, Palpation und Weichteiltechniken. Stuttgart: Thieme; 1998.

Zusman M. The meaning of mechanically produced responses. Australian Journal of Physiotherapy 1994; 1.

Index

ELSEVIER DVD-ROM LICENCE AGREEMENT

PLEASE READ THE FOLLOWING AGREEMENT CAREFULLY BEFORE USING THIS PRODUCT. THIS PRODUCT IS LICENSED UNDER THE TERMS CONTAINED IN THIS LICENCE AGREEMENT ('Agreement'). BY USING THIS PRODUCT, YOU, AN INDIVIDUAL OR ENTITY INCLUDING EMPLOYEES, AGENTS AND REPRESENTATIVES ('You' or 'Your'), ACKNOWLEDGE THAT YOU HAVE READ THIS AGREEMENT, THAT YOU UNDERSTAND IT, AND THAT YOU AGREE TO BE BOUND BY THE TERMS AND CONDITIONS OF THIS AGREEMENT. ELSEVIER LIMITED ('Elsevier') EXPRESSLY DOES NOT AGREE TO LICENSE THIS PRODUCT TO YOU UNLESS YOU ASSENT TO THIS AGREEMENT. IF YOU DO NOT AGREE WITH ANY OF THE FOLLOWING TERMS, YOU MAY, WITHIN THIRTY (30) DAYS AFTER YOUR RECEIPT OF THIS PRODUCT RETURN THE UNUSED PRODUCT AND ALL ACCOMPANYING DOCUMENTATION TO ELSEVIER FOR A FULL REFUND.

DEFINITIONS As used in this Agreement, these terms shall have the following meanings:

'Proprietary Material' means the valuable and proprietary information content of this Product including without limitation all indexes and graphic materials and software used to access, index, search and retrieve the information content from this Product developed or licensed by Elsevier and/or its affiliates, suppliers and licensors.

'Product' means the copy of the Proprietary Material and any other material delivered on DVD-ROM and any other human-readable or machine-readable materials enclosed with this Agreement, including without limitation documentation relating to the same.

OWNERSHIP This Product has been supplied by and is proprietary to Elsevier and/or its affiliates, suppliers and licensors. The copyright in the Product belongs to Elsevier and/or its affiliates, suppliers and licensors and is protected by the copyright, trademark, trade secret and other intellectual property laws of the United Kingdom and international treaty provisions, including without limitation the Universal Copyright Convention and the Berne Copyright Convention. You have no ownership rights in this Product. Except as expressly set forth herein, no part of this Product, including without limitation the Proprietary Material, may be modified, copied or distributed in hardcopy or machine-readable form without prior written consent from Elsevier. All rights not expressly granted to You herein are expressly reserved. Any other use of this Product by any person or entity is strictly prohibited and a violation of this Agreement.

SCOPE OF RIGHTS LICENSED (PERMITTED USES) Elsevier is granting to You a limited, non-exclusive, non-transferable licence to use this Product in accordance with the terms of this Agreement. You may use or provide access to this Product on a single computer or terminal physically located at Your premises and in a secure network or move this Product to and use it on another single computer or terminal at the same location for personal use only, but under no circumstances may You use or provide access to any part or parts of this Product on more than one computer or terminal simultaneously.

You shall not (a) copy, download, or otherwise reproduce the Product or any part(s) thereof in any medium, including, without limitation, online transmissions, local area networks, wide area networks, intranets, extranets and the Internet, or in any way, in whole or in part, except for printing out or downloading nonsubstantial portions of the text and images in the Product for Your own personal use; (b) alter, modify, or adapt the Product or any part(s) thereof, including but not limited to decompiling, disassembling, reverse engineering, or creating derivative works, without the prior written approval of Elsevier; (c) sell, license or otherwise distribute to third parties the Product or any part(s) thereof; or (d) alter, remove, obscure or obstruct the display of any copyright, trademark or other proprietary notice on or in the Product or on any printout or download of portions of the Proprietary Materials.

RESTRICTIONS ON TRANSFER This Licence is personal to You, and neither Your rights hereunder nor the tangible embodiments of this Product, including without limitation the Proprietary Material, may be sold, assigned, transferred or sublicensed to any other person, including without limitation by operation of law, without the prior written consent of Elsevier. Any purported sale, assignment, transfer or sublicense without the prior written consent of Elsevier will be void and will automatically terminate the Licence granted hereunder.

TERM This Agreement will remain in effect until terminated pursuant to the terms of this Agreement. You may terminate this Agreement at any time by removing from Your system and destroying the Product and any copies of the Proprietary Material. Unauthorized copying of the Product, including without limitation, the Proprietary Material and documentation, or otherwise failing to comply with the terms and conditions of this Agreement shall result in automatic termination of this licence and will make available to Elsevier legal remedies. Upon termination of this Agreement, the licence granted herein will terminate and You must immediately destroy the Product and all copies of the Product and of the Proprietary Material, together with any and all accompanying documentation. All provisions relating to proprietary rights shall survive termination of this Agreement.

LIMITED WARRANTY AND LIMITATION OF LIABILITY Elsevier warrants that the software embodied in this Product will perform in substantial compliance with the documentation supplied in this Product, unless the performance problems are the result of hardware failure or improper use. If You report a significant defect in performance in writing to Elsevier within ninety (90) calendar days of your having purchased the Product, and Elsevier is not able to correct same within sixty (60) days after its receipt of Your notification, You may return this Product, including all copies and documentation, to Elsevier and Elsevier will refund Your money. In order to apply for a refund on your purchased Product, please contact the return address on the invoice to obtain the refund request form ('Refund Request Form'), and either fax or mail your signed request and your proof of purchase to the address indicated on the Refund Request Form. Incomplete forms will not be processed. Defined terms in the Refund Request Form shall have the same meaning as in this Agreement.

YOU UNDERSTAND THAT, EXCEPT FOR THE LIMITED WARRANTY RECITED ABOVE, ELSEVIER, ITS AFFILIATES, LICENSORS, THIRD PARTY SUPPLIERS AND AGENTS (TOGETHER 'THE SUPPLIERS') MAKE NO REPRESENTATIONS OR WARRANTIES, WITH RESPECT TO THE PRODUCT, INCLUDING, WITHOUT LIMITATION THE PROPRIETARY MATERIAL. ALL OTHER REPRESENTATIONS, WARRANTIES, CONDITIONS OR OTHER TERMS, WHETHER EXPRESS OR IMPLIED BY STATUTE OR COMMON LAW, ARE HEREBY EXCLUDED TO THE FULLEST EXTENT PERMITTED BY LAW.

IN PARTICULAR BUT WITHOUT LIMITATION TO THE FOREGOING NONE OF THE SUPPLIERS MAKE ANY REPRESENTIONS OR WARRANTIES (WHETHER EXPRESS OR IMPLIED) REGARDING THE PERFORMANCE OF YOUR PAD, NETWORK OR COMPUTER SYSTEM WHEN USED IN CONJUNCTION WITH THE PRODUCT, NOR THAT THE PRODUCT WILL MEET YOUR REQUIREMENTS OR THAT ITS OPERATION WILL BE UNINTERRUPTED OR ERROR-FREE.

EXCEPT IN RESPECT OF DEATH OR PERSONAL INJURY CAUSED BY THE SUPPLIERS' NEGLIGENCE AND TO THE FULLEST EXTENT PERMITTED BY LAW, IN NO EVENT (AND REGARDLESS OF WHETHER SUCH DAMAGES ARE FORESEEABLE AND OF WHETHER SUCH LIABILITY IS BASED IN TORT, CONTRACT OR OTHERWISE) WILL ANY OF THE SUPPLIERS BE LIABLE TO YOU FOR ANY DAMAGES (INCLUDING, WITHOUT LIMITATION, ANY LOST PROFITS, LOST SAVINGS OR OTHER SPECIAL, INDIRECT, INCIDENTAL OR CONSEQUENTIAL DAMAGES ARISING OUT OF OR RESULTING FROM: (I) YOUR USE OF, OR INABILITY TO USE, THE PRODUCT; (II) DATA LOSS OR CORRUPTION; AND/OR (III) ERRORS OR OMISSIONS IN THE PROPRIETARY MATERIAL.

IF THE FOREGOING LIMITATION IS HELD TO BE UNENFORCEABLE, OUR MAXIMUM LIABILITY TO YOU IN RESPECT THEREOF SHALL NOT EXCEED THE AMOUNT OF THE LICENCE FEE PAID BY YOU FOR THE PRODUCT. THE REMEDIES AVAILABLE TO YOU AGAINST ELSEVIER AND THE LICENSORS OF MATERIALS INCLUDED IN THE PRODUCT ARE EXCLUSIVE.

If the information provided in the Product contains medical or health sciences information, it is intended for professional use within the medical field. Information about medical treatment or drug dosages is intended strictly for professional use, and because of rapid advances in the medical sciences, independent verification of diagnosis and drug dosages should be made.

The provisions of this Agreement shall be severable, and in the event that any provision of this Agreement is found to be legally unenforceable, such unenforceability shall not prevent the enforcement or any other provision of this Agreement.

GOVERNING LAW This Agreement shall be governed by the laws of England and Wales. In any dispute arising out of this Agreement, you and Elsevier each consent to the exclusive personal jurisdiction and venue in the courts of England and Wales.